AIDS UPDATE
2009

An Annual Overview of Acquired Immune Deficiency Syndrome

GERALD J. STINE, PH.D.

Department of Biology
University of North Florida, Jacksonville

Boston   Burr Ridge, IL   Dubuque, IA   Madison, WI   New York   San Francisco   St. Louis
Bangkok   Bogotá   Caracas   Kuala Lumpur   Lisbon   London   Madrid   Mexico City
Milan   Montreal   New Delhi   Santiago   Seoul   Singapore   Sydney   Taipei   Toronto

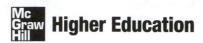

Higher Education

AIDS UPDATE 2009

Published by McGraw-Hill, a business unit of The McGraw-Hill Companies, Inc., 1221 Avenue of the Americas, New York, NY 10020. Copyright © 2009 by The McGraw-Hill Companies, Inc. All rights reserved. Previous edition © 2009. No part of this publication may be reproduced or distributed in any form or by any means, or stored in a database or retrieval system, without the prior written consent of The McGraw-Hill Companies, Inc., including, but not limited to, in any network or other electronic storage or transmission, or broadcast for distance learning.

Some ancillaries, including electronic and print components, may not be available to customers outside the United States.

This text is published by the **Contemporary Learning Series** group within the McGraw-Hill Higher Education division.

1 2 3 4 5 6 7 8 9 0 DOC/DOC 0 9 8

MHID 0-07-352759-9
ISBN 978-0-07-352759-8
ISSN 1081-5260

Managing Editor: *Larry Loeppke*
Senior Managing Editor: *Faye Schilling*
Developmental Editor: *Jade Benedict*
Editorial Coordinator: *Mary Foust*
Editorial Assistant: *Nancy Meissner*
Production Service Assistant: *Rita Hingtgen*
Permissions Coordinator: *Shirley Lanners*
Senior Marketing Manager: *Julie Keck*
Marketing Communications Specialist: *Mary Klein*
Marketing Coordinator: *Alice Link*
Senior Project Manager: *Jane Mohr*
Cover Designer: *Tara McDermott*

Compositor: *Lachina Publishing Services*
Cover Image: (Background Globe) © Corbis/R.F., (AIDS and Drig Testing Equipment) Getty Images/R.F., (Burning Candles) Getty Images/R.F., (Young Boy Lighting Candle in AIDS Ribbon) Copyright © 2007 by Sheyla Villena Gallardo/Global Health Council. www.globalhealth.org

www.mhhe.com

About the Author

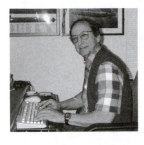

Gerald J. Stine is now Professor Emeritus at the University of North Florida, Department of Biology, in Jacksonville, Florida. He received his B.S. degree from Southern Connecticut University, M.A. at Dartmouth, Ph.D. at the University of Delaware, and did a postdoctoral study in radiation genetics at Oak Ridge National Laboratory, Oak Ridge, Tennessee. He continued his research at the University of Tennessee, Knoxville campus and published numerous scientific articles in recognized scientific journals. He then accepted a position at the University of North Florida. He has written 25 college-level textbooks, for example, *Biosocial Genetics*, *Human Genetics*, *The Sexually Transmitted Diseases*, and the *AIDS UPDATE* series. Large segments of his work in genetics and the sexually transmitted diseases have been used in five special project publications used in a number of universities nationwide.

This edition of *AIDS UPDATE* is the 18th. His interest in AIDS began with the June 5, 1981, publication of reports by the CDC and others about a strange new disease that affected *only* gay males. Dr. Stine regarded this announcement as utter nonsense. Early in 1983, a high-level member of the CDC gave a presentation in Jacksonville to some 300 people about this new disease (the virus was not yet isolated). The speaker said, "if you are heterosexual, male, a woman, or a child, you have nothing to worry about, this is a gay male disease." At that very moment Dr. Stine knew of heterosexual males, hemophiliacs, and several women and children with this disease! Restraining himself, he left

and began assembling his notes and learning about this new disease.

In 1988, he offered a new course called the "Biological and Medical Aspects of AIDS." He began writing his first book on AIDS in 1991, published in 1993. This was the first formal general purpose HIV/AIDS college-level textbook in the United States. He has continued to update for those needing the latest information on HIV/AIDS. The political and economic effects, pain, suffering, loss of life, and stigma due to HIV/AIDS continue.

Dr. Stine believes that AIDS, if it has not already, will soon be the worst transmittable viral or bacterial plague in human history. He has presented invited lectures on HIV/AIDS across the United States, in Canada, and in China. He received the Distinguished Alumni Award from his undergraduate college and presented the keynote address for the first Biotechnology Symposium held at Wuhan University, China. He was a member of the First Sino-American HIV/AIDS management symposium invited to China by the Chinese Medical Association. Dr. Stine is internationally recognized for numerous research publications and textbooks in the field of genetics, sexually transmitted diseases, and HIV/AIDS. He has prepared and published four professional brochures for genetic counseling and prenatal diagnostic testing while directing a prenatal genetic diagnostic center and is sought after by publishers to review manuscripts on genetics and HIV/AIDS. He has been consultant to seven college textbook companies. He is listed in the *American Men & Women of Science, Students International Directory of Scientists,* and *Who's Who in Technology Today.*

Contents

A Quarter Century of AIDS and Counting: A Humanitarian Crisis

June 5, 1981–June 5, 2009

"In the [28] years since the first case was reported, AIDS has changed the world. It has killed 22 million people and infected [35] million more. It has become the world's leading cause of death among both women and men ages 15 to 59. It has inflicted the single greatest reversal in the history of human development. In other worlds, it has become the greatest challenge of our generation."

Kofi Annan
Former Secretary General, United Nations

AIDS IS DIFFERENT FROM OTHER STORIES

Think of the major interdisciplinary, complex stories of our time; stories that are worldwide, ongoing, and urgent. Perhaps you think of climate change, famine, or nuclear proliferation. None of these is like the HIV/AIDS pandemic.

HIV/AIDS is a story of great breadth and sharp contrasts; covering it requires knowledge and sensitivity around personal issues such as sexuality, addiction, and social vulnerability. At the same time, it is a global story requiring a broad understanding of international politics, economics, scientific facts, and diverse cultural traditions. Interwoven with these strands of the HIV/AIDS story are the scientific, medical, and health-care stories which as an author, I must be able to "translate" these stories, events, and facts for you the student.

What complicates the presentations and explanations is the voluminous amount of difficult to interpret, tangled, intricate, complex, and perplexing, information available after 28 years of HIV/AIDS.

HUMANS AND HIV/AIDS

This is a political, medical, and social story about ourselves and the ways HIV/AIDS is moving through the world. HIV/AIDS is a deadly but preventable disease thriving in the human family, infecting or killing about 24 million of its members. It's a world in which HIV/AIDS has caused us to ask what kind of people are we? How did we get to this point? Where are we going? Can we for once find ways of compassion, humanity, and dignity for all men and women? Many people still believe AIDS is an African or Latin American disease and they blame both the people from these areas of the world for its spread. But they are not responsible for AIDS or HIV. The world is and until the world itself changes, HIV and AIDS will thrive in the human family for generations to come. There will be a very steep price to pay.

HOW DID IT ALL BEGIN?

June 5, 2006 was one of the most inauspicious anniversaries recognized in the United States. It marked the 25th anniversary of what would become the first case of AIDS in the United States; Michael S. Gottlieb didn't know it at the time, but when a 31-year-old man (also named Michael) was admitted to his hospital in 1981 with fever and weight loss, he was meeting the person who would become the first officially reported case in the global AIDS pandemic. Twenty-five years later, Michael or "Patient Zero" has long since died, but Gottlieb is still treating people with HIV. Since then, the United States has had the most severe HIV/AIDS pandemic of any developed country worldwide. The United States has the 10th largest HIV population. The other nine countries with higher HIV populations are in sub-Saharan Africa.

When this new disease was first recognized on June 5, 1981, the causative infectious agent was unknown. By 1983, AIDS cases had turned up in 28 nations. After it was determined in 1983 that the causative agent was a virus, the virus turned out to be unique even within its own classification of retroviruses. Since then, more has been learned about this retrovirus, the Human Immunodeficiency Virus (HIV), and in a shorter time span than is known about any other virus in human history. Nonetheless, this anniversary in no way marks the end of the Age of AIDS, although it may mark a new global beginning.

By the time HIV/AIDS emerged in the states of New York, California, Florida, Texas, and New Jersey, people were so terrified of this new disease that those afflicted by it were shunned by doctors, nurses, social workers, police officers, firemen, and the public at large. This ugly scenario began with the first report in the Centers for Disease Control and Prevention (CDC) June 5, 1981 edition of *Morbidity and Mortality Weekly Report* (MMWR).

Baffling Reports

In the June 1981 report, five young men, all active homosexuals, were treated for biopsy confirmed *Pneumocystis pneumonia* (PCP) at three different hospitals in Los Angeles, California. Two of the patients died. All five patients had laboratory-confirmed previous or concurrent Cytomegalovirus (CMV) infection and a candidal (fungal) mucosal infection. The authors of the report speculated that "some aspect of the homosexual lifestyle" or a "disease acquired through sexual contact" may have had a role in these unusual cases of PCP and also postulated that "a cellular–immune dysfunction related to a common exposure" may have been involved.

In July 1981, one month after CDC's first report, doctors from New York and California reported in MMWR 26 cases of the rare skin cancer, Kaposi's sarcoma, in 26 gay males ages 15 to 49. Several of these men also had Pneumocystis Jiraveci pneumonia (PCP) and Cytomegalovirus (CMV), and the authors cautioned "Physicians should be alert for Kaposi's sarcoma, PCP, and other opportunistic infections associated with immunosuppression in homosexual men," Although the disease was yet to be called AIDS, and the infectious agent was not yet discovered, some 200,000 people in the United States were already HIV infected, and they began dying with increasing numbers yearly until AIDS deaths peaked in 1995 at 55,000! In some social groups, the dead outnumbered the living. For example, from the San Francisco Gay Men's Chorus, there were 210 singers and 257 obituaries. Now nearly 28 years after the first reported case of AIDS and 25 years after the discovery of HIV as the cause of AIDS, effective control of the HIV/AIDS pandemic remains elusive. And, the three words echoing around the world are: **AIDS CRISIS WORSENS!**

In the modern world, 28 years seems a long time to be at war, but it is hardly surprising when the enemy is as elusive and pervasive as HIV. It has been 26 years since scientists first identified the cause of what was then a baffling new syndrome ravaging immune systems and destroying lives. Since then, AIDS has gone from being the scourge of relatively small groups, such as hemophiliacs, homosexuals, and intravenous-drug users in rich countries, to arguably the biggest threat to life and prosperity in the developing world. And we now know that no single research group or discipline will solve the puzzles of how to conquer HIV/AIDS. It is now clear that scientists were naïve to believe there would be an easy path from the discovery of HIV to the development of a vaccine.

ANTIRETROVIRAL DRUGS (ARVD)

The first Food and Drug Administration (FDA) approved ARVD was zidovudine (known as AZT) in 1987 but its toxic effect was, in effect, almost as bad as the disease. It was, however, a beginning. In 1995, with about 350,000 people dead from AIDS, the first of the protease inhibitors and nucleoside reverse transcriptase inhibitors were FDA-approved, and the death rate from AIDS dropped dramatically. From 2001 through 2008, the death rate has held steady at between 14,000 and 17,000 AIDS deaths per year. Through the 27th anniversary and counting, some 25 FDA ARVDs are being used to lengthen the lives of the HIV infected. Much has yet to be achieved concerning the arsenal of available ARVD because at least 20% to 40% of those infected cannot tolerate many of the drugs now available.

ORIGIN OF HIV

The best evidence through 2008 states that a virus called Simian Immunodeficiency Virus (SIV), found in chimpanzees in Africa, crossed into humans and changed its form to become a lethal agent in humans. This crossover is believed to have occurred around 1930, plus or minus about ten years. It is speculated that HIV arrived in the United States around 1968 and spread undetected throughout the 1970s.

SOCIAL IMPACT OF THE NEW DISEASE

Over the past 27 years and counting, AIDS activists and their supporters have forced sweep-

ing changes in how the U.S. blood supply is managed, the time frame used by the FDA for drug approval, and U.S. drug companies' search for new and improved antiretroviral drugs. They have also changed the rules on government-controlled marches and rallies. Socially, we have learned that antiretroviral drugs can prolong AIDS patients' lives; cultural changes for HIV prevention is very difficult; that Africa is still poor and vulnerable to HIV infections; that Asia is still in denial that millions of AIDS orphans have nowhere to turn; that celebrities have chosen more glitzy causes; and that now black and gay communities bury their dead quietly. America is allowing AIDS to be normalized like homelessness and poverty. The global AIDS crisis is not over; it has just begun. The statistics over the last 27 years are numbing beyond comprehension. Who can understand the meaning of 35 million people (ending 2009) throughout the world living with the virus? Or that HIV infection continues to increase throughout the world? It is only when people realize that at the end of 2009, 24 million people will have died of AIDS, or that a 15-year-old in South Africa has a 50:50 chance of dying of AIDS before the age of 30, that the horror begins to take on a human scale. The American perception of AIDS has gone through a cycle of meanings over the last 27 years. In the early days, there was no name for the disease; today we continue to ask how to cure it. In the early days there were major protests against the FDA and the medical and pharmaceutical companies. Today, there is quiet acceptance. The early demonstrators influenced basic research, the federal drug approval process, and the massive federal funding for a single disease. This disease as no other before it has changed the way people interact with their physicians, demand medical services, and take control of their own treatments regardless of illness. An entire generation has now been born that has never known an AIDS-free world. Children born with HIV have now themselves become mothers of newborns! The disease has changed the personal as well as the political—how we think and how we love, what we teach our children, and what words we say in public. More than anything else, HIV/AIDS has changed the way we view the threat of emerging diseases. Until HIV/AIDS, most of us thought of catastrophic plagues, such as the Black Death or the Spanish flu epidemic of 1918, as things of the past. We lost sight of the fact that every once in a while a new disease emerges. It happened with HIV/AIDS and it can happen again. Witness the current outbreaks of the Hanta, West Nile, SARS, monkeypox, and the avian flu viruses. AIDS also changed what it means to be a patient. People with AIDS stormed scientific conferences, banded together in ways no other patients ever had, helped revolutionize the process of testing experimental drugs, and inspired others. There is no question that breast cancer activism started because of AIDS activism. Those with cancer saw its success and decided to emulate it, deploying thousands of people to lobby for increased research funding.

HIV/AIDS also changed what it means to be gay in America. The images of gay men dying of this disease rendered them objects of sympathy and opened the doors to compassion. In the eyes of straight America, death gave gay men a humanity they had long been denied. Homophobia and attacks on gays became less acceptable. Although some argue that HIV/AIDS divided gays—positives from negatives—it seems more likely that a united gay community was forged in the crucible of HIV/AIDS. People facing mortality responded courageously and seized the chance to proclaim their identity. And it forced society's institutions—from hospitals that barred gay men from seeing their dying lovers to employers who denied them bereavement leave—to recognize gay relationships.

Over the last eight years, HIV/AIDS has increasingly become a disease of the black population in the United States. Of the 1.3 million people living with HIV/AIDS in the United States, about half are black.

Given the above facts about this disease, how will history judge out actions?

STOPPING HIV/AIDS

HIV/AIDS will not be stopped until people are prevented from contracting the virus which, in the absence of a vaccine, means forgoing risks including unprotected sex and injection drugs using contaminated needles. Twenty-seven years after the emergence of HIV, many governments still have not grasped the idea that simple preventive measures, such as providing condoms, sterile needles, and education have been shown to save lives and money. The greatest failure during this pandemic has been in prevention because many governments choose to ignore the subjects of sex and injection-drug use. Rumor, denial, and complacency remain the emotional cocktail that serves to numb people and their governments to the reality of HIV/AIDS. Half of all new HIV infections worldwide are occurring in those under age 25. AIDS cannot be stopped until young adults are protected and respected.

PREVENTION RESEARCH AND APPLICATION

The news—both good and bad—has come unceasingly. In 2005, a test-of-concept HIV vaccine trial began and in 2007 it was declared a failure. This is the third time a promising vaccine has failed. Vaccinology is hard work but it is beyond necessary, it is imperative. In December 2006, we learned that circumcision could reduce men's risk of HIV infection through vaginal sex. One month later, we learned that trials of the microbicide candidate cellulose sulfate would be halted because there appeared to be more infections in the active arm than in the placebo arm. And in July 2007, we learned that a major efficacy study of the diaphragm found no evidence that this particular cervical barrier reduced women's risk of infection.

We know that the field of HIV prevention research is years away from delivering even a partially effective vaccine or microbicide. The response to male circumcision itself, which is only partially protective, reminds us that the good news of circumcision comes with concern, questions, and ambivalence. Today's proven prevention strategies and the materials to enact them are not reaching the people who need them. For example, males in sub-Saharan Africa have access to three condoms a year and female condoms are almost nonexistent. Global tallies of new infections versus expanded treatment access shows that each year for every person who starts antiretroviral treatment, four people are infected with HIV. This ratio places an incredible strain on the fragile infrastructure available for HIV treatment and care.

AND THE REALITY IS

Mitchell Warren, AIDS Vaccine Advocacy Coalition (AVAC) Executive Director, said the following with regard to prevention strategies to prevent HIV/AIDS: "The truth is this: if the cure for AIDS were a glass of clean water, the world would still be hard pressed to bring the epidemic to a halt today. This virus thrives in places where the most basic elements of subsistence—clean water, shelter, food—are in shamefully short supply. It thrives in places where basic human rights—to dignity, health care, protection by the law—are equally scarce." (AVAC Report (2007). *Resetting The Clock*. New York (AVAC). Pages 1–64.)

BY THE NUMBERS

Nearly everywhere, HIV/AIDS is now the leading killer of young people in their most sexually active years. Sex, after all, remains the recreation of the poor. At the first international conference on AIDS in Africa that was held in Brussels before it was clear that AIDS was definitely caused by HIV, a scientist warned that "if AIDS turns out to be a sexually transmitted disease [as it is], it would spread across the world like a prairie fire." And it has. But, regardless of the large number of those who have died of AIDS and those infected, we still learn slowly. In 2009 in the United States, a significant number of people still believe that HIV is spread by kissing, by sharing a drinking glass, or from a toilet seat! In addition, the majority of people do not know that mother-to-child transmission is preventable and that other sexually transmitted diseases can increase your risk of becoming HIV infected.

On the 28th anniversary of HIV/AIDS, there will be about 1.9 million HIV infections in the United States, and about 610,000 of those infected will have died of AIDS. Worldwide, an estimated 24 million will have died of AIDS out of a total of 59 million HIV infected. About 50% are women! This disease will have orphaned some 14 million children worldwide. As we look back over the past 28 years of the HIV/AIDS pandemic there have been major changes since the early years when life after diagnosis largely amounted to a year or so of increasingly severe illness: frightful pneumonias, brain and eye infections, discolored-looking skin cancers, stark weight loss, and thrush, a fungal infection frequently so flagrant it oozed out of a person's mouth. New drugs now thwart these infections in modernized nations, but the vast majority of people across the world with HIV/AIDS continue to suffer these awful physical conditions.

HELP IS ON THE WAY

The United Nations

In 2001, in a precedent-setting special session, the first ever devoted to a public health issue, the UN General Assembly met and wrote its "Declaration of Commitment to a Comprehensive

Battle Against HIV/AIDS." This session is called "Global Crisis—Global Action." Most of the goals set out in this declaration targeted for 2003 and 2005 never materialized, or programs were tried and failed. But, this session of the General Assembly was an important turning point in the global response to HIV/AIDS. In June 2006, in acknowledgement of the 25th anniversary, a second special session of the UN General Assembly met to assess the progress made from the 2001 meeting and to determine what political statement must be made to further the global cause of AIDS. The 2006 Political Declaration calls for $23 billion to be spent on HIV/AIDS in 2010. But as we now know about $50 billion is needed. The Declaration also promotes the protection of human rights, gender equality, and the education and empowerment of women and young people, especially girls, to reduce their vulnerability to HIV, access to essential life-saving commodities, including male and female condoms, harm reduction related to drug use, safe blood supplies, and early and effective treatment of sexually transmitted infections (STIs).

Clearly the road to success in reducing HIV infections globally lies in the success of HIV prevention. To that end, recent advances in the production of an effective microbicide for vaginal and anal sex and the promise that circumcision holds for preventing the transmission of HIV are both positive steps for prevention. Even if the elusive vaccine can be found, its overall effect against HIV infections will be many years off, and because of global cultural views of handling a sexually transmitted disease, a vaccine may not be the final solution.

Each medical advance comes at a higher price and calls for more trained health-care workers, and in the most intensely infected areas, both money and manpower are scarce.

To bring HIV/AIDS under control in the quarter-century ahead, government leaders are going to have to see the pandemic for what it is and will continue to be—the most confounding public health problem in the world—and at long last give it the priority it deserves.

THE NEXT 25 YEARS

Just as no one was prepared for the holocaust of illness that was to come, no one can foresee what the full impact of 25 more years of this disease will entail, beyond knowing that the plight will be far worse, not better, as the nations with the largest populations, China and India, realize the full impact of HIV/AIDS.

Max Essex of the Harvard AIDS initiative said, "Just as the retrovirus that causes AIDS differs considerably today from the samples first studied 25 years ago, the virus will continue to change so much that 25 years from now it will bear virtually no resemblance to the HIV/AIDS virus types seen now. Its impact will change too." Will what we know about preventing current HIV infections be useless in 25 years?

Seth Berkley said that an HIV vaccine is the Holy Grail in curbing this plague. Like the chalice of legend, it has proved elusive. Its urgency is underlined by the fact that AIDS is on its way to killing as many people as the Black Death, the plague in the Middle Ages. But even if there is a vaccine, eradication of HIV is unlikely—HIV has a firm grip on the world. Yet, if a vaccine is not found, the increasing demands for antiretroviral drugs will be overwhelming and most likely will be available only to those who can afford them.

In the last decade, the international community has made great strides in expanding prevention, care and treatment programs but as AIDS marks its 28th year, the disease is outpacing our global response. The number of new HIV infections continues to climb globally.

Despite the advances in medical science against HIV/AIDS, the death toll over the next

25 to 50 years promises to far exceed the 30 to 40 million who died in the Black Plague of the 14th century or the 20 to 50 million who died during the 1918 Spanish flu pandemic.

WILL SUCCESS AGAINST HIV ALWAYS BE MARGINAL?

Does the next quarter century mark the endgame of this struggle between death and hope, or more repetitions of the cycle? Can treatment actually be delivered to all who need it? Will effective biological tools to prevent HIV infection be found? How will millions of deaths affect orphans, vulnerable youth, fragile cultures and global security? It does not bode well that patients in many states within our own borders languish on waiting lists for HIV medication.

There is great hope that current ARVD might prevent high-risk people from becoming infected (PrEP—pre-exposure prophylaxis). One of these, tenofovir, is being tested in several countries. Plans are to test it along with a second drug, emtricitabine. However, there is the risk that treatment will create a resistant strain or, as some critics claim, cause people to lower their guard and have more unprotected sex. There are also postexposure drugs that appear to prevent HIV from successfully infecting the exposed person. And, there is hope of having vaginal and anal microbicides to prevent HIV infection.

Efforts to find an effective vaccine, thus far, have failed. The International AIDS Vaccine Initiative says 30 vaccines are being tested in small-scale trials. Will there be a successful HIV vaccine available in the next 25 years? It is anybody's guess. As a preventive vaccine becomes less of a reality, more money and more efforts are being poured into prevention campaigns, but the efforts are uneven. Success varies widely from region to region and country to country.

During the next 25 years the spread of HIV/AIDS into the general populations of India and China will become a very frightening scenario. It has been estimated that by 2025, some 21 million people will die of AIDS in India and 15 to 18 million will die in China. And so the battle against HIV continues into the next 25 years.

HIV/AIDS

These diseases brought out our worst fears and we waged a war against ourselves as well as the virus. But ultimately this conflict has brought out great compassion and transformed the United States from a nation fraught with AIDS bigotry to one of understanding and concern for the infected and their families.

THE NEXT 25 YEARS MUST BE 25 YEARS OF HEALING, HELP, HOPE, AND SOLUTIONS

Tragically, the end of this global pandemic is nowhere in sight. We need a far more united coalition, united by a commitment to saving lives, even if we may have differences on tactics. We must spend our energy on fighting this epidemic, not on fighting each other. Surely one of the main lessons of these past 28 years is that when we are united we win; when we are divided, HIV wins. We must plan and act not just for today, but for the next 25 years. With every ounce of our intelligence, innovation, and determination, we must advance both social change and science in the fight against HIV/AIDS. The first decade of AIDS was defined by death and activism, the second by medicines and hope. The third decade must be one of finding a successful vaccine.

AIDS UPDATE 2009

WHY DO I WRITE ABOUT HIV/AIDS?

I began writing about a new disease, later called AIDS, in 1981, shortly after the Centers for Disease Control and Prevention issued the first of its reports. These writings were limited in scope because not much was known at the time. My writing then was for classroom use. Little did I know at the time the passion that I would develop about this disease. As the number of infected people and their deaths continued to rise, fear and discrimination reared their ugly heads because, in some cases, people are what they are, and, in other cases, because of the lack of available nonbiased educational material. At the time, in the mid-1980s, I felt a need to write, to help educate people about this disease, hopefully to answer questions and reduce the blatant discrimination occurring against those who already had the overwhelming burden of HIV disease. So, I began—I created a college-level HIV/AIDS course, taught it for several years, constantly shaping and reshaping the information necessary to help others learn the facts about this pandemic, and to destroy destructive myths. After I felt I had set the record straight in my classroom, I began writing HIV/AIDS college-level textbooks so that information on this pandemic could be shared more broadly.

There are many reasons I have not stopped writing about HIV/AIDS. First, because as Yogi Berra supposedly said, "It ain't over til it's over," and it "ain't" near over yet! Second, AIDS summons up the greatest themes in literature, among them sex, faith, and death—themes that are universal and unexpectedly permanent. Anyone who has lost a loved one to death, untimely or by nature, can read about AIDS and understand the emotional forces involved. Anyone who has taken care of someone who has been ill understands the need for compassion. Anyone who has faced death from a prolonged or life-threatening illness should be able to identify with those who suffer with AIDS. Anyone interested in uncovering acts of human kindness or, conversely, acts of despicable behavior can find them in writings about this disease.

But more than any of these reasons, my writing about AIDS is fueled by a need to do something, anything, to help. For the millions of people who are in pain and dying, I have little to offer except my writing. Although my only known risk factor was a blood transfusion in the mid-1970s, I cannot help but feel lucky that so far neither HIV/AIDS nor any other serious disease threatens my life or the lives of my wife and children. Is there a reason I have been spared to my present age when so many others have died? I write about AIDS, not just because I live but because it is part of our history. The AIDS pandemic has changed my feelings and attitudes toward people. I find myself more thoughtful and sensitive to others. AIDS has changed the world in some way for most everyone, and at least some of the information about this disease—its impact and repercussions—needs telling. So, I write about AIDS because someone needs to tell the story.

INTO THE NEW MILLENNIUM

The war on AIDS is still closer to the beginning than it is to the end, but I have never been more positive about the future for those who are HIV infected in the United States and other developed nations. The use of anti-HIV drugs in combination has led to a dramatic reduction in HIV-infected babies and AIDS-related deaths, as well as to a significant reduction in new AIDS cases and reductions in opportunistic infections. These events, along with new insight into the biology and pathology of HIV, may lead to a preventive vaccine and provide a shining light against a stark history of the first 28 years of a pandemic first reported in the United States in 1981.

With the creation of the Global Fund for HIV/AIDS, Malaria, and Tuberculosis in 2001, the G8 (group of eight industrial powers) founding of the International Global Fund for HIV/AIDS, and the decision by the world's largest antiretroviral manufacturers to dramatically lower drug costs to developing nations, there is now hope in those countries. However, the drugs are not yet free, and therefore are out of reach for millions of people living in poverty. But hope and help must begin somewhere—someone must first benefit before others can. **Let us pull together so that help, not just hope, will be available to all who need it!**

—Gerald Stine, Ph.D.

The information on HIV/AIDS within this text goes where the pandemic has taken us over the last 28 years and into the future. This information is not designed to replace the relationship that exists between you and your doctor or other health adviser. For all medical events/needs, consult with an appropriate physician.

AIDS IS A WAR THAT NO ONE WANTS TO LOSE BUT NO ONE YET KNOWS HOW TO WIN

• • • • • •

This book, as with my other seventeen HIV/AIDS college-level textbooks,
is also dedicated to
those who have died of AIDS,
those who have HIV disease, to those who care for them
and to
those who must prevent the spread of this plague—
EVERYONE, EVERYWHERE.

Preface

I hope that this 2009 edition of *AIDS UPDATE* will help you gain a clearer perspective on HIV and AIDS and the ways in which the disease both fuels widespread controversy and suffers under a silence that restricts some of the most important information about it. HIV/AIDS is a slow, progressive, and permanent disease. With the disease, there is no loss of infectivity, no development of either individual or group immunity, and no recovery. At present, there is no known biological mechanism that can stop the continuing expansion of the disease. The progressive increase in the pool of people carrying HIV, the virus that causes AIDS, will lead to an increase in the number of newly infected individuals. Until an effective vaccine can be developed or other interventions are at least moderately successful, the infection will continue to spread and will remain a crucial health issue. With the onset of this real human tragedy, we have been forced to learn about our social contradictions and examine our moral judgments. We have had some success in this venture, yet despite great improvements in our understanding of the scientific and social aspects of the disease, the AIDS crisis is not nearly over.

PURPOSE

While this volume is intended for use in college-level courses on HIV/AIDS and as a supplemental HIV/AIDS resource in medical and nursing schools, it is suitable for any situation in which information about the various aspects of HIV and AIDS is desired or required. This text reviews the most important infor-mation on all facets of HIV infection, HIV disease, and AIDS. It provides readers with a detailed background in the current biological, medical, social, economic, and legal aspects of this modern-day pandemic. Medical and social anecdotes bring a personal perspective to the worldwide HIV/AIDS tragedy, while other parts of the text detail the history of the pandemic. Special focus has been given to HIV transmission, including risk behaviors and means of prevention, and on the innumerable social issues surrounding this disease. Many of these issues are accompanied by open-ended questions to stimulate class discussions that help students reflect on what they have read.

IMPORTANCE

This book is important for two reasons. First, as educators, it is our job to expose our students to the new concepts in biology that are shaping humanity's future. To do that, we must expose them to new vocabulary, new methodologies, new information, and new ideas. It is my hope that this text will help in this endeavor. Second, because misinformation has increased the danger of the HIV/AIDS pandemic, this text attempts to counter common distortions and myths by presenting the most current, consistent, and scientifically acceptable information possible. The text also provides students with a strong conceptual framework for the issues raised by the HIV/AIDS pandemic so they will be better able to deal with new information as it arises.

During the 28 years since HIV/AIDS was defined as a new disease, more effort and money have been poured into research efforts surrounding HIV and AIDS than into any other disease in history. As a result, information on the virus that causes AIDS has accumulated at an unprecedented pace. The constant stream of new information about the changing social and scientific circumstances surrounding the disease makes it necessary to publish updated editions. The majority of references herein are dated between 1990 and 2008, with outdated information being replaced in each edition. What has been learned and what must still be learned to bring HIV infection, HIV disease, and AIDS under control is valuable information to all of us.

NEW TO THIS EDITION

This edition contains updated information and data in every chapter. Topics and content new to this edition include:

- Older data has been replaced by (a) estimated decreases in global number of people living with HIV; (b) number of people newly infected with HIV; and (c) number of deaths from AIDS. This decrease in global numbers was reported in the "2007 AIDS Epidemic Update" published by the World Health Organization (WHO) and the United Nations Program on AIDS (UNAIDS). This data has been updated to reflect the estimated numbers for 2008 and 2009 presented in this edition of AIDS UPDATE.

- Older data from the Center of Disease Control and Prevention (CDC) for the number of HIV infections in the United States have been replaced by an increase in numbers of HIV infections based on data collected from 33 states and 5 dependent areas which used confidential name-based HIV infection reporting beginning 2002 through 2006. These data were published in the CDC's "HIV/AIDS Surveillance Report 2006" but, was not published until March 2008. The estimated 2006 CDC data have been updated to reflect the estimated numbers for 2008 and 2009 and presented in this edition of AIDS UPDATE.

- Fourteen photographs, figures, line drawings, and tables are new to this edition, in addition to new Points of Information, Points of View, Boxes and Sidebars.

- Solid evidence that SIV_{CPZ} crossed into humans from chimpanzees and mutated into HIV.

- All states now report new HIV cases by name.

- New global data downsizing the pandemic is presented.

- Center of Disease Control and Prevention (CDC) recommends that all U.S. citizens, ages 13 to 64, be HIV tested.

- New data from the CDC showing a large increase in HIV infections is presented.

- The financial goals set out for the UN Global Fund for AIDS, Malaria, and Tuberculosis over the coming years are too large and not sustainable.

- An explanation of why HIV/AIDS is a unique and exceptional disease among all other diseases.

- PEPFAR, President Bush's five-year, $15 billion pledge to 15 nations to help stem HIV/AIDS, has been increased to $48 billion over the next five years (2009–2013).

SPECIAL FEATURES

- Each chapter begins with a **Chapter Concepts** section that allows students to preview the material and stay focused on key topics.

- A variety of **boxed essays** provide supplemental information on each chapter's topic. These features illustrate important events and information about HIV/AIDS, including stories from doctors and AIDS survivors, points of scientific note, and discussions of historical context that reveal how knowledge and perceptions of AIDS have evolved over time.

- **Discussion Questions** encourage students to think critically about difficult and controversial issues associated with HIV and provide a starting point for lively class discussions.

- **Further information** sources are listed at the end of relevant chapters. These Internet addresses and national hotline telephone numbers give students resources for additional information on prevention, therapy, healthcare providers, and specific focuses such as women, parents, children, and young adults.

- Chapter **Summary** and **Review Questions** provide students with a quick review of the key concepts of the chapter and help students test their understanding of the chapter's material. Answers appear in an appendix.

- A list of all **References** allows students to see the sources of all scientific and social data within the book, as well as to engage in further research on their own.

- A glossary of the more significant scientific and medical terms can be found in the back of the book.

- A multiple choice test bank and a DVD on HIV replication and the use of antiretroviral drugs to prevent replication is available for the instructors.

IN APPRECIATION

The help of the following organizations and people is most deeply appreciated: The Centers for Disease Control and Prevention (CDC), Atlanta, for use of slides and literature produced in their National Surveillance Report and the Morbidity and Mortality Weekly Report; from the *Sun Sentinel* of Ft. Lauderdale, Fla., Director of Photography Jerry Lower and Photo Archivist Britt Head for photographs out of the Caribbean; from the CDC, Richard Salik and Patricia Sweeney (Surveillance Branch); Robin Moseley, Patricia Fleming, Todd Webber (Division of HIV/AIDS Prevention); Barry Bennett, head of Retroviral Testing Services, for his permission and guidance on photographing HIV testing procedures at the Florida Health and Rehabilitation Office of Laboratories Services, Jacksonville, Fla.; Denise Reddington, Department of Health and Human Services, Washington, D.C.; PANOS Institute for their help in obtaining data on the economics of HIV/AIDS worldwide; personnel of the National Institute for Allergy and Infectious Diseases, the National Center for Health Statistics, Brookwood Center for Children with AIDS in New York; the George Washington AIDS Policy Center in Washington, D.C.; the National Institutes for Health; Hoffman-LaRoche Co., Abbott Laboratories, the Pharmaceutical Manufacturing Association; the National Cancer Institute; Pan American Health Organization; the Office of Technological Assessment; the Physicians' Research Network; BIO-RAD Laboratories; Teresa M. St. John, University of North Florida for illustrations; the individuals who have contributed photographs; the text reviewers whose work has been greatly appreciated; a special thank-you to Gilbertine Yadao who word-processed the updated material; Guy Selander, M.D., and Jack Giddings, M.D., who, over the years, have shared their medical journals with me; James Alderman, Mary Davis, Signe Evans, Cynthia Jordan, Paul Mosley, and Barbara Tuck—reference/research librarians at the University of North Florida; a very special thank-you to Sarah Phillips, head reference librarian at the University of North Florida, for her diligent commitment to assure the accuracy and timeliness of the information found throughout this book; to Michael Muyres for creating new photographic material used within this book; and to my wife Delores, who demonstrated a great deal of patience and understanding and gave up family weekends so the text could be completed on time.

This book has benefited from the critical evaluation of the following reviewers:

Dale J. Erskine
Lebanon Valley College

Kyle Funderburgh
UT Southwestern Medical Center at Dallas

Susan W. Gaskins
University of Alabama
Capstone College of Nursing

Deborah Gritzmacher
Clayton State University

Jacquelyn K. Westfall
The Ohio State University

Gerald J. Stine, Ph.D.
904-641-8979

gstine@unf.edu

gstine@bellsouth.net

A set of HIV/AIDS films for use with most chapters is available for the cost of copying and shipping. Contact the author via email.

Introduction: Histories of Global Pandemics, AIDS, Its Place in History, Overview of HIV/AIDS, International AIDS Conferences and Means of Remembering—the AIDS Quilt, Candlelight Memorial, and World AIDS Day

Awareness **OR**

Ignorance

Death **OR**

Survival

It's your choice, get the facts!

The Author

THREE WORDS ECHO AROUND THE WORLD: AIDS CRISIS WORSENS!

When AIDS first emerged as a recognized disease 27 years ago, few people could have predicted how the epidemic would evolve, and fewer still could have described with any certainty the best ways of combating it. Now, in the year 2009, it is known from experience that AIDS can devastate whole regions, knock decades off national development, widen the gulf between rich and poor nations, and push already-stigmatized groups close to the margins of society. Just as clearly, experience shows that the right approaches, applied quickly enough with courage and resolve, can and do result in lower HIV infection rates and less suffering for those affected by the pandemic. An ever-growing AIDS pandemic is not inevitable; yet, unless action against the pandemic is scaled up drastically, the damage already done will seem minor compared with what lies ahead. This may sound dramatic, but it is hard to play down the effects of a disease that stands to kill more than half of the young adults in the countries where it has its firmest hold.

HISTORY OF GLOBAL PANDEMICS AND EPIDEMICS

There has never been a time in human history when disease did not exist. The history of epidemics dates at least as far back as 1157 B.C. to the death of the Egyptian Pharaoh, Ramses V, from smallpox. Over the centuries, this extraordinarily contagious virus spread around the world, changing the course of history time and again. It killed 2000 Romans a day in the second century A.D., more than 2 million Aztecs during the 1520 conquest by Cortez, and some 600,000 Europeans a year from the sixteenth through the eighteenth centuries. Three out of four people who survived the high fever, convulsions, and painful rash were left deeply scarred and sometimes blind. Because victims' skin looked as if it had been scalded, smallpox was known as the "invisible fire." Even now, malaria in underdeveloped countries afflicts 300 million people, killing between 2 and 3 million each year. The problem is compounded by the development of drug-resistant malarial strains of protozoa. Thus epidemics are not new to humankind, but the fear they impose on each generation is.

How Is This History Relevant?

First, it is important to place HIV and AIDS in a longer-term context: Human populations have been devastated by pandemics before, and have survived. Some populations have even evolved genetically as a result. **Second,** humankind's civil, emotional, and spiritual evolution appears linked to pandemics: Each and every one of the major pandemics (especially bubonic plague or Black Death and Spanish flu) followed major social upheaval and ended during periods when new social structures were established. Such social changes included new value systems and, of course, improved social conditions such as water, housing, and sanitation methods. **Third,** the evidence of history suggests that when these pandemics are over, the development of civilization takes a dramatically different turn. The Bubonic plague accompanied the shift from force-as-law (military might—Roman Empire) to religious order (especially Catholicism), and also paralleled the breaking of the omnipotence of that same religious order, and the emergence of the Age of Reason (organized science and medicine). The Spanish flu accompanied the destruction of the all-pervasive class system and the emergence of communism, socialism, and capitalism as central global political and economic systems. An interesting area of speculation would be to consider whether these social evolutions would have occurred if these pandemics had not emerged.

The major recorded, pandemics (global) and epidemics (regional) that have devastated large populations are described in Table I-1.

FEAR, IGNORANCE AND CONDEMNATION: WHO IS TO BLAME?

During the Black Plague, instead of being concerned about providing care to the victims, people spent their time deciding how deep to dig the graves so that none of the horrid fumes would come up and infect others. It was determined that a grave should be six feet deep, and that is exactly how deep it is today. Plague victims were herded together into cathedrals to die or to pray for faith healing to save them. In fourteenth-century Germany and Switzerland, the Christians blamed the Jews for the outbreak of bubonic plague, believing that the Jews were poisoning the water—the very same water the Jews were drinking. As a result, entire communities of Jews were slaughtered. In the 1400s and 1500s, when syphilis was spreading across the world killing thousands, the Italians called it the French disease. Of course, the French called it the Italian disease. In the 1930s, cholera was considered a punishment for people unwilling to change their lives—the poor and the immoral. In New York the Irish were blamed. In the early twentieth century, polio in America was believed to be caused by Italian immigrants.

Placing Blame: Deja Vu All Over Again!

The history of epidemics teaches us, again and again, that blame is a central component of these events, whether it is cast upon socially ostracized groups of people, water supplies, politics, or religious or cultural beliefs. The sixteenth-century rise of Protestantism, especially Calvinism, increased public intolerance toward the ill. Victims of syphilis were condemned as targets of God's wrath and were ignored by many medical and charitable institutions. Religious artists often depicted Jesus striking down the unjust, raining murderous arrows down from heaven upon syphilis and those who suffered from bubonic plague. It was during this early modern period that the notion of "guilty" and "innocent" victims of disease arose.

The fear of HIV infection and AIDS and ignorance about this plague in our lifetime and its causes have also led to similar bizarre behavior and at times barbaric practices, strange rituals, and attempts to isolate those afflicted.

IMAGINE A WORLD WITHOUT AIDS

AIDS: Its Place in History

As the statistics on AIDS cases mounted, its identity as an inescapable plague seemed confirmed. It appeared to mimic the frightening epidemics of the past: cholera, yellow fever, leprosy, syphilis, and the plague. The history of AIDS—the history that seemed relevant to understanding the new pandemic—would be the history of the pandemics/epidemics of the past. Medical history suddenly gained new social relevance; policy analysts, lawyers, and journalists all wanted to know whether past pandemics/epidemics could provide some clues to the current crisis. How had societies attempted to deal with pandemics/epidemics in the past? The contemporary meaning of past plagues is read in the face of AIDS.

The AIDS pandemic is certainly one of the defining events of our time. There are stories to be told from it, stories of the people infected and affected by it—the well, the ill, the dying, and the survivors. There are the stories of scientific discovery, of HIV and viral mechanisms, and of genetic mysteries being understood. Then there are stories of scientific politics, claims and counterclaims, and the manipulating that goes on in the stratosphere of high-level science.

Table I-1   Plagues in History[1, 4, 5]

Disease	Dates	Place	Number Killed		Causative Organism	Time to Prevention/Cure (in years)
Measles	from 430 B.C.	Greece/Rome/World	Millions		Paramyxovirus	1712
Plague	542–1894	Europe/Asia/Africa	71 million		Yersinia pestis	580
Cholera	1826–1837	New Jersey	900,000		Vibrio cholerae	75
	1849	United Kingdom	53,293			
	1947	Egypt	11,755			
Tuberculosis	1930–1949	United States	1,000,000		Mycobacterium tuberculosis	85
	1954–1970		150,000			
Malaria	1847–1875	Africa/India	20 million +		Plasmodia	100
Scarlet Fever	1861–1870	United Kingdom	972 per million people		Streptococcus pyogenes	45
Polio	1921–1970	North America	37,000		Polio viruses Types I, II, III	40
Typhus	1917–1921	Russia	2,500,000		Rickettsias	25
Influenza	1918–1919	United States/Europe	21,640,000		Influenza virus	57
Smallpox	from 1122 B.C.	Europe (Middle Ages)	Hundreds of millions		Smallpox virus	3050
	1926–1930	India	423,000			
Gonorrhea	from 590 B.C. 1921–1992	United States	57,477		Neisseria gonorrhoeae	71
HIV/AIDS[2]			*Deaths*	*HIV Infections*	Human Immunodeficiency Virus	Treatments but no cure
	1981–2009	United States (estimated)[3]	610,000	1,900,000		
	1981–2009	Global (estimated)	24,000,000	59,000,000		

1. Historical time line on first suspected cases of the above diseases are: Plague, eleventh century B.C.; Cholera, 1781; Tuberculosis, 451 B.C.; Malaria, 1748; Scarlet Fever, 1735; Polio, 1894; Typhus, 1083; Influenza, 1580; Smallpox, 429 B.C.; Gonorrhea, 1768; Yellow Fever, 1647; HIV/AIDS, United States in the 1970s, in Africa, 1959.

2. Total AIDS data estimated through year 2009. Living in some state of HIV disease (9.4 million living with AIDS + 25.6 million with HIV disease = 35 million people living with HIV infection + 24 million dead = 59 million total HIV infections worldwide).

3. United States: of the estimated number of people infected with HIV, about 33% or 610,000 will have died through 2009.

4. Since 1977, 30 new pathogens have appeared, and 20 of the older pathogens have reemerged in drug-resistant forms. Humankind and microbes are engaged in a war of survival wherein both adapt to each other's every move.

5. HIV/AIDS is now second only to the bubonic plague or Black Death as the largest plague or pandemic in history. AIDS, the more preventable of the two pandemics, is expected to surpass the historical statistics of the bubonic plague!

AIDS Is a "Weapon of Mass Destruction!"

America's Secretary of State, Colin Powell, said in April 2004 that "HIV/AIDS is the greatest threat to mankind today, the greatest weapon of mass destruction on the earth."

The AIDS Pandemic Consists of Two Major Parts

The HIV/AIDS pandemic consists of two parts: one medical, the other social. HIV/AIDS infection has provoked a reassessment of society's approaches to public health strategy, healthcare resource allocation, medical research, and sexual behavior. Fear and discrimination have affected virtually every aspect of our culture. Both the medical challenge and, in particular, the social challenge will continue in the foreseeable future. **Arthur Ashe,** a world-class tennis player, so feared discrimination against himself and his family that he lived with AIDS for 3-1/2 years before he was forced to reveal he had the disease. Others, too many to count, have done likewise.

OVERVIEW OF HIV/AIDS

AIDS: A Big Disease with a Little Name, An Earthquake in Slow Motion

The global numbers of people who are HIV-infected along with those who have died from AIDS is almost incomprehensible and very difficult to express. (For the current number of AIDS cases and deaths, see Chapter 10). The numbers are too large to grasp and the implications too terrifying to contemplate. In addition, at this time the future appears grim: First, there is no near-term prospect of a vaccine. Second, existing drug therapies, though relatively effective, are too expensive for the vast majority of those infected. Third, those preventive interventions that can be effective in reducing the numbers of people becoming infected annually are not in place in countries most in need because the majority of the infected are undereducated and their countries still lack the infrastructure to deal with many infectious diseases, including AIDS.

What Is AIDS?

AIDS is defined primarily by severe immune deficiency, and is distinguished from virtually every other disease in history by the fact that it has no constant, specific symptoms. Once the immune system has begun to malfunction, a broad spectrum of health complications can set in. AIDS is an umbrella term for any or all of some 26 known diseases and symptoms. When a person has any of these diseases or has a CD4 or T4 lymphocyte count of less than $200/\mu L$ (microliter) of blood and also tests positive for antibodies to HIV, an AIDS diagnosis is given. (See Table 1-1 for a list of diseases.)

AIDS: A Human Affair

The history of AIDS is a human affair and is part of a cultural process of attempting to come to terms with a new and often terrifying series of events—of young people dying before their time, of the intermingling of sex and death—in a period in which the world itself is changing before our eyes.

The social meaning of the history of AIDS intimately touches upon ideas about sexuality, social responsibility, individual privacy, health, and the prospect of living a normal life span. Understanding how to respond to AIDS and how to think about this pandemic is important not only for what it reveals about the ways in which health policy is created in the United States and elsewhere, but also for what it implies about the human ability to meet the challenge of future emerging diseases and long-standing public health problems. The HIV/AIDS pandemic is a current and long-term public health problem worldwide.

AIDS is reversing decades of public health progress, lowering life expectancy, and significantly affecting international businesses. Lost productivity and profitability, the cost of sickness and death benefits, and the decline in a skilled workforce in the developing world will have economic effects worldwide. AIDS is affecting the military capabilities of some countries as well as international peacekeeping forces.

Lessons Learned from Other Pandemics/Epidemics

From the lessons of history it is difficult to conceptualize how the AIDS pandemic will be halted, let alone reversed, in the absence of a cheap curative drug or a cheap and effective preventative vaccine. The syphilis epidemic at the early part of the century displayed a similar kind of epidemiology to the present-day AIDS epidemic in the United States. The campaigns that were initiated then closely paralleled those in place at present for AIDS. There were vigorous educational programs to reduce high-risk sexual behavior, which were targeted at brothels and prostitutes as well as at military recruits to the U.S. Army. **Scare tactics** were spread through the use of posters, pamphlets, and radio—today it is television. Serological testing became mandatory before marriages could be licensed in certain states. However, these measures had little appreciable effect on the expansion of the syphilis epidemic. It was only the advent of a cheap, safe, and effective drug, penicillin, that eventually brought the epidemic under control.

One lesson learned from HIV/AIDS is that any disease that is occurring in a distant part of the globe may be in the United States, in your state, or in your town, tomorrow. Twenty or even 15 years ago one would not have expected to read that statement.

The advent of miracle drugs and vaccines that conquered the plagues of polio, smallpox, and measles led many people—including scientists—to believe that the age of killer diseases was coming to an end. HIV/AIDS ended that misconception.

AIDS: A UNIQUE DISEASE

The impact of this pandemic is unique. Unlike malaria or polio, previous modern pandemics, it mostly affects young and middle-aged adults. This is not only the sexually most active time for individuals, but also their prime productive and reproductive years. Thus the impact of HIV/AIDS is demographic, economic, political, and social. HIV/AIDS is a disease of human groups in its demographic and social impacts. In the most HIV-affected areas of the world, infant, child, and adult mortality is rising and life expectancy is declining rapidly. The cost of medical care for each infected person overwhelms individuals and households.

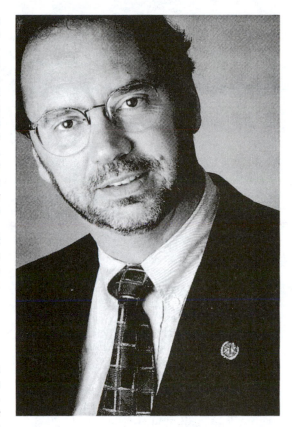

FIGURE I-1　Peter Piot, Executive Director of the Joint United Nations Program on HIV/AIDS (UNAIDS). He is a Belgian physician, microbiologist, and codiscoverer of the Ebola virus in 1976. He is the world's leading advocate for HIV/AIDS control and prevention. He will leave his UNAIDS position ending 2008 (1995–2008). *(Photograph courtesy of UNAIDS/Yoshi Shimizu)*

AIDS: A CAUSE OF DEATH

Peter Piot (Figure I-1), executive director of the United Nations Program on HIV/AIDS, speaking at the Thirty-Seventh Interscience Conference on Antimicrobial Agents and Chemotherapy, said "HIV has transformed the world, joining tuberculosis and malaria as a major cause of death worldwide. This epidemic won't be under control in any country until it is brought under control everywhere."

AIDS is the seventh leading cause of death among 1- to 4-year-olds, sixth among 15- to 24-year-olds, and second among 25- to 44-year-olds in the United States.

There is the expectation that parents will die before their children. Because of the HIV/AIDS epidemic, it is not working out that way for many thousands of parents. They are watching their children die in the prime of life.

The facts on HIV infection, disease, and AIDS that are presented in the following chapters, when understood, clearly place the responsibility for avoiding HIV infection on *you*. You must assess your lifestyle; if you choose not to be abstinent, you must know about your sexual partner and you must practice safer sex. **Never think that you are immune to HIV infection.**

ANOTHER ANNIVERSARY

June 5, 2009, will mark the beginning of the 28th year of the AIDS pandemic. No cure has been found and, although AIDS is now called a "manageable illness," people who are sick must make endless compromises to this disease. The AIDS pandemic forces people to face their mortality daily, for months and years.

A NEW ANNIVERSARY

March 21, 2008 marks the second annual National Native (American Indian, Alaska Native, and Native Hawaiian) HIV/AIDS Awareness Day.

National Native HIV/AIDS Awareness Day is an opportunity for Native people and others to create a greater awareness of the risk of HIV/AIDS to their communities; to remember those who have passed; to acknowledge those who are infected and affected by HIV/AIDS; to call for increased resources for testing, early detection, and increased options for treatment; and to eventually decrease the occurrence of HIV/AIDS among Native people.

May 19, 2009 marks the Third Annual Asia and Pacific HIV/AIDS Awareness Day. This is a federally funded national anti-stigma social marketing campaign called the "Banyan Tree Project." In 2008, 20 cities held events celebrating this day. Asian/Pacific Islanders in the U.S. account for about 1% of total HIV/AIDS cases.

Collectively, Asians and Pacific Islanders are among the fastest-growing racial and ethnic groups in the United States, and they represent an emerging risk group for HIV/AIDS. The enormous cultural diversity among Asians and Pacific Islanders in the United States poses significant challenges to HIV/AIDS prevention efforts. They represent many different nationalities and ethnic groups, and more than 100 languages and dialects, in addition to English, are spoken by members of this community.

INTERNATIONAL AIDS CONFERENCES

The International AIDS Conference is believed to be the single most important meeting on HIV/AIDS. The International AIDS Conference has been the timepiece of the pandemic. The venue, content, style, and mood of each meeting temporarily freezes in time the state of the worldwide HIV/AIDS pandemic.

LOOKING BACK I.1

TWO INTERESTING DETAILS FROM THE FIRST INTERNATIONAL AIDS CONFERENCE–1985

First, in the exhibit area there was a huge map of the United States that said on the top: "The Problem: AIDS. The Solution: Banish All Homosexuals." It had little pushpins on all the major cities of the United States indicating how many homosexuals lived in each. Second, then-Vice President George Bush addressed the assembly. As soon as he started to talk, he was shouted down. (Remember, this was seven years into the Reagan administration and it would be another year before Reagan uttered the word AIDS.) When people started to boo and shout, Bush stepped back from the podium a bit, turned around and said to the Secret Service agent standing behind him (thinking he was turned away from the microphone), "It must be a gay group." The words reverberated throughout the auditorium of the Washington Hilton.

In 1983, there were so few groups involved with HIV/AIDS research that they could stay in contact by telephone. As the virus spread, many countries became involved in HIV/AIDS research and clinical care. International, national, and state meetings were formed as a way to exchange new information. Since the first International AIDS Conference in 1985, the conferences have grown in size to the point that scientists questioned their usefulness.

As of 1994, the International Conference on AIDS is held every two years (Table I-2). The year 2000 Thirteenth International AIDS Conference was held in an underdeveloped nation for the first time. It was held in Durban, South Africa, a country where a significant proportion of the population has HIV/AIDS. Over 12,000 people attended this conference. The International AIDS Conferences are usually grim, but the Thirteenth International AIDS Conference was the grimmest yet, reporting death and infection rates that carry near-apocalyptic implications for the Third World, and particularly Africa.

The theme for this conference was "Breaking the Silence" but it is likely the conference will be remembered for the "Durban Declaration," a document signed by over 5000 physicians and scientists testifying to their belief that HIV causes AIDS. This declaration was created to convince the world that the experts in HIV research are certain that HIV causes AIDS. This document was to put those

Table I-2   International AIDS Conferences

Presented is a list of past International AIDS Conferences by month, year, and location. The number of *reported* AIDS cases and deaths are accumulative by year in the United States.

Number	Month	Year	Location	Deaths
1st	June	1985	Atlanta, Georgia	12,576
2nd	June	1986	Paris, France	24,686
3rd	June	1987	Washington, D.C.	41,088
4th	June	1988	Stockholm, Sweden	62,207
5th	June	1989	Montreal, Canada	90,000
6th	June	1990	San Francisco, California	121,536
7th	June	1991	Florence, Italy	157,000
8th	June	1992	Amsterdam, Netherlands	198,246
9th	June	1993	Berlin, Germany	243,627
10th	August	1994	Yokohama, Japan	298,496
11th	July	1996	Vancouver, Canada	381,896
12th	June	1998	Geneva, Switzerland	421,768
13th	July	2000	Durban, South Africa	463,905
14th	July	2002	Barcelona, Spain	497,630
15th	July	2004	Bangkok, Thailand	529,630
16th	August	2006	Toronto, Canada	561,630
17th	August	2008	Mexico City, Mexico	593,632 Estimated
18th	July	2010	Vienna, Austria	625,000 Estimated

Based on UNAIDS data, during the six days of the eighteenth conference, about 43,000 new HIV infections occurred and 35,000 people died of AIDS worldwide.

AIDS deaths are minimum estimates for the United States, based on data reported to the CDC, and updated. See Figure 10-6 for numbers of AIDS cases in each year.

UNAIDS Executive Director Peter Piot reported that between the Eleventh 1996 AIDS Conference and the Twelfth in 1998, 10 million people were infected with HIV! This, he said "represents a collective failure of the world." The rate of about between 2 million and 3 million new infections per year continues.

who, to this day, still do not believe HIV causes AIDS on notice that their beliefs are wrong. (More information on these HIV dissidents can be found in Chapter 2.)

The theme for the Seventeenth International AIDS Conference is, "Universal Action Now" (read Box 10.1, page 266, for important highlights from the seventeenth conference). The Eighteenth (XVIII) International Conference will be held in Vienna Austria from July 18 to 23, 2010.

MEANS OF REMEMBERING

Nothing visually communicates to the world the magnitude and loss more than the giant patchwork of memories, the **AIDS Quilt.**

The AIDS Memorial Quilt

The quilt was the idea of Cleve Jones, of San Francisco, who in 1985 feared AIDS would become known for the number of people it killed. He wanted a way of remembering the people, who were, in many cases, his friends.

During the eighth candlelight march in San Francisco, Jones asked fellow marchers to write on placards the names of friends and loved ones who died of AIDS. At the end of the march, Jones and others stood on ladders, above the sea of candlelight, taping these placards to the walls of the San Francisco Federal Building. The walls of names looked to Jones like a patchwork quilt.

Purpose and Dimensions of the Quilt

The purpose of the quilt is to educate. The AIDS Quilt is made up of individual fabric panels, each the size of a grave, measuring three feet by six feet, stitched together into 12 foot × 12 foot sections. In October 1987, the AIDS Quilt was first put on display on the mall in Washington, D.C. At that time it contained 1920 panels and covered an area larger than two football fields. It took less than two hours to

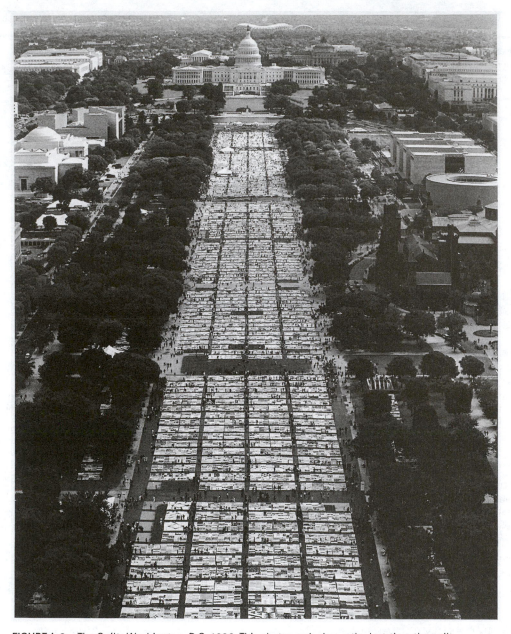

FIGURE I-2 The Quilt: Washington, D.C. 1996. This photograph shows the last time the quilt was displayed in its entirety on the capital mall, October 11–13. *(Photograph © AP/Wide World Photos)*

read all the names. In 1992 it took 60 hours. As of mid-2008 the quilt weighed about 60 tons with about 60,000 panels containing over 91,000 names representing about 16% of those who have died of AIDS in the United States (Figure I-2). Displayed in its entirety, it would cover over 45 football fields. It is the largest piece of folk art in the world and continues to increase in size daily. If the 3-by-6 foot panels were laid end to end, the quilt would stretch over 50 miles. There are about 50 miles of seams and 26 miles of canvas edging. There are panels from each of the 50 states and Washington, D.C. Each day new panels

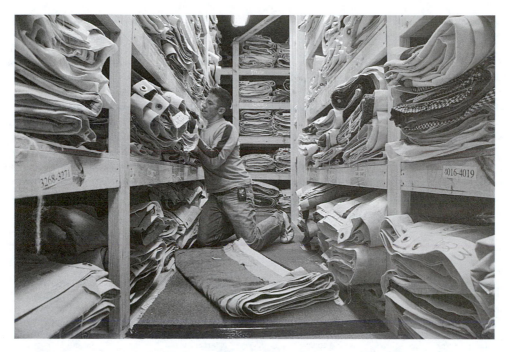

FIGURE I-3 Names Project Foundation person pulling out a block of the AIDS quilt from the storage bins in the Atlanta warehouse. (Photograph by Eric S. Lesser, with permission.)

arrive from across the United States and 37 foreign countries to be added to the quilt (Figure I-3). For those left behind, the panels represent an expression of love and a sign of grief—a part of the healing process.

Portions of the quilt tour in major cities. Over 20 million people have visited the quilt at thousands of displays around the world. Donations made for viewing the quilt are being used to support local Names Project chapters and their staffs.

Each panel has its own story. The stories are told by those who make the panels for their lost friends, lovers, parents, and children. The complete quilt was displayed in Washington, D.C., October 11–13, 1996, for the last time—it is too large to view again as a whole. It took 10 boxcars and a freight train to transport this work of art to the nation's capital.

By the end of 2009, over 600,000 Americans will have died from AIDS. If each of their names made up a separate panel, imagine the size of the quilt. If a name is read every 10 seconds, it would take over 62 days of calling names 24 hours a day!

A Reminder

People nationwide will celebrate the twenty-second anniversary of the AIDS Quilt on July 21, 2009. For more information about the Names Project's AIDS Memorial Quilt, call (404)688-5500, ext. 223; www.aidsquilt.org.

THE 25TH CANDLELIGHT MEMORIAL

The first candlelight march for AIDS occurred simultaneously in New York city and San Francisco in May 1983. The memorial march is now international. The International AIDS Candlelight Memorial honors the memory of those lost to AIDS, shows support for those living with HIV and AIDS, raises community awareness of HIV/AIDS, and mobilizes community involvement in the fight against HIV/AIDS. In 2008, the Candlelight Memorial was observed in about 1500 locations in 85 nations on every continent but Antarctica. The Candlelight march takes place on the third Sunday of May. (For additional information contact Sara Ann

Friedman, email: candlelight@ globalhealth.org or visit the website: http://www.globalhealth.org.)

WALKING TO CHANGE THE COURSE OF THE HIV/AIDS EPIDEMIC— UNITED STATES

The first **AIDS Walk** in America took place in Los Angeles, California, in 1985. The second AIDS Walk occurred in New York City in 1986. Since that time, HIV/AIDS volunteers in 43 other states have organ-ized AIDS Walks in numerous towns and cities within their borders (Table I-3; Figures I-4 and I-5). The purpose of the AIDS Walk event is **people, all kinds of people, from all walks of life, helping people!** The spin-off from these walks, due to their popular-ity, size, and ability to raise large sums of money, gave large numbers of people who may not have other-wise become involved in the HIV/AIDS crisis a voice so loud and resourceful that it enabled them to get the government's attention and helped promote new and different types of legislation recognizing the impact HIV/AIDS was having in the United States.

Table I–3   Aids Walks: United States 1985–2008: Forty–Five States, One Hundred and Fifteen Locations

Alabama	Illinois	Nebraska	Pennsylvania
Birmingham	Arlington Heights	Norfolk	Harrisburg
Alaska	Chicago	Grand Island	Philadelphia
Atlanta	Springfield	Lincoln	Pittsburgh
Arizona	Indiana	Omaha	Williamsport
Tucson	Evansville	Scottsbluff	Rhode Island
California	Fort Wayne	Nevada	Providence
Carson	Indianapolis	Las Vegas	South Carolina
East Bay	Iowa	New Hampshire	Myrtle Beach
Inland Empire	Central Iowa	Portsmouth	South Dakota
Long Beach	Des Moines	New Jersey	Sioux Falls
Los Angeles	Kansas	New Brunswick	Tennessee
Modesto	Lawrence	New Mexico	Knoxville
Orange County	Topeka	Albuqerque	Nashville
Palm Springs	Wichita	Santero	Texas
Sacramento Valley	Kentucky	Santa Fe	Austin
Santa Barbara	Louisville	New York	Dallas (Life Walk)
San Diego	Louisiana	Albany	East Texas
San Francisco	New Orleans	Binghampton	Houston
San Luis Obispo	Maine	Buffalo	Utah
San Bernardino	Augusta	Caribbean (Brooklyn)	Salt Lake City
Silicon Valley	Bagor	Hudson Valley	Vermont
Colorado	Brunswick	New York City	Burlington
Denver	Ellsworth	Rhode Island	Virginia
Connecticut	Portland	Rochester	Charlottesville
Hartford	Maryland	Syracuse	Washington
New Haven	Baltimore	Utica	Bremerton/Kitsap
Delaware	Michigan	North Carolina	County
Dover	Detroit	Charlotte	Olympia
Georgetown	Minnesota	Raleigh/Durham	Seattle
Wilmington	Minneapolis	Ohio	Tacoma
Florida	Missouri	Central Ohio	Washington, D.C.
Ft. Lauderdale	Central Missouri	Cincinnati	Wisconsin
Miami	Kansas City	Cleveland	Madison
Orlando	Ozarks/So. West	Oklahoma	Milwaukee
St. Petersburg	St. Louis	Oklahoma City	Wyoming
Tampa Bay	Massachusetts	Tulsa	Laramie
Georgia	Boston	Oregon	**CANADA**[1]
Atlanta	Worcester	Eugene	
Hawaii	Mississippi	Portland	
Honolulu	Jackson		
Kapiolani Park			

1. AIDS Saint John held its 15th Annual AIDS Walk For Life. These and other annual walks in communites across Canada have raised over $26 million since 1986 attracting over 500,000 people to walk.

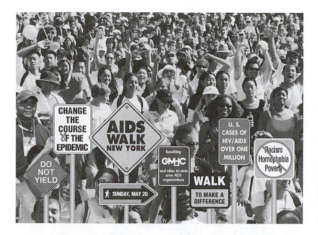

FIGURE I-4 **AIDS Walk New York.** In 2008, 45,000 people participated in the Walk, and they raised 7.05 million, the largest sum of money ever for an AIDS Walk. AIDS Walk SanFrancisco 2008 had 25,000 people participate and raised $4.6 million (over $70 million since 1987). (Photograph courtesy of Bert Champagne.)

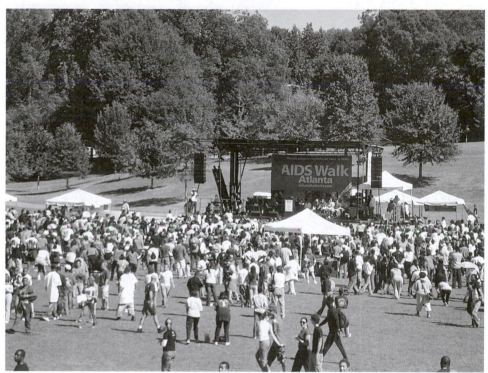

FIGURE I-5 **AIDS Walk Atlanta.** In 2008, about 9,000 people walked, raising about $650,000. (Photograph courtesy of Katerina Spasorska.)

The Beginning of AIDS Walks in America

When Craig Miller, Walkathon co-producer, first became involved in the 1985 AIDS Walk, this was still relatively early in terms of the public's awareness of the HIV/AIDS crisis. He said he was very nervous in organizing that first event. He and colleagues were concerned: Would the public really participate? Would we attract the thousands of people that we needed to make the event successful? Fortunately, the Los Angeles community did turn out in large numbers to support that first event. The event was hugely successful. Then, the Gay Men Health Crisis of New

York City asked if they would be willing to come to New York to help Gay Men Health Crisis get an AIDS Walk off the ground. This was also a very successful event, and from there, AIDS Walks began across the United States. Through 2008, over six million people had participated in these walks, raising over $350 million! Dollar for dollar, AIDS Walk monies have been put to more effective use at the grassroots level, helping organizations and people on the street, then any other form of money set aside to aid those infected with HIV.

BICYCLE RIDING TO CHANGE THE COURSE OF THE HIV/AIDS EPIDEMIC—UNITED STATES

The goals of the AIDS Bike Rides Across the United States are the same goals listed for AIDS Walks. It was more difficult to obtain information on bike riding HIV/AIDS events than for AIDS Walks. In a number of cases, earlier records of bike riding events were not kept or were unavailable. Table I-4 lists those for which data was found. Note that rides occurred in 24 states and the District of Columbia, most in 2007. Together, AIDS Walks and bike rides rose over $321 million dollars through 2007.

Four Other Means of Raising Money for HIV/AIDS in 2008

In February 2008, one event, Product Red Art Auction, raised $42.6 million for the Global Fund Programs in Africa. Also in February, the state of Illinois began a Red Ribbon Cash Lottery. The Illinois Department of Revenue expects the lottery to bring in $13 million annually. The money will be used to award grants within the state to help existing HIV/AIDS programs conduct education/prevention and free HIV testing. In May 2008, movie actress Sharon Stone hosted the 15th Cinema for AIDS gala, raising over $10 million. Singer Madonna raised $500,000 by auctioning off a private concert.

WORLD AIDS DAY: AN INTERNATIONAL DAY OF COORDINATED ACTION: A TIME TO RECHARGE AND RECONNECT

As in years past, rituals of candles and quilts coincide on World AIDS Day with the release of grave new statistics and heartrending personal stories—not only from distant countries but also from our own backyards. While humanitarian concerns demand that developed nations take action in the developing world, a growing apathy about the HIV pandemic in America helps perpetuate a pandemic that has already claimed over a 600,000 lives and counting.

The "Reading of Names" of those who have died of AIDS is a World AIDS Day vigil.

December 1 is now traditionally called World AIDS Day, a time of remembrance for those individuals who have died from AIDS, a time to assess the current status of the epidemic, and a time to evaluate the effectiveness of our efforts to control it. Now well into the third decade since the recognition of AIDS, it is estimated that about 59 million

---

LOOKING BACK I.2

WORLD AIDS DAY—LOOKING BACK— 22 YEARS LATER

In 1987, Jim Bunn, a press officer at the World Health Organization (WHO) in Geneva, conceived the idea of World AIDS Day (WAD) while editing a speech on AIDS for WHO's director-general. Bunn said that many world leaders avoided talking about AIDS at the time when it was a relatively new disease about which little was known. The idea of WAD was to cast a wide net, draw everybody in, and state that this is a worldwide problem. "We wanted to say to countries, if you don't have the signs of the epidemic in your country yet, you will. And you need to be aware of it and you need to be prepared for it." The WHO created a press kit for the first World AIDS Day on December 1, 1987 and sent it to media outlets and to community-based groups and nongovernmental organizations that were responding to the crisis. "Our hope was that this would become something that eventually the World Health Organization would have nothing to do with and it would take on its own life." That's exactly what happened. The event did garner its own momentum and raised public awareness of the disease. WAD encouraged activists to put pressure on governments to acknowledge and respond to the pandemic and helped foster the current worldwide acknowledgment of HIV/AIDS. Although the epidemic has changed over the past 22 years, Bunn believes that the annual observance is still important to remind people of the continuing problem, the need to care for those who are sick, the vulnerabilities of at-risk populations, and the need to raise money.

Table I–4   Aids Bike Rides Across the United States

			Money Raised
Alaska			
Fairbanks to Anchorage	AIDS Vaccine Ride 2000	August 20-21, 2000	$4.1 million
California			
San Francisco	1) 13th Annual Ron Wilmot Bike Ride	May 12, 2007	$18,000
	2) AIDS/Life Cycle	June 3-9, 2007	$11 million
Los Angeles	World's AIDS Day Bike Ride	December 1, 2007	
Colorado			
Colorado Springs	Pikes Peak Classic Century Ride	August 12, 2007	$13,000
Connecticut			
Hartford	CT AIDS Bike Tour	September 5-9, 2007	$32,000
Florida			
Key West	Smart Ride 4	March 30-31, 2007	$400,000
Georgia			
Atlanta to Athens	Action Cycling 200	March 20-21, 2006	$130,000
Hawaii	Paradise Ride	June 9-1, 2006	$200,000
Illinois			
Chicago	Ride for AIDS	June 2-3, 2007	$300,000
Kansas			
Shawnee	AIDS Bicycle Challenge	October 6, 2007	$18,000
Massachusetts			
Boston	Harbor to the Bay	September 15, 2007	$325,000
Boston to New York	AIDS Ride	June 20-23, 2007	$6.5 million
Provincetown to Stowe	Ride FAR	Since 1989 (1)	$1 million
Michigan			
Lansing	Life Ride 2007	June 16, 2007	Not available
Minnesota			
Minneapolis	Red Ribbon Ride	June 19-22, 2007	$700,000
Missouri			
Springfield	4th Annual Red Ribbon Ride	May 19, 2007	$47,000
New Jersey			
Bradley Beach	NJ Ride Against AIDS	September 28-30, 2007	$74,000
New Mexico			
Albuquerque	Tour De Bosque	June 30, 2007	$7,500
New York			
Ithaca	AIDS Ride for Life	September 15, 2007	$400,000
Niagara Falls to NYC	Empire State AIDS Ride	August 12-18, 2007	$348,000
North Carolina			
Raleigh	AIDS Walk & Ride	May 5, 2007	$149,779.49
Winston Salem	AIDS Action Ride	August 8-10, 2007	$2,420
Ohio			
Cleveland	Red Ribbon Ride	September 23, 2007	$61,630.86
Pennsylvania			
Gettysburg to NYC	Braking the Cycle	September 28-30, 2006	$409,000
South Carolina			
Lancaster	Dream Ride Lancaster	July 26, 2008	Not available
Texas			
Austin	Hill Country Ride for AIDS	April 28, 2007	$2.5 million
Dallas	Lone Star Ride 2007	September 29-30, 2007	$1.4 million
Vermont			
Burlington	7th Annual Champ Ride	June 9, 2007	Not available
North Ferrisburg	7th Annual Champ Ride	June 9, 2007	Not available
Washington			
Seattle to Portland	Ride to Fight AIDS	July 14-15, 2007	$50,000
Wisconsin			
Madison	ACT 5-AIDS RIDE	August 2-5, 2007	$296,000
Washington, D.C.	Tour de Friends	June 19-22, 2003	$2.6 million
		TOTAL	**$33,081,331**

(1) 1989 is the earliest ride listed; 26 rides listed in 2007.

people (by the end of 2009) will have been infected with HIV, clearly making this one of the worst epidemics of our time. Projections for 2005–2015 suggest that the situation will become even more serious as we reach about 90 million infected individuals.

December 1, 1988, was the first acclaimed *World AIDS Day* (WAD). The theme was "Join the Worldwide Effort." World AIDS Day is a day set aside to pay tribute to those who have AIDS and to those who have died of AIDS. For 2009 the theme will be "Stop AIDS: Keep The Promise." This theme will run through 2010. For information on World AIDS Day

2008, write 108 Leonard Street, 13th Floor, New York, NY 10013 or call (212)513-0303, or World AIDS Day Public Information Office, WHO-GPA, 1211 Geneva 27, Switzerland.

THE WORLD HEALTH AND UNAIDS ORGANIZATIONS

In January 2007, Margaret Chan began serving as director-general of the World Health Organization (WHO).

The WHO has established a global program on HIV infection and AIDS. The program has three objectives: to prevent new HIV infections, to provide support and care to those already infected, and to link international efforts in the fight against HIV infection and AIDS.

In 1995, the United Nations secretary-general chose Peter Piot to begin a Joint United Nations Program on HIV/AIDS (UNAIDS). Piot's job is to coordinate actions and reduce duplication among the 10 cosponsors of UNAIDS: United Nations Children's Fund (UNICEF), the United Nations Development Programme (UNDP), the United Nations Educational, Scientific and Cultural Organization (UNESCO), the United Nations Population Fund (UNFPA), the United Nations Office on Drugs and Crime (UNODC), the World Health Organization (WHO), the World Bank, the International Labor Organization, the World Food Programme, (WFP) and the United Nations High Commissioner for Refugees (UNHCR).

First Global AIDS Week: One Week–One Voice: May 18–24, 2008

In its first year (spring of 2006), the theme of Day 1 was "HIV in Marginalized Populations" (action: symbolic solidarity); Day 2 was "Behavior Change" (action: getting tested); Day 3 was "Access to Medications" (action: call-in campaign); Day 4 was "The Global and Local Disconnect" (action: provider shadowing opportunity); and Day 5 was "Taking Action" (action: Mosaic AIDS Variety Show Fundraiser). Thirteen countries participated. Thirty countries participated in 2008, the third annual event.

THE FUTURE

The history of HIV/AIDS is one of remarkable scientific achievement. Never in history has so much been learned about so complex an illness in so short a time. We moved into the new millennium, the third decade of AIDS, with hope and the determination to find better therapies and a vaccine. The task is formidable but it has to be done and it will be accomplished. The evolving story of the HIV/AIDS epidemic has been one of the major medical news events of the past 27 years. It is getting hard to imagine medicine or society without HIV/AIDS.

HIV/AIDS is a truly persistent global pandemic and will require a proportionate response to bring it under control. It is the plague of our lifetimes—and probably that of our children's lives as well. We already have people age 27 and younger who don't know what an HIV-free world is. They were born into this recognized pandemic (1981). To survive this pandemic, society must prevent the face of AIDS from becoming faceless. The chapters on HIV infection, HIV disease, and AIDS in this book will help bring widespread information on the virus into focus. The information within these chapters should also help eliminate many of the myths and irrational fears, or FRAID **(fear of AIDS),** generated by this disease. There is much work to be done by both scientists and society.

Perhaps a borrowed anecdote says it best:

> *As the old man walked the beach at dawn, he noticed a young woman ahead of him picking up starfish and flinging them into the sea. Finally catching up with the youth, he asked her why she was doing this. The answer was that the stranded starfish would die if left to the morning sun.*
>
> *"But the beach goes on for miles and there are millions of starfish," countered the old man. "How can your effort make any difference?"*
>
> *The young woman looked at the starfish in her hand and threw it to safety in the waves. "It makes a difference to this one," she said.*

(Adapted from *The Unexpected Universe* by Loren Eiseley. Copyright 1969, Harcourt Brace, New York)

Too easily we can become overwhelmed by the enormity of the AIDS pandemic. The numbers of patients and their constant needs have caused many to become paralyzed into inactivity and lulled into indifference. Like the old man, many ask "Why bother?"

For the sake of every individual living with HIV, we must focus on what each one of us can do. Each person can make a difference. Believing this, we are empowered to cope with the larger whole.

In June 2005, Peter Piot, head of the United Nations campaign to combat AIDS, said that "it is no longer realistic to hope that the world will meet its goal of halting and reversing the spread of HIV by year 2015." Robert Gallo, a leading HIV researcher and head of the University of Maryland's Institute of Human Virology, said "HIV/AIDS will be a problem for our children and our children's children." If by 2025, millions of people are still becoming infected with HIV each year, it will not be because there was no choice. It will not be because there is no understanding of the consequences of the decisions and actions being taken now, in the early years of the century. It will be because the lessons of the first 27 years of the epidemic were not learned, or were not applied effectively. It will be because, collectively, there was insufficient political will to change and/or halt the forces driving the HIV/AIDS pandemic. What politicians, institutions, communities, and individuals do today can change future, predictable scenarios of this pandemic." Such dire announcements actually increase the importance that everyone, everywhere become familiar with the various aspects of this global pandemic. For these reasons and many others each year, as this pandemic spreads across the globe, this book offers new insight into the many and varied aspects of HIV/AIDS. It provides much-needed information to students, their instructors, those that are HIV positive and negative, and the general public.

Valuable Stories

To aid in the understanding and acceptance of somewhat complex ideas and science in certain chapters, valuable **stories** provide first-hand testimony about the way research is done, its failures and successes, about the pain, suffering, and hardship endured by HIV-negative and -positive people as this disease impacts planet earth. Stories are mines of information, rich in memories and history, and this should be shared.

General Disclaimer

AIDS Update is designed for educational purposes only and is not engaged in rendering medical advice or professional services. The information provided through *AIDS Update* should not be used for diagnosing or treating a health problem or a disease. It is not a substitute for professional care. If you have or suspect you may have a health problem, consult your healthcare provider.

Librarians in Los Angeles and San Francisco Catalog HIV/AIDS Materials-January 2008

Librarians in Los Angeles and San Francisco have finished cataloging hundreds of thousands of HIV/AIDS documents and have made the documents available to the public. The **One National Gay & Lesbian Archives** received a $195,000 grant from the **National Historical Publications and Records Commission (NHPRC)** to catalog the materials. NHPRC also awarded a shared $170,000 grant to a library at the **University of California-San Francisco and the Gay, Lesbian, Bisexual and Transgender Historical Society.** It took three years for librarians to catalog the documents.

National AIDS Hotlines

♦ Centers for Disease Control and Prevention/National AIDS Clearing House, 1-800-458-5231.

♦ National AIDS, for the English-language service (open 24 hours a day, 7 days a week), call 1-800-232-AIDS (4636).

♦ The Spanish service (open from 8 A.M. to 2 A.M., 7 days a week) can be reached at 1-800-344-SIDA (7432).

♦ A TTY service for the hearing impaired is available from 10 A.M. to 10 P.M. Monday through Friday at 1-800-243-7889.

♦ National Prevention Information Network, 1-800-458-5231.

♦ National Herpes Hotline, 1-919-361-8488.

♦ National Native American AIDS Prevention, 1-510-444-2051.

♦ National Association of People with AIDS, 1-202-898-0414.

♦ National HIV Telephone Consultation Service for Health Care Professionals, 1-800-933-3413, San Francisco General Hospital, Bldg. 80, Ward 83, Room 314, San Francisco, CA 94110.

♦ HIV/AIDS Treatment Information Service, 1-800-HIV-0440 (448-0440), 9 A.M. to 7 P.M. Eastern time, Monday–Friday. 1-800-243-7012 Teletype number for the hearing-impaired, 9 A.M. to 5 P.M. Eastern time, Monday–Friday, Box 6303, Rockville, MD 20849-6303.

♦ AIDS Clinical Trials Information Service, 1-800-TRIALS-A 874-2572, 9 A.M. to 7 P.M. Eastern time, Monday–Friday. Information on clinical trials of AIDS therapies.

♦ National Gay and Lesbian Task Force AIDS Information Hotline, 1-888-843-4564.

♦ Gay Men's Health Crisis AIDS Hotline, 1-212-807-6655.

♦ National HIV/AIDS Education & Training Centers Program, 1-301-443-6364, Fax: 1-301-443-9887.

♦ AIDS National Interfaith Network, 1-202-546-0807, Fax: 1-202-546-5103, 110 Maryland Ave., NE, Room 504, Washington, D.C. 20002.

♦ National Hemophilia Foundation, 1-800-424-2634.

♦ Pediatric AIDS Foundation, 1-310-395-9051.

♦ National Pediatric HIV Resource Center, 1-800-362-0071.

♦ AIDSLINE via the National Library of Medicine. Free access via Grateful Med, obtained from NLM at 1-888-346-3656.

♦ National Institute on Drug Abuse Hotline, 1-800-662-HELP 1-4357.

♦ National Sexually Transmitted Diseases Hotline 1-800-227-8922.

♦ American Civil Liberties Union Guide to local chapters, 1-202-544-1076.

♦ AIDS Policy and Law, 1-215-784-0860.

♦ National Conference of State Legislatures HIV, STD and Adolescent Health Project, 1-303-830-2200.

♦ United States Conference of Mayors, 1-202-293-2352.

♦ Centers for Disease Control and Prevention, Public Inquiry, 1-404-639-3534.

♦ Food and Drug Administration, Office of Public Affairs, 1-301-443-3285.

♦ American Red Cross, Office of HIV/AIDS Education, 1-800-375-2040.

♦ World Health Organization, 1-202-861-4354.

Useful Internet Addresses

♦ AIDS Treatment Data Network, 1-800-734-7104, 611 Broadway, Suite 613, New York, NY 10012. http://health.nyam.org:8000/public_html/network/index:html, email: AIDS-TreatD@AOL.COM. A home page on the Internet for people with AIDS and their caregivers, it provides information on approved and experimental treatments for AIDS-related conditions. It also publishes a quarterly directory of clinical trials on HIV and AIDS in English and Spanish.

♦ AMA HIV/AIDS Information Center website (http://www.ama-assn.org) offers clinical updates, news, and information on social and policy questions. Cosponsored by Glaxo Wellcome Inc.

♦ Gay Men's Health Crisis (GMHC), website (http://www.gmhc.org) provides online forums hosted by GMHC representatives.

For additional help you may wish to consult with your college or community library. They may have access to the following AIDS-related data bases:

- AEGIS (AIDS Education Global Information System): http://www.aegis.org
- HIV Info Web: http://www.infoweb.org
- Kaiser Daily Global HIV/AIDS information: www.kaisernetwork.org
- Southern Africa AIDS Information Dissemination Service: www.safaids.org.zw
- Immunet: http://www.immunet.org
- Project Inform: http://www.projinf.org
- The Body: http://www.thebody.com/cgi/treatans.html
- HIVInSite: http://www.hivinsite.ucsf.edu/medical/tx-guidelines
- Search AIDSLINE, MEDLINE: http://www.igm.nim.nih.gov
- Vaccines: http://www.avi.org
- Women, children, healthcare workers, hemophiliacs, blind, deaf, and other affected groups: http://beaconclinic.org/website/groups
- AIDS/HIV statistics: http://www.avert.org/statindx.htm
- http://www.healthcg.com/hiv/links.html (provides linkage to nine major U.S. Guidelines for HIV Testing, OIs, Treatment, etc.)
- The Centers for Disease Control and Prevention's (CDC) National Prevention Information Network *(NPIN) Links:* http://www.cdcnac.org/hivlink.html and http://www.cdcnac.org/daynews.html
- National Institute of Allergy and Infectious Diseases (NIAID) online at: http://www.niaid.nih.gov

  Critical Path AIDS Project, a Philadelphia organization for people with HIV disease, provides another online source for the latest news in HIV disease prevention, research, clinical trials, and treatments. The publication's hot link leads to a directory of AIDS-related publications: (http://www.critpath.org)
- UNAIDS Global HIV/AIDS information: www.unaids.org
- WHO HIV/STI Surveillance: http://www.who.int
- European Center for the Epidemiological Monitoring of AIDS: http://www.ceses.org
- AIDS MAP Global HIV/AIDS information: www.aidsmap.com
- *Managing Desire: HIV Prevention Counseling for the 21st Century* targets the HIV test counseling community as well as the general consumer. The site is produced by Nicholas Sheon, the prevention editor of the *HIV Inside* website of the UCSF Center for AIDS Prevention Studies (http://hivsinsite.ucsf.edu) and an HIV test counselor at the Berkeley Free Clinic: (http://www.managingdesire.org)
- *AIDS* offers abstracts from recent issues: http://www.aidsonline.com

- *AIDS Weekly Plus* contains more than 35,000 articles on health-related topics. Full access is available by subscription: http://www.newsfile.com
- *AIDS Treatment News* posts the contents of every issue since the publication began in 1986: http://www.immunet.org/immunet/atn.nsf/homepage
- The *Bulletin of Experimental Treatment on AIDS (BETA)* published by the San Francisco AIDS Foundation, is free online: http://www.sfaf.org/beta.html
- *Treatment Issues,* published by the Gay Men's Health Crisis, provides free access to issues dating back to 1995: http://www.gmhc.org/aidslib/ti/ti.html
- *Project Inform* email (INFO@projinf.org), website, established in 1985 as a national, nonprofit, community-based HIV/AIDS treatment information and advocacy organization, serves HIV-infected individuals, their caregivers, and their healthcare and service providers through its national, toll-free treatment hotline: http://www.projinf.org
- The Synergy APDIME ToolKit is a user-oriented, electronic one-stop-shop of HIV/AIDS programming resources. Developed in collaboration with the University of Washington Center for Health Education and Research (CHER), the ToolKit contains five modules of the programming cycle covering Assessment, Planning, Design, Implementation Monitoring, and Evaluation: http://www.synergyaids.com/apdime/index.htm#

  The following is a sampling of general Internet resources for community research and HIV/AIDS information in Canada:
- Western Canada's largest AIDS group (in Vancouver, BC) has launched its redesigned website featuring online publications, a map of provincial resources, and links to over 100 AIDS websites. The website, published by the British Columbia Persons with AIDS Society, is one of the most popular sites in Canada and has operated for two years. The site carries information about:
  - *Treatments:* http://www.bcpwa.org/treat.htm;
  - *AIDS news:* http://www.bcpwa.org/news.htm;
  - *Organizational activities:* http://www.bcpwa.org/AboutBCPWA/board.htm; and
  - *Links:* http://www.bcpwa.org/Resources/links.htm
  - For more information: Pierre Beaulne, Developer, Communications and Marketing, British Columbia Persons With AIDS Society, mail to: pierreb@pace.org
- The Community-Based HIV/AIDS Research Program National Health Research and Development Program, Health Canada: http://www.hc-sc.gr.ca/hppb/nhrdp/cdr.htm
- The HIV/AIDS Aboriginal Research Program National Health Research and Development Program,

Health Canada: http://www.hc-sc.gr.ca/hppb/
nhrdp/abrfp.htm

♦ Community-University Research Alliances (CURAs),
Social Sciences and Humanities Research Council of
Canada: http://www.sshrc.ca/english/programinfo/
grantsguide/cura.html

♦ Canadian Strategy on HIV/AIDS:
http://www.hc-sc.gc.ca/hppb/hiv aids/

♦ Canadian HIV/AIDS Clearinghouse:
http://www.cpha.ca/clearinghouse e.htm

♦ Canadian AIDS Society: http://www.cdnaids.ca/

♦ Canadian Aboriginal AIDS Network:
http://www.caan.ca/

♦ Community AIDS Treatment Information Exchange:
http://www.catie.ca/

♦ Canadian HIV/AIDS Legal Network:
http://www.aidslaw.ca/

♦ Bureau of HIV/AIDS, STD and TB, Health Canada:
http://www.hc-sc.gc.ca/hpb/lcdc/bah/epi/epie.html

♦ Global Network of People Living With HIV/AIDS
(GNP+): email: gnp@gn.apc.org

♦ AIDS.org is Google's #1 resource for AIDS
information.

ACQUIRED IMMUNE DEFICIENCY SYNDROME (AIDS)

What do we know about AIDS? The next 14 chapters will present the many faces of the AIDS pandemic in the United States and other countries. Unlike people, the AIDS virus (HIV) does not discriminate; and it appears that most humans are susceptible to HIV infection, its suppression of the human immune system, and the consequences that follow. The viral infection that leads to AIDS is the most lethal, the most feared, and the most socially isolating of all the sexually transmitted diseases. We must, as a people, fight against AIDS, not against each other.

AIDS: Defining the Disease and Finding Its Cause

CHAPTER CONCEPTS

- The letters A, I, D, S (AIDS) are an acronym for Acquired Immune Deficiency Syndrome.
- AIDS is a syndrome, not a single disease.
- Cases of severe immune deficiency (AIDS) were found in five women between 1975 and 1981.
- The first cases of AIDS-related *Pneumocystis carinii* pneumonia (PCP) were reported by the Centers for Disease Control and Prevention (CDC) in June 1981, the first case of Kaposi's sarcoma in July 1981.
- Luc Montagnier discovered the AIDS virus in 1983.
- The first CDC definition of AIDS was presented in 1982 and expanded in 1983, 1985, and 1987, and again on January 1, 1993.

A= Acquired = means not inherited, develops after birth by contact with the disease-causing agent; in the case of AIDS, a virus received from someone else

I= Immune = an individual's natural protection against disease-causing microorganisms and viruses

D = Deficiency = a deterioration of the immune system

S= Syndrome = a group of signs and symptoms that collectively characterize a disease, for example, together they define AIDS as a human disease

OR

A notable timeline

In the history of human

Death, Devastation,

Suffering and Sorrow caused by HIV

DÉJÀ VU: A TIME OF AIDS

It was the best of times, it was the worst of times, it was the age of wisdom, it was the age of foolishness, it was the epoch of belief, it was the epoch of incredulity, it was the season of Light, it was the season of Darkness, it was the spring of hope, it was the winter of despair . . .

Charles Dickens, *A Tale of Two Cities*

THE NEW MILLENNIUM

Now into the third decade of AIDS, the disease HIV/AIDS remains a great challenge to public health, human rights, development, and national security. This is the first plague in the era of globalization. It has become the ultimate terrorist! The figures are truly alarming—over the last nine years, 2000 through 2009, about 22.5 million people will have become infected with HIV, bringing the total number of infections to about 59 million since the outbreak of this pandemic. While 95% of the cases are concentrated in developing countries, industrialized countries are experiencing about 100,000 new infections each year. By the end of 2009 about 24 million people will have died from AIDS worldwide. HIV/AIDS is devastating for the individual who may be infected, and its impact on communities and society at large is enormous. This disease disproportionately affects those population groups that are already vulnerable: children, women, the poor, the destitute, and millions of others whose life situations are further degraded by the denial of basic human rights. The majority of those infected are unable to afford the cost of effective health care. Clearly, political and economic solutions must be found if millions of lives are to be saved. Of all the promises the new millennium holds, of all the secrets it will tell, a cure or a vaccine for HIV disease will surely unfold among them. Nothing in recent history has so challenged our reliance on modern science nor emphasized our vulnerability before nature. We live with the Acquired Immune Deficiency Syndrome (AIDS) pandemic, witnessing its paradoxes every day. People living with the Human Immunodeficiency Virus (HIV) live with fear, pain, and uncertainty about the disease; they also endure prejudice, scorn, rejection, and despair. **This must change!**

AIDS: A DISEASE OR A SYNDROME?

AIDS has been presented in journals, nonscience magazines, newspaper articles, and on television as a disease. However, a disease is a pathological condition with a single identifiable cause. As we learned from the days of Louis Pasteur and Robert Koch, there is a single identifiable organism or agent for each infectious disease.

AIDS patients may have many diseases. Most AIDS patients have more than one disease at any given time. Each disease produces its own signs and symptoms. Collectively, the diseases that are expressed in an AIDS patient are referred to as a **syndrome.** The number of different diseases an AIDS patient has and the severity of their expression reflects the functioning of that person's immune system.

AIDS Was First Officially Reported in the United States in 1981. However AIDS Was in the U.S. Prior to the CDC Report of 1981

The first cases of AIDS in the United States were not in gay men. Five cases of extreme immune deficiencies were discovered between 1975 and 1981 in **heterosexual women.** They were reported by

Henry Masur (1982), then of Cornell, now of the National Institutes of Health (NIH). For puzzling reasons this report was not published until October 1982. One can ask, if this information had been published before the June 1981 report on severe immunodeficiency in gay men or the July 1981 *New York Times* report of "Rare Cancer Seen in 41 Homosexuals," would AIDS have become known as a gay disease? Given the 10- to 11-year incubation period, it is likely that HIV was in the U.S. by 1965 or earlier.

In January 1981, while Ronald Reagan was taking his first oath of office as president, doctors around the country were just discovering the pattern of symptoms and infections in patients that was to become a very new disease.

Initially, AIDS was reported by the CDC among homosexual males, most frequently those who had many sexual partners. Further study of the gay population led to the conclusion that the agent responsible for AIDS was being transmitted through sexual activities. In July 1982, cases of AIDS were reported among hemophiliacs, people who had received blood transfusions, and injection drug users. These reports all had one thing in common—**an exchange of body fluids.** In particular, blood or semen was involved. In January 1983, according to the CDC, the first cases of AIDS in heterosexuals were documented. Two females, both sexual partners of injection-drug users (IDUs), became AIDS patients. This was clear evidence that the infectious agent could be transmitted from male to female as well as from male to male. Later in 1983, cases of AIDS were reported in Central Africa, but with a difference. The vast majority of African AIDS cases were not among gay men but among heterosexuals who did *not* use injection drugs. This data supported the earlier findings from the American homosexual population: that AIDS is primarily a sexually transmitted disease. Also, the risk for contracting AIDS increased with the number of sex partners one had and the sexual behaviors of those partners. Early empirical observations on which kinds of social behavior placed one at greatest risk of acquiring AIDS were later supported by surveillance surveys, testing, and analysis.

FIRST REACTION TO AIDS: DENIAL

When the disease that would eventually be called AIDS first emerged in 1981, a few officials within agencies like the Centers for Disease Control and Prevention realized that a new infectious agent was at work and that it could well be spreading rapidly. They most cautiously tried to sound the alarm, but the nation was not ready to talk about subjects like **anal sex, needles,** and **condoms.** Among those most heavily in denial were gay men, who were most at risk. They were still enjoying sexual liberation won in the 1970s, and nobody was in a mood to call the party off, even as close friends and sexual partners began dying.

New York playwright Larry Kramer attempted to break through this denial in early 1983 with an article in a widely read gay magazine. Headlined "1,112 and Counting," Kramer warned: "If this article doesn't rouse you to anger, fury, rage and action, gay men have no future on this Earth."

As they turned their fears into political engagement, the activists confronted a Washington that resisted action. Blood banks denied that any extra precautions were needed to prevent transmission. AIDS was buried deep inside newspapers and seldom mentioned on television. The death of movie star

Rock Hudson in 1985 finally put AIDS on the front pages. But still, three young hemophiliacs, Ricky, Robert, and Randy Ray, were firebombed out of their Florida home when their neighbors learned they were HIV positive two years later.

Despite all of the evidence, over 10 years would pass before there was universal agreement that HIV caused AIDS and that HIV could not be transmitted by casual contact. People were, nevertheless, fired from their jobs across the country because of fears that they posed a threat to coworkers.

WHAT CAUSES AIDS?

In the Beginning, 1975, 1980, 1981, 1982

The appearance of AIDS in distinctly different populations, including women, young gay men, intravenous drug abusers, hemophiliacs, Haitians, infants, and blood transfusion recipients, argued for an infectious agent. But what kind of infectious agent would destroy the immune system of so many different groups of people?

There were very few facts, but many plausible theories about the causes of AIDS. Perhaps the cytomegalovirus (sito-meg-ah-lo-virus) had mutated to cause a more severe illness. Maybe the illness was related to "poppers" (amyl and butyl nitrite) and other drugs popular among gay men for enhancing sexual pleasure. One theory linked the origin of HIV to the 1970s, when government-sponsored hepatitis B vaccine experiments used thousands of gay men as guinea pigs in New York, Los Angeles, and San Francisco—the same cities that were the first to report AIDS cases. Some researchers thought the other sexually transmitted infections that many gay men contracted somehow overwhelmed the immune system to cause the mysterious disease. Government researchers suggested that sperm in the male bowel caused the disease, a theory that made little sense because homosexuality is probably as old as society. Few doctors immediately considered the possibility of a new infectious agent. Prior to the outbreak of this strange disease, infectious disease scientists arrogantly believed that virtually all diseases were known. It was just that many things were unknown about the individual diseases. In fact, an editorial in *The New England Journal of Medicine,* in December 1981 on possible causes of AIDS, disregarded and omitted the whole idea that AIDS might be caused by an unknown infectious agent! And in 1982, this journal refused to publish Michael Gottlieb's work on the very first cases of this new disease that devastated the immune system. The article was said to have been rejected because the disease was considered unusual and not of much importance!

Discovery of the AIDS Virus

Early in 1983, the agent that destroys an essential portion of the human immune system was identified by French scientists as a virus. From that point on there was a specific infectious agent associated with the cause of AIDS. The symptoms of viral-induced AIDS can begin *only* after one has been infected with a specific virus. This virus is now called the **Human Immunodeficiency Virus (HIV).** The viral-induced disease is referred to as HIV/AIDS because there are other reasons for a suppressed immune system, like congenital inherited immune deficiencies, exposure to radiation, alkylating agents, corticosteroids, certain forms of cancer, and cancer chemotherapy that also produce AIDS-like symptoms (Stadtmauer et al., 1997).

HIV/AIDS: This term is used to refer to three categories of diagnoses collectively: (1) a diagnosis of HIV infection (not AIDS), (2) a diagnosis of HIV infection and a later diagnosis of AIDS, and (3) concurrent diagnoses of HIV infection and AIDS.

President Ronald Reagan on AIDS

On September 17, 1985, President Ronald Reagan held his first press conference since the public disclosure three months earlier that actor Rock Hudson had AIDS. Up to that point, Reagan had never spoken publicly about the epidemic, despite the fact that the first cases of AIDS had been reported more than four years earlier and more than 12,000 people had been diagnosed. But things changed with the disclosure of Hudson's diagnosis; Americans who had never given the epidemic any thought were now confronted with the chilling notion that anyone—a Hollywood actor or even a child—could get AIDS.

Reagan's staff, anticipating questions on the subject, prepared him to respond. Just as they expected, he was asked whether, if he had school-aged children, he would send them to school with a child who had AIDS. "I'm glad I'm not faced with that problem today," Reagan answered. He expressed his compassion for "the child that has this," while stating as a given that "he is now an outcast and can no longer associate with his playmates and schoolmates." Reagan continued, "it is true that some medical sources had said that this cannot be communicated in any way other than the ones we already know and which would not involve a child being in the school. And yet medicine has not come forth unequivocally and said, 'This we know for a fact, that it is safe.' And until they do, I think we just have to do the best we can with this problem."

Reagan's answer left many public health and AIDS experts aghast. He had directly contradicted an advisory issued less than three weeks earlier by the federal Centers for Disease Control and Prevention (CDC), stating that "casual person-to-person contact as would occur among schoolchildren appears to pose no risk." But among those who must have been delighted with the president's answer was a 30-year-old attorney in the Office of the White House Counsel. Five days before the press conference, he reviewed the president's briefing materials and recommended the deletion of a sentence encapsulating the CDC's conclusion: "As far as our best scientists have been able to determine, AIDS virus is not transmitted through casual or routine contact." In a memorandum, the assistant counsel to the president explained, "I do not think we should have the president taking a position on a disputed scientific issue of this sort. There is much to commend the view that we should assume AIDS can be transmitted through casual or routine contact, as is true with many viruses, until it is demonstrated that it cannot be, and no scientist has said AIDS definitely cannot be transmitted." Exactly 20 years later, that lawyer, John G. Roberts, Jr., would sit before the U.S. Senate Judiciary Committee as the nominee for chief justice of the United States Supreme Court, and he then became a member of the Supreme Court.

By the end of 1985, over 900,000 people in the United States were infected with HIV and about 13,000 had died from AIDS. In 1987, when the president gave his first speech on AIDS, over 1 million people were HIV infected, and 76,000 men, women, and children had been diagnosed with AIDS, of which 40,000 had died of AIDS.

It took just two and a half years to find the cause of AIDS, HIV. It took another two years for blood tests to detect HIV to become commercially available. Once that occurred, the transmission of HIV through blood transfusions fell to almost zero in developed countries.

After years of insults and innuendos among scientists and in the press, President Ronald Reagan and French Prime Minister Jacques Chirac agreed to name as AIDS co-discoverers America's Robert Gallo and France's Luc Montagnier (mon-tan-yay). Naming co-discoverers was a political solution to end a dispute over patent rights covering the blood test for HIV.

HOW DOES HIV CAUSE AIDS?

Over time, HIV depletes a subset of lymphocytes called **T4 helper cells,** or **CD4+ cells,** that are essential in the production of cells necessary to cell-mediated immunity and in the production of HIV neutralizing antibodies (Figure 1-1). Cell-mediated

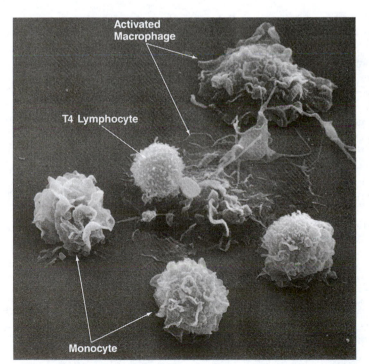

FIGURE 1–1 Normal Human T4 Lymphocytes, Monocytes, and Macrophages. Scanning electron micrograph of monocytes, macrophages, and a T4 or CD4+ lymphocyte, magnified 9000 times. These white blood cells are the targets of HIV infection. Note that the T4 lymphocyte (round cell, at the center) is adhered to a flattened macrophage. *(Photograph courtesy of Dr. M. A. Gonda)*

THE NEW YORK TIMES AND A.I.D.S., AUGUST 8, 1982

An article, "A Disease's Spread Provokes Anxiety," alerted its readers to the growing health crisis in the homosexual community that was baffling medical science. While the *Times* had previously reported on a disease causing opportunistic infections in gay men, this was the first time the term "Acquired Immune Deficiency Syndrome" or A.I.D.S. (the punctuation had not been dropped) appeared in a major newspaper. Later in 1982, the *Washington Post* joined the *Times* in reporting on the death of an infant who had received a blood transfusion from an AIDS-afflicted donor. With that, a second major national newspaper was officially in the business of covering the AIDS story.

THE CENTERS FOR DISEASE CONTROL (CDC): 1982/1983

Regardless of the fact that this new disease was increasing rapidly and killing all those who displayed the strange set of symptoms, the epidemiologists at the CDC in 1982 had other things to worry about: President Ronald Reagan was moving to reduce the size of the federal government, and CDC staff members were facing dismissal. Harold W. Jaffe, who scurried to stay employed, later went on to become chief epidemiologist for the center's AIDS team. Progress was also impeded by scientists who withheld information from health officials because they were competing against one another to be first to publish articles in medical journals that demanded exclusive information. Communication to the public was also poor. People had misplaced fears and misconceptions about the disease even after epidemiologists found, by late 1982, that this disease was transmitted through sex, blood transfusions, injecting drugs with contaminated needles and syringes, and from mother to child. Because health officials and journalists used the phrase "bodily fluids" instead of specifying semen, blood, and vaginal secretions, many people feared that they could contract AIDS from toilet seats or drinking fountains, or by eating at restaurants or going to school.

At a meeting of the World Health Organization (WHO) in Geneva in November 1983, it was clear that AIDS was a global health problem and that cases were occurring in many countries that had officially denied it. But these warning signs were disregarded.

---

immunity and antibodies are critical components of the human immune system. Without the ability to produce a sufficient number of immune-specific cells and immune-specific antibodies, the body is vulnerable to a large variety of infections caused by organisms and viruses that normally do not cause human disease. These infections create the symptoms and progression of illnesses that eventually kill AIDS patients. Thus AIDS begins with HIV infection. Technically it can be called **HIV disease, HIV T4 helper cell,** or **CD4+ cell disease,** but the popular press, scientists, and others still refer to HIV disease as AIDS. AIDS is the end stage of chronic HIV infection. **AIDS IS NOT TRANSMITTED, THE VIRUS IS.** People do not die of AIDS per se. They die of opportunistic infections, cancers, and organ failures brought on by the results of a failed immune system (see Chapters 5 and 6).

It is believed that eventually almost everyone who is *correctly* diagnosed with HIV/AIDS will die from AIDS. But not all who become HIV-infected will progress to AIDS. Estimates are that some 5% of the HIV-infected population will not progress to AIDS.

This implies that there is a percentage of the population that is resistant to HIV-associated immune system suppression. Since mid-1996, several genes that offer resistance to HIV infection have been identified. (See Chapter 4.)

Naming the Disease

Early in 1981, practically coincident with the report of the first cases of a new disease in the male homosexual community in the United States, there were reports of 34 cases of a new disease among Haitian immigrants to the United States and 12 cases of a disease previously unrecognized in Haiti—an aggressive form of **Kaposi's sarcoma** (kap-o-seez sar-ko-mah). Michael Gottlieb, who had identified the new disease that seemed to target gay men, found that although each of the cases was different, **all had one thing in common: Whatever was making the men sick had singled out the T lymphocyte cells for destruction.** Eventually the body's battered defenses couldn't shake off even the most harmless microbial intruder. The men were dying from what doctors termed opportunistic infections, such as **Pneumocystis pneumonia,** which attacks the lungs, and **toxoplasmosis,** which often ravages the brain.

THE CENTERS FOR DISEASE CONTROL AND PREVENTION REPORTS

In June 1981, the Centers for Disease Control and Prevention (CDC) first reported on diseases occurring in gay men that previously had only been found to occur in people whose immune systems were suppressed by drugs or disease [*Morbidity and Mortality Weekly Report (MMWR)*, 1981b].

The report stated that five young men in Los Angeles had been diagnosed with *Pneumocystis carinii* pneumonia (PCP) in three different hospitals. Because cases of PCP occurred almost exclusively in immune-suppressed patients, five new cases in one city at one time were considered unusual. The report also suggested "an association between some aspects of homosexual lifestyle or disease acquired through sexual contact and PCP in this population. Based on clinical examination of each of these cases, the possibility of a cellular immune dysfunction related to a common exposure might also be involved."

In July 1981, the CDC (*MMWR*, 1981b) reported that an uncommon cancer, Kaposi's sarcoma (KS), had been diagnosed in 26 gay men who lived in New York City and California. Between June 1, 1981, and May 28, 1982, the CDC received reports of 355 cases of Kaposi's sarcoma and/or serious opportunistic infection (OI), especially *Pneumocystis carinii* pneumonia (PCP), occurring in previously healthy persons between 15 and 60 years of age. Of the 355, 281 (79%) were homosexual (or bisexual) men, 41 (12%) were heterosexual men, 20 (6%) were men of unknown sexual orientation, and 13 (4%) were heterosexual women. Five states—California, Florida, New Jersey, New York, and Texas—accounted for 86% of the reported cases. The rest were reported by 15 other states. New York was reported as the state of residence for 51% of homosexual male patients, 49% of the heterosexual males, and 46% of the females. The median age at onset of symptoms was 36.0 years for homosexual men, 31.5 years for heterosexual men, and 29.0 years for women. Overall, 31% of all reported cases had onset before January, 1, 1981 (*MMWR*, 1981a; Masur et al. 1981).

These were unusual findings because KS, when it occurred, was usually found in older men of Jewish or

Italian ancestry. The sudden and dramatic increase in pneumonia cases, all of which were caused by a widespread but generally harmless fungus, *P. carinii,* and KS cases indicated that an infectious form of immune deficiency was on the increase. At first, the new disease was referred to as the "4 H disease" because the first cases of the disease were found among homosexuals, Haitians, heroin users, and hemophiliacs. Later this immunodeficiency disease was called **GRID** for **Gay-Related Immune Deficiency.** This new mysterious and lethal illness appeared to be associated with one's lifestyle. These early cases of immune deficiency heralded the beginning of an epidemic of a previously unknown illness. By 1982 and 1983, the disease was reported in adult heterosexuals and children. *Because a cellular deficiency of the human immune system* was found in every AIDS patient, along with an assortment of other signs and symptoms of disease, and because the infection was *acquired* from the action of some environmental agent, it was then named **AIDS** for **Acquired Immune Deficiency Syndrome.**

DISCOVERY OF THE AIDS VIRUS

There was no shortage of ideas on what caused AIDS. It was believed by some to be an act of God, a religious curse or penalty against the homosexual for practicing a biblically unacceptable lifestyle that included drugs, alcohol, and sexual promiscuity. The Reverend Billy Graham said "AIDS is a judgment of God." Jerry Falwell stated that AIDS is God's punishment, the scripture is clear, "we do reap it in our flesh when we violate the laws of God." Some believed AIDS was due to sperm exposure to amyl nitrate, a stimulant used to heighten sexual pleasure (Gallo, 1987). Others believed there was no specific infectious agent. They believed that certain people who *excessively stressed their immune systems* experienced immune system failure, and before it could recover other infections killed them. But many scientists who had expertise in analyzing the sudden onset of new human diseases thought the cause of this form of human immune deficiency was an infectious agent. They believed that the agent was transmitted through sexual intercourse, blood or blood products, and from mother to fetus. They also believed that this agent, which led to the loss of T4 or CD4+ cells, was smaller than a bacterium or fungus because it passed through a filter normally used to remove those microorganisms. This agent fit the profile of a virus.

In January 1983, **Luc Montagnier** (Mont-tan-yay) and colleagues at the Pasteur Institute in Paris isolated the virus that causes AIDS. (Hobson et al., 1991). In May of that year, they published the first report on a T cell retrovirus found in a patient with **lymphadenopathy** (lim-fad-eh-nop-ah-thee), or swollen lymph glands. Lymphadenopathy is one of the early signs in patients progressing toward AIDS. The French scientist (Figure 1-2) named this virus **lymphadenopathy-associated virus** (LAV) (Barre-Sinoussi et al., 1983).

Naming the Viruses that Cause AIDS: HIV-1, HIV-2

During the search for the AIDS virus, several investigators isolated the virus but gave it different names. For example, Robert Gallo (Figure 1-3) named the virus HTLV III (For the Third Human T Cell Lymphotropic Virus). Because the collection of names given this virus created some confusion, the Human Retrovirus Subcommittee of the Committee on the Taxonomy of Viruses reduced all the names to one: **Human Immunodeficiency Virus** or **HIV.** This term is now used worldwide.

In 1985, a second type of HIV was discovered in West African prostitutes. It was named HIV type 2 or **HIV-2.** The first confirmed case of HIV-2 infection in the United States was reported in late 1987 in a West

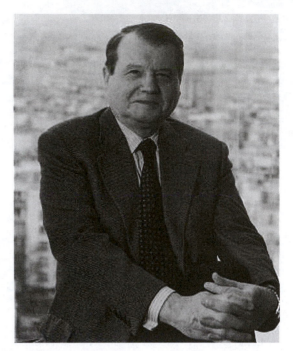

FIGURE 1-2   Luc Montagnier, President of the World Foundation for AIDS Research and Prevention. He is the co-discoverer of the Human Immuno-deficiency Virus (HIV), the cause of AIDS. He has co-founded two Centers for the Prevention, Treatment, Research and diagnosis of AIDS, one in the Ivory Coast and the other in Cameroon. His current studies are on the diagnosis and treatment of microbial and viral factors associated with cancers, neuro-degenerative and articular diseases. In 2008, he and colleague Francoise Barre-Sinoussi received the Nobel Prize in Medicine for their discovery of HIV.

African woman with AIDS. By December 1990, 16 additional cases of HIV-2 infection were reported to the CDC (*MMWR,* 1990). Beginning in 2008, a total of 136 HIV-2 infections have been reported from 22 states of the United States and the District of Columbia. Of the 136 infected persons, 102 are black and 78 are male. Ninety-five were born in West Africa, 19 in the United States (including 3 infants born to mothers of unspecified nationality), 3 in India, and 4 in Europe.

The region of origin was not identified for 15 of the persons. Twenty-eight have developed AIDS-defining conditions and 19 have died. These case counts represent minimal estimates because completeness of reporting has not been assessed; reporting varies from state to state according to state policy.

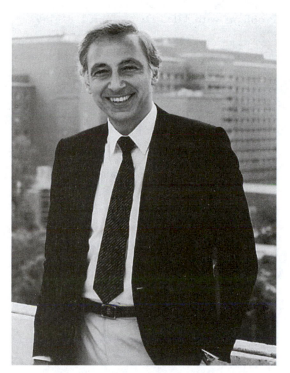

FIGURE 1-3   Robert Gallo, Director, Institute of Human Virology
Co-discoverer of the first human retrovirus and discoverer of HIV, developer of the first HIV blood test, director, Institute of Human Virology at the University of Maryland School of Medicine, he has received 27 honorary degrees and has twice won the Albert Lasker Award in Medicine, the most recognized award for biomedical science in the U.S.

First Reported Case of HIV-2 Infection

The earliest evidence of an individual exposed to HIV-2 comes from a case report on an infection most likely occurring in Guinea-Bissau in the 1960s. Anne-Mieke Vandamme of the Catholic University of Leuren in Belgium and colleagues believe that HIV-2 first moved into humans near the town of Canchungo in western Guinea-Bissau, since that is where the largest proportion of people carry it. The researchers calculate that HIV-2 jumped into humans in about 1940 for the A subtype and 1945 for the B subtype, a time when there were still Mangabey monkeys around Canchungo. A local fondness for eating the primates could have both wiped them out

and exposed people to mangabey viruses. In genetic terms, HIV-2 is much more closely related to the Simian Immunodeficiency Virus (SIV), a group of monkey viruses, than to HIV-1. Both HIV-2 and HIV-1 are said to have been derived from ancestral SIV variants that were from distinct regions and species and do not appear to be direct genetic descendants of each other (Marlink, 1996; Hahn et al., 2000). Clinically, what has been learned about HIV-1 appears to apply to HIV-2, except that HIV-2 appears to be less harmful (cytopathic) to the cells of the immune system, progressing to AIDS in only 20 percent of those infected and it reproduces more slowly than HIV-1. Because HIV-2 has now been found in 18 African countries with a prevalence of over 1%, the question is why is there no HIV-2 epidemic or pandemic similar to that caused by HIV-1? According to scientists working with HIV-2, most likely an epidemic has not occurred because of different behaviors of HIV-2 in relation to viral load. Surveys in West Africa found that HIV-2 never reaches a high viral load in the blood as found with HIV-1. Thus, it is reasoned that fewer HIV-2 cases means there are fewer to transmit to other people and fewer viruses to attack the immune system.

UNLESS STATED OTHERWISE, ALL REFERENCES TO HIV IN THIS BOOK REFER TO HIV-1 OR HIV.

DEFINING THE ILLNESS: AIDS SURVEILLANCE

The CDC reported that through 1983 there were 3068 AIDS cases in the United States and 1478 of these had died (48%). All demonstrated a loss of CD4+ or T4 lymphocytes, and all died with severe opportunistic infections. Opportunistic infections (OI) are caused by organisms and viruses that are normally present but do *not* cause disease unless the immune system is damaged. Clearly there was an immediate need for a name and definition for this disease so that a national surveillance program could begin.

Definitions of AIDS for Surveillance Purposes

The initial objective of AIDS surveillance was to describe the epidemic in terms of time, place, and individuals and to recognize immediately the changes in rate and pattern in the spread of AIDS.

The First Definition of AIDS: 1982

In order to establish surveillance, a system for monitoring where and when AIDS cases occurred, a workable definition had to be developed. The definition had to be *sensitive* enough to detect every possible AIDS patient, while at the same time *specific* enough to exclude those who may have AIDS-like symptoms, but were not infected by HIV.

In 1982, there was no *single characteristic* of AIDS that would allow for a useful definition for surveillance purposes. And so, the first AIDS surveillance definition was based on the **clinical description** of symptoms. The first of many criteria for the diagnosis of AIDS were: (1) the presence of a reliably diagnosed disease at least moderately predictive of cellular immune deficiency; and (2) the absence of an underlying cause for the immune deficiency or for reduced resistance to the disease (*MMWR*, 1982). Because the symptoms varied greatly among individuals, this was a poor first definition.

AIDS Definition Modified: 1982, 1985, 1987

The initial definition of AIDS was thus an arbitrary one, reflecting the partial knowledge of the clinical consequences that prevailed at the time. Various systems for classifying HIV-related illnesses have been revised since 1982 to take into account increasing knowledge about the spectrum of those illnesses. Had the whole picture of HIV infection and its clinical consequences been known in 1982, the term **"AIDS"** would not have been used. Instead, it would have been called **"HIV disease"** (or perhaps, following an older tradition, "Gottlieb's disease," after Mike Gottlieb, who first described it).

The 1982 definition was modified in 1983 to include new diseases then found in AIDS patients. With this modification, AIDS became reportable to the Centers for Disease Control and Prevention (CDC) in every state. In 1985 and 1987 additional diseases were included in the AIDS case definition.

Broadly speaking, the term **AIDS** may be understood as referring to the onset of life-threatening illnesses as a result of HIV disease that results from an HIV infection. AIDS is the end stage of a disease process that may have been developing for 5, 10, 15, or more years, for most of which time the infected person will have been well and quite possibly unaware that he or she has been infected.

Thus the number of AIDS cases reported from 1987 through 1992 reflects the revisions of the initial surveillance case definitions.

Problems with AIDS Definitions, 1981–1992

One major drawback to all the CDC AIDS definitions is the fact that through 1992, the Social Security Administration (SSA) used the CDC AIDS definition to determine disability. But all the definitions were primarily based on symptoms and opportunistic infections in men. Therefore, about 65% of women with HIV/AIDS symptoms were excluded from Supplemental Security Income (SSI) benefits. They were excluded because of failure to be diagnosed with AIDS by the CDC AIDS definition (Sprecher, 1991).

AIDS Redefined in 1993, 1994, 2000

On January 1, 1993, the newest definition of AIDS was put into the surveillance network. The reason for the new CDC definition was that epidemiologists felt the 1987 definition failed to reflect the true magnitude of the pandemic. In particular, it failed to address AIDS in women. Thus, the CDC expanded the AIDS surveillance case definition to include all HIV-infected persons who have less than 200 CD4+ or T4 lymphocytes/μL (microLiter) of blood, or a T4 lymphocyte percentage less than 14% of total lymphocytes. In addition to retaining the 23 clinical conditions in the 1987 AIDS surveillance case definition, the expanded definition includes (1) pulmonary tuberculosis, (2) invasive cervical cancer, and (3) recurrent pneumonia (Table 1-1). The **objectives** of these changes are to simplify the classification of HIV infection and the AIDS case reporting process, to be consistent with standards of medical care for HIV-infected persons, to better categorize HIV-related morbidity, and to reflect more accurately the number of persons with severe HIV-related immunosuppression who are at highest risk for severe HIV-related morbidity and most in need of close medical follow-up.

In 1994 pediatric case definitions were updated and in 2000 the surveillance case definition for HIV was revised to incorporate new laboratory tests.

Impact of the 1993 Definition

The expanded AIDS surveillance case definition had a substantial impact on the number of reported cases in 1993 (*MMWR*, 1993). Using this definition resulted in a substantial increase in the number of reported AIDS cases in all regions of the United States.

When compared to 1992 data the increase in reported cases in 1993 was greater among females (151%) than among males (105%). Proportionate increases were greater among blacks and Hispanics

Table 1-1 List of 26 Conditions in the AIDS Surveillance Case Definition

- ◆ Candidiasis of bronchi, trachea, or lungs
- ◆ Candidiasis, esophageal
- ◆ Cervical cancer, invasive[1]
- ◆ Coccidioidomycosis, disseminated or extrapulmonary
- ◆ Cryptococcosis, extrapulmonary
- ◆ Cryptosporidiosis, chronic intestinal (>1 month duration)
- ◆ Cytomegalovirus disease (other than liver, spleen, or nodes)
- ◆ Cytomegalovirus retinitis (with loss of vision)
- ◆ HIV encephalopathy
- ◆ Herpes simplex: chronic ulcer(s) (>1 month duration); or bronchitis, pneumonitis, or esophagitis
- ◆ Histoplasmosis, disseminated or extrapulmonary
- ◆ Isosporiasis, chronic intestinal (>1 month duration)
- ◆ Kaposi's sarcoma[2]
- ◆ Lymphoma, Burkitt's (or equivalent term)[2]
- ◆ Lymphoma, immunoblastic (or equivalent term)[2]
- ◆ Lymphoma, primary in brain[2]
- ◆ *Mycobacterium avium complex* or *M. kansasii,* disseminated or extrapulmonary
- ◆ *Mycobacterium tuberculosis,* disseminated or extrapulmonary
- ◆ *Mycobacterium tuberculosis,* any site (pulmonary[1] or extrapulmonary)
- ◆ *Mycobacterium,* other species or unidentified species, disseminated or extrapulmonary
- ◆ *Pneumocystis carinii* pneumonia
- ◆ Pneumonia, recurrent[1]
- ◆ Progressive multifocal leukoencephalopathy
- ◆ Salmonella septicemia, recurrent
- ◆ Toxoplasmosis of brain
- ◆ Wasting syndrome due to HIV

1. Added in the 1993 expansion of the AIDS surveillance case definition.

2. These are cancers.

(Adapted from the CDC, Atlanta.)

than among whites. The largest increases in case reporting occurred among persons aged 13–19 years and 20–24 years; in these age groups, a greater proportion of cases were reported among women (35% and 29%, respectively) and were attributed to heterosexual transmission (22% and 18%, respectively).

Problems Stemming from Changing the AIDS Definition for Surveillance Purposes

Each time the definition of AIDS has been altered by the CDC, it has led to an increase in the number of AIDS cases. In 1985, the change in definition led to a 2% increase over what would have been diagnosed prior to the change. The 1987 change led to a 35% increase in new AIDS cases per year over that expected using the 1985 definition. The 1993 change resulted in a 52% increase in AIDS cases over that expected for 1993. Such rapid changes alter the baseline from which future predictions are made and make the interpretations of trends in incidence and characteristics of cases difficult to process. **For the first time because of the 1993 AIDS definition, one could be diagnosed with AIDS and remain symptom-free for years (become HIV positive and have a T4 or CD4+ cell count of less than 200).**

Summary

Much continues to be written about HIV/AIDS. Some of it, especially in lay articles, has been less than accurate and has led to public confusion and fear. **HIV infection is not AIDS. HIV infection is now referred to as HIV disease. AIDS is a syndrome of many diseases,** each resulting from an opportunistic agent or cancer cell that multiplies in humans who are immunosuppressed. The new 1993 CDC AIDS definition will allow, over the long term, earlier access to federal and state medical and social services for HIV-infected individuals.

Review Questions

(Answers to the Review Questions are on page 425.)

1. The letters A, I, D, and S are an acronym for?

2. Is AIDS a single disease? Explain.

3. When was the AIDS virus discovered and by whom?

4. In what year did the CDC first report on a strange new disease that later was named AIDS?

5. Name one different acronym for HIV.

6. How many times has CDC changed and expanded the definition of AIDS? In what years?

7. What is one major advantage of the new CDC AIDS definition for the HIV-infected?

2 What Causes AIDS: Origin of the AIDS Virus

CHAPTER CONCEPTS

- AIDS dissidents say AIDS is not caused by HIV infection.
- HIV/AIDS scientists say AIDS is caused by HIV infection.
- An unbroken chain of HIV transmission has been established between those infected and the newly infected.
- HIV is believed to have crossed into humans from chimpanzees.
- A viral precursor to HIV may have entered humans 300 years ago or in the early 1900s.
- A third new HIV strain is found.
- The earliest AIDS case to date was reported in 1959.

THE CAUSE OF AIDS: THE HUMAN IMMUNODEFICIENCY VIRUS (HIV)

The unexpected appearance and accelerated spread of an unknown lethal disease soon raised two important questions: **What** is causing the disease? **Where** did it come from? These questions will be answered.

This section has a subtitle that states that AIDS is the result of HIV infection. However, 26 years after the identification of HIV as the cause of AIDS (1983–2009) there are still a relatively small number of scientists and nonscientists who claim that HIV does *not* cause AIDS. For a balanced HIV/AIDS presentation, this claim will be presented first.

HIV Does Not Cause AIDS: A Minority Point of View

Throughout the HIV/AIDS pandemic, there have been skeptics who have challenged or dissented from the most widely held beliefs of the world's best HIV/AIDS scientists. The scientists' belief, based on overwhelming scientific data, that HIV does cause AIDS is the conventionally accepted wisdom worldwide. Those who do not accept the scientific data about HIV/AIDS are referred to as "AIDS dissidents" or "AIDS denialists." They contend that there is no connection or link between HIV and AIDS. They contend that HIV/AIDS is the greatest medical hoax in history!

Fronted locally by ACT UP/San Francisco, a renegade chapter long ago disowned by the rest of the AIDS activist movement (and not to be confused with ACT UP/Golden Gate, which respects most conventional AIDS research), members have repeatedly plastered the Castro district with stickers reading, "AIDS Is Over," and "Don't Buy the HIV Lie." (Figure 2.1). In May and June 1999, the Los Angeles-

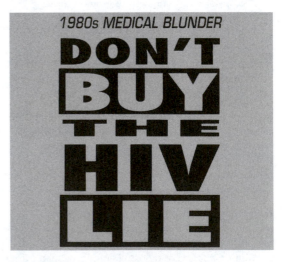

FIGURE 2-1 The image HIV/AIDS dissidents still support! (Image courtesy of Smith TC, Novella (2007) HIV Denial in the Internet Era. PLS Med4(8): e256.)

based dissident group Alive & Well ran a series of full-page ads in several gay/lesbian and alternative papers, including the *Bay Area Reporter, Bay Times,* and *Bay Guardian,* arguing that AIDS is not contagious, HIV is harmless, and that HIV/AIDS drugs are the real danger. The first of the ads states that, "What we have experienced for 20 years is not a sexually transmitted epidemic but a tragic medical mistake. Contrary to popular beliefs, AIDS is not a new disease, AIDS is a new name given by the Centers for Disease Control (CDC) to a collection of 29 old illnesses and conditions. . . . These illnesses and conditions are called AIDS only when they occur in persons who also have certain protective, disease-fighting proteins called antibodies in their blood." In her book, *What If Everything You Thought You Knew About AIDS Was Wrong?,* Christine Maggiore elaborates, "None of these diseases appear exclusively in those who test (HIV) positive. . . . All 29 indicator diseases have established causes and treatments unrelated to HIV." AIDS, in other words, isn't an epidemic at all; it's a phony construct. Maggiore, who tested HIV positive in 1992, has never taken antiretroviral drugs, remains relatively symptom-free and believes that those who have died of AIDS actually died from prescription or recreational drugs, or fear. Her explanations for the global AIDS pandemic: In Africa, people are dying at the same rate as before; in America, people are victims of the prescription drugs.

Who Is Christine Maggiore?

(The following information was abstracted from the *Los Angeles Times* article, "A Mother's Denial, a Daughter's Death," by Charles Ornstein and Daniel Costello, September 2005.)

Her background commands attention. She is an engaging, articulate woman. She owned her own clothing company. She presents talks on HIV at local schools, health fairs and has appeared on TV shows presenting her dissident or anti-HIV views about AIDS. Her disbelief that HIV causes AIDS is in line with the beliefs of University of California–Berkeley biology professor Peter Duesberg, whose well-publicized dissident views on AIDS (presented below) place him outside the mainstream of scientific beliefs that HIV does cause AIDS. She founded Alive and Well Alternatives, a nonprofit group that challenges common assumptions and scientific facts about HIV/AIDS. (See Box 2.1)

Disbelieving Scientists (HIV/AIDS Dissidents)

Scientist Peter Duesberg is perhaps the most vocal in his concern that the scientific community is investigating the wrong causative agent. Duesberg is a molecular biologist at the University of California at Berkeley and a member of the National Academy of Sciences. Duesberg has advanced his anti-HIV/AIDS hypothesis at great expense to himself. He states that "I have been excommunicated by the retrovirus-AIDS community with noninvitations to meetings, noncitations in the literature and nonrenewals of my research grants, which is the highest price an experimental scientist can pay for his convictions."

In 1971 at age 33, Duesberg co-discovered cancer-causing genes in viruses. In the March 1987 issue of *Cancer Research,* he published "Retro-viruses as Carcinogens and Pathogens: Expectations and Reality." The article provoked a great deal of scientific discussion and received a lot of popular press coverage. In the article Duesberg argues that there is *no evidence* that HIV causes AIDS. He has published additional articles in *Science* (1988) and in the *Proceedings of the National Academy of Sciences* (1989) stating that HIV is not the cause of AIDS. In short, Duesberg suggests that there is no single causative agent, that the disease is due to one's "lifestyle." He marshals arguments to support his theory that, in the United States and probably in Europe, AIDS is a collection of noninfectious deficiencies predominantly associated with drug use, malnutrition, parasitic infections, and other specific risks. To read more on Duesberg, see the Wayt Gibbs article, "Dissident or Don Quixote?" in the August 2001 *Scientific American.*

Duesberg believes the tests that detect HIV antibodies are useless. In the June 1988 issue of *Discovery* he said, "If somebody told me today that I was antibody positive, I wouldn't worry one second. I wouldn't take Valium. I wouldn't write my will. All I would say is that my immune system seems to work. I have antibodies to a virus. I am protected."

In June 1990, Robin Weiss and Harold Jaffe wrote a critical refutation of Duesberg's theory that HIV cannot be the cause of AIDS. Duesberg's response suggested that he was unaware of published data that clearly answer the questions he raises concerning HIV involvement in AIDS. For example, one of Duesberg's major points is that no one has

BOX 2.1

CHRISTINE MAGGIORE, PROMINENT HIV DISSIDENT, LOSES DAUGHTER TO AIDS?

According to the literature (some references provided below), the events of 2005 put an entirely new spotlight on Christine Maggiore's beliefs on HIV/AIDS. In May, her 3-year-old daughter, Eliza Jane Scovill, died from an apparently sudden and unexpected illness. Several weeks prior to Eliza Jane's death, Maggiore stated that her two children were in excellent health. Neither son Charles or Eliza Jane were HIV tested to this point in time.

TIMELINE TO ELIZA JANE'S DEATH (EXTRACTED FROM THE *LA TIMES* ARTICLE)

- The first hint that Eliza Jane was ill came at the end of April 2005 when she developed a runny nose showing yellow mucus.
- On April 30, Maggiore took her daughter to a pediatrician. The doctor found the girl had clear lungs, no fever, and adequate oxygen levels.
- May 5, Maggiore sought a second opinion from another pediatrician. During an interview with this pediatrician, he said that he suspected there was an ear infection but believed it could be resolved without antibiotics. In a follow-up call, he said Eliza's parents told him that she was getting better. Some time after that, Maggiore asked a Denver physician, who was visiting Los Angeles, to examine her daughter. This physician said he found fluid in her right ear drum.
- May 14th, the Denver physician examined her again and prescribed the antibiotic amoxicillin.
- May 15th, Eliza Jane vomited several times and was pale. While Maggiore's husband was on the phone with the Denver physician, Eliza Jane stopped breathing and "crumpled like a paper doll."
- May 16th, Eliza Jane died early in the morning at Van Nuys hospital. It was reported that neither hospital staff nor the coroner were told that the mother was HIV positive. Maggiore said that she was never asked about her HIV status.

According to interviews and records and after some time interval, the Los Angeles medical examiner declared the cause of death to be "AIDS related pneumonia."

On December 10, 2005, Christine Maggiore, whose daughter allegedly died of AIDS-related pneu-monia appeared on *ABC News Primetime* to share her reasons for not testing her children for HIV. She maintained that Eliza Jane died of an allergic reaction to antibiotics. Her son Charles tested HIV negative after his sister's death. Maggiore continues to question the coroner's findings. In a November 2005 article in "The Body" (www.thebody.com), the question was asked, "Is it right, is it fair, for a child to pay with her life for this level of arrogance on the part of the parent? Surely, the word denial has seldom had a more clear definition than what is seen here. Ms. Maggiore and her partner face a terrible dilemma in their grief. They are faced with acknowledging the possibility they have been horribly wrong. If they acknowledge error, they must accept responsibility for the loss of their daughter. A denialist dilemma indeed."

In the April 2006 edition of *POZ Magazine*, Bob Lederer stated in his article, "Dead Certain," that several months after Eliza Jane died, James K. Ribe, MD, senior deputy medical examiner at the Los Angeles County coroner's office, pronounced that her death had been caused by *Pneumocystis carinii* pneumonia (PCP), one of the most common and fatal opportunistic infections associated with HIV, and her death was declared to be AIDS-related. Slides of cells from Eliza Jane's lung showed microscopic evidence of colonies of *Pneumocystis carinii*. The autopsy report also described the presence of HIV core proteins in the brain, which was diagnosed as HIV encephalitis. **The coroner's office would not confirm to *POZ Magazine* whether it had actually tested her blood for HIV infection or HIV antibodies.** However, according to other published reports, Eliza Jane's T4 or CD4+ cell counts were in the normal range. It would appear that the blood test for HIV would be crucial to the coroner's statement that Eliza Jane died of AIDS.

Some Reference for Information about Christine Maggiore and Daughter Eliza Jane's Death:

Lederer, Bob (2006). Dead Certain? *POZ Magazine*, April edition. pp. a18–23. www.poz.com.

Project Inform Perspective (2005). Project Inform: A Denialist Dilemma. November issue. www.thebody.com/pinf/nov05/aids_denialists.html?rn128h. pp 1–6.

Ornstein, Charles, et al. (2005). A Mother's Denial, a Daughter's Death: [Home Edition]. *Los Angeles Times.* Los Angeles, CA. September 24. p. A.1.

BOX 2.1 (*continued*)

For a transcript of the December 2005 *ABC Primetime* interview with Christine Maggiore, go to www.transcripts.tv. For a copy of ABC News Home Video call 1-800-505-6139 or go to ABCNews at datapakservices.com.

Farber, Celia (2006). A Daughter's Death, A Mother's Survival. Los Angeles City Beat. August 3. pp. 1–10. www.lacitybeat.com.

ABCNEWS (December 8, 2005). Did HIV-Positive Mom's Beliefs Put Her Children at Risk? Coroner says 3-year-old died of AIDS; her mother and another doctor dispute that. abcnews.go.com/primetime/print.

yet shown that hemophiliacs infected with HIV progress to AIDS. The data on matched groups of homosexual males and hemophiliacs, which show that *only* those infected with HIV develop AIDS, have been available for a number of years (Weiss et al., 1990).

Duesberg's arguments and disagreements with the vast majority of prominent scientists who have researched the causal agent of AIDS are many. But they pale when placed next to the overwhelming evidence that leaves no doubt in the opinion of most scientists that HIV causes AIDS (see Andrews, 1995; Cohen, 1993; Moore, 1996).

Based on an August 1992 report in *Newsweek,* a father discussed his decision, based on Duesberg's claims, to counsel his infected hemophiliac son to avoid zidovudine (ZDV) treatment. This situation is similar to what happened when desperate cancer patients followed the advice of a credentialed academician who recommended vitamin therapy as the cure for cancer. Based on such advice, some people failed to undergo truly effective therapy.

DISCUSSION QUESTION: Is Duesberg's opinion on this issue inadvertently harmful to humans? To the scientific process? Will the use of his idea, that HIV does not cause AIDS, provide a course of action that will stop the Acquired Immune Deficiency Syndrome?

Others Join Duesberg's Belief that HIV Does Not Cause AIDS

In 1996, Duesberg's book, *Inventing the AIDS Virus,* was published and in 1998 he and David Rasnick published a paper, *"The AIDS Dilemma: drug diseases blamed on a passenger virus."* Through 2008, it appears that Duesberg still believes that HIV does not cause AIDS. He believes that HIV is just another opportunistic agent (Duesberg, 1993, 1995a, 1995b; Moore, 1996). With each new scientific report, it becomes

more difficult for Duesberg to maintain his position. Regardless of the reports that newborn infants with HIV got HIV *only* from HIV-infected mothers and progress to AIDS while noninfected newborns from the same mothers do not progress to AIDS and that some 50% of HIV-infected hemophiliacs have developed AIDS *yet no* HIV-negative hemophiliac has ever developed AIDS (Darby et al., 1995; Levy, 1995; Sullivan et al., 1995). In addition, Duesberg claims that the drug AZT (zidovudine) causes AIDS. What does he make of the AIDS Clinical Trials Group (ACTG) Protocol 076 that demonstrated AZT treatment of women during pregnancy and delivery reduced transmission from mother to infant from 25% in the placebo-treated mothers to 8% in those who received AZT (Connor et al., 1994)?

For those who wish to know more on the rebuttal of Duesberg's arguments, read the study reporting on the death rate among HIV-positive and HIV-negative British hemophilia patients (Baum, 1995; Darby et al., 1995; Editorial, 1995). For more by Duesberg see his Web page, www.duesberg.com. Also see www.garynull.com.

Impact of HIV/AIDS Dissident Thinkers on the President of South Africa

David Rasnick, an American chemist, is a leader of the HIV/AIDS dissidents in the United States. He is also the person who is thought to be, at least partially, responsible for South African President Mbeki's belief that HIV does not cause AIDS. In February 2002, Rasnick and South African computer science Professor Philip Machanick, who believes that HIV causes AIDS and that the antiretroviral drugs are not as toxic as Rasnick says, have agreed, after a heated exchange of letters, to a challenge. The date, at this time, has not been set. But should this bizarre game of chicken occur, the scenario will go something like this: Rasnick

BOX 2.2

SCIENCE TAKES BACKSEAT TO POLITICS: SOUTH AFRICAN PRESIDENT THABO MBEKI SAYS HIS GOVERNMENT HAS A RIGHT/OBLIGATION TO DOUBT WHETHER HIV CAUSES AIDS

Beginning in March 2000, two tragedies began unfolding simultaneously in South Africa. The first is epidemiological, with millions of men, women, and children infected with HIV destined to develop AIDS. The second is political, with President Thabo Mbeki (Figure 2-2) seriously entertaining a discredited view that challenges the role of HIV as the cause of AIDS. Together, the tragedies may well increase the AIDS pandemic in South Africa. The outcome can only be measured in untold suffering, death, and orphans.

DENIAL THAT HIV CAUSES AIDS

President Thabo Mbeki and other HIV dissidents believe that if HIV exists it does not cause AIDS. The disease AIDS does not exist. There is no epidemic nor are there deaths from AIDS. There is just mass hysteria caused by a conspiracy among pharmaceutical multinationals, aided and abetted by political and medical self-interest.

Orthodoxy—People who believe HIV causes AIDS have demonstrated a rapidly expanding foundation of scientific and medical understanding that rests upon a detectable virus, and have documented evidence of the impact of this virus on the human immune system. There is an impressive array of leading scientific names—the signatories to the Durban Declaration include many Nobel laureates.

Believing in the orthodox position suggests that things can be done to prevent people from becoming HIV-infected and dying of AIDS.

Belief in the dissident view tends to suggest that because HIV does not cause AIDS, there is no epidemic; nothing needs to be done. People are dying of diseases exacerbated by poverty, as they have always done. It is simply that these are being recorded more often. There is no infectious agent at work, in South Africa or in the world, causing a new and different disease!

IT'S TIME TO FISH OR CUT BAIT?

HIV either causes AIDS or it does not, and the answer must come from science—not politics! The reasons supporting HIV as the cause of AIDS are too numerous to list here, but many of those reasons are found in this chapter and in Chapter 10 (see HIV/AIDS statistics for Africa).

In April 2002, President Mbeki began to distance himself from the AIDS dissidents. Mbeki has decided to cut informal contact with them and communicate with them only when the advisory panel meets.

WHEN LIFE GIVES YOU LEMONS, THEY CAN'T BE USED TO TREAT AIDS!

In July 2003 the South African Cabinet instructed Health Minister Manto Tshabalala-Msimang to develop a plan, to make antiretroviral drugs available to all HIV-infected people, and she did. In 2005 the health minister told a National Conference on AIDS in South Africa that the nation should be focused on other diseases—cancer, diabetes, and other communicable diseases—not just AIDS. In 2007 she repeated her stand that antiretroviral drugs are not the answer to treating people living with HIV or AIDS, nutrition is the answer. She advocates a diet of beetroot, garlic,

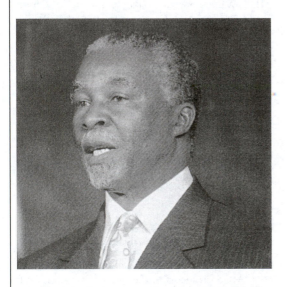

FIGURE 2-2 South African President Thabo Mbeki. In September 2003, Mbeki said he did not know anyone with HIV infection or AIDS. It is believed that members of his staff died of AIDS. In September 2008, Mbeki resigned his position and was replaced by interim president Kgalema Motlanthe. *(Photograph© AP/World Photos)*

BOX 2.2   (*continued*)

lemon juice, and olive oil. The health minister said, in mid-2005, "Raw garlic and a skin of the lemon—not only do they give you a beautiful face and skin, but they also protect you from AIDS." ·

At the 2006 16th International AIDS Conference, 81 internationally renowned HIV/AIDS scientists petitioned President Mbeki for his health minister's resignation. His response was to appoint a committee to oversee Tshabalala-Msimang's national HIV policy. And this committee set a five-year plan to prevent new HIV infections and the widespread use of antiretroviral therapy. In August 2007 Mbeki fired his deputy health minister, Nozizwe Madlala-Routledge, who believes HIV causes AIDS.

In early 2008, after growing pressure from frustrated activists, the policy committee of the National Health Council ordered that South Africa's HIV-positive pregnant women would now have access to medication that could further reduce the risk of passing the virus to their babies. They will receive the more effective dual therapy of zidovudine and nevirapine instead of a single antiretroviral treatment. In September 2008 along with Mbeki's resignation, his health minister Manto T-Msimang was replaced by Barbara Hogan who believes that HIV causes AIDS.

DISCUSSION QUESTION: What if you were president of a country in which 1 in 9 people were infected with a virus that you were told would kill them unless they were treated with exceptionally expensive medications that will always be outside the range of your healthcare system finances? Add to that a mandate from your country's constitution guaranteeing each citizen the right to health care. And, half its citizens, over 20 million, live below poverty level. And add to that the absolute need for clean water, decent highways, new schools, hospitals, fire departments, farming equipment, and many other services needed to run your country. What would you do? Might you search for a way to deny that HIV is a major factor in AIDS so that money saved could be better used elsewhere? Offer pro/con discussion.

will intentionally infect himself with HIV to prove that it does not cause disease, and Machanick will take drugs to prove they are not toxic. Under the agreement, Rasnick will inject himself with HIV on television and the two will meet annually to compare health status. It is doubtful that the action of this challenge will ever occur. Machanick is never going to get a doctor to prescribe him medication for a disease he doesn't have and Rasnick stipulated that he be injected with a highly purified virus, a condition that is impossible to meet. Results, if any, will be offered after they occur.

EVIDENCE THAT HIV CAUSES AIDS

It has been firmly established that there is a high correlation between HIV infection and the development of AIDS. With respect to establishing HIV as the causative agent of AIDS, look at some of the evidence that concludes that HIV infection and AIDS are invariably linked in time, place, and population group.

1. The one common denominator is the presence of HIV within the entire range of people with this particular disease: individuals who are HIV positive over time will have symptoms of HIV disease. Individuals who are HIV negative will not.

2. The virus has been identified by electron microscopy inside and on the surface of T4 cells only in HIV-positive and AIDS patients.

3. Recent work by Bruce Patterson and Steven Wolinsky has shown that the genetic material of HIV (HIV DNA) can be found in as many as 1 in 10 blood lymphocytes of persons with HIV disease (Cohen, 1993).

4. Antibodies against the virus, viral antigens, and HIV RNA are found only in HIV-positive and AIDS patients.

5. There is an absolute chronological association between the emergence of AIDS and the appearance of HIV in humans worldwide.

6. There is a chronological association of HIV-positive individuals who progress to AIDS. Significantly, in the years before AIDS, people with hemophilia had never been noted to be particularly susceptible to the more obvious fungal infections, such as candida esophagitis, common to AIDS patients and others with low-lymphocyte type immune deficiency. After 1984, this type of AIDS-associated opportunistic infection and immune failure rapidly became the single most common cause of death in people with hemophilia in America.

SUPREME COURT OF SOUTH AUSTRALIA, JANUARY 2007

For the Defense

A medical physicist at Royal Perth Hospital, Eleni Papadopulos-Eleopulos, and emergency room doctor Val Turner gave testimony at the Supreme Court of South Australia during an appeal by a man convicted of exposing three women to HIV. Asked by the prosecutor whether "you would have unprotected vaginal sex with an HIV positive man," Ms. Papadopulos-Eleopulos replied "anytime." She and Val Turner were the lead expert witnesses for Andre Chad Parenzee, 35, who was convicted in February 2006 on three counts of having unprotected sex with three women despite knowing he was HIV positive. He infected one of them. His mother has spent $250,000 on her son's defense. Papadopulos-Eleopulos and Turner's key claim is that HIV has never been isolated and identified as a retrovirus, that HIV is the result of the misinterpretation of laboratory phenomena and experiment, and that HIV is not sexually transmitted or the cause of AIDS. Ms. Papadopulos-Eleopulos said AIDS is a disease that results from the oxidizing of the inside of the body and from repeated exposure to semen resulting from passive anal intercourse. HIV is not a virus and cannot be transmitted from one person to another during sex.

The judge asked her to consider the good record of antiretroviral drugs in extending the lives of HIV/AIDS patients. He asked her, "Is it your evidence that it is a waste of resources to give antiretrovirals to pregnant women?" "Yes," she said.

For the Prosecution

The prosecutor asked seven eminent HIV/AIDS scientists to give rebuttal testimony. In short, all experts testified that the Perth group's testimony was wrong! One of the scientists who testified was Robert Gallo (Figure 1-3). Robert Gallo, along with Luc Montagnier (Figure 1-2), discovered HIV, and Gallo created a blood test for HIV in 1985. Robert Gallo said, "I can't believe that this case occupies the time of the court—it is absurd." He described the defense testimony as "beyond stupid, sad, deeply nonsensical, and extremely wrong." He suggested the defense witnesses, members of the HIV dissident study circle the Perth Group, were using the case as a ploy to advance their theories. He lost patience with defense lawyer Kevin Borick's provocative questioning of the accuracy of HIV tests. Gallo said, "You are driving me nuts with this . . . for God's sake." Gallo said, "No one knows more about HIV testing than me." Gallo said that his work had contributed to the cleansing of HIV from Australia's donor blood supply in the late 1980s. "I don't expect a thank you, but I don't expect to be provoked to that degree."

Conclusion:

The judge dismissed defense claims that HIV did not exist. Andre Chad Parenzee's appeal was dismissed. He was convicted on three counts of endangering life and was sentenced to nine years in prison.

The rise in total mortality in people with hemophilia was sudden: Death in this population, which had been stable in 1982 and 1983, suddenly increased by a factor of approximately 900% in the first quarter of 1984. This increase was consistent with an epidemic, or some new very toxic contamination of the clotting factor supply. Mortality figures in hemophilia patients also showed something else important, that the new deaths of the late 1980s, by virtue of all being diagnosed with AIDS, demonstrated that most or all of them occurred in people with hemophilia who were HIV positive. Since these deaths accounted for almost the entire new increase in mortality, it could be inferred that the mortality rate for HIV-negative people with hemophilia did not increase much in the 1980s, if at all (Harris, 1998).

7. Hemophiliacs from low- and high-risk behavior groups were equally infected from HIV-contaminated blood factor VIII concentrates.

8. Studies of blood transfusion-acquired AIDS cases have repeatedly led to the discovery of HIV in the patient as well as in the blood donor.

9. With the exception of persons who had their immune systems suppressed due to genetic causes or by drug therapy, prior to the appearance of the virus, there were no known AIDS-like cases. The virus has been isolated worldwide—but only where there are HIV-positive people and AIDS patients.

10. An HIV-positive identical twin born to an HIV-positive mother developed AIDS, but the HIV-negative twin did not.

11. Only HIV-positive mothers transmit HIV into their fetuses and only these HIV-positive newborns progress to AIDS. HIV-negative newborns from HIV-positive mothers *do not get* AIDS!

12. Drugs developed specifically to inhibit the replication and/or maturation of HIV, thereby lowering the level

of HIV found in HIV-infected people, have delayed the onset of HIV disease and, for HIV-infected pregnant women, have decreased the birth of HIV-infected infants in the USA by 90%.

13. If HIV does not cause AIDS, how do HIV dissenters explain the positive effects of drugs used to affect the early and late stages in the life cycle of HIV that have lowered viral load to unmeasurable levels in the blood? And what of those with HIV disease and AIDS who have been virtually restored to life and who are now back at work? Or, how do they explain the positive effects offered by HIV phenotype- and genotype-resistant drug testing?

14. Finally, there have been numerous reports in the literature on HIV-Infected Individuals (homosexual, bisexual, and heterosexual) transmitting the virus to their sexual partners and both eventually dying of AIDS. *The unbroken chain of HIV transmission between prostitutes and their customers, between injection-drug users sharing the same syringe, from infected mothers to their unborn fetuses, and so on all lead to the inescapable conclusion that HIV does cause AIDS.*

In short, Koch's postulates have been satisfied: HIV disease meets all four criteria.

1. The causative agent must be found in all cases of the disease. (It is.)

2. It must be isolated from the host and grown in pure culture. (It was.)

3. It must reproduce the original disease when introduced into a susceptible host. (It does.)

4. It must be found in the experimental host so infected. (It is.)

In summary, HIV is the singular common factor that is shared between AIDS cases in gay men in San Francisco, well-nourished young women in Uganda, hemophiliacs in Japan, and children in Romanian orphanages. The identification of HIV as the causative agent of AIDS is now firmly accepted by scientists worldwide.

The HIV/AIDS Surveillance Report, CDC, MMWR 1999; 48 (RR13): 1 provides abundant evidence that HIV causes AIDS. Questions and Answers at the end of this document address the specific claims of those who assert that HIV is not the cause of AIDS.

The Durban Declaration Admonishes HIV Dissidents—A statement signed by over 5000 HIV/AIDS scientists and physicians from 50 countries and 5 continents was released to the press on July 1, 2000

(www.nature.com). Their statement that HIV causes AIDS is their answer to those who believe otherwise. They believe the evidence that HIV causes AIDS is clear, concise, exhaustive, and unambiguous. To conquer AIDS, everyone must understand that HIV is the enemy. (The Durban Declaration can be found at http://www.eurakalert.org/releases/hte-uncc063000.html. The evidence that HIV causes AIDS can be found at http://www.thebody.com/niaid/hivcauseaids.html.)

In short, the dissidents, belief is an example of a myth masquerading as a topic for discussion. The vast majority of HIV/AIDS scientists and medical personnel may feel as George Orwell stated in his book *1984,* "What can you do against the lunatic ... who gives your arguments a fair hearing and then simply persists in his lunacy?" *HIV DOES CAUSE AIDS!*

DISCUSSION QUESTION: You have just read some of the evidence for and against HIV being the cause of AIDS. Assuming you agree with the vast majority of HIV/AIDS investigators worldwide that HIV does cause AIDS, do you think there comes a time at which dissenters should forfeit their right to make claims on other people's time and trouble by the poverty of their arguments and by the wasted effort and exasperation they have caused? NOW discuss the value of the dissenter. NOW discuss the danger of the dissenter's information or claims.

ORIGIN OF HIV: THE AIDS VIRUS

Clarification of the Term "Origin of HIV"

Scientists are searching for the source of HIV or HIV-like ancestor. Finding this source will give us the origin of HIV as it pertains to where and in which animal the virus was housed prior to entering humans. But it does not mean the beginning of the virus per se—that will most likely never be known.

Tracking the origins and early history of a newly recognized disease is more than just an academic exercise. Unless we understand where HIV came from we run the risk of new emergencies, and unless we understand the ecology that allowed it to spread, we will be unable to control newly identified diseases. A classic example of tracking a source of a disease and the local epidemic it caused is John Snow's investigation of the cholera epidemic in Golden Square,

London, in 1854; his removal of the handle of the Board Street pump contained the outbreak.

Cholera is caused by a spiral-shaped microorganism called *vibrio cholerae,* which is carried in the cholera-infected person's feces and is transmitted to others via *vibrio cholerae*–contaminated water or food. Removing the handle from the pump stopped people from drinking or using the contaminated water—epidemic over!

More than virtually any other disease, AIDS has generated myths and far-fetched theories about its origin, its causes, and even its very existence. These are probably linked to fear and denial prompted by a virus that is fatal, incurable, and sexually transmitted—and can infect people for years before they show any signs of illness.

Why Do Scientists Want to Know Where HIV Originated?

The object of determining the origin of the AIDS virus is to gain insight into how the virus may have evolved the unique set of characteristics that enable it to destroy the human immune system. Such information will offer valuable clues as to how rapidly the virus is evolving and how to combat it and perhaps help prevent future viral plagues.

In the modern era of diseases like the bird flu (avian influenza), Ebola, and SARS, the question of what launches new epidemics and pandemics is extremely important. The somewhat shocking answer is that we actually know nothing about the factors that launch animal viruses into epidemics or pandemics. Equally important is the question of why most animal viruses fail to launch sustained human-to-human transmission. These are critically important questions that are being bypassed.

Is HIV a New or Old Virus?

The terms "new" and "old" are relative to time and age. Viruses known, say less than 50 years, are generally considered new. Whether a virus is considered new or old is of considerable importance.

If, for example, HIV is a new virus, say less than 30 years old, the many different varieties of HIV now infecting people worldwide probably evolved from a common ancestor sometime after World War II. New varieties can be expected to continue evolving at a frightening pace for several more decades, possibly producing new strains of the virus that are even more dangerous than those now infecting people. This could mean that vaccines now being developed based on current virus strains may not be useful in 10 to 20 years. But, should the known strains of the virus prove to be hundreds or thousands of years old, it might be possible that the current types of HIV are in a state of global balance and most likely they would not offer scientists any shocking evolutionary surprises in the future.

Some Ideas on the Origin of HIV: UFOs, Biological Warfare, Cats, and Other Ideas

UFOs—Fear stimulates the imagination. Out of human fear have come some rather strange explanations for the origin of the AIDS virus. Early reports had unidentified flying objects (UFOs) crashing to Earth and releasing a "new organism" that would wipe out humanity.

Biological Warfare—There were frequent reports in the Soviet press linking AIDS with American biological warfare research. The Soviets agreed in August 1987 to stop these reports (Holder, 1988).

Ethnic Cleansing: **Conspiracy Beliefs**—There are also reports of extremism, as in the case of Illinois State Representative Douglas Huff of Chicago who told the *Los Angeles Times* that he gave over $500 from his office allowance fund to a local official of the Black Hebrew sect to help the group investigate its claim that Israel and South Africa created the AIDS virus in a laboratory in South Africa. Huff said AIDS is "clearly an ethnic weapon, a biological weapon" designed specifically to attack nonwhites (*CDC Weekly,* 1988). Kenyan ecologist and the 2004 Nobel Prize Winner, Wangari Maathai said in 2004 that HIV was created by scientists "for the purpose of mass extermination. We know that developed nations are using biological warfare, leaving guns to primitive people. AIDS is not a curse from God to Africans or the black people. It is a tool to control them designed by some evil-minded scientists." A few days after this statement, in another interview, she said "HIV was deliberately devised to destroy black people."

In January 2005, according to results of a study released by the Rand Corporation and Oregon State University, nearly half of 500 black Americans ages 15 to 44 responding to a telephone survey said they believe that HIV is man-made, with approximately 12% saying they believe HIV was created and spread by the CIA and nearly 27% saying that AIDS was produced in a government laboratory. In addition, about 16% of respondents agreed that the government created HIV to control the black population, and about 15% agreed with a statement saying that AIDS is a form of genocide against African-Americans. Over half, 53.4%, said they believed that there is a cure for AIDS but it is being withheld from the poor (Bogart et al., 2005).

Domestic Cats—Still another myth to surface is that the AIDS virus came from domestic cats. Because of its similarities to human AIDS, feline immunodeficiency virus has been called "feline AIDS." The cat retrovirus may damage cats' immune systems, leaving the animals vulnerable to opportunistic infections *or* it may cause feline leukemia. However, the cat virus has never been shown to cause a disease in humans.

Other Ideas—The origin of HIV has been attributed to HIV-contaminated polio, smallpox, hepatitis, and tetanus vaccines; the African green monkey; African people; their cattle, pigs, and sheep—and the United States CIA. With respect to the use of HIV-contaminated vaccines, a number of articles suggest that early monkey kidney cultures used to produce the polio vaccine carried HIV. Review of the literature offers *no* evidence that this occurred. The argument for the safety of the polio vaccine lies in the absence of any AIDS-related diseases among the hundreds of millions of persons vaccinated worldwide (Koprowski, 1992).

The Mystery Continues

The origin of HIV remains a mystery and may never be proven to everyone's satisfaction. Some of the scientific theories include the introduction of HIV into humans through (a) the use of HIV-contaminated polio vaccine from the late 1950s into the early 1960s, or (b) the worldwide introduction of disposable plastic syringes that were used and reused and reused until they were too short and blunt for sharpening. This means that serial passing of a precursor virus to HIV could change through the use of unsterilized needles and syringes into HIV. There is also (c) the cut hunter theory where the virus, e.g., SIVcpz (the theoretical precursor to HIV), would have a natural transfer via the handling of blood or chimpanzee tissue and body parts during the slaughter of these animals.

For many scientists, regardless of theory, there is still something missing, an explanation of how SIV (Simian Immunodeficiency Virus), a harmless infection in humans for perhaps thousands of years, suddenly becomes HIV and lethal. There is no evidence that people contract HIV or AIDS from monkeys (HIV-2) or chimpanzees (HIV-1). And SIV does not cause an AIDS-like illness in monkeys or chimpanzees. There is the possibility that an SIV/HIV evolving hybrid has remained in the human population for hundreds if not thousands of years until such

---

POINT OF INFORMATION 2.1

SCIENTISTS REPORT ON EARLIEST AIDS CASES

The first recorded AIDS case in America was that of a 15-year-old male prostitute who demonstrated Kaposi's sarcoma and died in 1969. Frozen tissue samples contained HIV antibodies. These findings were reported at the Eleventh International Congress of Virology in August 1999.

The first documented case of AIDS in Europe was seen in a Danish surgeon who had worked in Zaire. She died in 1976.

The first documented case of AIDS in Africa occurred in 1959.

Some Information on the African Case

Scientists have pinpointed what is believed to be the earliest known case of AIDS—an African who died in 1959. The scientists looked for signs of HIV in 1213 blood samples that were gathered in Africa between 1959 and 1982. They found clear signs of the virus in one taken from a Bantu man who lived in Leopoldville, Belgian Congo—what is now Kinshasa, Republic of Congo—in 1959. Scientists compared the genes from the 39-year-old sample of HIV with current versions of HIV. They realized that if they had an old sequence of HIV genes it would serve as a yardstick to measure the evolution of the current HIV. HIV has mutated over the years to form 11 distinct subtypes, lettered A through K. One of these, subtype B, is the dominant strain in the United States and Europe, while subtype D is most common in Africa. The family tree of HIV looks like a bush with the various subtypes forming the limbs. Scientists believe the 1959 HIV is near the trunk, around the point where the subtypes B and D branch off and that this virus is an ancestor to B and D. These data suggest that all HIV subtypes evolved from one introduction of HIV into people, rather than from many crossovers from animals to humans, as some have speculated.

time that the final genetic transformation or evolution of SIV into HIV occurred. After all, humans have hunted, handled, and eaten primates for thousands of years. Recent laboratory accidents have shown that SIV can infect humans. Even though at the moment no identifiable disease has been associated with the SIV/human infections, such accidents have demonstrated the potential for cross-species or zoonotic (a disease acquired from a vertebrate animal) transmission of HIV-related viruses. Why not believe the same for the origin of HIV-1?

That being said, some of the current scientific ideas on the origin of HIV are presented. The answer to the origin of HIV is important because scientists have no idea of what it takes to launch animal viruses into human epidemics or pandemics. And the occurrence of other viral human epidemics and pandemics is only a matter of time as the world waits for the next avian flu or SARS epidemic/pandemic.

Some Scientific Ideas on the Origin of HIV

Vanessa Hirsch and colleagues (1995) presented evidence that a virus isolated from a species of West African monkey, the Sooty Mangabey (an ash-colored monkey), may have infected humans 20 to 30 years ago. They believe this virus subsequently evolved into HIV-2. Hirsch et al. studied a virus known as the Simian Immunodeficiency Virus (SIV) that infects both wild and captive Sooty Mangabey monkeys (SIVsm). They molecularly cloned and sequenced the DNA of the virus and constructed an evolutionary tree of the several known primate immunodeficiency viruses. This tree showed SIVsm to be more closely related to HIV-2 than to HIV-1.

Gerald Meyers of Los Alamos National Laboratory states that SIVsm and HIV are so closely related that when HIV-2 is found in a human, it may be the Sooty Mangabey virus. However, HIV-1 does not sufficiently resemble HIV-2 or SIVsm, thus HIV-1 probably did not evolve from SIVsm/HIV-2. The prevailing theory for HIV-1 is that humans were first infected with HIV-1 through direct contact with precursor HIV-infected chimpanzees. The chimpanzee-to-human scenario is easier to accept than humans infecting chimpanzees.

Be a Virus, See the World

Albert Osterhaus of Erasmus University Rotterdam, The Netherlands, believes that *all* human viral infec-tious diseases ultimately have an animal origin, and natural transfer of these infections is a common event in animal populations.

The Current Theory on HIV Origin: A Chimpanzee (cpz)

Beatrice Hahn and colleagues (1999; 2000; 2003; 2006) from the University of Alabama at Birmingham say they have gathered sufficient evidence to believe the origin of HIV-1 in humans to be a cross-species transmission from a particular subspecies of chimpanzee—meaning that a simian virus closely related to HIV moved from chimpanzees to humans, and later mutated into its current form (Figure 2-3).

Hahn presented three lines of evidence in support of their thesis. First, the genes of **SIVcpz** isolates cluster on evolutionary trees according to their chimpanzee subspecies or origin, either *Pan troglodytes troglodytes* from West Africa or *Pan troglodytes schweinfurthii* in East Africa. By sequencing parts of the virus's genetic material, the scientists found that more segments of the simian and human virus overlapped than had been identified in three previous simian viruses isolated in recent years from other chimpanzees.

Second, all known HIV-1 strains, including the M group that accounts for about 99% of all HIV-1 infections, as well as the O group and the N group, form a genetic cluster with the West African chimpanzee viruses. This clustering is also geographic and consistent with the likely equatorial Central African origin of HIV-1 (Figure 2-4). Hahn said she had initially been equally ready to accept the idea that chimps had gotten HIV from humans, rather than vice-versa. However, a third line of evidence convinced her that HIV-1 was introduced into the human population from at least three cross-species transmissions from chimpanzees—she found evidence of genetic recombination among the SIVcpz strains of the *troglodytes'* lineage.

In addition, scientists in the United States found evidence in chimpanzees that SIVcpz is found in East Africa as well as West Africa, suggesting that not only is the virus widely distributed in Africa, but that continued hunting of the species for food and keeping the animals as pets could result in another outbreak of an AIDS-like disease. These data document, for the first time, that humans are continuously exposed to an unprecedented variety of SIVs through the consumption of bush meat (Santiago et al., 2002; Peeters et al., 2002; Kalish et al., 2005).

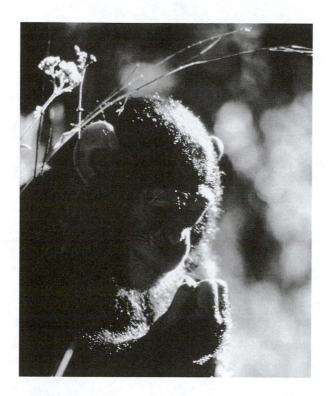

FIGURE 2-3 Photograph of *Pan troglodytes troglodytes*. This photograph was taken in the Gabon region of Africa where the sole species of *Pan troglodytes* is found. Their numbers are declining rapidly due to the "bush meat" trade—their slaughter and selling of their body parts. (*Photograph courtesy of Karl Ammann, wildlife Photographer*)

The question that remains is, where did SIVcpz come from?

In mid-2006, Hahn and colleagues reported on their detection of SIVcpz antibodies and nucleic acids in fecal samples from wild-living *P.t. troglodytes* apes in southern Cameroon, where prevalence rates in some *troglodytes* communities reached 29% to 35%. By sequence analysis of the endemic SIVcpz strains, they traced the origins of pandemic (group M) and non-pandemic (group N) HIV-1 to distinct, geographically isolated chimpanzee communities. These findings establish *P.t. troglodytes* as the natural reservoir of HIV. Hahn said, "Chimpanzees acquired their infections like humans did, by hunting and consuming naturally infected primates." The authors of the study also postulate that, "given the extensive genetic diversity and phylogeographical clustering of SIVcpz now recognized, and the vast areas of west central Africa not yet

sampled, it is quite possible that still other SIVcpz lineages exist that could pose risks for human infection and prove problematic for HIV diagnostics and vaccines." This study, "Chimpanzee Reservoirs of Pandemic and Non-pandemic HIV-1," was published in the *Science* journal, website at Science Express (doi. 10.1126/science. 1126531).

Is the Search for the Origin of HIV Over?

It is nice to think that the issue of HIV origin has been solved. However, time will tell if Hahn's current effort will be the final word on the subject. Some questions still remain. Why, for example, does HIV-1 appear to be so benign in chimpanzees, as has been shown in numerous infection experiments over the years? For scientists, the new chimpanzee finding is just as much a beginning as an end. Although researchers may have

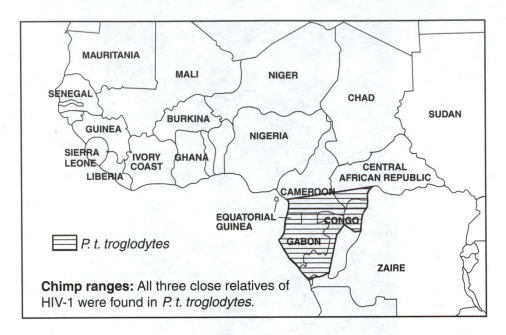

FIGURE 2-4   Geographic Ranges of one Subspecies of Chimpanzee *Pan troglodytes*. *(Adapted from Hahn, 1999)*

the best evidence so far that HIV came from chimpanzees, no one can yet say how the virus became lethal to humans. Chimpanzees share over 98% of the genes that exist in humans, yet they don't get AIDS. So which of the remaining genes protect chimpanzees from an infection that has turned out to be almost universally fatal in people? Also, researchers are still investigating how, after taking root in just a few people, HIV gradually traveled all over the world.

How Often Did SIVcpz Cross Over into Humans?—Researchers now believe that AIDS-like viruses moved from chimp to human more than once, creating different strains of HIV. This means a vaccine against one strain of HIV may not control a new epidemic. As it turned out, *Pan troglodytes troglodytes* live in the region of Africa where HIV-1 was first recognized. Since there are three separate groups of HIV-1 (M, O, and N), the scientists believe that HIV-1 crossed into people from chimps at least three times. Hahn said that SIV appears to have dwelled in primates for hundreds of thousands of years before turning into the deadly human virus, HIV. Hahn believes hunting, which exposes people to

excessive amounts of blood during slaughter, allowed precursor HIV to infect humans.

Why Do Chimpanzees Resist HIV Infection?—With regard to the question of why chimpanzees resist HIV infection, in late 2002 Dutch investigators presented a theory that an AIDS-like epidemic killed large populations of chimps about 2 million years ago. The survivors of this viral (SIVcpz-like?) eradication were selected for survival because they carried the genes necessary to resist the viral infection. Over the years, this genetic selection gave rise to chimpanzees that are resistant to viruses closely related to HIV, for example SIVcpz and HIV itself.

DISCUSSION QUESTION   If humans become infected with SIVcpz from chimpanzees, where or how did the chimpanzees get SIVcpz? Elizabeth Bailes and colleagues (2003) believe that SIV-infected monkeys gave rise to SIVcpz through monkey to monkey cross-species SIV transmission and recombination among slightly genetically different SIV to produce SIVcpz. Because chimpanzees feed on these monkeys, they become SIVcpz-infected, much like humans who consumed the SIVcpz-infected chimpanzees. Thus, chimpanzees and humans acquired their versions of the pre-HIV virus the same way—by killing and eating animals infected with similar viruses.

Where Did HIV Begin to Circulate Among Humans?—According to Nicole Vidal and colleagues (2000), because of the unprecedented degree of HIV-1 group M genetic diversity found in the Democratic Republic of Congo (9 of the 11 different group M subtypes), the HIV-1 pandemic must have originated in Central Africa.

Daniel Vangroenweghe (2001) states that the earliest cases of HIV infection and AIDS in the 1960s and 1970s occurred in Congo-Kinshasa (Zaire), Rwanda, and Burundi. These countries appear to be the source of HIV group M epidemic, which then spread outward to neighboring Tanzania and Uganda in the East, and Congo-Brazzaville in the West. Then it spread to Haiti. Hundreds of single men from Haiti participated in the UNESCO educational program in the Congo between 1960 and 1975, and it is believed, that they returned to Haiti infected with HIV.

Do We Know How HIV Got Into the United States?

Michael Worobey said at the March 2007 Fourteenth Conference on Retroviruses and Opportunistic Infections (CROI) that Haiti has the oldest HIV epidemic outside Africa and provided the source for the strain of HIV seen in North America and Europe. Worobey said that an international team of researchers found that the type of HIV most prevalent in Haiti, the United States, and Europe—HIV-1 group M, subtype B—moved from Africa to Haiti around 1966. HIV spread around Haiti before a single migration of the virus took it out of Haiti to the U.S. by 1969 and then worldwide between 1969 and 1972. The research also suggests that HIV-1 group M originated comparatively recently, probably no earlier than the early 20th century (Worobey et al. 2007; Gilbert et al. 2007).

The exact circumstances surrounding the emergence of the strain of HIV in the U.S. and Europe have long been the subject of debate. Investigators from the U.S., Denmark, and the United Kingdom recovered complete HIV-1 env gene sequences from samples obtained from five Haitian AIDS patients between 1982 and 1983 who were recent migrants to the United States. To test the hypothesis that subtype B has a Haitian origin, they conducted phylogenetic analysis of samples obtained from these patients and of a further 117 samples obtained from patients in 19 different countries using the analysis of the gag gene sequence from the different viral samples. A U.S. or non-Haitian origin for subtype B was strongly rejected in favor of a Haitian origin.

When Did HIV Begin to Circulate Among Humans?—Scientists do have some idea when the virus began to circulate among people. From looking at samples of HIV taken at different times and in different parts of the world, researchers have constructed a type of genetic clock for HIV-1. The speed of the clock is determined by how much the virus changes over time. A key to setting this clock came with the discovery of the two oldest known HIV infections, one found in 1959 in a man, the other in a woman in 1960 who lived in what is now Congo. After the AIDS epidemic began, both frozen samples were thawed and screened for the presence of HIV. In 2008 Michael Worobey and colleagues compared the genetic data from the older HIV with samples from newer HIV. They concluded that HIV has been circulating in humans since 1908 or earlier!

Continued Evolution of HIV in Humans?—Possible *good* news (?) is that HIV would, after killing millions of humans, become a harmless passenger as most likely its precursor SIV did thousands of years ago in chimpanzees. The bad news would be that HIV is evolving into a virus that is more easily spread and/or becomes more lethal. Time will tell.

SUMMARY ON THE ORIGIN OF HIV

In summary, there are at least three ideas on the possible origins of the AIDS virus: (1) It is a human-made virus, perhaps from a germ warfare laboratory; (2) it originated in the animal world and crossed over into humans; and (3) HIV has existed in small, isolated human populations for a long time and, given the right set of conditions, it escaped into the larger population. Computer modeling of DNA sequence in HIV and SIVsm and the recent work of Beatrice Hahn and colleagues suggests that HIV evolved within the last 100 to 300 years. So for now, the question remains: Is AIDS a new disease or an old disease that was late being recognized—so late that

VIRUSES CROSSING FROM PRIMATES INTO HUMANS

Although it may appear odd that distinct strains of HIV should have colonized humans from different animal species on different occasions, natural cross-species transfer has occurred frequently for other retroviruses, not just HIV. There is also a precedent with the flaviviruses, yellow fever and dengue, and with malaria. *Plasmodium falciparum* malaria, arising in Africa, is closely related to the parasite of chimpanzees, whereas *P. vivax* came from Asian monkeys.

WHY HAS HIV SHOWN UP NOW—IS THIS A NEW VIRUS?

Based on scientific evidence, different SIV strains apparently crossed into humans several times during the twentieth century. There may have been many earlier introductions or precursor HIV into humans but, like Ebola or Lassa fever viral outbreaks, they may only have occurred locally, temporarily, and soon vanished. What helped HIV to become endemic, and group M to become epidemic, might have been the huge expansion of needle and syringe use in the mid-twentieth century during periods of mass vaccination and injecting antibiotic use, as suggested by Preston Marx and colleagues (2001). In other words, it is not the cross-species transfer event that is new or different but the social conditions and medical practices that allowed the evolving HIV eventually to adapt to sexual transmission which allowed for its survival in humans. Strains of SIV most likely crossed into humans around 1900, plus or minus about 15 years. So, yes, this is, according to scientists, a new virus!

rounds of HIV replication presented humans with new HIV mutations, some of which were to become lethal. In the 1960s, war, tourism, and commercial trucking forced the outside world on Africa's once isolated villages. At the same time, drought and industrialization prompted mass migrations from the countryside into newly teeming cities. Western monogamy had never been common in Africa, but as the French medical historian Mirko Grmek notes in his book, *History of AIDS* (1990), urbanization shattered social structures that had long contained sexual behavior. Prostitution exploded, and venereal diseases flourished. Hypodermic needles came into wide use during the same period, creating yet another mode of infection. Did these trends actually turn a chronic but relatively benign infection into a killer? The evidence is circumstantial, but it's hard to discount.

Summary

The AIDS virus was discovered and reported by Luc Montagnier of France in 1983. Identifying the virus that caused the immunosuppression that caused AIDS allowed for AIDS surveillance definitions that began in 1982. The recent recognition of non-HIV AIDS cases is not unexpected and can be explained. Presently, there is no new threat of another AIDS-causing biological agent.

The recent work of Beatrice Hahn and colleagues may have pinpointed the reservoir of a precursor HIV-like virus in the chimpanzee, *Pan troglodytes troglodytes*.

HIV was transported into the United States in the early 1970s by men who became HIV infected while working in the Congo.

Review Questions

(Answers to the Review Questions are on page 425.)

1. What may be the strongest evidence for saying that AIDS is caused by HIV?

2. Where did HIV originate and where did the first HIV infections appear?

3. Those who do not believe HIV causes AIDS are referred to as _____.

4. **Name** the woman (mother) who does not believe HIV causes AIDS and **name** the 3-year-old daughter who is said to have died from AIDS.

we will never know its true source, the origin of HIV? Continued investigations may answer these questions.

Has HIV Always Caused a Lethal Disease—AIDS?

An additional question to where HIV came from is whether it has always caused disease. From the study of human history, as it relates to human disease, scientists have numerous examples that show that as human habits change, new diseases emerge. Regardless of whether HIV is old or new, history will show that social changes, however small or sudden, have most likely hastened the spread of HIV. Increased

5. Name the scientist who is the leading advocate of the idea that HIV does not cause AIDS.

6. The president of South Africa is _____.

7. Have Koch's postulates been satisfied in the laboratory under defined conditions that HIV is the causative agent of AIDS? Explain.

8. Is HIV a new or old virus?

9. Is it HIV or SIV that causes a disease in chimpanzees?

10. Name the scientist who appears to have the best evidence that HIV is a new virus and crossed from an animal into humans.

11. In what country was the first currently documented case of HIV infection found, and in what year?

Biological Characteristics of the AIDS Virus

CHAPTER CONCEPTS

- Retroviruses are grouped into three families: oncoviruses, lentiviruses, and foamy viruses.
- HIV is a lentivirus.
- HIV contains nine genes; its three major structural genes are GAG-POL-ENV.
- HIV contains 9749 nucleotides, its genetic code.
- Six HIV genes regulate HIV reproduction, and at least one gene directly influences infection.
- HIV RNA produces HIV DNA, which integrates into the host cell to become proviral DNA.
- Genome-wide scan reveals 273 human proteins that HIV uses to complete its life cycle.
- HIV undergoes rapid genetic changes in infected people.
- The reverse transcriptase enzyme is very error prone.
- HIV causes immunological suppression by destroying T4 helper or CD4+ cells.
- HIV is classified into major (M), outlier (O), and new (N) genetic subtypes. Type M is responsible for 99% of HIV infections worldwide.

VIRUSES NEED A HOST CELL IN ORDER TO REPRODUCE

Viruses are microscopic particles of biological material, so small they can be seen only with electron microscopes. A virus consists solely of a strip of genetic material (nucleic acid) within a protein coat.

Viral genomes (DNA and RNA that contain the genetic information to replicate) are very small and contain few genes compared to living cells. With their limited coding capacity, viruses must enter host cells and must borrow or hijack cellular proteins to complete their replication.

VIRUSES ARE PARASITES

Viruses are parasitic agents; they live inside the cells of their host animal or plant, and can reproduce themselves *only by forcing the host cell to make viral copies*. The new virus leaves the host cell and infects other similar cells. By damaging or killing these cells, some viruses cause diseases in the host animal or plant. Many viruses that infect humans are never eradicated. Ex-

amples of viruses that persist for the life of the individual include *herpes simplex* virus, cytomegalovirus, Epstein–Barr virus, and *varicella zoster* virus. These viruses typically do not cause progressive disease but are held in check by a protective immune response. Genetically, viruses are the simplest forms of "life-like agents"; the genetic blueprint for the structure of the **Human Immunodeficiency Virus (HIV)** is 100,000 times smaller than that contained in a human cell. The complete sequence of 9749 nucleotides that form the genetic code for HIV have been identified and their arrangement sequenced (mapped).

Scientists have produced a great deal of information about HIV over a relatively short time. In the history of medical science, the immediate involvement of so many scientists followed by the rapid identification of the causative agent of AIDS is equaled only by the rapid identification of the SARS virus in 2003. More is known about HIV than about the viruses that cause such long-standing human diseases such as polio, measles, yellow fever, hepatitis, flu, and the common cold. Humankind is fortunate that HIV began spreading through the human population as a pathogen in the mid- to late-1970s. By then scientists had discovered and begun to exploit the molecular aspects of biology. Molecular methodologies necessary to begin the immediate molecular study of HIV were in place to define and refine our knowledge of viruses and, in particular, to learn about HIV.

VIRUSES SPECIFIC TO CELL TYPE

1. **Viruses are very specific with regard to the types of cells they can enter/reproduce.** Not all viruses can attach to or enter all cells. Humans survive in a world full of viruses that *only* enter or reproduce in a variety of bacteria, protozoa, fungi, and higher forms of plant and animal life. It appears that most of these viruses are harmless to humans—if they enter the body they cannot reproduce in human cells—they do not cause human damage. For those viruses that do enter human bodies from animals such as pigs, chickens, rabbits, mice, cows, monkeys, etc. that cause a human disease, most are very specific as to which cells in a human body they can enter/reproduce and damage. For example, the flu virus enters the human respiratory tract cells. Epstein-Barr virus infects cells in the nose and throat. The hepatitis viruses enter liver cells, but each of the hepatitis viruses causes a different degree of human cell damage over time. Some cause a more immediate disease—for example, hepatitis A virus—while hepatitis B or hepatitis C may not cause significant cell damage for years. Polio virus enters cells of the human nervous system that are different from those cells of the nervous system that herpes virus invades. HIV enters and reproduces in cells of the human immune system.

2. **Why do different viruses enter specific cell types?** Each of the viruses that causes human disease does so by finding a cell type that carries a receptor molecule (a protein or a protein attached to a sugar molecule) that *fits* with a projection of a surface molecule of a given virus—much like the key to a lock. That's why specific viruses are known to be associated with certain types of human tissue. For example, there are viruses that attach only to the receptors of heart, gut, eyes, throat, liver, and other specific human cell tissues. Find a way to block either the human cell receptors (CD4, CXCKR-4, and CCKR-5—to which HIV attaches) without harming the cell or to block the given viral receptor (in HIV it's gp120), and one has a therapy for the given viral disease.

RETROVIRUSES

Some viruses belong to the Retroviridae. Some members of this family have proven to be valuable tools in molecular biology research; their ability to import foreign genes into cells has been explored as a possible vehicle for gene therapy. Retroviruses also are potent disease agents, associated with arthritis, systemic lupus erythematosis, and a form of leukemia in adult humans, and they infect and cause a deadly immunodeficiency syndrome in humans: AIDS.

Data that researchers have gathered during years of work comparing the genetic makeup of SIVs and HIV have shown that while primate species infected with SIVs are the long-time natural hosts to those viruses, humans are not the natural hosts of HIV.

There are three subfamilies of retroviruses, two of which are associated with human disease: **oncoviruses** (cancer-causing) and **lentiviruses** or slow viruses, of which HIV-1 and HIV-2 are members. **Spumavirus** is the third group but is not known to be associated with human disease. As a lentivirus, HIV has genetic and morphologic similarities to other animal lentiviruses such as those infecting cats (Feline Immunodeficiency Virus), sheep (visna virus), goats (caprine arthritis-encephalitis virus), and nonhuman primates such as chimpanzees (Simian Immunodeficiency Virus or SIV).

The retroviruses and in particular the lentiviruses have presumably been present for thousands of years. Modern sociodemographic changes and other human factors have allowed rapid mutating (changing) lentiviruses, such as HIV, to find new niches and host populations in which to reproduce. Now let us review some of the characteristics of HIV, the virus that causes AIDS.

DESCRIPTION OF HIV; HOW IT ATTACHES TO A HOST CELL AND BUDS OUT OF THE CELL

As can be seen in Figure 3-1, the virus is a sphere measuring 1000 Å or 1/10,000 mm in diameter. The cone-shaped core in a spherical envelope is the dominant feature. Within the cone-shaped core there are two identical strands of viral RNA, each coupled to a molecule of transfer RNA (tRNA) that serves as a primer for reverse transcription of viral RNA into viral DNA. In order for HIV to replicate, it **must** make a DNA copy of its RNA. It is the DNA genes copied from HIV RNA that allow HIV to replicate! Also present with the RNA are an integrase, a protease, and a ribonuclease enzyme. The released virus is processed internally by HIV protease to form the characteristic dense lentivirus core. Most HIV appear to have initiated

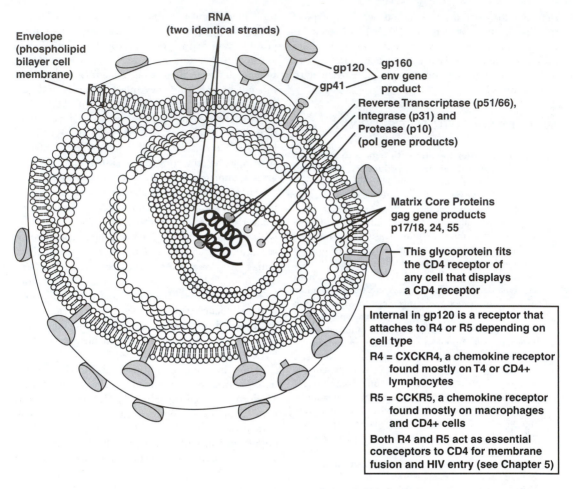

FIGURE 3-1 Human Immunodeficiency Virus. It infects cells by a process of membrane fusion that is mediated by its envelope glycoproteins (gp120 gp41, or Env) and is generally triggered by the interaction of gp120 with at least two cellular components: CD4 and a coreceptor belonging to the chemokine receptor family (CXCKR-4 or R4 and CCKR-5 or R-5). For an excellent review of chemokine receptors and HIV infection, see McNieholl et. al. 1997.

DNA synthesis prior to completion of budding and maturation. Actual maturation of HIV takes place after it buds out of the cell (see Figure 3-3 and Figure 4-9). The membrane of HIV is derived from the host cell. HIV gains the membrane while budding out or exiting the cell (Figure 3-2). The membrane, acquired from its host cell, consists of two lipid (fat) layers impregnated with some human proteins, for example Class I and Class II human lymphocyte antigen complexes important for controlling the immune response (Figure 3-3). The external viral membrane also contains molecules of viral glycoproteins (gp)—a sugar chain attached to protein. Each glycoprotein appears as a spike in the membrane. Each spike consists of two parts: one

is **gp41,** which contains a coiled-up protein and extends through the membrane. On interaction between the HIV envelope and T4 cell coreceptors (CD4/chemokine receptors R4 and R-5), the gp41 coiled protein is unsprung and like a harpoon, it pierces the cell membrane, initiating the first step in HIV infection. The second part, **gp120,** extends from the end of gp41 to the outside and beyond the membrane (the numbers 41 and 120 represent the mass of the individual gps in thousands of daltons). As a complete unit, **gp41** plus **gp120** is called **gp160.** These two membranes or **envelope proteins** play a crucial role in binding HIV to CD4 protein molecules found in the membranes of several types of immune system cells.

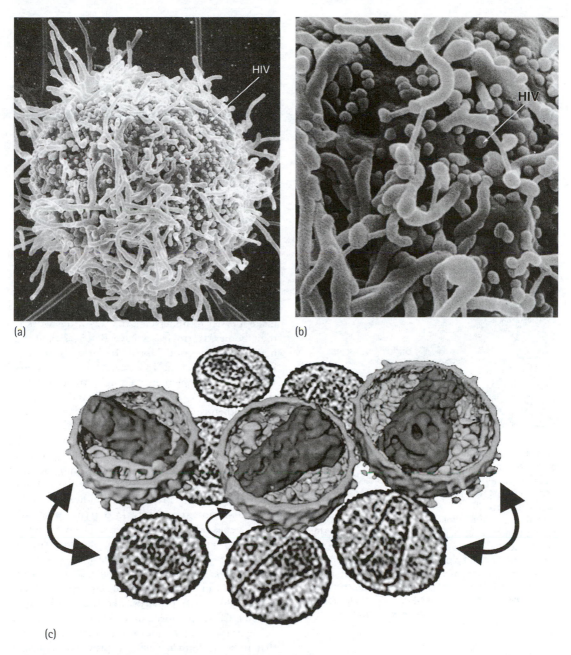

(a)

(b)

(c)

FIGURE 3-2 Viral Replication in Human Lymphocytes. Scanning electron micrograph of HIV-infected human T4 lymphocyte. (a) A single cell infected with HIV showing virus particles and microvilli on the cell surface (magnified 7000 times). (b) Enlargement of a portion of the mountain-like cell surface in (a) showing multiple virus particles budding out of the cell surface (magnified 20,000 times). As each HIV exits the cell, it leaves a hole in the cell membrane. (c) Core Assembly: Insights from Three-Dimensional Reconstruction of HIV. CRYO-ELECTRON TOMOGRAPHY REVEALS THE VIRAL MORPHOLOGY AND CORE FORMATION INSIDE THE CAPSID OF HIV AS SHOWN IN PHOTOGRAPHS a and b (Briggs et al., 2006). (Photographs a and b courtesy of K. Nagashima, Program Resources, Inc., NCI-Frederick Cancer Research and Development Center. Photograph c courtesy of Brigg, J. A., Grunewald, K., Glass, B., Forster, F., Krausslie, H. G., and Fuller, S. D. (2006). "The Mechanism of HIV-1 core assembly: insights from three-dimensional reconstructions of authentic virions," *Structure* 14, 15–20.)

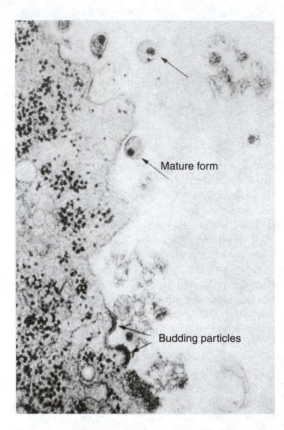

FIGURE 3-3 Budding and Mature Retroviruses. HIV buds from infected cells only at special points on the cellular membrane known as "lipid rafts." The rafts are rich in cholesterol. Without the cholesterol HIV cannot fuse with new CD4+ or T4 cells (Hildreth, 2001). This is a photograph of HIV taken by electron microscopy. Note the difference between the free or mature HIV and those that are just budding out through the membrane of a T4 helper cell. This cell came from an HIV-infected hemophiliac. Closely observing the mature HIV, one can make out the core protein area surrounded by the cell's membrane (virus envelope). *(Courtesy of the Centers for Disease Control and Prevention, Atlanta)*

Full-length HIV RNA is complexed with capsid proteins, and the nucleocapsid is transferred to the cell surface membrane at envelope-containing sites.

HUMAN IMMUNODEFICIENCY VIRUS (HIV): ITS LIFE CYCLE

Retroviruses are so named because they *reverse* the usual flow of genetic information within the host cell in order to reproduce themselves. In all living cells, normal gene expression results from the genetic information of DNA being copied into RNA (Figure 3-4). The RNA is translated into a specific cellular protein. In all living cell types, the directions for protein synthesis come from the species' genetic information contained in its DNA:

$$DNA \rightarrow RNA \rightarrow Protein\ Synthesis$$

THE HIV LIFE CYCLE

Understanding how HIV works inside the human cell gives scientists important clues about how to attack it at its most vulnerable points. Knowing the secrets of how the virus functions and reproduces itself—a process called its life cycle—can help scientists design new drugs that are more effective at suppressing HIV and have fewer side effects. For people with HIV, knowing how HIV works can make it easier to understand the way drugs work in their bodies. Retroviruses have RNA as their genetic material—not DNA! In brief, retrovirus RNA is copied, using its reverse transcriptase enzyme, into a complementary single strand of DNA (Figures 3-5, 3-6). The single-strand retroviral DNA is then copied into double-stranded retroviral DNA (this replication occurs in the cell's cytoplasm). At this point the viral DNA has been made according to the instructions in the retroviral RNA. This retroviral DNA migrates into the host cell nucleus and becomes integrated (inserted) into the host cell DNA. A recent study indicates that the viral DNA integrates only into transcriptionally active genes. The integrated viral DNA is now a **provirus.** From this point on, the infection is irreversible—*the viral genes are now a part of the cell's genetic information and will be replicated.* In this respect, HIV can be considered an acquired dominant genetic disease! A provirus, like the "mole" in a John Le Carre spy novel, may hide for years before doing its specific job. But for HIV, there is evidence that in some human cells the provirus begins to produce new copies of HIV RNA immediately after becoming a provirus or shortly thereafter.

Before the HIV provirus's genes can be expressed, RNA copies of them that can be read by the host cell's protein-making machinery must be produced. This is done by **transcription.** Transcription is accomplished by the cell's own enzymes. But the process cannot start until the cell's RNA polymerase is activated by various molecular switches located in

Central Dogma

Prior to 1970, cell biologists thought that genetic information flowed only in one direction.

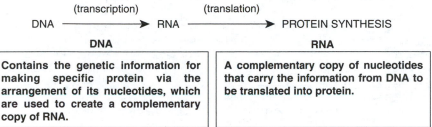

DNA	**RNA**
Contains the genetic information for making specific protein via the arrangement of its nucleotides, which are used to create a complementary copy of RNA.	A complementary copy of nucleotides that carry the information from DNA to be translated into protein.

Reverse of Central Dogma

In 1970 the reverse transcriptase enzyme (RT) was found in a virus. These viruses became known as retroviruses.

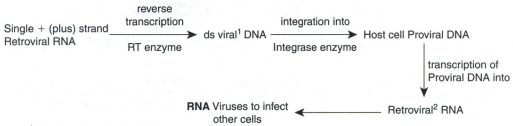

[1] ds = Double-stranded DNA

[2] If the RNA transcribed is spliced, RNA base sequences are rearranged. This RNA = messenger RNA and is used to make retroviral protein. If RNA transcribed is not spliced, it becomes the RNA genome of the new virus.

FIGURE 3–4 Retroviral Flow of Genetic Information. The general directional flow of genetic information in all living species is from DNA, where the information is stored, into RNA, which serves as a messenger for the construction of proteins that are the cells' functional molecules. This unidirectional flow of genetic information has been referred to as the "Central dogma" of molecular biology. In the 1960s, Howard Temin and colleagues discovered an enzyme that copied RNA into DNA, a reverse of what was normally expected, thus the name *reverse transcriptase.*

two DNA regions near the ends of the provirus: the **long terminal repeats.** This requirement is reminiscent of the need of many genes in multicellular organisms to be "turned on" or "off" by proteins that bind specifically to controlling sequences.

Production of Viral RNA Strands or RNA Transcripts

Within the host cell nucleus, proviral DNA, when activated, produces new strands of HIV RNA. Some of the RNA strands behave like messenger RNA (mRNA), producing proteins essential for the production of HIV. Other RNA strands become encased within the viral core proteins to become the new viruses. Whether the transcribed RNA strands become mRNA or RNA strands for new viruses de-

pends on whether or not the newly synthesized RNA strands undergo complex processing. RNA processing means that after the RNA is produced, some of it is cut into segments by cellular enzymes and then reassociated or **spliced** into a length of RNA suitable for protein synthesis. The RNA strands that are spliced become the mRNA used in protein synthesis. The unspliced RNA strands serve as new viral strands that are encased in their protein coats (capsids) to become new viruses that bud out of the cell (Figure 3-5).

Two distinct phases of transcription follow the infection of an individual cell by HIV. In the first or early phase, RNA strands or transcripts produced in the cell's nucleus are snipped into multiple copies of shorter sequences by cellular splicing enzymes. When they reach the cytoplasm, they are only about 2000 nucleotides in length. These early-phase short

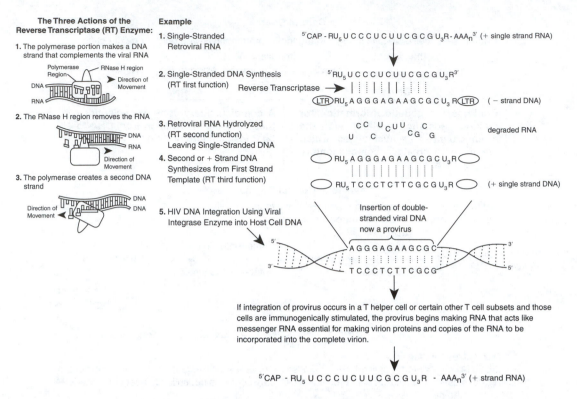

FIGURE 3–5 Proposed Production and Function of Retroviral Provirus. Note the reverse transcriptase enzyme has three functions: **(1)** to act as an RNA-dependent DNA polymerase transcribing single-stand DNA from viral RNA; **(2)** to demonstrate RNase H activity (RNase H is a subunit of the RT enzyme) by hydrolyzing the retroviral RNA off the RNA-DNA complex; and **(3)** to act as a DNA-dependent polymerase and transcribe the second DNA strand complementary to the first DNA strand. The process of viral RNA transcription is complex. When completed, the viral RNA gives rise to the formation of either linear or circular molecules of proviral DNA. Each end of the provirus contains an identical long series of terminal-repeating nucleotides or LTRs. LTRs are not a part of the viral genome. Although retroviral DNA integration is considered to be the normal route for RNA virus reproduction, retroviral reproduction may occur without proviral integration (see Figure 3–6).

transcripts encode only the virus's **regulatory proteins;** the structural genes that constitute the rest of the genome are among the parts that are left behind. In the second or late phase, two new size classes of RNA—long (unspliced) transcripts of 9749 nucleotides making up the new viral genome and medium-length (singly spliced) transcripts of some 4500 nucleotides—move out of the nucleus and into the cytoplasm. The 4500 nucleotide transcripts encode HIV's structural and enzymatic proteins (Greene, 1993).

Experimental results reported by Somasundaran et al. (1988) showed that when lymphoid cell lines or peripheral blood lymphocytes were infected with a laboratory strain of HIV, up to 2.5 million copies of

the viral RNA were produced by cells; and within three days of infection, up to 40% of the total protein synthesized by the cells was viral protein. This is an unprecedented takeover for a retrovirus that typically makes only modest amounts of RNA and protein.

Much of what HIV does after entering the host cell or while integrated as a retroprovirus depends on the activity of its genes.

HOW HIV ESCAPES THE INFECTED CELL

This is a primary example of how a virus, in this case, HIV, uses living cells to achieve its mission—to infect,

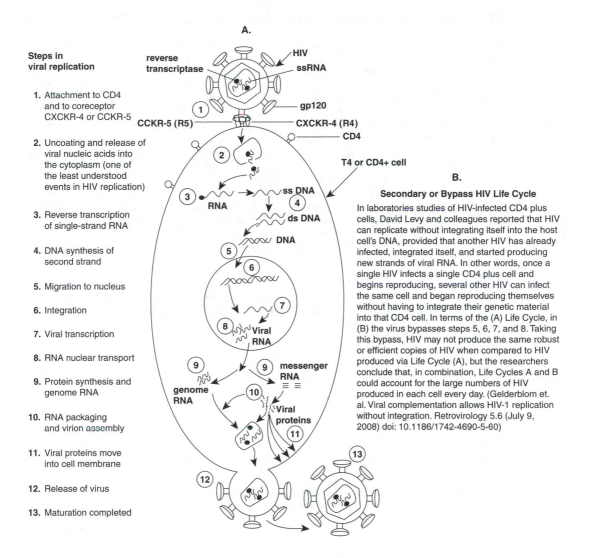

A.

Steps in viral replication

1. Attachment to CD4 and to coreceptor CXCKR-4 or CCKR-5

2. Uncoating and release of viral nucleic acids into the cytoplasm (one of the least understood events in HIV replication)

3. Reverse transcription of single-strand RNA

4. DNA synthesis of second strand

5. Migration to nucleus

6. Integration

7. Viral transcription

8. RNA nuclear transport

9. Protein synthesis and genome RNA

10. RNA packaging and virion assembly

11. Viral proteins move into cell membrane

12. Release of virus

13. Maturation completed

reverse transcriptase

HIV
ssRNA

gp120

CCKR-5 (R5)   CXCKR-4 (R4)
                          CD4

T4 or CD4+ cell

ss DNA
RNA
ds DNA
DNA

Viral RNA

messenger RNA

genome RNA

Viral proteins

B.

Secondary or Bypass HIV Life Cycle

In laboratories studies of HIV-infected CD4 plus cells, David Levy and colleagues reported that HIV can replicate without integrating itself into the host cell's DNA, provided that another HIV has already infected, integrated itself, and started producing new strands of viral RNA. In other words, once a single HIV infects a single CD4 plus cell and begins reproducing, several other HIV can infect the same cell and began reproducing themselves without having to integrate their genetic material into that CD4 cell. In terms of the (A) Life Cycle, in (B) the virus bypasses steps 5, 6, 7, and 8. Taking this bypass, HIV may not produce the same robust or efficient copies of HIV when compared to HIV produced via Life Cycle (A), but the researchers conclude that, in combination, Life Cycles A and B could account for the large numbers of HIV produced in each cell every day. (Gelderblom et. al. Viral complementation allows HIV-1 replication without integration. Retrovirology 5.6 (July 9, 2008) doi: 10.1186/1742-4690-5-60)

FIGURE 3-6 (A) Primary of Expected Life Cycle of HIV in a T4 or CD4+ Lymphocyte. On average, the life cycle of HIV in an infected T4 cell is about two days. This means that one HIV in one person in one year can produce about 180 generations of HIV. The lifetime of HIV in the blood is about six hours. After fusion of viral and cellular membranes, the inner part of HIV, called the **core**, is delivered into the cell cytoplasm. Uncoating of the core occurs, releasing two identical RNA strands, accompanying structural proteins and enzymes necessary for HIV replication. HIV RNA is then copied into HIV DNA, which is then transported into the cell's nucleus for insertion or integration into the host cell's DNA. This feature of the virus life cycle is essential for the spread of HIV in vivo, because it allows infection of nondividing cells such as monocytes and terminally differentiated macrophages and dendritic cells. There is still some confusion as to whether HIV becomes a latent infection once HIV DNA becomes inserted or integrated into the host DNA. Evidence indicates that whether HIV is latent depends on the tissue that one is investigating. For example, in the T4 lymphocytes within the lymph nodes, HIV is constantly being replicated, while some T4 lymphocytes in the blood carry HIV in the latent state. (B) Secondary or Bypass HIV Life Cycle.

PROTEINS THAT COULD BE USED TO HALT THE PRODUCTION OF HIV ARE IDENTTIFIED

The life cycle of HIV is very complex, yet it only produces 15 proteins. Clearly, HIV depends on multiple host-cell proteins to successfully complete its life cycle. This implies that there are many proteins that remain to be discovered. Finding these proteins may spotlight novel drug targets for use in antiretroviral therapy. In January 2008, Stephen Elledge and colleagues published an HIV research paper that Robert Gallo, head of the Institute of Human Virology in Baltimore, Maryland, and founder of the first HIV antibody test said was "destined to become one of the key HIV papers of this decade, if not longer." Using cutting-edge molecular techniques, Stephen Elledge and colleagues found that HIV relies on 273 human proteins to do its work. Of these so-called HIV

dependency factors (HDFs), only 36 had been discovered to this time. Their discovery was made using a genome-wide scan of human DNA, specifically 21,000 human genes that encode proteins. The research team effectively short-circuited or blocked all 21,000 genes one at time using RNA interference screens (RNAi) and then asked if HIV could complete its life cycle. By a process of elimination, they isolated those genes that HIV uses to complete its life cycle. The most immediate challenge is to elucidate the molecular details of how these 273 HDFs interact with HIV. Currently, the authors can only suggest possible connections. But what a great starting point! (Cohn, 2008).

---

replicate, and exit a cell. In October 2001, Jennifer Garrus and colleagues reported on how HIV takes over the human cell's normal processes in order to leave a cell. This discovery could lead to new drugs to control HIV disease in those who are HIV-infected. In a key part of their study, scientists crippled the cells' machinery by silencing a gene that normally makes the protein (Tsg101) necessary for HIV to escape or bud out of the cell. Thus, clusters of connected HIV particles were stuck at the cell membrane and could not get out. The new study showed the Tsg101 protein within cells acts as a key link to the budding process. One part of Tsg101 protein connects to an HIV protein while another part of the Tsg101 protein links to other proteins within a cell—proteins the virus uses to exit the cell. Shutting down the means by which HIV leaves the cell means that other susceptible cells will not become infected. Blocking Tsg101 protein after a person becomes infected could keep the virus from spreading to other cells. These scientists speculate that many other viruses may use the same exit pathway. After 27 years, scientists still do not know just how HIV kills cells bearing a CD4 protein and scientists still do not know why T4 or CD4+ cells fall from about 1000 per microliter of blood to less than 100 per microliter of blood over a 10-year period while viral loads may remain constant or show an enormous increase over a short time interval. And in many people, the relationship of viral load to the rate of their disease progression is questionable at best.

BASIC GENETIC STRUCTURE OF RETROVIRAL GENOMES

The first retrovirus was isolated from a sarcoma (a cancer) in chickens by Peyton Rous in 1911 and was named the Rous sarcoma virus. The basic genetic structure of the Rous sarcoma virus and all animal retroviruses is the same. They all contain retroviral RNA sequences that code for the same three genes abbreviated GAG, POL, and ENV. Flanking each end of the retroviral genome is a sequence of similar nucleotides called long terminal repeats or redundancies (LTRs).

$$5' = \underset{\text{LTR}}{\underline{\text{GAG POL ENV}}} = 3'$$

Some of the animal retroviruses such as the Rous sarcoma virus contain an additional **oncogene** (ONC) that, along with its LTRs, causes a rapid form of cancer in chickens that kills them in one to two weeks after infection. Without the **onc** gene the virus causes a slow, progressive cancer.

Retroviral Genome of HIV

What sets the HIV genome apart from all other known retroviruses is the number of genes in HIV and the apparent complexity of their interactions in regulating the expression of the GAG-POL-ENV genes (Figure 3-7).

The Nine Genes of HIV—The HIV genome contains at least nine recognizable genes that produce at

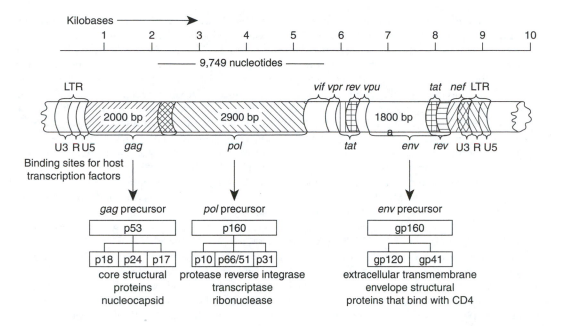

FIGURE 3-7 Genome of HIV. Nine of the genes making up the HIV genome have been identified. They are positioned as shown. Five are essential for HIV replication and six control reproduction (see text for details). The maxtrix protein, p17, forms the outer shell HIV, lining the inner surface of the viral membrane. Key functions of p17 protein are: orchestrates HIV assembly, directs GAG p55 protein to host cell membrane, interacts with transmembrane protein, gp41, to retain envelope-coded proteins within HIV, and contains a nuclear localization signal that directs HIV RNA integration complex to the nucleus of infected cells.

least 15 individual proteins. These proteins are divided into three classes: (1) GAG, POL, and ENV, the three major **structural** proteins; (2) Tat and Rev, the two **regulatory** proteins; and (3) Nef, Vif, Vpu, and Vpr, the four **accessory** proteins. Five of the nine genes are involved in regulating the expression of the GAG-POL-ENV genes.

The letters **GAG** stand for group-specific antigens (proteins) that make up the viral nucleocapsid. The GAG gene codes for internal structural proteins, the production of the dense cylindrical core proteins (**p24,** a nucleoid shell protein with a molecular weight of 24,000), and several internal proteins, which have been visualized by electron microscopy. The GAG gene has the ability to direct the formation of virus-like particles when all other major genes (POL and ENV) are absent. It is only when the GAG gene is nonfunctional that retroviruses (HIV) lose their capacity to bud out of a host cell. Because of these observations, the GAG protein has been designated the virus particle-making machine (Wills et al., 1991).

The **POL** gene codes for HIV enzymes, protease (p10), the virus-associated polymerase (reverse tran-

scriptase) that is active in two forms, and endonuclease (integrase) enzymes. The integrase enzyme cuts the cell's DNA and inserts the HIV DNA. Evidence from retroviral deletion studies shows that the loss of LTRs on the 3′ side of the POL gene stops viral DNA integration into the host genome. However, nonintegrated DNA, without its LTRs and integrase enzyme, can still produce new viruses. This clearly demonstrates that viral DNA integration is not essential for viral multiplication even though integration is the normal course of events (Dimmrock and Primrose, 1987).

The regulation of HIV transcription appears to be intimately related to the onset of HIV disease and AIDS. Thus interruption or inactivation of the POL gene would appear to have therapeutic effects.

The **ENV** gene codes for HIV surface proteins, two major envelope glycoproteins (gp120, located on the external "spikes" of HIV and gp41, the transmembrane protein that attaches gp120 to the surface of HIV) that become embedded throughout the host cell membrane, which ultimately becomes the **envelope** that surrounds the virus as it "buds" out. Studies on how HIV kills cells have revealed at least one way in which the envelope glycoproteins enhance T helper cell death. The envelope glycoproteins cause the formation of **syncytia;** that is, healthy T cells fuse to each other, forming a group around a single HIV-infected T4 or CD4+ cell. Individual T cells within these syncytia lose their immune function. Starting with a single HIV-infected T4 helper cell, as many as 500 *uninfected* T4 helper cells can fuse into a single syncytium. Continued creation of these syncytia could deplete a T4 cell population.

Several studies have demonstrated that the appearance of syncytium-inducing (SI) HIV strains during the chronic phase of HIV disease heralds an abrupt loss of T4 or CD4+ lymphocytes and a clinical progression of the disease. Although the SI phenotype is detected in many patients with AIDS, it has also been isolated from individuals who have not gone on to an early development of AIDS. However, the marked decrease in the T4 lymphocyte counts after shifting from non-SI (NSI) to SI strains as well as the negative effect SI strains have on primary HIV infection suggests that their appearance may not be just a consequence, but the actual cause of immune system alterations (Torres et al., 1996).

The Six Genes of HIV that Control HIV Reproduction—Collectively, the six additional HIV genes tat and rev (regulatory genes), and nef, vif, vpu, vpr (auxiliary genes) working together with the host cell's machinery actually control the reproductive retroviral cycle: adhesion of HIV to a cell, penetration of the cell, uncoating of HIV genome, reverse transcription of the RNA genome producing proviral DNA and immediate production of new viral RNA, or the integration of the provirus and later viral multiplication. The six genes allow for the entire reproductive scenario—from infection to new HIV—to occur in 5 to 6 minutes in dividing cells. Currently there are no drugs that target a regulatory gene or its products. (Jouvenet et al., 2008)

Gene Sequence—The HIV proviral genome has been well characterized with regard to gene location and sequence, but the function of each gene is not completely understood. The genes for producing regulatory proteins can be grouped into two classes: genes that produce proteins essential for HIV replication **(tat** and **rev)**, and genes that produce proteins that perform accessory functions that enhance replication and/or infectivity **(nef, vif, vpu,** and **vpr)** (Rosen, 1991).

Gene Function—Each end of the proviral genome contains an identical long sequence of nucleotides, the long terminal repeats. Although these LTRs are not considered to be genes of the HIV genome, they do contain regulatory nucleotide sequences that help the six regulatory/auxiliary genes control GAG-POL-ENV gene expression. For example, the **vif** gene is associated with the infectious activity of the virus. Currently, the predominant view is that vif acts at the late stages of infection to promote HIV processing or assembly (Potash et al., 1998).

The **tat** gene, (transcription activator) is essential for HIV infection of T4 cells and HIV replication (Li, 1997; Stevenson, 1998). It is one of the first viral genes to be transcribed. The tat gene produces a trans-activator protein, meaning that the gene produces a protein that exerts its effect on viral replication from a distance rather than interacting with genes adjacent to **tat** or their gene product. **Tat** contains two coding regions or exons—areas that contain genetic information for producing a diffusible protein—which, through the help of the LTR sequences, increases the expression of HIV genes, thereby increasing the production of new virus particles. The tat protein interacts with a short nucleotide sequence called TAR located within the 5′ LTR region of HIV messenger RNA (mRNA) transcripts (Matsuya et al., 1990). Once that tat protein binds to the TAR sequence, transcription of the provirus by cellular RNA polymerase II accelerates at least one thousandfold.

The **rev** gene (regulator of expression of viral protein) selectively increases the synthesis of HIV structural proteins in the latter stages of HIV disease, thereby maximizing the production of new viruses. It does this by regulating the splicing of the HIV RNA transcript (cutting out nucleotide sequences that exist between exons and bringing the exons together) and transporting spliced and unspliced RNAs from the nucleus to the cytoplasm (Patrusky, 1992; Fritz et al., 1995).

The **nef** (negative effector) gene produces a protein that is maintained in the cell cytoplasm next to the nuclear membrane. It is believed **nef** functions by protecting the cell from dying, allowing the cell to continue producing HIV. Several antigenic forms of nef protein have been found, which suggest multiple activities of nef within HIV-infected cells (Kohleisen et al., 1992; Sagg et al., 1995). Olivier Schwartz and coworkers (Cohen, 1997) showed that **nef** can prompt cells to yank down from their surfaces a molecule known as the major histocompatibility complex (MHC), which displays viral peptides to the immune system. The group predicted that this "down-regulation" of MHC would make HIV-infected cells resistant to cytotoxic T cell killing (Collins et al., 1998) (see Chapter 5).

In August 2001, Yuntao Wu and colleagues reported that after HIV RNA manufactures a DNA copy, but prior to its integration into the cell's DNA, the HIV DNA stimulates the production of **tat** and **nef** viral proteins. These proteins awaken T4 cells out of their dormant state. Once the T4 cells are activated, they become vulnerable to nuclear invasion by HIV DNA, allowing the virus to integrate into the T4 cell DNA structure. Not only will the activated T4 cell allow HIV DNA to enter the nucleus and insert itself into human DNA, an activated T4 cell produces a higher rate of HIV RNA replication (Wu et al., 2001).

The functions of the **vpr** gene, which codes for a **v**iral **p**rotein **R,** is associated with the transport of cytoplasmic viral DNA into the nucleus. Vpr is also involved in steroid production that in turn helps produce HIV, is required for the efficient assembly or release of new HIV viruses, and stops T4 cell division. Although vpr protein is not needed for HIV to reproduce in T4 or CD4+ cell cultures, it appears to be very important for HIV to reproduce in macrophages. Vpr can induce CD4+ cell death even when the cells are not HIV-infected and is also poisonous to cell mitochondria, which may be important in killing cells that are HIV-infected. It has recently been shown that HIV-infected people who are long-term nonprogressors to AIDS have a mutant or nonfunctional form of the vpr gene (Lum et al., 2003).

Vif or the Viral Infectivity Protein—Vif is produced using one of the smallest and least understood of the nine genes that make up HIV. In 2002, scientists probing the secrets of Vif reported two startling developments. They found that human cells contain a powerful enzyme, a cytidine deaminase known as APOBEC3G (pronounced APPO-beck) that can stop the production of HIV. Simultaneously, they discovered that HIV itself has overcome this natural defense by using Vif protein to neutralize that enzyme. It has been shown that as HIV buds out of a cell it carries the APOBEC enzyme, that is, the enzyme stows away inside the new virus. When HIV infects a new cell and begins making genetic copies of itself, APOBEC becomes active, causing HIV to mutate at such a rapid pace that resulting HIV copies are inactive. But HIV then produces Vif protein that destroys APOBEC—HIV's solution to survival! Some HIV/AIDS scientists believe that those findings are the most important new information in HIV/AIDS research since the identification of HIV in 1983. Once scientists gain an understanding of how Vif blocks this protective enzyme, they can devise tests to measure how well a potential new drug interferes with that process. Presumably a chemical that disables Vif from producing its protein or prevents it from attacking APOBEC could become a potent antiretroviral drug.

Vpu has two important functions in the life cycle of HIV. Vpu codes for a **v**iral **p**rotein **U** that destroys the CD4 protein within the T4 lymphocyte. This helps in the assembly and release of HIV from the cell. Vpu also has the important function of interfering with host cell proteins that cause new HIV to cluster on the cell's membrane surface. Cellular proteins called tetherins to tether or hold the new virus on the membrane, stopping the release of that virus into the body. Vpu proteins block this tethering action. Vif, Vpr, and Vpu appear to be necessary for HIV to replicate.

Of the HIV proteins, tat, rev, and nef are termed *early* proteins because their production results from the cutting and splicing of full-length HIV mRNA; vif, vpu, and vpr are termed *late* proteins because their production results from unspliced or single-spliced mRNA.

In summary, HIV/AIDS researchers have picked apart the AIDS virus, decoding its 9 genes and isolating its 15 proteins. Now they are trying, piece by piece, to understand how these components work together to produce one of the most lethal microbes in history. As biologists learn what makes HIV tick, they get new ideas about how to destroy it.

How Genes Store Genetic Information and the Importance of Mutations or Change Within Genes— Genes store the information necessary for creating living organisms and viruses. In sexually reproducing organisms, the information is stored in the form of DNA organized into structures called chromosomes. Apart from sex cells (eggs and sperm) and mature blood cells, every cell in the human body contains 23 pairs of chromosomes. One of each pair is inherited from the mother, the other from the father. Each chromosome is a packet of compressed and twisted DNA. Genes are sections of DNA containing the blueprint for the whole body, including such specific details as what kind of receptors cells will have, for example, CD4, CD8, R4, R-5, and so on.

DNA is made up of a double-stranded helix held together by hydrogen bonds between specific pairs of bases. The four bases A, T, G, and C (adenine, thymine, guanine, and cytosine) bond to each other in fixed and complimentary patterns that give humans and other species their individuality. If a gene is thought of as a sentence, and the nucleotides in DNA as letters, a change or mutation of only one letter can affect the entire sentence or the information the DNA gives the cell. To get an idea of how many mutations can occur in a cell, consider that humans have about 3.2 billion base pairs, in their haploid or 23 chromosomes, that make up about 35,000 genes or sentences that contain the information that makes a human. There are about a million differences between your 3.2 billion-letter DNA alphabet and that of another person. The kind, number, and sequence of nucleotides (bases) in human DNA and that of other species is much greater. Another way of saying this is that the closer a species resembles a human or vice-versa, the closer will be the DNA base sequences.

For example, the DNA base sequence in a chimpanzee is about 98% identical to humans. That means the difference between human DNA and chimpanzee DNA is only a base sequence difference for about 60 million base pairs out of 3.2 billion human base pairs.

Importance of Genetic Stability to a Species—The individual or collective characteristics (phenotypes) of any virus, cell, or multicelled organism depend on the expression of their genes and the interaction of gene products within a given environment. From a biological point of view, changes in phenotype (observable characteristics) that are inheritable are by definition genetic changes. Such changes occur due to changes in the kind, number, and sequence of bases in DNA. Base changes may occur by addition, substitution, and deletion. These changes are referred to as **genetic mutations.** Genetic mutations provide biological heterogeneity and genetic diversity (similarity as a species but dissimilarity with regard to certain characteristics). Investigations on the rate at which genetic mutations occur in living species indicate that DNA is a stable molecule with relatively low mutation rates for any given gene. Because of low mutation rates within the DNA of a species's gene pool (all the genes that can be found in the DNA of a species) and selection pressures by a slowly changing environment, species evolution is constant but very slow.

Genetic mutations in the strain of an organism or virus produce genetic and phenotype **variants** (different members) of that strain. Regardless of the rate at which mutations occur, *they are genetic mistakes*—they are not intentional, they just happen by chance. Most mutations or genetic mistakes either make no

difference to an organism or virus (silent mutations) or they cause a change. Few genetic mistakes within a stable environment improve the species. After all, the species arrived at this point in time via genetic and environmental selection pressures—those with the best constellation of genes survived to reproduce those genes. In species that produce large numbers of offspring, genetic mistakes that are lethal or lead to an early death are of little consequence to the species. A genetic mistake that improves the chance of survival and reproduction is retained.

Genetic Instability of HIV—A virus like HIV can produce hundreds of replicas within a single cell. Genetic mistakes during viral replication produce variant HIVs. In biological economic terms, HIV replicas are inexpensive to make. Even if most of these mutant HIV replicas are inactive or throwaway copies, it makes little if any difference to the HIV per se. However, if a few HIV replicas received environmentally advantageous mutant genes, these HIV mutants would survive as well as or better than the parent HIVs. Both parent HIV and mutant HIV can reproduce in the same cell and exchange genes. Over time, only the most fit mutant or variant HIVs are transmitted among people and undergo still further genetic changes. These variant HIVs could, with sufficient accumulative genetic changes, become a new type of HIV—for example, an HIV-3.

Investigations of some of the RNA viruses revealed relatively high mutation rates. Thus some of the RNA viruses are our best examples of evolution in "real" time. Because of their high error rate during replication they show, as expected, both high genetic diversity and biological heterogeneity in their host, and a rate of evolution about a million times faster than DNA-based organisms (Nowak, 1990). HIV, in particular, fits this category. Heterogeneity of HIV is reflected by: (1) the difference in the kinds of cells variant HIV infects; (2) the way different HIV mutants replicate; and (3) the way different variants of HIV harm infected cells.

It is now known that HIV is capable of enormous genetic flexibility, which allows it to become resistant to drugs, to escape from immune responses, and to avoid potential HIV vaccines. What is not known are all the factors contributing to viral diversity in individual infections. Clearly the high error rate of the reverse transcriptase (because this enzyme lacks a 3′ to 5′ exonuclease proofreading ability, that is, it cannot correct mistakes once they are made) and the high turnover rate in infected cells generate vast numbers of different virus mutants. The diversity of newly produced variants, however, is shaped by a combination of mutation, recombinations of HIV RNA, and selection forces. The main selective forces that have been proposed to drive HIV diversity are the immune response, cell tropism (cell types most likely to attract HIV), and random activation of infected cells. At the time of seroconversion a person may carry a homogeneous virus population, but then diversification occurs as HIV infects many different cell types and tissues in the body (Bonhoeffer et al., 1995).

For further information on HIV evolution, diversity, and HIV disease progression, see Chapter 7, Box 7.2.

GENETIC REVOLUTION

Genetic revolution occurs when an organism or virus such as, say, SIV leaves one host (chimpanzee), enters a new host (humans), and rapidly diversifies its genes in an attempt to interpret and adapt to its new environment, as when SIVcpz became HIV in humans. As HIV continued to replicate or reproduce, it became more fit to survive in humans. That fitness occurs in two ways, through mutation or change in individual nucleotides making up the genes, and through recombination, a process in which there are large exchanges of sections of HIV diploid RNA.

FORMATION OF GENETIC RECOMBINATION IN HIV

HIV, like all retroviruses, is diploid. Each viral particle contains two RNA strands, each full length and able to replicate. No other virus families, RNA or DNA, are diploid. Typically both RNA strands in a retroviral particle derive from the same parent provirus. However, if an infected cell simultaneously harbors two different proviruses, one RNA transcript from each provirus can be encapsidated into a single virion. When this virion subsequently infects a new cell, the reverse transcriptase may jump back and forth between the two RNA strands so that the newly synthesized retroviral DNA sequence is recombinant between that of the two RNA strands. All subsequent progeny virions will be of this recombinant genotype.

If two RNAs with sequence differences are co-packaged in one virion, a mosaic HIV genome containing genetic information from both RNAs could be generated, yielding novel viral genomes. Recombination can also salvage genetic damage or detrimental mutations in one RNA strand by adopting genetic information from the other RNA strand. Thus, recombination may not only introduce genetic diversity, it may also serve as a repair mechanism for the HIV genome (Jetzt et al., 2000).

Mutations create the changes in the genetic material of HIV, but recombination quickly reshuffles these changes.

Forming a recombinant HIV is the same concept as a plant or animal hybrid. The hybrid or new species has picked up genetic information from two distinctly unrelated parents. For example, each of us is a recombinant. Each parent has its own genetic information, and the children are their recombinants. So recombination is a natural process. For us, the process doesn't usually produce large genetic changes. For HIV, the recombination process can produce tremendous change in a single replication cycle. In the case of HIV intersubtype recombinants, each parent is a different subtype, the recombinant picks up part of its genetic information from one parent, apart from the other. They are also genetic hybrids.

Thomas Folks and colleagues (2004), from their results of studies on short gene regions found in serum samples collected in Kinshasa in the mid-1980s, showed that 37% of HIV strains represented recombinant types of HIV. Thus, they proposed that the HIV pandemic was well established in Central Africa by the early 1980s and that some recombinant HIV most likely seeded the early global pandemic.

Completing the Picture on Producing HIV Genetic Variability: HIV Subtypes or Clades

Michael Sagg and colleagues (1988) examined the generation of molecular variation of HIV by sequential HIV isolates from two chronically infected people. They found 39 distinguishable but highly related genomes (HIV variants). These results indicate that HIV heterogeneity occurs rapidly in infected individuals and that a large number of genetically distinguishable but related HIVs rapidly evolve in parallel and coexist during chronic infection. That is, whenever a drug or the immune response successfully attacks one variant, another arises in its place. Pools of genetically distinct variants that evolve from the initial HIV that begin the infection are often referred to as **quasispecies** (Delwart et al., 1993; Diaz et al., 1997). However, even though a person possesses diverse quasispecies of HIV, only a very narrow population (perhaps only one) of HIV is transmitted from mother to child or between sexual partners (Derdeyn et al. 2004).

Additional evidence indicates that some HIV genetic variants demonstrate a preference (tropism) as to the cell type they infect. This means that one genetic change may allow the virus to enter cells that were once immune to the virus. Also, a report by Helen Devereux and colleagues (2002) states that a wide variety of quasispecies circulate in each individual and that there may be HIV evolving independently in different body compartments. The rapid genetic change, which results in altered viral products, makes it very difficult to design a vaccine or drug that will be effective against all HIV variants. To date, HIV drug-resistant mutants have been found for all FDA-approved nucleoside and nonnucleoside analogs and protease inhibitors used in the treatment of HIV-infected people and AIDS patients! (Chapter 4 presents a discussion of currently used drug therapies for HIV/AIDS.)

HIV Antigenic Variation—This refers to differences in a protein that occur as a result of changes in HIV RNA/DNA. Each variation of protein produced elicits the production of a different antibody. Such protein changes occur, for example, as a result of changes in the HIV GAG-POL-ENV genes. Antibodies are made against the different GAG-POL-ENV gene proteins, but the antibodies made against the ENV gene protein appear to be the most important. These antibodies neutralize the envelope glycoproteins that seem to be an essential part of HIV's infecting process. The ENV gene is subject to the most frequent mutations, producing HIV with different envelope glycoproteins within a given individual.

It now appears that HIV can constantly change its surface antigenic composition, thereby allowing it to escape antibody neutralization. Thus, HIV mutations allow the virus to persist in the presence of an immune response. This immune selection viral phenomenon is not new. It is what the influenza virus does yearly so that last year's vaccine will not protect people from this year's variation. However, HIV differs from viruses such as influenza. Influenza and many other viruses do not have an RNA to DNA replication step so they are not as mutable as the retroviruses. Because of the error-prone reverse transcriptase enzyme used by the retroviruses, the possibility of genetic change far exceeds that for any other known nonretroviral human pathological virus.

DISTINCT GENOTYPES (SUBTYPES/CLADES) OF HIV-1 WORLDWIDE BASED ON ENV AND GAG PROTEINS

HIV is actually an umbrella term for two genetically distinct types of virus: HIV-1 and HIV-2. HIV-1 embraces three genetically distinct groups: M, N, and O. Of these, group M viruses, the ones that are perhaps most studied and are known to be most responsible for infections worldwide, have been subdivided into 11 genetically distinct subtypes, identified by letters A through K. Genetic analyses of HIV-2, the less virulent form of HIV, have yielded six subtypes, identified as A through F.

As stated previously, this book is about HIV-1 or HIV. In order to better understand globally circulating strains of HIV, HIV investigators have placed, based on genetic diversity, the various HIV strains into three major groups, **M,** for the **main** HIV genotypes or **clades** found in different populations, and groups **O** (outlier) and **N** (nonmajor, nonoutlier) for HIV genotypes or clades that are significantly different from those in the **M** group.

Group M HIV causes over 99% of the world's HIV/AIDS. **Group O** and the more recently discovered **Group N,** cause less than 1%.

Group M Subtypes or Clades

There are 11 subtypes or clades of group M: A, B, C, D, E, F, G, H, I, J, and K. The M subtypes have been analyzed with respect to the differences between them based on the variations found in their GAG and ENV proteins (Robertson et al., 1995).

Within a subtype, envelope gene sequences vary from 7% to 12%. Between subtypes the genetic variation is up to 30%. There is the belief that a vaccine against one subtype won't offer protection against the rest. (For discussion of HIV vaccines see Chapter 9 on prevention). Subtypes B and E together make up about 14% of HIV infections worldwide. Subtypes A, C, and D make up about 84% of HIV infections.

The 11 different M subtypes or clades and O have been globally mapped (geographically located) in Figure 3-8 (Brix et al., 1996; Workshop Report 1997). This figure demonstrates the dissemination of the different subtypes from 1990 through 2006. Clearly, subtype B, closely related to subtype D, predominates in the Americas although in Brazil, Argentina, and Uruguay substantial proportions of infections are caused by F subtype or BF recombinant viruses. Apart

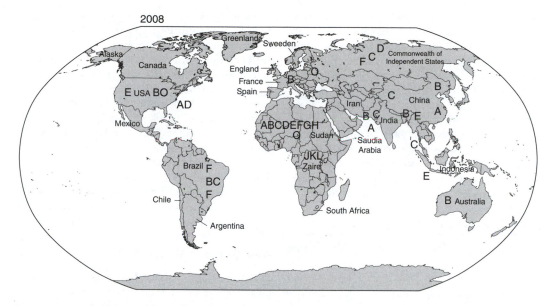

FIGURE 3-8 Global Distribution of the 11 M subtypes and O in 2008 in Areas of Highest Prevalence. Clearly this global map shows that HIV subtypes are no longer continent based—all subtypes are now present on all continents. No satisfactory explanation exists for the skewed worldwide distribution of HIV-1 subtypes. The worldwide spread of viral subtypes makes it clear that a world vaccine will be required, that is, one that is not subtype specific. None appears to be on the horizon, although large-scale trials with existing envelope vaccines are underway in some developing countries *(Brodine et al., 1997 updated; Taylor et al. 2008)*

from these three countries, infections with non-B genetic forms are unusual; however, recently, it was reported that env subtypes A, C, and H had been identified in 5 of 11 samples in Cuba. The identification of diverse non-B subtypes in Cuba is not unexpected, considering that large numbers of Cuban military and civilian personnel had been stationed in the 1970s and 1980s in Angola, a country neighboring the Democratic Republic of Congo (DRC), where the highest group M diversity is found, and that many of the early cases of HIV infection in Cuba were detected among these individuals. The explosive epidemic in Southeast Asia is chiefly attributable to subtype E. There are ample documented introductions of subtypes C, E, and F from endemic areas into the United States and the Western Hemisphere. Subtype C now accounts for about 40% of *new* HIV infections worldwide—particularly in China and India. There is no one subtype that is representative of this global pandemic.

International Genetic Subtypes

Numerous groups have shown an increase in intermixing of HIV genetic subtypes in multiple international locales. HIV subtypes A, B, C, D, F, G, and H have appeared throughout Europe; B, F, C, and D have been found in Brazil; one-third of new infections in Germany are non-B; 15% of infections in a New York City hospital are non-B; increasingly, E is found among injecting-drug users in Thailand, from 24% subtype E in 1991 to 44% in 1995, and among heterosexual risk groups, a change from 86% subtype E in 1991 to 98% in 1995; and group O has been detected in at least 12 African countries, France, Spain, and in the United States, as well as M/O dual infections. In South Africa, there is spreading of subtypes B and D throughout the homosexual population and C/E throughout the heterosexuals studied. The impact of this is an increasing spread of non-B subtypes into previous B areas, which has significant implications for vaccine development.

Subtypes Related to Transmission Route

While the current geographic distribution of subtypes is generally acknowledged to have arisen from accidents in viral trafficking, the perpetuation of these patterns may be due to the affinity of certain subtypes for certain targets. Max Essex of Harvard has studied

Langerhans cells as a target of viral entry for subtypes E and C. He has proposed that Langerhans cells, prevalent in the female genital tract, are less hospitable to subtype B. He concluded that non-B subtypes are dominant in countries where the major mode of HIV transmission is through heterosexual contact and that this is due to the greater accessibility of subtypes E and C through the Langerhans cells. In China, in a large group of injection-drug users, a recombinant subtype AB was found to the exclusion of other subtypes. It is estimated that over half of all HIV infections worldwide are from subtype C. It is the most common subtype found in Southern Africa, China, and India.

Global Predominant HIV-1 Subtypes

A. W. Africa, E. Africa, Central Africa, East Europe, Mideast
B. N. America, Europe, Mideast, E. Asia, Latin America
C. S. Africa, S. Asia, Ethiopia
D. E. Africa
E. S.E. Asia

HIV-2 primarily West Africa.

Do HIV Subtypes or Clades Influence the Response to Antiretroviral Therapy?

This question is urgent, since only 12% of global infections are caused by the most studied subtype, B, and 50% of prevalent HIV infections and 47% of all new HIV infections are caused by subtype C. This discrepancy in the availability of clinical data for non-B subtype is exacerbated by the fact that, until the past few years, antiretroviral treatment has been largely unavailable in many countries with non-B subtypes of HIV.

HIV RNA Recombination

Robertson and colleagues (1995) reported that eight of the group M subtypes appear to have been involved in recombination with each other, giving rise to genetic hybrids. These studies raise questions of whether a vaccine that works against one of the subtypes will work against a subtype hybrid.

Group O Subtypes

Group O contains at least 30 genetically different subtypes of HIV. Group O subtypes are referred to as **"outliers"** because their RNA base sequence is only 50% similar to the known genotypes of the M group. The O variants have been known since 1987 but have been found mainly in Cameroon, Gabon, and surrounding West African countries that, to date, have only been marginally affected by AIDS. Group O viruses were of concern primarily because their divergence from group M was sufficient to miss their detection by ELISA HIV testing. (The ELISA test is discussed in Chapter 13.) Seven people in France were identified with group O HIV in 1994. The first documented case of group O HIV infection in the United States was found in April 1996 in Los Angeles. By the beginning of 2003, only three cases of HIV subtype O infection had been reported in the United States. This subtype was found in a Los Angeles County woman and a Maryland woman; both came into the United States from Africa. HIV subtype O is not routinely tested for in the United States.

New Group N Subtype?

In August 1998, Francois Simon and colleagues reported the discovery of a *new* HIV-1 isolate that *cannot* be placed in the M or O subtype category. The authors suggest that the new isolate be classified as group **N** for **"new"** or **"non-M non-O."** The new isolate, designated **YBF30**, was found in a small number of people in the West African nation of Cameroon. The first isolate was from a 40-year-old woman who died of AIDS. This virus is similar to SIV (cpz-gab) and it either branched with the SIV strain or between it and HIV-1 group M. The authors state that future strains of SIV (cpz) could be found and strains that are closely related to YBF30 might circulate among Cameroonian chimpanzees.

SIV retroviruses are endemic in many species of primates but usually don't cause disease, which makes them natural hosts for what are known as lentiviruses or slow-acting viruses. But when they cross the species barrier into a new host like humans, these viruses may become pathogenic, causing illness. Based on evolutionary studies, researchers think SIV has existed in sub-Saharan Africa for thousands of years, adapting to several species including the African green monkey and Sooty Mangabey. There are six closely linked strains of SIV. Chimpanzees carry at least three different viral predecessors of HIV-1 that gave rise to groups M, O, and N. Sooty Mangabeys carry an ancestor of HIV-2.

Simon's discovery of group N also raises other critical questions and challenges. Looking ahead, how many other SIV strains may have crossed the species barrier? Should we be mass screening for this new virus N or increasing surveillance of the other SIV strains? What about the human recombinant viruses? How well are we tracking them?

FIRST CONFIRMED CASES OF HIV GROUP O–CAUSED AIDS

A Norwegian sailor died of AIDS in 1976 at the age of 29. His wife and youngest daughter, born in 1967, also died of AIDS. The members of this Norwegian family represent the earliest confirmed cases of AIDS and the first case of HIV type O infection. The first symptoms appeared in 1966 in the sailor, in 1967 in his wife, and in 1969 in their daughter. Between 1961 and 1965 he traveled the world's oceans, calling at ports in all six inhabited continents. On his first voyage, which began in August 1961 just after his fifteenth birthday, he worked as a kitchen hand on a Norwegian vessel that sailed down the West African coastline, calling at ports in Senegal, Liberia, Cote d'Ivoire, Ghana, Nigeria, and Cameroon. A gonorrheal infection during this trip shows that he was sexually active. He returned home in May 1962, and never returned to Africa. No known evidence suggests that the sailor was bisexual, which means that sexual contact with a woman is the most straightforward explanation for his infection. This would suggest that HIV group O has been circulating in that part of Africa for at least 36 years.

Second Confirmed Cases of HIV Group O–Caused AIDS?

The second case of group O infection found in the literature is the second child of a French barmaid from Reims, who died in 1981. The child's clinical history is highly suggestive of neonatal AIDS. In 1992 a group O virus was isolated from the mother, who by then had AIDS.

Summary

HIV is a retrovirus. It has RNA for its genetic material and carries reverse transcriptase enzyme for making DNA from its RNA. HIV, using its enzyme, copies its genetic information from RNA into DNA, which becomes integrated into host cell DNA and may remain silent for years, or until such time as it is activated into producing new HIV. HIV contains at least nine genes; three of them, GAG-POL-ENV, are basic to all animal retroviruses. The six additional genes are involved in the infection process and regulate the production of products from the three genes. HIV, because of its error-prone reverse transcriptase enzyme, mutates at an unusually high rate. With time, many mutant HIV variants can be found within a single HIV-infected person. A vaccine against one mutant HIV may not work against a second—like the vaccines made yearly against different mutant influenza viruses.

A new group of HIV has been identified, group N.

Review Questions

(Answers to the Review Questions are on page 425.)

1. Why is HIV called a retrovirus?

2. What are the three major genes common to all retroviruses? How many additional genes does HIV have?

3. Why are retroviruses, and HIV in particular, believed to be genetically unstable? Give two reasons for your answer.

4. What is believed to be the major reason for the high rate of genetic mutations in HIV production?

5. All of the following are HIV accessory genes except

   (a) tat   (b) env   (c) vpr
   (d) rev   (e) vpu

6. HIV contains _____ nucleotides and _____ genes.

   (a) 9/10,331   (b) 8/9746   (c) 6/9000
   (d) 3/8000   (e) 9749/9

7. Name the error-prone HIV enzyme that is a major cause of HIV mutants.

   (a) reverse holozyme   (b) reverse integrase
   (c) reverse transcriptase   (d) reverse spiral case
   (e) reverse nuclease

8. HIV is very specific with regard to the types of cells it can enter.

   (a) True   (b) False

9. HIV attaches first to the following receptor on a T lymphocyte:

   (a) CD5+   (b) CD4+   (c) CD28+
   (d) CD8+   (e) CD9+

10. How many RNA strands does HIV contain?

   (a) 3   (b) 1   (c) 2   (d) 4   (e) 5

11. Name the three major genes of HIV.

12. In general, about how many CD4+ cells are in a microliter of blood?

13. What role does the vif gene play in HIV survival in an infected cell?

14. What two processes occur during the replication of HIV that gives HIV a chance to survive changing environmental conditions?

15. Group M has how many subtypes of clades and which subtypes causes most of the infections in the United States, in China and in India, and heterosexual South Africa?

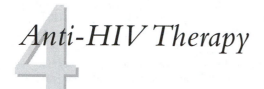

Anti-HIV Therapy

I plan on keeping on trucking. I plan on doing great. I wouldn't be this way without the medicines and theoretical advances and technology. And I haven't gone through half of the drugs yet, and that makes me happy. But it is a hard disease to have.

18-year-old U.S. woman, infected since birth, name withheld by request.

We are constantly humbled by the devastation that something so small, HIV, can cast upon something so large, a human. This chapter provides no final answers; there is no curative therapy, no truly outstanding therapies (drugs that benefit all HIV-infected without major side effects) against HIV, and, with the number of expensive anti-HIV drugs that are available, debate continues about the details on which drugs offer the best combination therapy and on the standard of care for HIV/AIDS patients. Because some 95% of HIV-infected people develop AIDS, and because 90% of all *new* HIV infections are occurring in developing nations, an inexpensive, easily taken, nontoxic, effective HIV-directed therapy is essential. Physicians need a drug that works against HIV as antibiotics once worked against a large variety of disease-causing bacteria.

ANTI-HIV THERAPY

The ideal solution would be to prevent HIV from causing an infection. Then anti-HIV therapies would not be necessary. However, there are no means available to stop HIV from entering the body and infecting a limited number of cell types—primarily those cells displaying CD4 protein antigen receptor sites. Following HIV infection, there is a depletion of cells carrying the CD4 protein, especially the **T lymphocyte (T4) cells of the human immune system.** (See Chapter 5 for an explanation of cell types in the human immune system and their function.) With T4 or CD4+ cell loss (lymphocytes carrying the CD4 protein), over time immunological response is lost. Loss of immunological response leads to a variety of opportunistic infections (OIs). The suppression of the immune system and increasing susceptibility to OIs and cancers give HIV/AIDS a multidimensional pathology. (OIs are presented in Chapter 6). Because HIV/ AIDS is a multidimensional syndrome, it is unlikely that a single drug will provide adequate treatment or a cure.

An ideal goal for HIV drug investigators would be to find a drug that excises all HIV proviruses from the cell's DNA. It is very unlikely that this kind of drug will soon, if ever, be available. Alternatively, the elimination of all HIV-infected cells might be of comparable benefit, as long as irreplaceable cells are not totally lost through the process. In essence, this is the goal that the human immune system sets for itself, yet falls short of reaching, in the vast majority of HIV-infected individuals.

In the absence of a curative weapon, therapies must be designed to prevent the spread of the virus in the body. Most of the FDA-approved anti-HIV therapies are presented in this chapter.

The Dark Age of Anti-HIV Therapy

Between the years 1981 and 1987, when hundreds of thousands in the United States and millions worldwide had already become HIV infected and many thousands had already died, there were no effective drug therapies against HIV. Physicians offered anything and everything they thought held promise, agents like suramin, Isoprinosine, and a host of treatments pushed by "quacks" who said they knew how to treat this new illness. This was truly an **age of darkness across Planet Earth.** Even in March 1987 when researchers tried zidovudine (ZDU aka AZT)—a long-abandoned cancer treatment drug, a nucleoside—the atmosphere that prevailed was still one of trying anything that might help. Luckily, this drug slowed the replication of HIV, and everyone immediately took notice. However, it was like a three-act play: Acts I and II were over, and the scientists still had no idea if they had had any value. Act III put them on the road to investigating nucleosides as anti-HIV medications—but it took another four years before a second antiretroviral drug, didanosine (DDI), reached the market and another four years to market the first protease inhibitor. This began the final scene of Act III. The advent of highly active antiretroviral therapy (HAART) is described here.

Can HIV Infection Be Cured? Can HIV Be Eradicated from the Body?

An effective cure means cleansing the body of the HIV. To find a cure, HIV incorporation into human DNA and subsequent reproduction of new virus must be understood. Without interference, the **HIV provirus** will remain in host-cell DNA for life. The provirus can, at any time, become activated to mass produce HIV, which leads to cell death and eventually to the individual's death. As of this writing, there is no way to prevent either the HIV proviral state or to stimulate proviral activation, a necessary condition for HIV removal from host cell DNA.

What Would It Take to Cure HIV Infection?

To cure HIV infection would require one of two options: Kill every single infected cell in the body and destroy all viruses floating outside of those cells in the human bloodstream and in other infected tissue, or spare the infected cells but destroy the viruses hidden inside human DNA without damaging human genes in the process. So daunting are these tasks, so far beyond the current intellectual level of biological sciences, that the search for a cure effectively ended on the day in 1983 when French scientist Luc Montagnier announced his discovery that AIDS was caused by a retrovirus. Through 2009 an estimated 59 million people will have been infected with HIV. The number of people cured via therapy—zero. Science has yet to discover a genuine cure for any viral disease, though it is possible to restrain some infections through the use of drugs and vaccinations.

HIV ERADICATION UPDATE—2008

As presented, to date, current antiretroviral therapy only suppresses the viral life cycle, the production of new HIV, without eradicating the HIV provirus. However, Indrani Sarkar and colleagues (2007) write about their construction of an enzyme or recombinase that effectively exercises or cuts the integrated proviral HIV DNA out of the human chromosome! The researchers used their carefully constructed recombinase, called "Tre," to remove all traces of HIV from cultured human cervical cells over a three-month period. This is the first demonstration, ever, of the actual removal of the integrated HIV provirus from a human cell. The scientists plan, over the next several years, to test the Tre enzyme on mouse chromosomes to see if they can precisely remove segments of mouse DNA without damaging their chromosomes. Accomplishing that, they will move on to testing Tre or other constructed enzymes on HIV-infected humans. The largest obstacle to potential human use will be its safe and effective introduction into the different HIV-infected cell types in the human body, beginning with the CD4-infected cells. However small this first step may be, its footprint is large, and this research offers promise about tomorrow.

ANTIRETROVIRAL THERAPY (ART) DRUGS WITH FDA APPROVAL

Most Americans have no direct contact with the U.S. Food and Drug Administration (FDA), but their lives literally depend on the effectiveness of the agency. Charged with assuring the safety of specific foods and all medicines, the FDA has oversight of 25% of the U.S. economy. One of the FDA's key functions is approving and monitoring prescription drugs—a job that is particularly crucial for people with HIV infection or other life-threatening diseases. The FDA is the American Gold Standard of endorsement! (See Point of Information 4.1.)

Gold Standard of Therapy

The **gold standard** for determining the efficacy (effectiveness) of a new treatment is that it alters the disease in a way that is beneficial to the patient. Therefore, the end points most often used in clinical trials of therapies for a disease such as HIV/AIDS include prolongation of life or the extension of time to a significant disease complication.

But studies using these end points require large numbers of patients and/or the passage of considerable amounts of time. **Surrogate markers** (that is, physiological measurements that serve as substitutes for these major clinical events) can eliminate this problem if their validity and correlation with clinical outcome in people can be confirmed. The use of surrogates has the potential to shorten the duration of clinical trials and expedite the development of new therapies.

Major Surrogate Markers Used to Evaluate ART

The **T4 or CD4+ immune cell number** and **viral load** (the number of HIV-RNA strands in blood) are the two most studied and commonly used surrogates (alternates) for clinical efficacy of anti–HIV therapies. They are imperfect measurements, however, because changes in T4 or CD4+ cell number per microliter of blood (a very, very small drop) and RNA strands per milliliter of blood are only partially explained by the effects of therapy. T4 or CD4+ cell counts exhibit a high degree of day-to-day variation in individuals, and methods used to count these cells are difficult to standardize.

THE DRUG DEVELOPMENT, APPROVAL PROCESS, AND CLINICAL TRIALS

In the United States, drug discovery and FDA approval currently takes an average of 12 to 15 years and costs about $400 million (from the laboratory to the drugstore). In 1996, Merck & Co. claims to have spent $1 billion over 10 years to bring the protease inhibitor **Crixivan** to market! The odds against a new drug making it to the market are about 10,000 to 1. The clinical trial process for a drug usually includes 3$\frac{1}{2}$ years of preclinical testing using laboratory and animal studies and 6 years of studies (clinical trials) in humans. **Phase I** includes 20 to 80 healthy volunteers and takes about a year to test the drug's safety. **Phase II** takes about two years and involves 100 to 300 persons with the disease to assess the drug's effectiveness and to look for side effects. **Phase III** of clinical trials lasts about three years and includes 1000 to 3000 patients to verify effectiveness and identify adverse reactions of a drug. Phase IV is the post marketing phase. These trials are used to determine long-term safety and efficacy of the approved drug. Since 1989 the FDA has allowed Phases I and II to be combined to shorten the approval process on new medicines for serious and life-threatening diseases. It now takes about 18 months for a drug to go through the review process for approval by the FDA. About one in five medicines that begin a clinical trial is approved for consumer use.

Global annual drug research and development spending is about $70 billion, but only 10% of that money goes to research on diseases that account for 90% of the world's infections.

THE HIV/AIDS DRUG MARKET

The ART market is estimated to be about $11 billion a year by 2015. The $350 billion American pharmaceutical industry has been investing over $1 billion a year since the late 1980s to bring new and improved HIV drugs to market. Since 1987, a new FDA-approved antiviral drug has entered the market on average of every 9.4 months.

Beginning in 2009, 84 companies had 85 medicines and vaccines for AIDS and AIDS-related conditions in testing. This is in addition to 85 HIV and HIV-related FDA-approved medicines already on the market.

The most difficult part of presenting anti-HIV therapies to the public is the analysis of the incredible amount of new information continuously coming out in the scientific literature and attempting to make sense out of some very contradictory findings (*The Drug Development and Approval Process,* Pharmaceutical Manufacturers Association, December 1998 updated).

Clinical Trials

A clinical drug trial is a government-funded and organized study of an experimental or unproven drug to determine the drug's safety and efficacy (whether or not it works). Drug trials for HIV/AIDS, sponsored by the Food and Drug Administration (FDA), are organized into the AIDS Clinical Trial Group (ACTG). Guidelines are set to determine how the ACTGs may be run and who is eligible to participate. Taking part in a trial may entitle persons to receive medical examinations and checkups and to have their overall health monitored. For many people with AIDS, the ACTGs are the only means of access to certain potentially lifesaving drugs, and the only form of health care they may ever receive. Historically, FDA policy on admitting women into clinical trials has been confusing and discriminatory at best. Until recently, the FDA had an outright ban on all women of childbearing potential from participation in early stages of drug trials. In March 1994, FDA took two important steps to ensure that new drugs are properly evaluated in women. First, it provided formal guidance to drug developers to emphasize its expectations that women would be appropriately represented in clinical studies and that new drug applications would include analyses capable of identifying potential differences in drug actions and value between the sexes. Second, the agency altered its 1977 policy to include most women with childbearing potential in the earliest phases of clinical trials.

The Disconnect Between CD4+ Cell Count and Viral Load with Regard to Their Clinical Benefits (see Snapshot 4.1)

Recent investigations have shown that there is a T4 cell level and viral load level **disconnect.** This means that viral suppression by itself does not always predict immunological and clinical benefit. T4 cell counts and viral load can be clearly dissociated during treatment: T4 cells can increase in the presence of a high viral load, remain stable, or drop. **Clinical benefit** is more closely associated with the level of T4 cells rather than viral load. Recent data support the hypothesis that T4 cell depletion during HIV infection occurs largely as a result of the immune system's inability to generate new mature cells, and that the main effect of antiretroviral

A QUICK TAKE ON THE IMPORTANCE OF VIRAL LOAD AND C4+ CELL COUNTS IN IMMUNE-DISCORDANT PEOPLE

First, there really is a disconnect, as presented, between CD4+ cell count and viral load, or immune-discordance. Which is more important in determining the disease progression in an HIV-positive immune-discordant person? Both viral loads and CD4+ cell counts are important parameters of HIV disease progression. However, knowing the viral load can help a person understand the likelihood that their T-cell count is going to drop. If the CD4 cell count is 400 and the viral load is high, the doctor gets concerned because that means that likely, over the next year or two, the CD4 cell count is going to drop more quickly than that of someone who comes in with a CD4 cell count of 400 but has a very low viral load. Think about the viral load as the engine that is driving the CD4 cell count decline. The more viruses, the lower the CD4 cell count. Like foxes and rabbits: The virus is the fox, and your CD4 cells are rabbits. The more foxes, the quicker the rabbits are going to disappear, so the foxes must be reduced. This was the paradigm for a long time. This model is based on data that are now about 12 years old. However, new studies looked at the viral load before people started therapy and looked at CD4 cell counts in groups of individuals from different clinics across the country. The studies showed that when you place people's data into large groups, the viral load does seem to predict what happens to people in general but not what happens in individual patients. Researchers found that when they looked at people who had high viral loads and low viral loads, some of the people with low viral loads saw their T-cell counts drop quickly, while some of the people who had high viral loads saw their T-cell counts drop slowly. Yes, there was an overlap between patients, but, for individual patients, the viral load didn't do very well at predicting how quickly their T-cell count would drop. Thus, if individual patients with similar viral loads were grouped together, generally their CD4 cell count dropped at a different rate than that of another group of people who had a viral load at a different level. So if you had a group of people who had a high viral load, their CD4 cell count would tend to drop more quickly than that of people who had, as a group, a low viral load. But when investigators reviewed the data of individuals, that viral load–to–CD4+ count relationship did not exist. These are important studies because they help clinicians understand that each patient has to be treated individually.

therapy is to help restore the immune system's ability to produce new T4 cells. (Perrin et al., 1998; Telenti et al., 1998; Deeks et al., 1999; Clark et al., 1999; Hellerstein et al., 1999; Rodriguez et al. 2006)

THE HIV MEDICINE CHEST: ART DRUGS RECEIVING FDA APPROVAL

The evolution of treatment for HIV should be considered one of the most important accomplishments in the history of modern medicine. The introduction of protease inhibitors in the mid-1990s, along with insights into viral dynamics and the importance of using multiple active agents in combination, marked the beginning of the highly active antiretroviral therapy (HAART) era and substantially improved survival rates for individuals infected with HIV. In less than two decades, 25 unique antiretroviral therapies in more than 30 different formulations have been developed—a feat virtually unparalleled in the history of medicine.

A Delicate Balance

For most HIV medicines to work properly, their bloodstream levels must be precise. Too much, and they're too toxic. Too little, and they fail to keep the virus in check.

The number and kinds of HIV drugs, their recommended mixtures, and their timing and dosage change almost continuously. This can be a source of tremendous confusion for patients and medical practitioners alike.

Drug Interactions

Taking other prescription drugs, non-prescription (over-the-counter) or recreational drugs, herbal products, or even food can course large changes in the amount of the drug in your bloodstream. This is called a drug interaction. Everyone taking antiretroviral (ARV) drugs should be very careful about drug interactions. Their doctor should know about ALL drugs and supplements they are taking.

From March 1987 through 2008, 25 individual anti-HIV drugs and 6 combination drugs have received

Table 4-1 Choices: Anti Retroviral Therapy (ART); Nucleoside Analogs, Non-Nucleosides, Protease Inhibitors, Entry Inhibitors, and Integrase Enzyme Inhibitors.

Name	FDA Approved	Cost/Year[a]
Nucleoside analog (reverse transcriptase inhibitor)		
Zidovudine, ZDU (Retrovir)/AZT	March 1987	$4,340.18
Didanosine, ddI (Videx)	October 1991	$3,686.85
Zalcitabine, ddC (Hivid)	June 1994	$3,013.89
Stavudine, d4T (Zerit)	June 1994	$4,061.28
Lamivudine, 3TC (Epivir)	November 1995	$3,818.75
Combivir (Zidovudine/lamivudine)	September 1997	$7,940.61
Abacavir (Ziagen)	December 1998	$4,930.75
Trizivir (Ziagen/Retrovir/Epivir)	November 2000	$12,895.71
Tenofovir (Viread)[b]	October 2001	$5,198.00
Emtricitabine (Emtriva)	July 2003	$3,625.56
Truvada (emtricitabine/tenofovir)	August 2004	$9,683.45
Epzicom[d] (Epivir/Ziagen)	August 2004	$10,151.88
Atripla (Sustiva/Viread/Emtriva)	July 2006	$13,800.00

Nucleoside analog reverse transcriptase inhibitors are potent in combination with other drugs; used alone, they lead to HIV resistance. *ZDV (AZT), d4T, 3TC,* and *abacavir* penetrate the blood-brain barrier. Common side effects: lactic acidosis. *Seven* new nucleoside analogs are in some phase of testing in the United States.[c]

Non-nucleoside compounds; (non-nucleoside reverse transcriptase inhibitors)		
Nevirapine (Viramune)	June 1996	$4,395.36
Delavirdine (Rescriptor)	April 1997	$3,842.13
Efavireuz (Sustiva, Stocrin)	September 1998	$5,258.69
Etravirine (Intelence)	January 2008	$9,766.68

Non-nucleoside analog reverse transcriptase inhibitors (NNRTIs, or non-nukes) may interact with other *cytochrome p450-processed drugs:* protease inhibitors, oral contraceptives, etc. NNRTIs have a mixed ability to penetrate the blood-brain barrier. Common side effect: mild rash. Some doctors build up drug doses slowly to avoid rash; the other worry is that dose building increases risk of drug resistance.

Protease inhibitor drugs		
Saquinavir mesylate (Invirase)	December 1995	$5,233.39
Ritonavir (Norvir)	March 1996	$9,001.32
Indinavir (Crixivan)	March 1996	$6,310.46
Nelfinavir (Viracept)	March 1997	$8,641.23
Saquinavir (Fortovase)	November 1997	$2,954.93
Amprenavir (Agenerase)	April 1999	$4,372.71
Keletra (Lopinavir/Norvir)	September 2000	$8,040.05
Atazanavir (Reyataz)	June 2003	$9,959.88
Fosamprenavir (Lexiva)	October 2003	$7,800.00
Tipranavir (Aptivus)[d]	June 2005	$3,340.68
Darunavir (Prezista)	June 2006	$9,125.00

Protease inhibitors (PIs) are very potent and may interact with other drugs using cytochrome p450 metabolic pathways. Potentially life-threatening if taken with Seldane, Hismanal, Propulsid, Halcion, or Versed. Avoid rifabutin, Nizoral, rifampin. Poor absorption may affect potency. Common side effects: liver toxicity, hypoglycemia, flatulence, bloating, lipodystrophy (fat distribution). Seven new protease inhibitors are now in some phase of testing in the United States. In addition, there are at least 28 other antiretroviral drugs being investigated.

NEW DRUG CLASSES

Entry Inhibitors—bar HIV from entering immune cells		
T-20 (Enfuvirtide, Fuzeon)	March 2003	$20,000 (WAC)[c]
Maraviroc[e] (Selzentry, the first CCR5 co-receptor inhibitor)	August 2007	$13,200
FP21399		
PRO 542 and 140		
TNX-355, —CXCR4		
receptor blockers AK6:02 Glaxo		
873180—CCR5 blocker		
Integrase Inhibitors -prevents HIV DNA from entering human DNA		
Raltegravir (MK 0158)[e]	October 2007	$12,133.08

Continued

[a] Cost is based on average prescription prices as found in Jacksonville, FL., pharmacies, 2008.

[b] Tenovir is the first nucleotide analog approved for HIV treatment. It blocks HIV replication similar to the nucleoside analogs.

[c] Atazanavir is the first once-a-day PI for use with other anti-HIV drugs. Fuzeon, on launch day (USA) 2003, cash and carry price was $2,200/month or $26,400/year. In 2006 the price was $2,335/month or $28,020/year. Wholesale acquisition cost (WAC) was $20,000. In May 2003, of the 142 largest insurers, 94% agreed to cover Fuzeon, as have Medicaid programs in 48 states.

[d] Prevent the viral proteins from assembling into the HIV capsid that houses viral RNA, enzymes, etc.

There are now drugs that interfere with at least 9 different mechanisms in the process by which HIV attaches itself to specific cell types, enters them, enters the cells' DNA, makes copies of itself, and exits the cell.

[e] Maraviroc is the second FDA entry inhibitor drug. Raltegravir is the first FDA HIV integrace enzyme inhibitor drug. Both drugs will be used in salvage patient therapy, that is, patients resistant to current antiretroviral therapy. TNX-355 is a monoclonal antibody against CCR5.

FDA approval for use in persons infected with HIV. There are at least 31 FDA-approved drugs when combination pills and reformulations are included. Other drugs have been FDA-approved for **expanded access use** where standard regimes have failed (Table 4-1).

Seven of the 25 FDA-approved noncombination anti-HIV drugs are nucleoside (nuk–lee–o–side) analogs (each drug resembles one of the four nucleosides, nucleosides containing adenine, thymine, guanine, and cytosine that are used in making DNA). One is a nucleotide analog. Five are non-nucleosides. All 13 are **reverse transcriptase inhibitors** (RTIs). Ten drugs are HIV-**protease** (pro-tee-ace) inhibitors. Two are HIV entry inhibitors and one is an integrese inhibitor. Cellular targets of these drugs can be seen in Figure 4-1. In addition to large numbers of drug choices, there is the problem of eating or not. That depends on the ART one is taking.

Drugs Taken with Food

A stomach full of food usually means acid and fats are present. Stomach acids—secreted when food is present—are needed to dissolve and absorb the protease inhibitor (PI) Reyataz (atazanavir). Most PIs, including Viracept (nelfinavir), Aptivus (tipranavir), Norvir (ritonavir), and Invirase (saquinavir) are fatlike molecules that need to be emulsified with dietary fats for our mostly watery bodies to be able to absorb them.

Drugs Taken on an Empty Stomach

Food in the stomach slows the transit of drugs, increasing their absorption. But some drugs are absorbed properly only if they can get through the stomach quickly, so no food is best. For example, Sustiva (efavirenz) gets into your bloodstream well enough without food; fat-laden food causes too much to be absorbed, which increases the risk of side effects. Stomach acid chews up Videx before it can slip from the gut into the bloodstream. "EC" means it's coated to withstand those acids. If the drug lingers in the stomach waiting for food to be digested, the protective coating will be destroyed and too little of the drug will reach the small intestine. Crixivan (indinavir) also is absorbed best if it passes through the stomach quickly.

FDA-APPROVED NUCLEOSIDE/ NON-NUCLEOSIDE ANALOG REVERSE TRANSCRIPTASE INHIBITORS AND PROTEASE INHIBITORS

All the known mechanisms by which HIV impairs the human immune system depend on HIV reproduction. Therefore, the development of anti-HIV replication drugs would appear to be a positive first step in controlling HIV reproduction.

Targets of Antiretroviral Drugs: Generalized Scheme

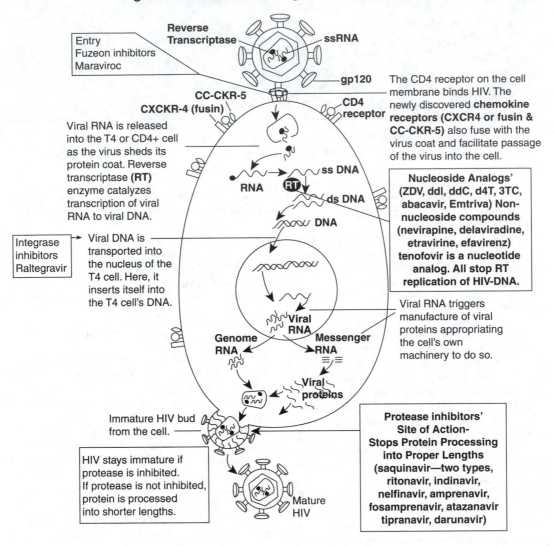

Entry
Fuzeon inhibitors
Maraviroc

Reverse Transcriptase

ssRNA

gp120

CC-CKR-5
CXCKR-4 (fusin)

CD4 receptor

The CD4 receptor on the cell membrane binds HIV. The newly discovered **chemokine receptors (CXCR4 or fusin & CC-CKR-5)** also fuse with the virus coat and facilitate passage of the virus into the cell.

Viral RNA is released into the T4 or CD4+ cell as the virus sheds its protein coat. Reverse transcriptase **(RT)** enzyme catalyzes transcription of viral RNA to viral DNA.

RNA

RT

ss DNA

ds DNA

DNA

Nucleoside Analogs' (ZDV, ddl, ddC, d4T, 3TC, abacavir, Emtriva) Non-nucleoside compounds (nevirapine, delaviradine, etravirine, efavirenz) tenofovir is a nucleotide analog. All stop RT replication of HIV-DNA.

Integrase inhibitors
Raltegravir

Viral DNA is transported into the nucleus of the T4 cell. Here, it inserts itself into the T4 cell's DNA.

Viral RNA

Genome RNA

Messenger RNA

Viral RNA triggers manufacture of viral proteins appropriating the cell's own machinery to do so.

Viral proteins

Immature HIV bud from the cell.

HIV stays immature if protease is inhibited. If protease is not inhibited, protein is processed into shorter lengths.

Mature HIV

Protease inhibitors' Site of Action- Stops Protein Processing into Proper Lengths (saquinavir—two types, ritonavir, indinavir, nelfinavir, amprenavir, fosamprenavir, atazanavir tipranavir, darunavir)

FIGURE 4-1 The diagram shows five classes of FDA-approved antiretroviral drugs used in therapy. These drugs attack five different targets. All 25 FDA-approved individual antiretroviral compounds are represented with respect to their anti-HIV activity. The nucleoside analogs act early after infection, while the protease inhibitors act later in the HIV life cycle, after viral proteins have been synthesized into long strands. Those strands of amino acids contain the individual HIV proteins that become functional after they are cut into their appropriate amino acid sequence lengths. NOTE: The enzyme integrase is required for HIV DNA to enter human DNA. Drugs called integrase and **maturation inhibitors** are in development. (See Table 4-1.)

Each of the eight nucleoside/nucleotide analogs, sometimes referred to as **nukes,** on entering an HIV-infected cell interferes with the virus's ability to replicate itself (Figure 4-2). That is, when any of the eight nucleoside/nucleotide analogs are incorporated into a strand of HIV DNA being newly synthesized, it stops further synthesis of that DNA strand. The nucleoside analog stops the HIV enzyme, reverse transcriptase, from joining the next nucleoside into position.

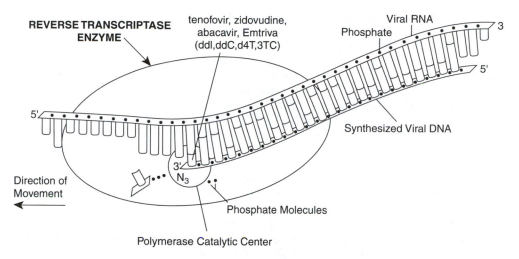

REVERSE TRANSCRIPTASE ENZYME

tenofovir, zidovudine, abacavir, Emtriva (ddI,ddC,d4T,3TC)

Viral RNA

Phosphate

3

5'

Synthesized Viral DNA

Direction of Movement

N_3

Phosphate Molecules

Polymerase Catalytic Center

FIGURE 4-2 Incorporation of FDA-Approved Nucleoside/Nucleotide Analogs Preventing HIV Replication. Zidovudine (ZDV) is a synthetic thymidine analog that is widely used in the treatment of HIV disease and AIDS. HIV-RT is 100 times more sensitive to ZDV inhibition than is the **human transcriptase.** The incorporation of zidovudine-triphosphate into HIV DNA by the action of HIV reverse transcriptase terminates DNA chain extension because polymerization or the incorporation of the next nucleotide adjacent to the azide N_3 group cannot occur. Similar blockage of DNA replication occurs when FDA-approved ddI, ddC, d4T, or 3TC are used. Abacavir is the first 2' deoxyguanosine analog to be used.

Focus on the Eight Nucleoside/Nucleotide Analogs (NRTIs)

Each of the eight drugs has limited effectiveness as a **monotherapy.** The principal limitations are: (1) they are not 100% effective in stopping HIV reverse transcriptase from making HIV DNA; (2) positive clinical effects are short-term, they are not sustained; (3) each drug has its own set of toxic side effects; (4) individually they do not delay the onset of AIDS; and (5) HIV rapidly becomes resistant to each of them.

Antiretroviral Therapy (ART) and Side Effects—No Free Lunch

ART, just like medicines for high blood pressure, cholesterol, or even acne, can cause side effects. It is common for patients to experience some side effects when starting ART. The good news is that most of these side effects get better or go away in time. The body has to adjust. Still, it is very important to take ART on time every day. Some side effects may not show up until you have been on the medicine for a long time. In some cases, the side effects may be related to the class or group of ART they are in. Some of the side effects are presented within each class of ART drugs presented.

Side Effects

Each of the eight nucleoside/nucleotide reverse transcriptase inhibitors (NRTIs) is associated with severe to moderate side effects. For example, zidovudine causes anemia (lowered blood cell count), nausea, headache, and lethargy and inhibits mitochondrial DNA replication in humans (de Martino, 1995); didanosine causes peripheral neuropathy (PN) (a burning pain or pins and needles-like sensation in hands and feet) and pancreatitis (a dangerous swelling of the pancreas) and is very hard for people with poor appetites to take; zalcitabine causes PN and mouth ulcers; stavudine causes PN; and lamivudine causes hair loss and PN. Many experience nightmares.

Collectively, some 15% of HIV-infected people cannot tolerate the nucleoside/non-nucleoside antiretroviral drugs. Even those who can tolerate the drugs are time-limited and right now according to Anthony Fauci, director of the National Institute of Allergy and Infectious Diseases, about 80% of those on drug therapy are running out of time.

USE OF NON-NUCLEOSIDE ANALOG REVERSE TRANSCRIPTASE INHIBITORS

Non-nucleoside reverse transcriptase inhibitors (NNRTIs), sometimes referred to as **non-nukes,** are a structurally and chemically dissimilar group of antiretrovirals that can be used effectively in triple-therapy regimes. The mechanism of action of NNRTIs is distinct from that of nucleoside analogs, even though both *prevent* the conversion of HIV RNA into HIV DNA. Nucleoside RT inhibitors constrain, or stop, HIV replication by their incorporation into the elongating strand of viral DNA, causing chain termination. In contrast, NNRTIs are not incorporated into viral DNA but inhibit HIV replication directly by binding noncompetitively to RT. NNRTIs at first appear to offer hope. All five tested did inhibit the RT-HIV enzyme (atevirdine, delvaridine, loviridine, nevirapine, and etravirine). But this inhibition was short-lived because HIV-resistant mutants for each of the non-nucleoside RTIs were found within weeks of their use. Combination therapies using, for example, zidovudine and nevirapine, have shown some success but it turned out that various drug combinations do not extend survival time. But they do extend the asymptomatic period! The primary advantage of using NNRTIs in therapy is to delay the use of protease inhibitors. But, they are associated with liver damage.

The key to future success in using the reverse transcriptase inhibitors (RTIs) is finding RTIs that work in cells that are not undergoing division. Most RTIs currently in use work only in cells that are dividing (dividing cells must replicate their DNA).

FDA-APPROVED PROTEASE INHIBITORS

Recall from Chapter 3 that some HIV genes code for **reverse transcriptase** (RT), **integrase,** and **protease** enzymes. Later on in the reproductive cycle of HIV a specific **protease** is required to process the precursor GAG and POL proteins into mature HIV components, GAG proteins, and the enzymes integrase and protease (Erickson et al., 1990). If protease is missing or inactive, noninfectious HIV are produced. Therefore, inhibitors of protease enzyme function represent an **alternative** strategy to the inhibition of reverse transcriptase in the treatment of HIV infection (Figures 4-3 and 4-4).

As research progressed, scientists found that HIV protease is distinctly different from human protease enzymes, so a drug that blocks HIV protease should not affect normal human cell function. This means that HIV protease blockers are specific to HIV protease. By 2009, some 20 HIV protease-inhibiting drugs were under study, 6 were in clinical trials, and 10 had received FDA approval.

Problem: at least 15% of people must give up protease inhibitors because of severe side effects. About 15% of people do *not* respond to protease inhibitors, and new reports indicate that protease inhibitors are failing to suppress HIV replication in over half of those people in treatment from one to three years (Valdez et al., 1999; Clough et al., 1999). HIV is an impressive enemy. In late November 2003, Megan O'Brien and colleagues reported that over 50% of AIDS patients on first line therapy (taking anti-HIV drugs for the first time, two nukes and a PI) changed or stopped taking their drugs during their first year! The major reason was gastrointestinal problems followed by fatigue and changes in body composition.

PROTEASE INHIBITORS

In 1988, protease inhibitors with potent and selective antiretroviral activity in cell culture were identified, but the insolubility, poor oral absorption, and rapid liver metabolism of candidate drugs delayed the identification of suitable therapeutic agents until 1992. The **protease inhibitors,** made up of a small number of amino acids (up to 15), bind to the protease active site and inhibit the activity of the enzyme. This inhibition prevents cleavage of the long HIV proteins, resulting in the formation of immature *noninfectious* viral particles. There are 10 PIs currently in use (see Table 4-1 for their names and costs).

FDA-Approved Combination Therapy Drugs/Costs

Six drug combinations have been FDA-approved. Combivir is a combination of nucleosides zidovudine and lamivudine. *The cost is about $662/month.* Kaletra is a protease inhibitor combination containing lopinavir/Norvir. *The cost is about $667/month.* Trizivir is the first to contain three nucleoside analogs—Ziagen (abacavir), Retrovir (zidovudine or AZT), and Epivir (3TC); *the cost of Trizivir is about $1080 per month.* Truvada is a com-

A. Why HIV Protease is Essential for HIV Replication

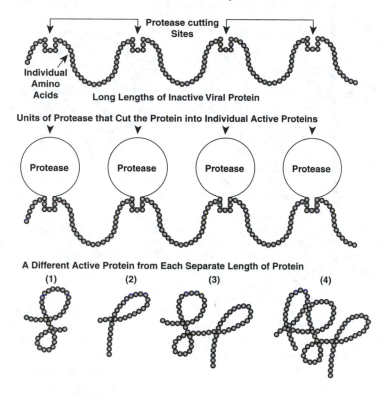

Protease cutting Sites

Individual Amino Acids

Long Lengths of Inactive Viral Protein

Units of Protease that Cut the Protein into Individual Active Proteins

Protease   Protease   Protease   Protease

A Different Active Protein from Each Separate Length of Protein

(1)   (2)   (3)   (4)

FIGURE 4–3   Representation of Protease and Protease Inhibitors. (A) The function of HIV protease is to release the individual replication enzymes, core proteins, and envelope proteins so that HIV can develop into mature, infective HIV. (B) Blocking the production of these essential HIV proteins using protease inhibitors produces immature, noninfective HIV. The action (cutting of protein lengths into active HIV components) of HIV protease occurs during and just after HIV buds out of the cell. Also see Figure 4-4.

B. How HIV Protease Inhibitors Inhibit Viral Protease Function

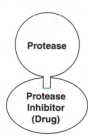

Protease

Protease Inhibitor (Drug)

A Protease Inhibitor Binds to the Cutting Site of the Protease. The Inactivated or Blocked Protease Cannot Cut the Protein.

bination of the nucleosides emtricitabine and tenofovir. *The cost is about $796/month.* Epzicom (Epivir/Ziagen) costs about $846/month (see Table 4–1).

Seeking The Perfect Pill: Once A Day

Gilead Sciences and Merck have joined forces to create the first once-daily pill containing two classes of anti-retroviral drugs. This is the sixth combination drug for use in the U.S. The pill is a fixed combination dose of Atripla (tenofovir and emtricitabine) and efavirenz, two nucleosides with one non-nucleoside reverse transcrip-

tase inhibitor. At the right price this pill may become a standard treatment worldwide. In July 2006, the FDA approved the three-drug, once-a-day, fixed-dose tablet to be used in the 15 countries funded by PEPFAR (see Chapter 14 for explanation of PEPFAR).

The Continuous Debate on the Use of Protease Inhibitors

Protease inhibitors have been hailed as lifesaving anti-retroviral drugs since their general use debut in 1996. But there is a major rift in the HIV/AIDS community

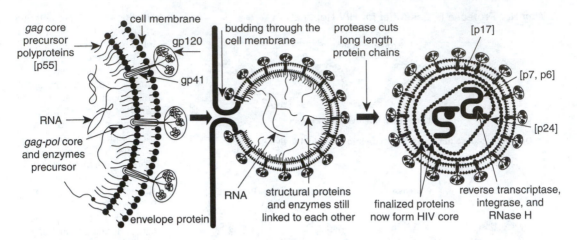

FIGURE 4-4 Representation of HIV Assembly. During the budding process, the viral GAG and GAG-POL polyproteins assemble at the cell membrane together with viral RNA to form immature HIV. These polyproteins are then cleaved by the HIV-coded protease enzyme to provide the structural and functional (enzyme) proteins essential to form the *mature*, infectious viral core. *(Adapted from Vella, 1995)*

concerning their use as new information emerges. The new drugs have saved people's lives, that's true. But the new drugs have also killed people. That's also true! They have damaged and deformed some people so badly that although they are alive, they say they wish they were dead. Drug cocktails comprised of protease inhibitors—now considered to be the standard treatment for infected patients who are both sick and healthy—have caused many to suffer liver damage, kidney failure, strokes, heart attacks, and other devastating side effects that are deemed inevitable by advocates of the new retroviral treatments, but called horrific and unnecessary by opponents. According to Joseph Sonnabend, a former HIV/AIDS physician at St. Luke's–Roosevelt Hospital Center, "There is absolutely no question whatsoever that protease inhibitors have helped people. But they've probably hurt more people than they've helped. The people for whom benefit has been proven beyond a doubt are really sick people who would have died without them. But the target population for the drug therapy are those that are still healthy, and these people will almost certainly have their lives damaged by these drugs."

ENTRY INHIBITORS AND PROBLEMS

Entry inhibitors make it possible for the first time to stop HIV from entering a cell. Thus, there are now drugs to target HIV before and after it enters a cell!

(Figure 4-1). Fuzeon was FDA-approved in 2003 but has the drawback of being an injection drug. In August 2007, **Maraviroc** or **Selzentry** was FDA-approved. This is the first member of a new class of oral drugs in more than a decade—meaning it can be taken by mouth. This entry inhibitor targets the R5 (CCCR5) receptor in the CD4+ T lymphocytes or T4 cells. An inhibitor of the R5 receptor was long sought because it was shown **not** to be vital to health and survival (see Snapshot 4.2).

Problem 1

Selzentry will only be effective against CD4+ cells using the R5 receptor. It will not be effective against HIV that target the R4 receptor (and will have a limited effect against HIV with the ability to target both receptors). Because R4-targeting HIV is more common in people who have been infected with HIV for several years, the people who are most likely going to be using Selzentry will be those whose CD4+ cells are displaying the R5 receptor or a mixture of R5 and R4 receptors. A new laboratory test, Monogram Bioscience's Trofile tropism assay (to determine if R5 is present on the person's CD4+ cells) will be necessary before Selzentry can be used. Even among patients who begin Selzentry treatment with R5-tropic HIV, there is the possibility that their virus will switch to the R4 receptor during therapy, meaning that the addition of Selzentry will no longer have any signifi-

A MYSTERY SOLVED: THE HUNT FOR THE ELUSIVE BLOOD HIV-INHIBITING PROTEIN

In 1996, U.S. and European researchers writing in several science journals said a **small group of Caucasian** gay men carry a gene mutation that provides natural protection against HIV. As a result of these studies, scientists realized that HIV carries out its damage by first attaching to a receptor on the surface of CD4+ cells, much as a key enters a lock. This receptor was called CCCR5 or R5. It turned out that R5 was necessary for HIV to successfully enter a CD4+ lymphocyte. This critical finding led groups of scientists to search for a drug that could bind with R5, blocking HIV entry. After an 11-year race among three drug companies, Pfizer released the first oral entry inhibitor drug. This drug, in a sense, mimics the genetic defect wherein the R5 mutation blocks the production of R5 cell receptor. So if the receptor is there but blocked, the end result is the same—HIV cannot bind to the cell's receptor. The drug is called maraviroc; its trade name is Selzentry. Pfizer expects to generate over $300 million in sales by 2011.

HIV Integrase Inhibitors and Problem

From reports at the 2007 14th Conference on Retroviruses and Opportunistic Infections, two HIV integrase inhibitory drugs have been tested and found to have excellent activity against HIV replication. The integrase enzyme of HIV is essential for HIV DNA to become incorporated into the cell's DNA. Blocking this enzyme stops HIV DNA integration and thus the formation of HIV. Merck's inhibitor **raltegravir** (ral-tegra-veer), or Isentress, was FDA-approved in late 2007. Gilead's integrase inhibitor, was called **elvitegravir** (el-vy-tegra-veer), not yet FDA approved, appears to allow early HIV resistance to occur. Both integrase inhibitors are to be used in conjunction with other antiretroviral therapy in patients who are failing to benefit from that therapy.

Problem

Independent work by developers of the two leading integrase inhibitors offered evidence that resistance to one integrace inhibitor may mean resistance to other, integrase inhibitors.

cant benefit. It is not uncommon for HIV to switch from using R5 to R4 receptors during the course of the disease. Much like drug-resistance testing, tropism testing can be ordered by a healthcare provider if Selzentry treatment failure is suspected. Tropism tests cost between $1,400 and $2,000.

Problem 2

It is not yet known how often resistance to CCR5 drugs will happen and what level of resistance will put patients at risk of possible disease progression though the emergence of virus that prefers the second coreceptor on CD4 cells, CXCR4(R4). Ample research shows that growth of a R4-using viral population forecasts a more rapid CD4 decline.

INTEGRASE INHIBITORS

In October 2007, the FDA approved the first integrase inhibitor, raltegravir (trade name Isentress). This is the first in a new class of HIV drugs.

What Are Integrase Inhibitors?

Integrase is one of three viral enzymes necessary for HIV DNA replication. Integrase does what the name implies; it integrates (blends) HIV DNA, its genetic material, into the DNA of human CD4 cells. This blending of DNA makes it possible for the infected cell to make new copies of HIV. By interfering with integrase, the integrase inhibitors prevent HIV/DNA from integrating into the CD4 cell, thus stopping HIV replication.

Why Are Integrase Inhibitors Important?

Integrase inhibitors are a new class of HIV medication. They target a new step in the HIV life cycle. Because they target new life cycle steps, even the most drug-experienced HIV patient should benefit from integrase inhibitors. In other words, because integrase inhibitors target HIV differently than existing HIV medications, most HIV-positive patients should benefit from integrase inhibitors to some degree. Integrase offers a new option for patients with an extensive HIV-medication history or HIV resistance.

Maturation Inhibitors

Maturation inhibitors disrupt processing of the viral GAG protein by preventing the conversion of the capsid precursor (p25) into the mature capsid protein (p24). Although maturation inhibitors target the same enzymatic step as protease inhibitors, their methods of action differ. The lead candidate in the maturation inhibitor class is bevirimat (formerly PA-457) (Table 4-1).

DEVELOPMENT AND SELECTION OF HIV DRUG-RESISTANT MUTANTS

Development of Drug-Resistant Nucleoside Analog Mutants

HIV reverse transcriptase, the enzyme that copies (transcribes) HIV RNA into HIV DNA, is *unable* to edit or eliminate transcription errors during nucleic acid replication. Because there is no repair or correction of mistakes (as occurs in human cells), there are about one to five mutations in each new replicated HIV DNA/HIV RNA strand (Coffin, 1995). This means that each new virus is different from all other HIV that is being produced because new virus is being produced at a rate of 1 billion to 10 billion per day! There will be 1 billion to 10 billion new HIV mutants produced each day in one person. Thus, virtually all possible drug mutations, and perhaps many combinations of mutations to drugs, are generated in each patient daily (Ho et al., 1995; Wain-Hobson, 1995; Wei et al., 1995; Hu et al., 1996; Mayers, 1996).

DEVELOPMENT OF HIV DRUG-RESISTANCE TO PROTEASE INHIBITORS

HIV resistance to all ten PIs has been found in clinical trials. The development of HIV resistance to PIs is a major concern. For example, recent studies (Schmit et al., 1996) found that long-term (one year) use of **ritonavir** is associated with the production of at least nine different mutations that make HIV resistant to ritonavir. These ritonavir-resistant mutants also demonstrated cross-resistance to both **indinavir** and **saquinavir.** John Mellors (1996) reported that within 12 to 24 weeks after indinavir therapy, at least 10 different HIV-resistant indinavir mutations occurred and five HIV saquinavir-resistant mutations occurred with the use of the individual drugs. Cross-resistance to ritonavir occurred in *at least* 19 isolates of HIV-indinavir resistant mutants.

Selection of Drug-Resistant Mutants

Based on the large number of mutant HIV produced in any one person, it is not surprising that HIV emerges with resistance to drugs used in antiretroviral therapy. Such strains are referred to as **drug-resistant mutants.** HIV drug-resistant mutants are selected to reproduce most effectively under conditions of selective pressure exerted by the presence of the drugs. Those HIV able to resist the drugs continue to multiply; those that are sensitive to the drugs are destroyed (Figure 4-5).

The Demise of Monotherapy

Prior to 1987 antiretroviral therapy was an unknown. People became infected with HIV and were diagnosed with AIDS, on average, 10 years later. They died of AIDS, on average, three years after their AIDS diagnosis. This, however, is no longer true. In developed countries like the United States, available antiretroviral drugs are extending lives beyond what we can currently predict. Twenty-two years ago (1987) the first

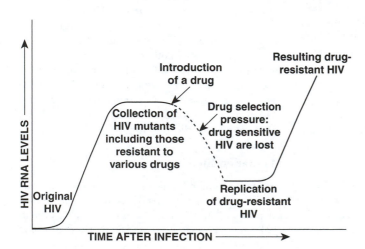

FIGURE 4-5 Enrichment of Drug-Resistant HIV. The development of drug-resistant HIV variants in an individual limits available treatment. This drug-resistant HIV is transmitted such that the recipient becomes infected with one or more drug-resistant HIV variants.

antiretroviral drug, zidovudine (AZT as it is often referred to), entered the fight against HIV replication. The infected person took 12 pills per day—two pills every four hours around the clock. Unknown to patients and physicians at the time, the zidovudine dosage being prescribed was too high and proved toxic for some people. Some died prematurely. Others became resistant to zidovudine because HIV needs more than one drug to suppress it. The use of zidovudine and newer antiretrovirals as single agents had to stop.

But, it took seven years before David Cooper, an AIDS-drug therapy researcher, declared 1995 the year of the "demise of monotherapy for HIV and the rise of combination drug therapy" (Simberkoff, 1996; Stephenson, 1996). The **standard of therapy** became and was that *all* ART drugs must be used in combination and that each combination include two nucleoside reverse transcriptase inhibitors and a protease or a nonnucleoside inhibitor. The use of three or more drugs in combination is referred to as **HAART** or **Highly Active Anti-Retroviral Therapy.** HAART is a collection of different drugs, each with its own side effects. The HAART era really began in March of 1996 after the FDA approved ritonavir and indinavir, two protease inhibitors, which dramatically shifted medication strategies: According to the newest U.S. treatment guidelines (May 2006), the recommended regimens are Combivir or Truvada or Kaletra (see Table 4–1). The goal of using HAART is to suppress HIV replication or viral load. As a result of a large reduction in HIV, fewer T4 or CD4+ cells become infected and die, so the end result is more CD4+ cells remain to divide. Thus, it appears that HAART causes an increase in T4 or CD4+ cells over time, but the increase is not from an increase in new CD4+ cell production. Rather, the increase is due to cell division of existing CD4+ cells saved by HAART drugs.

Antiretroviral Therapy (ART) Saves Lives!

In 2006, Rochelle Walensky and colleagues reported that ART and OI therapies have, since 1989, saved about 3 million to 5 million years of life in the United States. Their data come from estimates of adults with AIDS receiving the recommended standard of care in the year of diagnosis. Rochelle and colleagues also found that zidovudine (AZT) and Retrovir treatment averted about 2860 new cases of HIV infection in infants, which resulted in another 186,790 years of life granted. The survival benefit would have increased to 277,150 years had all pregnant HIV-infected women received zidovudine. They say that if those who don't know they have HIV/AIDS were found and treated, it could mean another 2 million years of life saved! Rochelle said that "this kind of survival benefit far exceeds that which can currently be achieved for patients with other chronic diseases, including chemotherapy for breast cancer, bypass surgery for coronary artery disease, and bone marrow transplantation for non-Hodgkin's lymphoma." She estimated that ART can lengthen the life span of persons with AIDS by nearly 15 years.

Antiretroviral Therapy Is Expensive

(See Table 4–2 and Point of Information 4.3.) The cost of ART is expensive, as shown in a study on annual expenditures per patient at an HIV outpatient clinic (Chen et al., 2006). In Table 4–2, antiretroviral therapy represented 56% of the overall costs; however, the improvement in clinical status associated with successful antiretroviral therapy, as demonstrated by increases in CD4 cell count, led to a reduction in healthcare expenditures in other areas. In particular, the sickest patients (CD4 cell count <50 cells/μL) require eight times more nonantiretroviral medication expenditures and six times more hospitalization expenditures than do the healthiest patients (CD4 cell count >350 cells/μL). The most striking finding in this study, however, was the low expenditures for healthcare services provided by HIV physicians and clinics. Taken together, these findings demonstrate the relative cost of care in a fashion that informs policy makers, payers, and healthcare administrators.

To quantitate the reduction in expenditures associated with an increase in CD4 cell count, they assessed the impact of changes in CD4 cell count strata on annual expenditures during the year-long

---

LOOKING BACK 4.1

THE ERA OF HAART—1996

Steven Deeks of San Francisco General Hospital (SFGH) said in 1996 that "everybody hailed the three drug cocktail or Highly Active AntiRetroviral Therapy (HAART) as the major breakthrough to that time." Everyone at SFCH was placed on HAART. People who were lying on their deathbeds in the hospital got up and walked out. Many people at the time were so euphoric that they quickly, too quickly, believed that HIV was conquered—HIV was no longer a problem! Then in 1997, Deeks said, "We realized the tremendous benefit of HAART was only happening in half of our patients!"

BOX 4.1

PROTEASE INHIBITORS: EXTENDING LIFE; THE DOWNSIDE OF THIS GIFT—RECOVERY?

THE LAZARUS EFFECT: A RETURN TO FUNCTIONAL STATUS

In November 1995, one man in his late forties wrote his obituary—he had been fighting off HIV disease, then AIDS, for over 13 years. In another case, the man's T cell count was zero. He was on oxygen and morphine. Funeral arrangements were made, and his friends and family were on a death vigil. They are but two examples of several thousand men, beginning in 1999, all under age 50, who had given up hope—they believed they were a short step away from death. Some ran up huge debts—maxed out all their credit cards and gave lavish gifts. Some regretted the way they had lived or not lived to this point, some became very angry, some made peace with themselves and others, but *all* felt death was imminent. *Then it happened*—the results of combination therapies using nucleoside and non-nucleoside reverse transcriptase inhibitors and protease inhibitors *dropped viral load counts* to unmeasurable or undetectable levels in people with HIV disease and AIDS patients. And, those with significantly lowered viral loads demonstrated surprising recovery—their T4 cells rebounded in some cases from below 200 back up to 500 or more. These "AIDS cocktails," as the combination therapies were soon called, gave people with AIDS a new chance at a productive life for the first time since the beginning of the pandemic in the United States in 1981.

CAN THERE BE A DOWNSIDE TO SUCH A MIRACLE?

Of course the most tragic downside is the fact that not all who would benefit from the drug cocktail can tolerate the drugs or afford them—but that is not the issue that is relevant to the question per se. No, this question pertains to a downside, if any, for people who can tolerate the drugs and have access to these drugs.

WHAT KIND OF PROBLEMS EXIST?

Guilt

Many who now feel "new" again feel *guilty* because these drugs are not available to all who need them—the poor and the uninsured in the United States and those in underdeveloped nations.

Reestablishing Relationships

Depending on how long and how severe the illness, the affected became more or less isolated—even "best" friends stopped calling or dropping by. Some who also had AIDS died, while some were too sick to care or mourn them; but now that they have recovered? **What now? At the beginning of year 2009, about 650,000 people in the United States were on anti-HIV therapy, which includes protease inhibitors. These drugs are not yet deemed necessary to the other 600,000 HIV-infected in the United States. To date they are mostly unavailable in developing nations.**

Ability to Work Again—Loss of Disability Pay

Disability insurance has been a cocoon of safety for many now experiencing "new" life. Traditionally, people with AIDS received disability checks until death. But suddenly it is not so certain that this will be the case. People who were expected to die are going to be coming back. Nobody is prepared for this. Now that drug cocktails have extended life expectancies, it is expected that these people will be reevaluated and lose their disability payments. They will have to go back to work.

Across the United States, AIDS groups are deluged with calls from patients who are excited, confused, or frightened about the prospect of ending disability status and returning to work. In Miami, a psychologist has begun weekly seminars on résumé writing and job interviews for AIDS patients who have not worked in years. At AIDS Project Los Angeles, counselors field 100 calls each week on return-to-work issues.

POLITICAL DOWNSIDE

As scientists dare ask whether HIV eradication may be possible in some people in the near future (two to five years), the press may be promising more than the scientists can deliver, but the press can and does influence political will. If the political will to fight this disease **weakens** due to the **premature declaration of victory,** this may be the greatest downside of all!

---

period of observation. Compared with patients who remained in the same level of CD4 cell counts, patients who moved to a higher level during the year had lower annual expenditures, whereas patients who moved to a lower level experienced higher ex-

penditures. Because antiretroviral drugs improve CD4 cell counts, these findings further demonstrate the clinical and economic benefit of antiretroviral therapy among patients for whom therapy is currently recommended.

Table 4–2 Mean Annual Expenditure per Patient by Cost Component and CD4 Cell Count Category for 635 Patients from the University of Alabama at Birmingham HIV Outpatient Clinic.

CD4 cell count category	No. of patients	Cost per Patient per Year (% of Total Cost) by Cost Category					
		Total cost	Antiretroviral medication	Nonantiretroviral medication	Hospital costs	Other outpatient costs[1]	Physician/clinic costs
<50 cells/μL	62	$36,532 (100)	$10,855 (30)	$14,882 (41)	$8353 (23)	$1909 (6)	$533 (1)
50–199 cells/μL	99	$23,864 (100)	$11,862 (50)	$6,685 (28)	$3369 (14)	$1416 (6)	$532 (2)
200–349 cells μL	143	$18,274 (100)	$11,935 (65)	$3,452 (19)	$1186 (7)	$1365 (7)	$336 (2)
>350 cells/μL	331	$13,885 (100)	$9,407 (68)	$1,855 (13)	$1408 (10)	$930 (7)	$285 (2)
All	635	$18,640 (100)	$10,500 (56)	$4,240 (23)	$2342 (13)	$1199 (6)	$359 (2)

[1] Other outpatient costs include outpatient radiological examinations, laboratory tests, procedures, and home health care. (Source Ray Chen and Colleagues, *Clinical Infectious Diseases,* 2006)

Bruce Schackman and colleagues (2006) studied costs as they related to lifetime cost of medical care of HIV-infected adults using current ART. They estimated the monthly medical cost for people with HIV, from the time of beginning appropriate care (begin ART with a T4 or CD4 cell count of less than 350) until death, to be $2,100 on average. The projected life expectancy for these individuals, if they remained in optimal HIV care, was estimated to be 24.2 years, and the lifetime-per-person HIV-care cost was calculated to be $618,900. Seventy-three percent of the cost is antiretroviral medications, 13% inpatient care, 9% outpatient care, and 5% other HIV-related medications and laboratory costs. For patients who initiate ART with CD4 cell count at <200/[mu]L, projected life expectancy is 22.5 years, and the cost is $567,000. Results are sensitive to drug manufacturers' discounts, ART efficacy, and the use of enfuvirtide for salvage therapy. Given the CDC's projection of 40,000 new HIV infections each year over the last 17 years, the total cost per year would be $618,000 × 40,000 or $24.8 billion for future treatment costs for any given year! In 2006, the CDC raised the estimated number of new HIV infections for that year to 56,300. There have been over 56,000 infections per year from at least 2002.

The Function of HAART: Suppression of HIV Replication and Restoration of Immune Competence

The function of HAART is to suppress HIV replication regardless of the number of drugs used. The reasoning is to keep the viral load low so that sexual transmission of HIV becomes unlikely, and to prevent HIV mutation by reducing its ability to replicate. A number of clinical trials have demonstrated that only about half the patients placed on HAART, for the first time, are able to achieve maximal suppression—undetectable or less than 50 copies of HIV RNA per milliliter of blood. Where HAART works, most people reduce their viral load to 50 copies within 24 to 32 weeks. Less is known about the long-term durability of this suppression. Of those who achieve this undetectable viral load, the majority will experience a viral rebound during the first year of therapy and most everyone will experience the rebound if they stop taking the drugs (Back, 2001). In 2007 the CDC reported that 40% or about 468,000 people living in the United States who should be receiving ART are not getting it. Of these, beginning in 2007, about 25% or 278,000 of those people were not receiving ART. Worldwide, at the beginning of 2009, of the 34 million people living with HIV, about 10 million people in developing nations need antiretroviral drugs now. The WHO's goal, based on a 3 by 5 policy, was to have 3 million people in Africa and Asia on therapy by year 2005. The goal failed by over one million. The new goal is universal access to ART by 2010. It appears that this goal will not be met.

According to the Institute for Health Sector Development, London, between 12 million and 18 million people would benefit from antiretroviral therapy (ART). This is between two and three times WHO estimates. And this raises serious concerns about how ART is going to be delivered on the global scale.

HOW COMBINATION DRUG THERAPY CAN REDUCE THE CHANCE OF HIV DRUG RESISTANCE

Combination drug therapy works because a single strand of RNA, the genetic material of HIV, must be a multiple mutant, that is, it must carry a genetic change to become resistant to *each* new drug used. So, the greater the number of drugs used, each capable of stopping HIV replication, the greater the number of genetic changes that must occur in a single RNA strand of the virus. For reasons of explanation, say that the chance of change in one nucleotide of HIV for resistance to a single drug occurs in one RNA strand during the production of 10,000 (10 thousand) or 1×10^4 such strands. This is a reasonable figure! Then to have a second nucleotide mutation occur in that same single strand for resistance to a second drug, again at 1×10^4 means that only one RNA strand in 100 million or 1×10^8 would carry both genetic changes. For three separate nucleotide mutations occurring in one RNA strand then, it would be $(1 \times 10^4) \times (1 \times 10^4) \times (1 \times 10^4)$ or only one RNA strand out of 1,000,000,000,000 (1 trillion) would carry a resistance to all three drugs at the same time. But as small as this number is, recall that 1 billion to 10 billion genetically different RNA strands are produced each day in one individual. **In short, HIV can change or mutate at every nucleotide or base daily!** Also, individual RNA strands can exchange nucleotides in a process called recombination. This increases the chance of multiple resistant RNA strands. This is why it is so important to slow the replication of HIV—fewer rounds of replication mean fewer RNA strands, thus fewer possibilities of producing HIV that are resistant to AIDS drug cocktails (Figure 4-6). Current AIDS drug cocktails, especially those using one or more protease inhibitors, quickly and significantly reduce HIV replication—this is why people on these combination therapies must take them on schedule, in prescribed doses, and maybe for the rest of their lives.

Multidrug Cocktails: Success Breeds Danger

Multidrug cocktails work well initially because they are attacking the strains of HIV that are least resistant to the drugs. But the result of that success is to en-

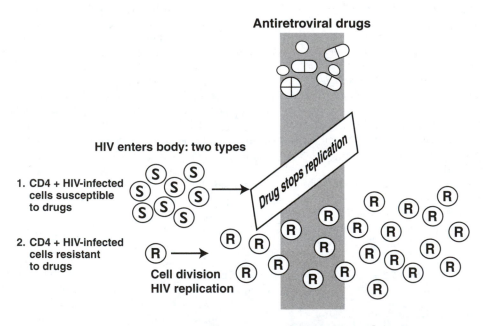

FIGURE 4-6   Drug-Resistant Variants Become Predominate.

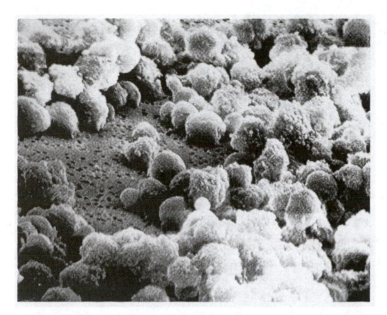

FIGURE 4-7 Production of HIV. Each dark hole in the T4 cell membrane represents the emergence of one new HIV that came off the membrane and is loose in the body. Each HIV-infected T4 cell is producing about 3000 to 4000 viruses at any time. Each HIV in this photograph is genetically different from any other HIV being released from this T4 cell and most likely genetically different from any other HIV in the body. T4 or CD4+ cells live for about 80 days in a healthy person and about 25 days in an AIDS patient. (*Source: Courtesy of the Centers for Disease Control and Prevention, Atlanta*)

courage the rapid spread of HIV strains that are highly resistant to the drugs, which could give rise to a new and even more dangerous AIDS epidemic among people most at risk for the disease (Figure 4-7).

Several separate research investigations, using two new types of sensitive diagnostic tests, found evidence suggesting that about 30% of individuals newly infected with HIV are carrying forms of the virus that are already resistant to one of the 25 drugs, and 14% are resistant to two of the drugs used in American combination therapy. In Great Britain, 13% of the HIV infected are resistant to three of the main classes of antiretroviral drugs.

Mutations that confer resistance to nucleoside analog reverse transcriptase inhibitors, non-nucleoside reverse transcriptase inhibitors, and protease inhibitors have all been identified in HIV-infected Americans who have never been treated with antiretroviral drugs.

In summary, the frequency of genetically variant HIV within an HIV population is influenced by the mutation rate, fitness of the mutant to survive, the size of the available HIV pool for genetic recombination, and the number of HIV replication cycles.

Coinfection and Superinfection

Coinfection—This is an infection with at least two genetically different strains of HIV from the **same** clade or group, for example clade B. (Not to be confused with coinfection meaning infected with two completely different viruses like HIV and HCV or hepatitis C). In February 2000, the first documented case of **HIV coinfection** was reported at the Seventh Conference on Retroviruses and Opportunistic Infections. An HIV-infected male became infected with a second strain of HIV, one more aggressive than the HIV he carried. He acquired the second strain from a different sexual partner who harbored the variant HIV. Prior to his second infection he demonstrated good health. His health declined markedly after he acquired the second infection.

Superinfection—This is an infection by strains of HIV from **different** clades or subtypes, for example A and E or B and C.

At the 2004 Eleventh Conference on Retrovirus and Opportunistic Infections, investigators from Los Angeles and San Diego presented evidence that the annual rate for superinfection in their studies was 5%.

HIV TREATMENT REGIMEN FAILURE

Regimen failure occurs when the anti-HIV medications being taken do not adequately control HIV replication. There are three basic types of regimen failure:

Virologic failure: Regimens should lower the amount of HIV in the blood to undetectable levels.

IT'S THE STIGMA THAT KILLS!

This is a story about Lance C. Hogue, Jr. He is an HIV Clinical Nurse Practitioner Specialist who has been working in the area of HIV/AIDS services since 1983. In 2001, he was diagnosed with HIV, the end result of an occupational injury in the hospital emergency room.

"Suddenly, my life changed 100%. My family, a group of well-educated doctors, teachers, business folk, etc. whom I always thought of as hip on most things were clearly not. My mother forbade me to tell anyone (I now realize as a result of her own shame). My family knew that I had been attacked by a psychotic, suicidal, drug-addicted HIV-infected patient. He attempted to kill me in order to escape and have a cigarette. Some months later I sero converted. I will never forget that day because I told my mother and she said, "You will not tell anyone in the family." I was so taken aback by the test results and everything I had been through that day, I just said okay. As time went on and I was fired from my job—where I had been awarded the Nurse of Year three years in a row—for not returning to work due to both physical and mental complications, I was able to finish graduate school four days after being given my surprise HIV diagnosis. I very quickly realized I was going to have to take care of myself and that wasn't going to be easy. I became more isolated and suddenly alone. I was very ill; eventually my CD4 cell count dropped to 50. At this point I immediately went to ART and in time went into the "Lazarus syndrome" having prepared for death and rebounding because of ART. I became very depressed, feeling like life's best was past me. I called friends, many long-term friends; they had wondered what had happened to me. Where had I disappeared to? I told them one by one what had happened. We cried on the phone, many rushed to see me, fearing the worst. Because of ART, I had little energy to care or do much of anything except take my drugs and visit the toilet!"

Mother's Reaction Regrettably Altered My Behavior—"Out of respect for my mother's wishes, I did not tell anyone in the family that I was HIV positive. I led a double life with untold agony in each."

He went to therapy once a week for several years, mostly because of the commitment he made to his mother. He said, "I struggled for months in therapy with this, was I depriving my family of the right to know or was it my personal business? Was there a need for them to know? What if things got worse? Would they be angry if I told them? Would they be

angry if I didn't? Who do I need to be thinking about? I'm sick as a dog and here I am worried about what others think. Now if I had cancer as they initially thought I had, it would all be okay. But it wasn't cancer, no one bothered to call, no one asked questions. Silence was the operative mode in the family.

One day in 2002 while my mother was visiting I observed behaviors like not sitting on my toilet seat, drinking from my cups or glasses, not wanting to eat food I prepared, etc. I guess I was taking in all of this feeling like I was some kind of alien or something and when I had told her she blew up! Her only words to my situation were, "It's not all about you anymore." She packed her bags and walked out, not be heard from again. That was June 2, 2002. Funny thing is, I haven't heard from one family member, either, other than an e-mail telling me to stop treating my mother so badly and that she loved me. But no one in the family knows all I have gone through, how I lost everything, and how I almost died more than once. How I later went on to fight colorectal cancer in 2003 and 2005, how I lived for all of these years having to go on disability and medical assistance and food stamps and lose all my dignity. And who pays for the $2,600 in drug bills and who pays the health insurance, what it was like to be on food stamps, how the social services worker didn't care that my medical insurance got cut off by accident by computer and I couldn't get care, or how Medicare kicked me out of the program due to a computer glitch and I couldn't get my HIV meds two days before I was about to travel for the holidays, or how I felt traveling over the U.S. border with HIV meds fearing they'd find them and refuse me entry back into the U.S., and it goes on and on."

A Welcome Surprise—"I remember in 1993 in an inner city hospital, working in a psychiatric unit, with a drug addict who was very angry and depressed over the stigma-related things her family did, like burn the sheets after she slept over, make her eat on paper plates and use plastic utensils, etc. She told me that her family are good Baptist folks who go to church every day. But she said, 'I'm angry with God, but I can't be. It's not okay to be angry, that is a sin.' I shared with her that I felt that anger was as okay to share as she shares happiness or sorrow, so I'm sure that any God would be okay with her expressing her feelings. The next day she awakened and made an incredible turn that dumbfounded the doctors that had tried her on numerous medications. I believe my words, as simple as they were, gave her permission to do as she felt she needed, and she was able to move on to forgiving herself and moving on in life."

Lance's Decision—"I decided I needed to do what I needed, too, which was take care of myself if I was going to outlive this virus or it was going to eat me alive. I made that decision months after my therapist told me, 'I don't think you're going to make it. The virus is eating you alive and you internalize stigma, depression, and isolation.' "

His Return—Because ART reduced his viral load and his CD4 cell count has increased, he feels about whole again. He has returned to the HIV community and is involved in his local community in state-level planning, traveling, and teaching, in addition to attending the Presidential Council on HIV and international HIV/AIDS conferences as an advocate.

He said, "I have kept every pill bottle I have ever been given since I have been on HIV medications, and I have kept the pharmacy receipts for those bottles. I have two huge trunks of bottles and boxes on wheels." (Figure 4-8)

As a public health expert on HIV, he is constantly asked to give presentations about HIV/AIDS. He takes his trophies (all bottles/boxes) in a trunk with him. It does make the point! Beginning in 2009, Lance Hogue is enjoying excellent health and providing people from all walks of life important information on HIV/AIDS.

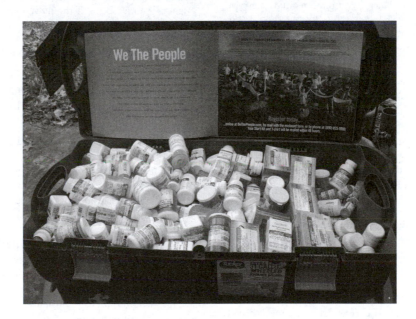

FIGURE 4-8 Trunk containing antiretroviral prescription drug vials and boxes accumulated over seven years, seven months. A 35-gallon container holds this patient's entire history of ART through 2008. His reduced cost is $239,615 or $2,633.13 per month. Retail cost is $299,518. The cost is for prescription drugs only. They do not include hospital care or other forms of HIV/AIDS patient care. (Source: Lance C. Hogue, Jr., with permission.)

Virologic failure has occurred if HIV can still be detected in the blood 48 weeks after starting treatment or if it is detected again after treatment had previously lowered the viral load to undetectable.

Immunologic failure: An effective regimen should increase the number of CD4 cells in the blood or at least prevent the number from going down. Immunologic failure has occurred if the CD4+ count

CAN AN HIV DRUG PREVENT HIV INFECTION—PRE-EXPOSURE PROPHYLAXIS (PrEP)?

Will a Pill a Day Prevent HIV Infection?

PrEP is an experimental, unproven strategy that aims to reduce the risk of acquiring HIV through the use of a once-daily antiretrovirals in HIV-negative people. As the new report (Anticipating the Results of PrEP Trials: A powerful new HIV prevention tool may be on the horizon. Are we prepared?) notes, by mid-2009 there could be more people enrolled in PrEP trials than in vaccine and microbicide efficacy trials combined. Perhaps the closest precedent for pre-exposure prophylaxis is the use of the antiretroviral drugs AZT, nevirapine, and/or other of these drugs to **prevent** mother-to-child transmission of HIV during pregnancy, delivery, and during breast-feeding.

In 1995, scientists from Gilead and the University of California at Davis published studies in the journal *Science* that showed that a preventive shot of Viread (tenofovir) could block HIV from infecting monkeys (monkeys can be infected with HIV but there is no progression to AIDS as in humans). But it wasn't clear that the drug would block sexual transmission of the virus in people.

A number of HIV/AIDS physicians in New York, San Francisco, and Florida began giving Viread to people who believed they might have been exposed to HIV. Although none of these people became HIV positive at the time, it is not hard evidence that Viread can prevent HIV infection or HIV transmission—still, the possibility is intriguing, and interesting enough for the National Institutes of Health, Centers for Disease and Prevention, and Bill and Melinda Gates Foundation to fund three separate human studies of the drug to determine whether the drug can prevent HIV infection. The Gates Foundation has awarded a $6.5 million grant to fund a randomized, placebo-controlled clinical trial to evaluate whether Viread is effective at reducing the risk of HIV infection. The trial includes 2000 volunteers in Ghana, Nigeria, and Malawi. All of the study participants received "safer" sex counseling and condoms even though their use may make it more difficult to prove whether the drug works to prevent HIV. In addition, the CDC granted $3.5 million to fund a third study examining the drug's safety as a preventive among sexually active men who have sex with men in San Francisco and Atlanta. The race is on; if the prevention trials are a success, there will be a large number of people who would demand Viread.

In 2006, two additional drugs were added for the prevention of HIV infection, Emtriva (emtricitabine) and a combination pill of Viread/ Emtriva called Truvada. Some physicians are now prescribing Truvada for both pre- and post-HIV exposure. However, the results of these clinical trials are not available at this writing.

---

decreases below the initial count before starting therapy or does not increase above the initial count within the first year of therapy.

Clinical failure: Clinical failure has occurred if there is an HIV-related infection or a decline in physical health despite at least three months of anti-HIV treatment.

Virologic failure is the most common kind of regimen failure. People with virologic failure who do not change to an effective drug regimen usually progress to immunologic failure within about three years. Immunologic failure may be followed by clinical failure. Clinical failure results in the use of third line regimens.

Third Line Regimens: Salvage, Mega, or Giga HAART Therapy

Under current definition, a treatment-experienced, or so-called salvage HIV-infected patient, is one who has failed at least three HIV regimens that include at least one drug from each approved drug class. Salvage therapy is the use of substitute drugs that will continue to suppress viral replication when standard therapy fails. There is no "single recipe" for salvage therapy. Although the HIV salvage population is on the rise as the life expectancy of patients with HIV increases, they are still underrepresented in new clinical trials because sponsors of new drugs do not expect the drugs to be effective in salvage patients. The reasons that HIV drug regimens lose their effectiveness are as varied as the patients who are undergoing treatment with them. Treatment failures, which can occur in up to 60% of patients, can develop in those with a prolonged history of sequential HIV therapy because of built-up resistance. They also can occur in patients who fail to comply with their prescribed therapy or who are given a poorly suited regimen at the outset.

The Kitchen Sink—By early 2009 over 40,000 patients in America developed resistance to the three main HIV drug classes. Clearly some of the drugs were being recycled in a variety of new combinations. The try-anything approach—the kitchen sink!

In mid-2006, darunavir or Prezista was FDA approved to be used along with ritonavir (ritonavir slows the metabolism of Prezista) and at least two other anti-HIV drugs, but only in HIV-infected adults who have tried and failed other anti-HIV drug regimens. At the moment, it appears that Prezista is effective against strains of HIV resistant to the other protease inhibitors.

How Many People Are on Salvage Therapy?

The number of HIV-infected persons in America and Europe requiring salvage therapy is increasing rapidly. In America, between 30% and 50% of those in therapy are now in salvage therapy. Because these therapies are not proving effective, deaths due to AIDS are increasing. Fifteen percent who fail salvage therapy die within three years.

Throughout the developed world, 1 in 10 AIDS patients now requires salvage therapy because they carry HIV resistance to the drugs. About 1 in 50 of these patients is resistant to all 25 FDA-approved antiretroviral drugs. In 2002, French scientists began to use mega HAART or giga HAART therapy for those with limited treatment options. The theory behind using a larger number of drugs is that not all the virus in a person's body is going to be resistant to all the drugs. By using many drugs with different mechanisms of blocking HIV from reproducing, it may still be possible to achieve a potent anti-HIV effect. This salvage or rescue regime consists of the following drugs: three to four nucleoside reverse transcription inhibitors (NRTIs), hydroxyurea, one or two non-NRTI, and three to four protease inhibitors. Continued studies will determine the safety and effectiveness of mega/giga HAART therapies.

Genotypic and Phenotypic Drug Resistant/Susceptibility Profiles

Determining the specific drug-resistant and drug susceptibility profiles for a strain of HIV can be very useful in order to establish when a change in therapy will best suit the patient and, if necessary, to begin a plausible salvage therapy.

Genotypic Analysis

Establishing a list of genetic mutations or changes in HIV or RNA related to drug resistance is called genotypic analysis and indicates a given HIV's genetic resistance to a given drug. Each HIV genetic change or mutation to a drug is listed by a license-plate-looking name such as "K103N," which means that none of the nonnukes will work in the patient. Note that when HIV becomes resistant to one drug, it can, at the same time, become resistant to others that function in the same manner (cross-resistance). The suspected degree of drug resistance, as suggested from genotypic analysis, can be measured directly by adding the drug in question to an HIV-cell culture and determining the HIV's ability to reproduce.

Phenotypic Analysis

A virus-culture-drug assay is called phenotypic analysis. A check is made to see if HIV's resistance to a given drug correlates to a given genetic mutation and if other mutations offer a cross-resistance to that drug. In this way, drugs that work against the different HIV mutants can be used in salvage therapy.

Phenotypic results are easier to interpret than genotyping results because they do not require the expert interpretation of complex mutation patterns. The drug susceptibility data provide information for the clinician to select a treatment effective against the viral population circulating in the patient's blood. The main use of phenotypic assays at present is to identify those antiretroviral drugs that still retain activity against the patient's virus. They are also useful to detect transmission of drug-resistant virus and to monitor HIV patients during early viral rebound. In essence, phenotypic testing provides information to target antiretroviral therapy against the predominant HIV variant in the patient.

However, phenotype testing is very expensive at $800 to $1,000 per test. Because of the time element (about two to five weeks) and cost, such testing is not readily available to the patient. Thus, patients rely on the cheaper (about $400 to $500) and faster (one week) genotypic testing. Most third-party payers do not cover these tests. Genotype analysis is now available through five commercial laboratories and phenotype testing in two.

In general, resistance tests can't predict which drugs will work—only the ones that don't—which is why they're mostly recommended to help people whose regimens are failing. As with viral load tests, it's critical to be consistent about which tests you use. For now, most often, the decision to change drug therapy is based primarily on increases in viral load.

VIRAL LOAD: ITS RELATIONSHIP TO HIV DISEASE AND AIDS

Viral load refers to the number of HIV RNA strands in the blood plasma or serum of HIV-infected persons (a discussion of HIV RNA production is provided in Chapter 3; also see referenced material, Jurriaans et al., 1994; Henrard et al., 1995; Goldschmidt et al., 1998). In general, two to six weeks after HIV exposure, infected individuals develop a high level of blood plasma HIV RNA. Methods now exist to quantitate the amount of HIV RNA in the blood plasma or serum of HIV-infected people. (**Plasma** is a transparent yellow fluid that makes up about 55% of blood volume. Removing fibrinogen and blood clotting factors from plasma results in **serum**.) The reduction of viral load with the use of antiretroviral drugs can slow the destruction of the immune system. Viral load is also an indicator of viral replication. For measurement of viral load, see Chapter 13.

The Purpose of HIV Viral Load Testing

If a patient is not taking anti-HIV drugs, his or her viral load will be monitored during regular clinic visits to provide clues about the likely course of HIV disease if left untreated. Among people with the same T4 or CD4+ cell count, those with higher viral loads tend to have more rapid disease progression than those with lower viral loads.

Physicians recommend viral load testing for the following reasons:

◆ to help you make decisions about starting or changing drug treatment for HIV;

◆ to find out your risk for disease progression;

◆ to show how well your drug regimen is working;

◆ to help determine your HIV disease stage.

Undetectable Viral Load

An undetectable viral load has been proposed as the gold standard of HIV treatment by the guidelines used in the past few years. Suppressing viral load below the limits of detection results in the greatest reduction in the risk of death or illness. Undetectable viral load is one of the aims of antiretroviral therapy. However, the definition of "undetectable" viral load is constantly changing as the technology used to measure viral load improves. An undetectable viral load result indicates that a specific viral load test cannot find any HIV in a given blood sample. An undetectable result does not mean that the blood is free of HIV. In fact, most people with undetectable viral load have HIV in their blood, as well as in tissue, and bodily fluids. For each viral load test, there is a lower limit of detection—a limit below which it is not possible to measure the amount of HIV present. Samples with very low levels of HIV, for example below 50 copies/ml, are described as having a viral load that is undetectable, or below the level of detection. The higher an individual's viral load before starting treatment, the greater the reduction in viral load required to bring it down to undetectable levels. For this reason, some clinicians recommend more aggressive treatment to people with very high viral load compared to people with lower viral load (Palmer et al., 2008).

When Is Viral RNA Found in the Plasma?

HIV RNA strands are present during *all stages* of the disease, and the viral load increases with more advanced disease (Piatak et al., 1993; Saksela et al., 1994). Following infection with HIV, there is usually a rapid increase of HIV proteins and RNA followed by a lengthy period of viral RNA replication at lower but measurable amounts (Figure 4-9). In well-characterized groups with known dates of HIV seroconversion, a high viral load immediately after seroconversion (Mellors et al., 1995) and at three years after seroconversion (Jurriaans et al., 1994) appear to be strong predictors of HIV disease progression.

MEDICAL COMPLICATIONS ASSOCIATED WITH ANTI-HIV DRUG THERAPIES (ART)

The term "medical complications" is used herein to describe clinical problems in the management of HIV infection. Most doctors now agree that not everyone infected with HIV needs to take antiretroviral drugs. But everyone with HIV does need medical monitoring and care and access to treatment when and if appropriate. Because those taking antiretroviral treatment have had a fraction of the death rate of those without treatment does not necessarily mean that one's chance of survival will be correspondingly increased by antiretrovirals. The reduced death rates reflect the benefit of treatment for those who have needed and responded to it. (Bozzette et al., 2001; Freedberg et al., 2001).

For those who think AIDS is over—it is not.

For those who think the drugs are working well—they do for some people, for a number of years.

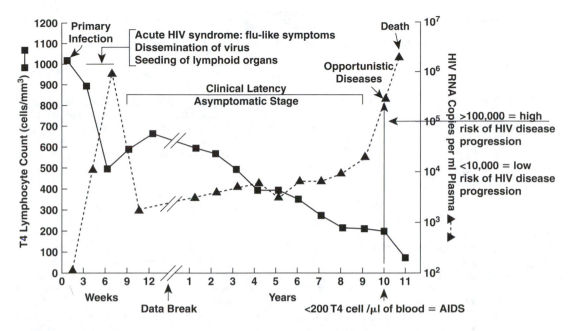

FIGURE 4-9 Clinical Course of HIV Disease as Related to T4 Cell Count and Level (number of HIV RNA Copies (Viral Load) in Plasma. In an Average Patient Without Antiretroviral Therapy: Primary Infection to Death. During primary infection (the time period between infection and development of HIV antibody), HIV RNA levels spike (*triangles*) and HIV disseminates throughout the body. This is followed by an abrupt drop in measurable HIV RNA in the blood (probably due to the production of HIV antibody), followed by a steady rise in HIV RNA until death. Over these same time periods, there is a continuous loss of T4 cells (*squares*). Note that the asymptomatic stage can be quite long—on average about 10 to 12 years, at which time T4 cell counts drop and HIV RNA copies increase to levels where there is high risk of opportunistic infections.

Side Effects of HAART

AIDS really is not yet manageable if it is not survivable. Rounding out what has been learned about anti-HIV drug toxicity is that HIV drugs are implicated in lipodystrophy, heart problems, bone loss (hip replacement), intercellular malfunctions called mitochondriosis (my-toe-con-dree-o-sis), lactic acidosis, and liver and kidney dysfunction and failure. Mitochondriosis is mitochondrial dysfunction—some side effects include fat redistribution syndrome, commonly referred to as lipodystrophy. "Lipo" (short for lipodystrophy) is an umbrella term for the gain or loss of fat where you weren't quite expecting it. (See Point of Information 4.3, page 94.) Additional side effects associated with mitochondrial toxicity that interrupts cellular energy production that leads to fatigue are shortness of breath, weight loss, rapid heartbeat, hair loss, numbness and pain in the hands, arms, feet, and legs, muscle disease, heart disease, inflammation of the pancreas, increased blood

acidity, and kidney irregularities. Add in various opportunistic infections and the drug toxicities required to treat them, and one finds many surviving AIDS patients have become antiviral and antibiotic multidrug resistant. These AIDS patients require stronger and more toxic remedies month after month and year after year. Ultimately one eventually dies, either from infection or from complications from treatments.

The leading cause of HIV/AIDS-related death in the United States now that ART is available to most is HIV-associated liver failure, cardiovascular events, diabetes, and a variety of cancers.

Management of HIV/AIDS: Treat Early, Treat Late?

Building the Ship as It Sails—There are at least three major decisions that have to be made early in the management of HIV/AIDS patients. The **first** is when to begin antiretroviral therapy, the

MY PROBLEMS OR SIDE EFFECTS ASSOCIATED WITH TAKING MY ANTIRETROVIRAL MEDICINES

by Jonathan Kivett, 2007

So I am starting on my pile of pills. Two Kaletra, an AZT, two Invirase, Bactrim. Add to the mix a Claritin and a couple of Tylenol for the inevitable headaches. I will wash it down with a teaspoon of Mepron (for my PCP), and make sure I eat a full high-fat meal with it. The meds have made my taste buds interpret anything as metallic. I'm bitching, I know. Worst part? I isolated myself from anyone who might want to come over and hang out, mainly because Kaletra gives a person gas beyond my capacity to articulate. It's the worst stuff, that's why forensic examiners dab Noxema or Menthol ointment under their nose before unzipping a body bag. It's like being an over inflated bag of humiliation. But I digress.

Thing is, I have a viral load well over 500,000. I have roughly 40 T4 or CD4+ cells left to play with. My round of *pneumocystis carinii* pneumonia (PCP) has left me weak, tired, skinny, and far closer to the other side of the dirt than I would prefer. I would love to have more time to research the meds, to wait for the next development, to fundamentally change my life, my personality, address the myriad of issues which have historically impacted my adherence to and management of the highly effective, yet highly toxic meds available for HIV treatment. Many of the meds I have tried in the past have been reformulated, re-configured, made easier to tolerate and at lower doses. Many more meds, including some great integrase inhibitors, are set to be released in 2007. But, time, though, is a luxury I don't seem to have. When I asked my doctor what the difference was between starting a med regimen NOW and waiting till sometime in 2007, waiting for the new stuff, he just looked at me and shook his head. I have lost about a hundred T4 cells since I started getting sick in August. Don't have a hundred more to lose. Zero, apparently, is not a good number at which to start HAART therapy. And he said point-blank that I would not be in good shape if I waited. So he put me on this older regimen (with an added extra PI boost of Invirase) to tide me over, hoping I would start reconstructing a semblance of an immune system, and beat back that viral load while we all wait. Wait for the better drugs to become available.

But while I wait, I stare at my pile of pills. Twenty-one pills a day, not counting the liquid PCP treatment/preventative or the clonazepam that helps me to sleep at night. The cost of these meds, if one is paying full retail, is staggering. I am looking at over three thousand dollar's worth of medication per month. Add to that the monthly doctor visits and lab work, and my survival retails for around four thousand dollars per month. The only way I can receive these drugs, this treatment, is by remaining impoverished and at the mercy of governmental assistance. This does not escape my emotional attention, and the sense of shame and stigma is sometimes just a little more than I can easily bear.

Ten of these pills carry side effects which range from the annoying to the debilitating. My favorite rooms in the apartment are the bed and the bathroom. Old Kaletra gave me scarcely controllable explosive diarrhea seventeen times a day. A new formulation of Kaletra shaves that down to ten times a day, give or take my amount of caloric intake or the stupid notion that I could walk to the laundry room and back. The AZT gives me anemia, headaches and fevers. In order to maintain my existence, I know I am sacrificing my health. So for the time being, each time I put the pile of pills in front of me, I cringe. They are nasty, horrible tasting things. But something in me wants to live just a touch more than it wants to die.

My adherence sucks. My history with the meds sucks. But whatever I have done, I have turned what could have, maybe SHOULD have been a plummet into the earth into a semi-controlled glide just staying on this side of the grass. It's taken me a LONG time to get really sick, and my failed attempts, a month here, three months there, to adhere to therapy have bought me time. Time for the next big thing to come out, time for the research to move just ahead of my virus and its destination, my death. Time for me to embark on crazy stuff that everyone does, from self-medication to serial dating to growing older, gaining gray on my hair and some perspective in my heart.

But time is up.

So I gag down the pills in hope of feeling JUST a little better. Staying alive a little longer. I settle in for an evening of television, ferret cuddling, extended moments to the bathroom and horrible gas. I pour some more Coke Zero out of the can. I wait for the foam to settle before taking the glass to my lips. Giving it time.

Giving time to the both of us.

(Jonathan spends his better days writing and playing with his ferrets.)

second is which drugs to use to initiate treatment, and the **third** is how long to administer a given therapy.

Clinicians face a dilemma of choice when advising asymptomatic patients with established HIV infection on when to begin highly active antiretroviral therapy (HAART) and what drugs to use. Begin early, some researchers advise, because later there will be a higher virologic hurdle to overcome. Begin later, others recommend, and save potent drugs until the patient's immune system begins to fail. If therapy is started too early, cumulative side effects of the drugs used and the development of multidrug resistance may outweigh the net benefits. If therapy is started too late, increases in disease progression and mortality outweigh the benefits (Table 4-3).

In order to assess the very best time to initiate antiretroviral therapy, one needs to know the goal of antiviral therapy. Most HIV/AIDS physicians would agree that the goal is multidimensional: to prolong life while improving the quality of life; to suppress HIV replication to the limits of detection for as long as possible; to select the best possible therapy for the individual; and to minimize costs and side effects to drug therapy. With these goals in mind, and the drugs available to suppress HIV replication and extend life with quality, the first question remains "When should one begin antiretroviral therapy?"

U.S. Department of Health and Human Services (DHHS) Guidelines and International AIDS Society-USA (IAS-USA) Recommendations for the Use of Antiretroviral Therapy (May 2006, October 2006, updated November 2008)

There are no "one size fits all" treatment guidelines. Over the last 12 years it has been learned that antiretroviral therapy is becoming more individualized.

In general, the DHHS guidelines and IAS-USA recommendations are the most aggressive on when to start therapy, followed by French guidelines. The Brazilians are the least aggressive, recommending dual nucleoside therapy for those with earlier disease and lower viral loads. Overall, the various guidelines involve expensive strategies that can only be used in more developed countries, or in the wealthier sectors of less developed countries.

The current guidelines now list T4 or CD4+ count below 350 cells/mm^3 as the most significant

---

Table 4–3 Risks and Benefits of Early Versus Delayed Initiation of Antiretroviral Therapy

Benefits	Risks
EARLY THERAPY	
Control of viral replication may be easier to achieve and maintain	Drug-related reduction in quality of life
	Greater cumulative drug-related adverse events
Possible delay or prevention of immune system compromise	Earlier emergence of drug resistance if viral suppression is suboptimal
Lower risk of resistance with optimal viral suppression	Limitation of future antiretroviral treatment options
Possible decreased risk of HIV transmission	
DELAYED THERAPY	
Avoid negative effects on quality of life	Possible risk of irreversible immune system depletion
Avoid drug-related adverse events	Possible greater difficulty in suppressing viral replication
Delay emergence of drug resistance	Possible increased risk of HIV transmission
Preserve maximum number of future drug options when HIV disease risk is highest	

(Adapted from U.S. Department of Health and Human Services, 2002 updated.)

The optimal time to initiate antiretroviral therapy in asymptomatic HIV-infected patients with CD4+ cell counts above 200/μL of blood is not known and remains a controversial issue. At the Tenth Conference on Retroviruses and Opportunistic Diseases, Martin Hirsch provided an excellent summary of the current data. Patients do not do as well on HAART if they start when their CD4+ count is <200 cells/μL or viral load is >100,000 cells/mL, so it is clear that therapy should be started before patients reach these benchmarks. However, the T4 or CD4+ count above 200 cells/μL at which therapy should be started is unclear, and opinions will likely change as therapy becomes more convenient, tolerable, and less toxic.

RESULTS OF VIRAL LOAD AND QUESTIONS PEOPLE ASK

RESULTS OF VIRAL LOAD TESTS

Results of viral load tests can range from almost zero to over a million; low numbers mean fewer viruses in the blood and less active disease; high numbers mean a more active disease.

RELEVANCE OF VIRAL LOAD TESTING

Researchers are still trying to decide on the important values for viral load. In general, though, results can be interpreted as follows:

HIV Viral Load Result	Interpretation Death within 6 years
5000 or fewer	6%
10,000 or fewer	18%
10,000 to 30,000	35%
Over 30,000 copies	70%

Experimental viral load tests can now detect as few as 5 to 20 RNA strands/mL. Current tests in use measure between 50 and 400 RNA strands/mL.

DETECTABLE VERSUS UNDETECTABLE LEVELS OF HIV RNA

Detectable

The lower a person's viral load, the less likely they are to progress to AIDS. The effectiveness of anti-HIV drugs is usually measured in terms of the percentage of people who achieve viral loads below 50 and 400 copies/mL after a set period of time. For example, a *trial will* find out how many people on a particular drug combination are below 50 copies after six months of treatment.

Undetectable

Many individuals have an undetectable level of HIV RNA in their blood after taking combination therapy. But undetectable RNA levels do not mean that the person is cured or no longer infectious. An undetectable RNA level means that too few RNA strands are present to measure. The number of RNA strands is below the level of tests of sensitivity.

Achieving undetectable viral loads is now the gold standard for successful HIV treatment. The more rapidly one's viral load becomes undetectable and the longer it remains suppressed, the better the chance for long-term survival. A measurable viral load after it was once undetectable is regarded as a sign of drug failure. Never reaching undetectability is also considered a drug failure for that person.

Jane Simoni and colleagues (2003) reported that, on average, only 50% of AIDS patients on antiretroviral therapy (HAART) achieve HIV RNA levels below detection limits. The major reason for not doing so is patients' poor adherence to medical regimens (see Point of Information 4.3). A few studies have shown that some people have maintained undetectable levels of HIV for the past 13 years. Not everyone achieves undetectable levels.

TYPICAL QUESTIONS ABOUT VIRAL LOAD

1. **What is the viral set point?** The viral set point represents an equilibrium between the virus, which wants to replicate, and the host, which tries to control or contain the replication (viral reproduction is about equal to viral clearance). It appears that each patient establishes his or her own set point within two to six months after initial infection with HIV. HIV drugs appear to alter the set point for HIV by reducing its ability to replicate. This helps lower the body viral load and gives the body a chance to restore some of the lost immune function.

2. **What is the cost of a viral load test? Does insurance pay for it?** Beginning 2009, a viral load test cost between $150 and $250. Some insurance policies pay for the test.

3. **If a viral load test result was 12,000 and six months later it is 18,000, is the change important?** Viral load may rise and fall without any change in health. The rule of thumb is that viral load change is not significant unless it more than doubles.

4. **How often should viral load be measured?** Measuring viral load every four months, at the same time T4 or CD4+ cells are measured, has been suggested.

5. **Can viral load be associated with determining anti-HIV therapy?** Measuring viral load about four weeks after changing antiretroviral medications can be useful for finding out whether the new treatment is working.

6. **A person's T4 cells had been between 400 and 600 for several years, and suddenly his viral load rose to 50,000 and his physician recommended drug therapy. Why?** Research suggests that people with viral loads over 10,000 are at higher risk for the progression of HIV disease, regardless of T4 or CD4+ cell counts.

MONETARY REASONS FOR PRODUCING ANTIRETROVIRAL DRUGS

From a drug developer's standpoint, AIDS must be the most attractive disease on earth. There are five obvious reasons: (1) the drugs are very expensive, (2) many patients are privately insured because they are healthy and working, (3) thanks to advocacy groups the government pays for drugs for many people who can't afford them, (4) the drugs don't cure anybody, and (5) they appear to be necessary for a lifetime! Where else in American medicine is there a population of uninsured patients of whom 79% have access to HIV/AIDS antiretroviral drug therapy that costs between $12,000 and $20,000 a year? Is there anywhere else in American medicine where such expensive health care has been made available to the poor and disenfranchised populations? According to the U.S. Department of Health and Human Services, 60% of those needing HAART therapy receive it.

ECONOMICS OF PRODUCING ANTIRETROVIRAL DRUGS

In 1998, the markets for HIV/AIDS therapeutics totaled more than $2 billion in U.S. revenues and according to industry consultants Frost & Sullivan (http://www.frost.com), these markets are projected to reach $20 billion ending 2009. These figures represent revenues derived from the following HIV drug product classes: protease inhibitors (PIs), nucleoside reverse transcriptase inhibitors (NRTIs), and non-nucleoside reverse transcriptase inhibitors (NNRTIs).

DEATH PREVENTION PROFITS

In 1995 there were 55,000 AIDS-related deaths. Using the new antiretroviral drugs, in 1996 the number of deaths fell to 38,000. By 1998 deaths dropped to 18,000, and by 2002 to about 17,000. Using 1995 as a baseline for number of deaths, each year thereafter the fewer that died, the greater the number that must continue to take the drugs for the rest of their lives. Until there are preventative and therapeutic vaccines, or some form of cure available, the number of drug consumers continues to grow. In the United States an estimated 56,000 plus new HIV infections now occur each year. Why wouldn't a company commit itself to producing HIV/AIDS drugs? Tony Casper (2000) reported that the profits on antiretroviral drugs are enormous. He gave the following examples: In 1999, Glaxo Wellcome made $589 million on $4.1 billion of Combivir (AZT + 3TC) sales. Profits between 1997 and 2001 for AZT, about $800 million; for 3TC about $1.6 billion; for ddl about $400 million and for d4T $1.4 billion. Yielding to political and foreign competitive drug production and pricing, the world's major drug companies like Boehringer, Glaxo SmithKline, Roche, Merck, and Bristol-Myers Squibb have drastically lowered their drug pricing policies in the underdeveloped nations in Africa and Asia. They say that their prices are near to or at cost.

---

threshold to consider in deciding when antiretroviral treatment is recommended, or should at least be offered to the patient. All HIV-positive individuals who are symptomatic or are aymptomatic and have a CD4+ count below 200 cells/mm^3—irrespective of the viral load—should be receiving antiretroviral treatment. Patients with a CD4+ count above 200 cells/mm,^{3} but below 350 cells/mm,^{3} should be offered treatment, irrespective of the viral load, although this is still considered to be a controversial recommendation. Entering 2009, the long-term benefits of when to start antiretroviral therapy are still being discussed. At best, the different studies on the subject lead to confusion because similar studies have produced conflicting/contradictory results. This point was clearly presented at the 14th Conference on

Retroviruses and Opportunistic Infections in February 2007 and again in the January 2008 Department of Human Services Guidelines.

Antiretrovirals Not to Be Used!

Important in the updated guidelines is the list of antiviral drugs and drug combinations that should not be offered at any time. Theoretically, a physician has over 15,000 separate three-drug combinations available to him. But many of the combinations will be harmful. The question is which? (25 FDA-approved drugs used in combinations of three at a time equals 25^3 equals 15,625 possibilities.)

The new guidelines also caution against the use of interrupted therapy. They also provide information

CURRENT PROBLEMS USING ANTI-HIV THERAPY

First, Duration: Many patients ask how long they will have to continue therapy; how long will they have to be harnessed to pills and doctors?

Second, Adherence or Compliance: You don't have to like them, you just have to take them! Healthcare providers have been dealing with the issue of client **adherence** or **compliance** for centuries. The medical literature shows that it is difficult for patients to adhere to even the simplest treatment regimens. Factors associated with poor adherence include unstable housing, mental illness, and major life crises. Also adding to adherence problems are pill burden, pill size, frequency and timing of dose, dietary and/or water requirements or restrictions, liquid formulations, unpleasant drug taste, adverse events, storage requirements, number of prescriptions, and other factors such as the number of co-payments, refills, and medication bottles. **Adherence** to a drug regimen means taking all the prescribed anti-HIV drugs at the scheduled times and not missing any doses. Any time people are asked to change and/or maintain new behaviors to treat an existing condition or to prevent a threatened one, there is a good chance that they will not comply, consistently and correctly, to the prescribed activities. **The Achilles heel of anti-HIV therapy:** Skipping only a few pills can trigger the emergence of drug-resistant strains of HIV. This could create a condition worse than the initial infection because the drug-resistant virus could overwhelm the individual taking the drugs and anyone else to whom the individual transmitted the virus.

Playing Doctor: There is a present danger that the behavior of underdosing (not taking enough) or partial compliance (taking the drug when they feel like it) or patients who modify their dosage regimens—to extend their prescription—may create HIV strains resistant to all currently available drugs. The major reason given by HIV-positive people on anti-HIV therapy for missing doses was, I FORGOT! (33%).

Stephen Beeker and colleagues (2002) report a mean overall adherence rate of only 53% among a population of over 3700 Medicaid recipients. Barely one-quarter of subjects achieved an adherence rate of 80% or higher, and adherence was worst among those aged 18–24 years.

Class Adherence Experiment: For an HIV class experience on adherence at the University of North Florida, 50 students aged 18–24 were asked to take either three or four different-colored M & M candies representing four different antiretroviral drugs, at three specified times per day between six in the morning and midnight for three days (Friday through Sunday). They were given the colored M & Ms and a dosing schedule sheet to record their compliance. After completion of the experiment, class compliance at 100%, 90%, 80%, and 70% was zero! Their overall comment—now we can better relate to what it must be like for those who must be compliant.

DISCUSSION QUESTION: Do you think the results would be much different in your college or university HIV/AIDS class?

Clearly much more needs to be done to improve rates of adherence, or many patients will be embarking on a rapid route to resistance and treatment failure.

Third, Drug Costs in America: Larry Kramer, a cofounder of Gay Men's Health Crises, states that the cost of his drugs to combat AIDS, which do not include a protease, amounts to about $19,000 a year; this does not include visits to his doctor or the batteries of blood tests he routinely requires. *A New York Times* article estimated that drugs for someone with symptomatic AIDS cost about $70,000 a year. In response, a New York University adjunct law professor and gay-rights advocate wrote a letter to the editor saying that his drugs cost $84,000 a year using protease inhibitors; the annual drug cost can exceed $150,000. At these prices, how many of the nation's HIV infected will be able to afford proper HIV therapy? AT THESE PRICES PEOPLE HAVE TO CHOOSE WHETHER TO PAY RENT, BUY FOOD, OR PAY FOR THEIR MEDICINE—SOME CHOICE! MANY PEOPLE WITH HIV/AIDS TURN TO VIATICAL OR LIFE INSURANCE SETTLEMENTS

The viatical industry started in 1989 because people with AIDS were becoming bankrupt due to their medical expenses. Selling a life insurance policy is called viatification. If you want to sell a life insurance policy, you can sell it directly to a viatical investment company (Figure 4-10). A viatical investment company finds investors who want to buy life insurance policies, and it finds people who want to sell their policies. The company pays the person selling their policy a percentage of the policy's value, and when the person dies, the company receives the life insurance benefits and pays the investors. Before potent antiviral medications were available, viatical companies paid as much as 85% of a policy's face value. Since the introduction of effective therapies, offers have fallen to around 30% of face value. Peo-

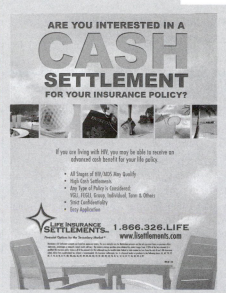

FIGURE 4-10 Viatification—Selling a Life Insurance Policy. (*Courtesy Life Insurance Settlements*)

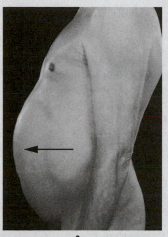

FIGURE 4-11 Protease Paunch—Also Referred to as Crix Belly. This lipid disorder (lipodystrophy) occurs in many patients using protease inhibitors for anti-HIV therapy. In addition to the visual effects of antiretroviral therapy, there are a number of dangerous side effects—see text for details. (*Photograph courtesy of Dr. David Cooper*)

ple with HIV/AIDS are living longer, so the investors must wait longer for payment.

Fourth. Effectiveness of Antiretroviral Therapy Causing Complacency Among High-Risk Groups: Success using ATR has led to complacency with regard to high-risk sexual behavior, which in turn has resulted in a rise in numbers of new HIV infections. Regardless of whether the ARTs are effective in blocking HIV replication, there is evidence that HIV-infected people are more susceptible to a number of cancers and other health conditions that are considered rare in the general population. This occurs because the virus causes nonrepairable damage to the immune system.

Fifth, side effects: The paradox of HIV treatment is that sometimes the cure feels worse than the disease, especially when treatment begins before symptoms arise. Sometimes the cure also looks worse than the disease. For example, abnormal fat redistribution or **lipodystrophy,** can appear at a time when a person's HIV might otherwise be invisible—both to others and to him or herself. Lipodystrophy occurs particularly on the abdomen—central obesity, referred to as the **protease paunch** (Figure 4-11)—and on the back between the shoulder blades, called **"buffalo hump"** (Figure 4-12) and may include a loss of fatty tissue in the arms, legs, and face. Women may experience narrowing of the hips and breast enlargement. HIV-infected children placed on HAART therapy also experienced lipodystrophy (Vigan et al., 2003).

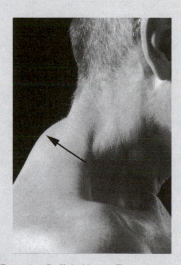

FIGURE 4-12 Buffalo Hump. The enlargement of a cervicodorsal fat pad. Buffalo hump develops after the use of protease inhibitors for anti-HIV therapy. In addition to the visual effects of antiretroviral therapy, there are a number of other dangerous side effects—see text for details. (*Photograph courtesy of Dr. David Cooper*)

BOX 4.2

TESTING OF ANTI-HIV DRUGS FOR POST-EXPOSURE PREVENTION (PEP)

The Forum—A woman has sex with her HIV-positive husband and the condom breaks. A woman is raped by a man who is HIV-positive. A child is sodomized by an HIV-positive male. A prison guard is bitten by an HIV-positive inmate. A couple has unprotected sex—a one-night stand. These were some of the cases brought up by experts as they debated whether doctors should be prescribing AIDS drugs as a morning-after or *Post Exposure Prophylaxis* or prevention (PEP) treatment for those exposed to HIV.

In mid-October 1997, San Francisco became the first city in the United States to offer new PEP drugs to individuals trying to prevent HIV infection.

TIMING IS EVERYTHING

72-Hour Window—The standard of practice for about four years at most medical centers is to offer antiviral drugs promptly when healthcare workers of AIDS patients are stuck with needles or come into contact with body fluids from infected patients. New federal guidelines recommend ART drug treatment using three antiretroviral drugs each day for 28 days, starting no later than 72 hours after exposure.

Resources—The following resource is available for consultation regarding HIV PEP: PEPline http://www.ucsf.edu/ hivcntr/Hotlines/PEPline Telephone: 1-888-448-4911

About 80% of U.S. health-care workers are female and many of them are of child bearing age. PEP would appear to be a very important procedure for them.

As of the beginning of 2009 about 1500 American healthcare workers have received PEP care—20 have become HIV positive, but they admitted to continuing to practice high-risk behavior. Regardless, over the past 14 years, PEP has become the standard of care for occupational exposure to HIV.

Treatment Guidelines—In 1998, the CDC issued guidelines for the use of PEP by people in the health-care setting (occupational exposure to HIV). In 2005,

the CDC issued guidelines for the use of PEP for everyone else.

What Are Disadvantages of PEP?—One of the biggest fears about PEP is that people will return to unsafe sexual and drug-using practices if they believe that PEP will prevent them from becoming infected. There is some evidence that treatment advances, including PEP, may be leading to increasing incidence of unsafe sex in the United States. For example, rates of gonorrhea among men who have sex with men have recently increased for the first time since the early 1980s. There is a wide spectrum of situations to consider, but there are no absolutes when it comes to the right choices regarding PEP. PEP after HIV exposure is recommended because of the knowledge that in some cases it works. It is well recognized that the use of ZDV in pregnant women dramatically reduced vertical transmission of HIV to newborns. It is therefore conceivable that the use of antiretroviral medication following sexual exposure to HIV will also be effective. However, studies to date remain controversial (Pinkerton et al., 2004 updated).

Caution—Clearly this is not a morning-after pill. The treatment is not foolproof, but it offers an important safety net to prevent HIV infection in certain cases. It shouldn't be considered a substitute for more reliable ways to avoid getting infected with HIV, such as abstinence, monogamy, or condom use. Epidemiologist Lisa Grohskopf of the CDC's Division of HIV/AIDS Prevention said studies have shown that an antiretroviral drug regimen cut the risk of HIV infection by 80% in healthcare workers exposed on the job. The CDC said that PEP is not recommended for habitual drug users who share needles or for people who frequently engage in risky sex. Those people would have to take antiretroviral drugs practically nonstop, which the health agency does not endorse.

DISCUSSION QUESTION: With your current knowledge about HIV/AIDS, if you knew that you had just been exposed to HIV would you ask for immediate therapy? Why?

on the use of drug combination pills and on testing for HIV drug resistance. The latest update to the guidelines includes recommendations for which antiretroviral drugs should be used during pregnancy in order to reduce the transmission of HIV from mother to fetus/newborn.

The Future for HAART–SMART?

The National Institute of Allergies and Infectious Disease (NIAID) was funding a $120 million study to resolve which is the best HAART strategy—Hit Early-Hit Hard, Hit Later-Hit Carefully or Hit and Run, that is, Interrupted Therapy.

The main study questions in SMART were:

1. Is it better to *Use* antiretroviral drugs continuously to keep the amount of virus in the blood as low as possible regardless of CD4+ cell count? or,
2. Is it better to *Wait* and *Not use* antiretroviral drugs during times when the CD4+ count is higher than 250 and the risk of becoming ill is low?

THE SMART TRIAL WAS CANCELLED ON JANUARY 11, 2006.

Reason: The independent Data and Safety Monitoring Board showed that participants who took their antiretroviral drugs on an irregular basis were more than twice as likely to experience increased disease progression to AIDS or death compared with those on a daily treatment regimen. Patients taking episodic drug treatments also were more likely to experience cardiovascular and kidney complications as well as liver disease. In other words, the study teaches that interrupting therapy and tolerating low CD4 cell counts is a very bad idea! However, it should be noted that the cessation of SMART does not necessarily mean that all treatment strategies involving interruptions of antiretroviral therapy are dangerous, just that the specific approach employed by the SMART study design was less successful at preventing clinical events than continuous treatment. There is good scientific data suggesting that individuals who initiate therapy with relatively high CD4+ cell counts can safely interrupt therapy.

NOVEL DRUGS

Peptides and AntiSense Drugs as the Next Possible Antiretroviral Therapy

Tropical frogs have specialized granular glands in the skin that produce and store packets of peptides, small protein-like molecules. In response to skin injury or alarm, the frogs secrete large amounts of these antimicrobial peptides onto the surface of the skin to combat pathogens like bacteria, fungi and viruses (Van Compernolle et al., 2005). Scientists at Vanderbilt University screened 14 antimicrobial peptides from a variety of frog species for their ability to block HIV infection of CD4+ cells. They found several peptides that inhibited HIV infection without harming the immune cells. They speculated that the peptides destroyed HIV by creating holes in the

envelope, covering HIV, interrupting the integrity of the developing virus.

A second peptide was found in human blood, called **virus-inhibitory peptide** (VIRIP). The peptide has a chain length of 20 amino acids. Frank Kirchhoff and colleagues (2007) say that this peptide, in a test tube, inhibited 60 strains of HIV from infecting T4 lymphocytes. Like the antiretroviral drug Fuzeon, VIRIP inhibits HIV entry by interacting with gp41, a protein on the surface of HIV.

Further research using both the frog and human peptides will be continued.

Antisense Drugs

These are a mirror image of part of the HIV genetic code. The drug locks onto HIV DNA to prevent it from functioning. One antisense drug, HGTV43 by Enzo Therapeutics, is starting phase II trials.

VIRxSYS is testing a gene therapy product, VRX496, in a phase II trial. The product involves modifying a patient's own CD4 cells with an antisense factor and then reintroducing them to the patient.

The Once-a-Month Pill

Researchers are now working on a once-a-month pill to suppress HIV replication. If such a pill or injection can be achieved, it would be of significant benefit to those who use pre- and post-exposure ART.

DISCLAIMER

Knowledge about HIV/AIDS changes rapidly. This textbook is designed for educational purpose only and is not engaged in rendering medical advice or professional services. The author does not accept any responsibility for the accuracy of the information or the consequences arising from the application, use, or misuse of any of the information contained herein, including any injury and/or damage to any person or property as a matter of product liability, negligence, or otherwise. No warranty, expressed or implied, is made in regard to the contents of this material. Verify all information independently. This material is not intended as a guide to self-medication. The reader is advised to discuss the information provided here

GLOBAL AVAILABILITY OF HIV DRUG THERAPY

Table 4–4 Antiretroviral Drug Coverage for People with HIV/AIDS in Highly Affected
Countries, 2008

Estimated % of Antiretroviral Drug Coverage of Those Who Need Them

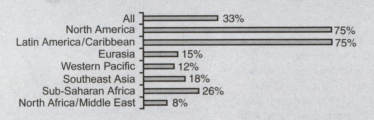

All	33%
North America	75%
Latin America/Caribbean	75%
Eurasia	15%
Western Pacific	12%
Southeast Asia	18%
Sub-Saharan Africa	26%
North Africa/Middle East	8%

Estimated number receiving ART, 3.3 million.

Estimated number who need ART, 9 to 10 million.

Adapted from Kaiser Education Tutorials. *Current State of the Global HIV/AIDS Epidemic,* 2006 updated.

The goal of the world Health organization is to have 10 million people on antiretrovirals by 2010.

THINKING POSITIVE, BUT WHAT IF?

For the first 27 years (1981–2008) of this pandemic, people have been told that AIDS kills. But now various organizations, the WHO, NIH, UNAIDS, and others are saying to the globally HIV infected that you can now live with this disease. The attempt here is to repackage and remarket a still-lethal disease into one with which if people will just educate themselves and find a source of anti-retroviral drugs globally, all will be well in the world of HIV/AIDS. The push in this message is to tell everyone their health is in their hands. With the latest estimates, that 9 to 10 million people who need antiretroviral drugs have little if any access to them, the new message may be meaningless. **First,** although about one million people began ART in 2008, there were 2.5 million new HIV infections. For every person going into treatment, about two or three are going to the back of the line. **Second,** while new medicines and improved services help people infected with HIV/AIDS live longer and more productive lives for those in the developed nations that can access them, the economic burden is high. This means that HIV is not just a health issue, it's also an issue in economics. Antiretroviral regimens can cost from $25,000 to over $100,000 per year.

LATE TREATMENT, NO TREATMENT, AND ADHERENCE

Despite ever-widening access to ART, the Joint United Nations Program on HIV/AIDS (UNAIDS) estimates that through 2008 only 21 countries provided antiretrovirals to at least 50% of people who needed them. Yet in the world's developed countries, even those with universal free access, surprisingly large numbers of people start treatment late, never get started, or have a hard time sticking with their regimens (schedules).

UNITED STATES: CHANGING ATTITUDES

From 1981 into 2009, the American public's attitude toward HIV infection has changed from terror to apathy. In many minds, HIV disease is considered a chronic disorder requiring doctor's appointments, medication, and intensive care, much like the deadly disease diabetes. With the variety of treatments available for HIV-positive patients today, success is measured in years instead of months. Life expectancies for the HIV infected have increased steadily from 1996 due to aggressive antiretroviral treatments such as HAART. The psychological effects of life-lengthening drug therapy are now very positive, allowing a patient who feels hopeless to begin to embrace the future. It is very important that the public understand that, although treatable, HIV is still a transmittable disease with no cure. With the increasing number of HIV strains becoming resistant to the current antiretrovirals, it is not too difficult to imagine this pandemic starting over. Still, the success the developed world is experiencing has created a backlash in the underdeveloped nations.

GLOBAL ANGER: POLITICS AND PEOPLE

In many parts of the world, entire societies are comprised of families surviving on less than $2 a day. And these societies are besieged by HIV/AIDS.

Widening gaps in access to antiretroviral drugs, creating glaring differences in life expectancies for America's HIV-infected population versus the vast majority of AIDS-affected people in the world, have become pivotal sources of global political anger. Resentment is building in both middle-income and poor nations; as the wealthiest nine nations thrive, the poorest nations witness the evaporation of previous development gains, rising foreign debts, and rising mortalities. Resentment can translate into support for anti-Europe and anti-Americanism in many forms. In 2004, the imams of northern Nigeria, for example, convinced mothers to shun polio vaccination for their children, on the premise that America put HIV in the vaccine—a successful propaganda campaign that has so far spawned a resurgence of crippling polio epidemics in Nigeria and at least 16 other predominately Muslim nations. Though many pharmaceutical companies have fought to protect high pricing schemes and patents at the expense of global access to affordable medicines, American firms have taken the brunt of the blame and are the target of a special anger bent on ignoring European and American medical patent rights in all their forms.

TREATMENT OPTIONS

With at least 25 antiretroviral drugs available in the United States and other developed nations, there are many options to explore. But treatment options in the developing world are limited, and the question of when to switch may ultimately be determined by what is available to switch to. For some, depending on which country they live in, there may be one first-line regime that is routinely prescribed because it is generally safe and effective, easy to dispense, and affordable to use in mass treatment programs. A second-line therapy, if one is available, will likely be much more expensive, and may be withdrawn due to futility once it has failed. For patients in these settings a second chance could be their last chance.

with a doctor, pharmacist, nurse, or other authorized healthcare practitioner and to check product information (including package inserts) regarding dosage, precautions, warnings, interactions, and contraindications before administering any drug, herb, or supplement discussed herein.

Summary

New results in the field of HIV therapy have given HIV-infected persons new hope in their battle against HIV disease and AIDS. First, combinations of nucleoside analogs were shown to have a clinical benefit (prolonged survival and fewer AIDS-defining events) when given to symptomatic individuals. Next came the demonstration of the extraordinary capability of protease inhibitors. The introduction of the protease inhibitors is the most powerful intervention against HIV to date. Marked reductions in viral load, striking clinical improvement, and reduction in mortality have been observed among patients able to take these medications *properly*. Whether to initiate protease inhibitor therapy in the very early stages of HIV disease is controversial.

Neither protease inhibitors, nucleoside, or non-nucleoside inhibitors work for all HIV-infected persons; the reasons for this lack of efficacy are not completely understood. Long-term adverse effects of protease inhibitors are beginning to show.

Antiviral drugs have certainly shown tremendous success in reversing the trend of HIV infection that leads to disease. But with up to 40% of treated individuals now showing HIV strains that are strongly resistant to anti-HIV drugs, the reality of the dangerous cellular reservoirs of HIV must be better understood.

Looking at the problem of resistance, it's now known that unless the virus is virtually eliminated from the blood—again, an unlikely prospect—it's only a matter of time before a viral mutant emerges that is resistant to therapy. Current estimates are that the virus mutates once each time it copies itself—over 1 billion times a day. It's like going to Las Vegas. HIV just keeps spinning its bases (its genetic building blocks), looking for a jackpot.

Over the past year, progress in HIV has continued to resemble an electrocardiogram. The sharp dips represent difficult roadblocks that have blunted our hopes for a cure. The peaks mark scientific breakthroughs and new approaches used to bring HIV under control. As we enter the year 2009 and move through the new millennium, the overall picture remains mixed and varies greatly among individuals battling the virus. But there are many reasons to be optimistic and even excited about the state of research, at least from a scientific point of view, without losing sight of the real battles to be faced. In 2006, 2007, and 2008, several exciting new antiretrovirals emerged from the research laboratories. Atripla, a once-a-day nucleoside combination pill which has fewer side effects and drastically reduced adherence problems, became available in 2006 along with a very effective new protease—darunavir (Presista). In 2007 a second very effective entrance inhibitor was FDA-approved, maraviroc (trade name Selzentry), which blocks the R5 receptor on CD4+ cells. Also, the HIV integrase inhibitor Raltegravir received FDA approval. In 2008 etravirine, a new non nucleoside drug, received FDA approval.

Concerns about serious drug side effects and drug resistance linked to long-term use of HIV combination therapies have replaced optimism, causing a growing number of people on therapy to reconsider the benefits versus the risk of potent antiviral therapies and to seek alternative approaches. In response, pharmaceutical manufacturers have worked to simplify drug regimens and create more potent, less toxic products. It appears now that HIV/AIDS scientists and clinicians may have been a bit too optimistic about what the drugs could do. Today the treatment community is unanimous about one thing: The next generation of drugs must be more powerful and easier to take. They should also improve the problems associated with the present generation of drugs, such as toxic side effects, resistance, dosing, absorption, and bioavailability (the active part of a drug that's available to fight the virus).

At the moment, current treatments are inadequate. HAART has given people time, but it has not provided a cure. At best, antiretroviral drugs have slowed disease progression. The drugs are complicated to administer, require close medical monitoring, and can cause significant side effects. They are also very costly and, as a result, are inaccessible to the majority of people living with HIV/AIDS in underdeveloped nations.

Some AIDS Therapy Information Hotlines

For HIV/AIDS treatment information, call:

The American Foundation for AIDS Research: 1-800-39AMFAR (392-6237)

AIDS Treatment Data Network: 1-800-734-7104

AIDS Treatment News: 1-800-TREAT 1-2 (873-2812)

National HIV Treatment: 1-800-822-7422

For information about AIDS/HIV clinical trials conducted by National Institutes of Health and Food and Drug Administration-approved efficacy trials, call:

National AIDS Clinical Trials Information Service (ACTIS): 1-800-TRIALS-A (874-2572)

For more information about HIV infection, call:

Drug Abuse Hotline: 1-800-662-HELP (4357)

Pediatric and Pregnancy AIDS Hotline: 1-212-430-3333

National Hemophilia Foundation: 1-212-219-8180

Hemophilia and AIDS/HIV Network for Dissemination of Information (HANDI): 1-800-42-HANDI (424-2634)

National Pediatric HIV Resource Center: 1-800-362-0071

National Association of People with AIDS: 1-202-898-0414

Teens Teaching AIDS Prevention Program (TTAPP) National Hotline: 1-800-234-TEEN (8336)

General information:

English: 1-800-332-2636

Spanish: 1-800-344-7432

TDD Service for the Deaf: 1-800-243-7889

General information for healthcare providers:

National Clinician's Post Exposure Treatment: 1-888-448-4911

HIV Telephone Consultation Service: 1-800-933-3413

Review Questions

(Answers to the Review Questions are on pages 425-426.)

1. Can HIV infection be cured?

2. What is a surrogate marker?

3. From _____ 1987 through 2007 _____ individual and combination anti-HIV drugs were FDA-approved.

4. How many FDA-approved anti-HIV drugs are nucleoside or nucleotide analogs?

5. How do nucleoside analogs inhibit HIV replication?

6. What are the two major problems in the use of nucleoside and non-nucleoside analogs in HIV therapy?

7. What is HIV viral load? What can its quantitative measurement reveal?

8. Name the ten protease inhibitors that have FDA approval for use in the United States.

9. How do non-nucleoside drugs inhibit HIV replication?

10. Briefly describe the focus of HIV combination drug therapy.

11. After starting antiretroviral therapy, what is an acceptable target for viral load that indicates the therapy is effective?

    A. 5000 copies/mL
    B. 5000–10,000 copies/mL
    C. 10,000–15,000 copies/mL
    D. No acceptable target level has been set.

12. Which of the following statements is correct regarding HIV pathogenesis?

    A. HIV contains two copies of the viral DNA genome.
    B. Viral polyproteins are cleaved by protease.
    C. The RNA copy is integrated in the host-cell chromosome.
    D. gp120 envelope glycoprotein facilitates entry of HIV core particle into the cell's cytoplasm.

13. Some medical centers are offering drug therapy that may be able to:

    A. cure AIDS
    B. help prevent HIV infection shortly after exposure
    C. effectively treat HIV/AIDS without side effects
    D. prevent HIV infection
    E. prevent AIDS

14. HIV escapes the effects of HIV antiretroviral drugs by _____.

    A. gobbling up the chemicals
    B. disguising itself as an immune cell
    C. pretending to be a harmless virus
    D. changing its genetic makeup

15. When HIV mutates in response to a drug, it can cause _____.

    A. the virus to become less "fit"
    B. the drug to become less effective
    C. other drugs to become less effective
    D. all of the above

16. Single mutations are _____ worse than a group of mutations.

    A. always
    B. never
    C. sometimes
    D. none of the above

17. When your virus becomes resistant to a drug in your drug combination, your _____ may go up.

    A. temperature
    B. CD4 cells
    C. doctor bills
    D. viral load

18. True or False: Resistance is an all-or-nothing deal—the drugs work perfectly or not at all.

19. A high genetic barrier to resistance means a drug requires _____ to reduce its effectiveness.

    A. multiple viral mutations
    B. a single viral mutation
    C. experimental gene therapy
    D. cross-resistance with another drug in the same class

20. True or False: Mutations take years to develop, so missing one day's dose of meds will not contribute to resistance.

21. Cross-resistance is a problem for which class of drugs? _____

    A. protease inhibitors
    B. nukes
    C. non-nukes
    D. all three classes

22. Which of the following is not an important issue when choosing a drug regimen? _____

    A. potential side effects
    B. easy dosing schedule
    C. high genetic barrier
    D. All three are important.

23. What is the name of the newest entry inhibitor anti-retroviral drug? _____

24. True or False: ART has lowered the number of deaths in the United States.

25. Highly active antiretroviral therapy (HAART) is less than ideal because

A. it does not eliminate latent HIV infection.
B. its cost is too great for 90% of AIDS sufferers.
C. it often has severe side effects.
D. some HIV strains are resistant to it.
E. All of the above.

5 The Immunology of HIV Disease/AIDS

For most, immunity is simply there when it's needed, like the umbrella sitting by the door. But the immune system's elegance—honed by millions of years of warfare with invaders of every kind—shouldn't be confused with simplicity. The immune system is a thing of beauty—subtle enough to distinguish dangerous invaders like viruses from benign interlopers such as food; clever enough to recognize when the body's supposedly friendly cells turn cancerous and should be eliminated. But the immune system can also go seriously awry. When it begins attacking healthy tissues, the result can be any one of 80 autoimmune diseases such as lupus or rheumatoid arthritis. It's the price we pay for having such a dynamic, finely balanced system.

THE IMMUNE SYSTEM

All living organisms are continually exposed to substances that are capable of causing harm. Most organisms protect themselves against such substances in more than one way—with physical barriers, the skin for example, or with chemicals that repel or kill invaders. Animals with backbones, **vertebrates,** have these types of general protective mechanisms, but they also have a more advanced protective system called an **immune system.** The immune system is a mind-numbing, incredibly complex network of organs containing cells that recognize foreign substances in the body and destroy them. Like a security force, it protects vertebrates against pathogens, or infectious agents, such as viruses, bacteria, fungi, and other parasites.

Although there are many potentially harmful pathogens (agents that cause diseases), no pathogen can invade or attack all organisms because a pathogen's ability to cause harm requires a susceptible victim, and not all organisms are susceptible to the same pathogens. For instance, the virus that causes AIDS is strictly a human pathogen; it does not cause a disease in any other animal. Similarly, humans are not susceptible to the viruses that cause canine (dog) distemper or feline (cat) leukemia. This is because the cells in different animals carry their own specific receptors or protein fragments wherein each **receptor** on a given cell only allows a specific cellular product or environmental agent to attach.

An Explanation of the Importance of Cell Receptors

In the study of cells, the term **receptor** is used to describe any molecule that interacts with and subsequently holds onto some other molecule. The receptor is like the hand, and the object held by the hand is commonly called the **ligand.** The interaction between the receptor and ligand implies **specificity;** a receptor known to bind with substance X would not normally bind with a different substance. For example, a two-slotted electrical wall outlet is a receptacle (receptor) for a two-pronged plug (ligand). A three-pronged plug will not fit into this receptacle. Depending on the type of two-slotted receptacle, even some two-pronged plugs may not fit.

Where Are Cell Receptors Located?

Receptors can be found inside a cell, and especially embedded within all the membranes that a given cell may have. In humans, there are organ systems present, and a given receptor may be found associated only with a particular type of cell that comprises a particular type of tissue that makes up a particular organ.

What Do Receptors Do?

Receptors are critical to the life of all cells, whether the cells represent an animal, a plant, a fungus, or a bacterium. Every function, response, interaction, pathway, process, and other term you might think of that concerns the moment-to-moment existence of a cell is controlled by various receptor/ligand-induced systems. Essentially, you are what your genetically coded

receptors allow you to become. In Chapter 3, there is an explanation of receptors that restrict the types of virus that can attach to certain cell types. In particular the ligand, in this case HIV, attaches almost exclusively to the CD4 (protein) receptor on a specific population of T lymphocytes (T4 or CD4+ lymphocytes).

Function of the Immune System

A man dies because his body rejected a heart transplant; a woman is crippled by rheumatoid arthritis; a child goes into a coma that is brought on by cerebral malaria; another child dies of an infection because of an immunodeficiency; an elderly man has advanced hepatic cirrhosis caused by iron overload. These five clinical situations are diverse, yet all have one thing in common: a malfunction of the human immune system.

The immune system filters out foreign substances, removes damaged and dead cells, and acts as a security system to destroy mutant and cancer cells. It is composed of a number of specialized cells, several organs, and a group of biologically active chemicals. The human immune system is like a jigsaw puzzle—many parts come together to form an overall defense against disease-causing agents. If parts of the immune system are missing or damaged, illness may occur due to an immune deficiency.

Separating Friend from Foe: How the Immune System Decides

Skin prevents disease-causing agents from entering the body. But they can enter through body openings, cuts, or wounds. Whether the invader is a life-threatening bacterium or a relatively harmless cold virus, your immune system must control it—if it does not, the harmless may become the harmful! A single infectious microorganism or virus that survives and multiplies may cause a severe illness. Some infectious agents resemble the body's own cells. How do immune cells know which to attack and which to ignore? The answer is, once an agent enters the body, it triggers an **immune response** if the body does not recognize the substance or agent as a part of itself or **"self."** All body cells have special molecules, called **class I proteins,** on their membranes that are like flags or barcodes with the word "self" on them (Figure 5-1). The cells of the immune system try to destroy anything present in the body that is not carrying the self molecules—anything that is **"nonself."** Nonself is any substance or agent that triggers the creation of antibodies (very specific body

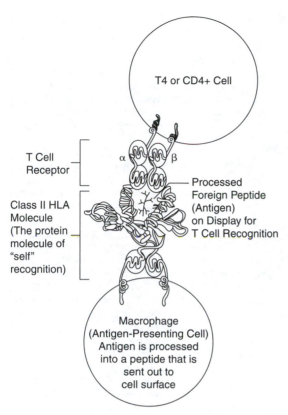

T4 or CD4+ Cell

T Cell Receptor

α   β

Class II HLA Molecule (The protein molecule of "self" recognition)

Processed Foreign Peptide (Antigen) on Display for T Cell Recognition

Macrophage (Antigen-Presenting Cell) Antigen is processed into a peptide that is sent out to cell surface

FIGURE 5-1 Interaction Between a Human Leukocyte Antigen "Self" Protein (HLA), a Foreign Peptide (Antigen), and a T Cell Receptor. The diagram represents the trimolecular interaction of a processed antigen into a peptide that is being presented on the surface of the antigen-presenting cell to a T4 cell. The presence of the class II HLA self identity marker and the presence of the foreign peptide stimulate the T4 cell into action. *(Adapted from Sinha, 1990)*

proteins that react against [*anti*] anything foreign that gets into the [*body*].) Such nonself substances are called **antigens.** Antigens may be whole viruses or organisms or parts of viruses, organisms, or their products.

In general, most cellular organisms that damage cells do so from the outside by producing toxic chemicals or in some way externally interfering with the cell's metabolism. But viruses invade or enter different cell types, forcing them to produce viral replicas at the expense of the cells' own essential metabolic functions. Gradually, like a machine wearing out, host cells start to malfunction and die. The best thing a virus can do is find a host cell that does not die and

that can produce replicas indefinitely. In a biological time frame, new disease-causing viruses are often very deadly to new hosts. If a new virus strain is too deadly, it kills its host before other hosts are infected, and the ensuing epidemic dies out. For example, the **Ebola virus** makes its victims very weak shortly after infection and kills them in 7 to 14 days. This virus kills quickly and vanishes. Its origin is still unknown. Over biological time, successful viruses like the human herpes virus and their new hosts learn to accommodate each other. This will most likely happen with human-HIV associations, but how many people over how many years will have to die before human cells learn to accommodate HIV is unknown. Perhaps it will never happen. Smallpox virus has been infecting humans for thousands of years and has never been accommodated by humans.

Cooperation and Coordination Within the Human Immune System

The basic premise of the immune system is simple: to coordinate the activities of various cell types in order to provide extended, if not lifelong, protection against disease-causing pathogens. Usually, this cooperating system works flawlessly, quashing diseases before they can kill their host and sparking an immunity to provide protection against future attacks. Sometimes, however, the system fails and infection and disease prevail—and there is no greater example of this than HIV, a pathogen that almost always succeeds in circumventing and manipulating the body's immune defense to facilitate its own survival.

HUMAN LYMPHOCYTES: T CELLS AND B CELLS

The hallmark of the human immune system is its ability to mount a highly specific response against virtually any foreign entity, even those never seen before in the course of evolution. It is able to do this because of the number of different kinds of cells called lymphocytes. The human immune system contains about 2 trillion (2×10^{12}) lymphocytes, but a relatively small number when compared to the 100 trillion cells in the body (see Box 5.1, Figure 5-4). Most mature lymphocytes recirculate continuously, going from blood to tissue and back to blood again as often as one to two times per day. They travel among most other cells and are present in large numbers in the thymus, bone marrow, lymph nodes, spleen, and

CLASS I AND CLASS II PROTEINS

THE HUMAN LEUKOCYTE ANTIGEN (HLA)

This system is, in some respects, the immunological equivalent of a sophisticated alarm system. Human Leukocyte Antigen (HLA) molecules are produced within human cells and act as receptacles for fragments of cellular or foreign (for example, viral) proteins. The HLA molecules then display these fragments on the outside of the cell; a single cell is typically adorned with several hundred thousand different HLA-peptide complexes. This process allows circulating T cells to survey the HLA complexes for signs of any foreign substances that might indicate the presence of a pathogen. HLA molecules are divided into two major classes (I and II), which are recognized by different subsets of T cells. The CD8 molecule on CD8+ or T8 T cells interacts with class I HLA molecules. Likewise, the CD4 molecule on CD4+ or T4 cells interacts with class II molecules. In both cases, the substance associated with the HLA molecule is recognized by a structure on the T cell called a T cell receptor (TCR). The critical aspect of the HLA system for immunity is that both class I and II molecules come in hundreds of different versions, dependent on the HLA genes inherited from our parents. The precise shape and size of an HLA molecule governs its ability to associate with a diverse array of substances (most often a peptide or short length of amino acids) and to present them to T cells. HLA molecules thus exert a profound influence on the body's ability to mount a broad and effective T cell response to any given pathogen.

More Detail on HLA

There is a series of some 40 different genes located on human chromosome 6 that is referred to as the *Human Leukocyte Antigen (HLA)* or as the **major histocompatibility** (tissue type) **complex (MHC).** The genes in this region produce a series of proteins that are *almost* unique to the individual. Because these proteins belong to the individual, they would be recognized as foreign or as an *antigen* when placed in another human, for example, as in a transplanted heart (transplantation antigens). Almost all cells in an individual have a sample of their own HLA proteins or transplantation antigens located on the surface of each cell's membrane. Thus, a person's transplantation antigens are recognized as **self-proteins** by his or her immune system. Such HLA proteins are referred to as **class I** (type 1) tissue compatibility proteins. These proteins cause transplant graft rejections. With minor exceptions, there is not much of your body tissue that would not be rejected if placed in another human body because your class I proteins would be recognized as foreign by the recipient

body's immune system. But how does the recipient's immune system recognize these class I proteins as foreign? Answer: By using a second class of HLA proteins, **class II.** Relatively few human cell types carry this protein on their cell membranes. All such cells carrying the class II protein are derived from a monocyte–macrophage cell series, which includes macrophages located in the lung, liver and spleen, dendritic cells of the gut, skin, spleen and lymph nodes, Langerhans cells of the skin, and microglial cells of the nervous system.

The class II protein, located on the membrane of these cell types, allows these cell types to act as the body's police force. These cells *digest* foreign protein into smaller products. Some of these products, a small series of amino acids or **peptides,** are then escorted to the cell surface alongside a molecule of the class II protein. In this way, the cells carrying a class II protein serve up or present the foreign substance or antigen alongside or adjacent to the class II protein or "self molecule" so that immune system cells, notably the T4 cells and B cells, can sense the presence of the foreign protein and initiate an immune response against it—the activation of a variety of immune system attack cells (cytotoxic T cells, killer T cells) and the production of very specific antibodies.

In medically important viral infections, **neutralizing antibodies** are generated within 6 to 14 days. In contrast, such protective antibodies generally appear 50 to 150 days after infection with HIV and the hepatitis B virus (HBV) in humans (Pianz et al., 1996).

PROCESSING "FOREIGN" PROTEIN AND LOADING OF THEIR PEPTIDES ONTO CLASS I AND CLASS II MOLECULES

Protein processing and loading of peptides onto class I molecules that are carried out to the cell membrane is taking place all the time in most body cells. There is always plenty of material to feed the processing machinery, because worn-out, damaged, and misfolded internal proteins are continuously being degraded and replaced by new ones.

By contrast, the processing of proteins from outside the cell and the loading of peptides onto class II molecules are normally restricted to B cells, macrophages, and dendritic cells, which are very efficient at taking in material. Although most class I and class II molecules form complexes with peptides derived from proteins inside and outside the cell, this demarcation is by no means absolute.

As a consequence of protein processing, the surfaces of a body cell become adorned with peptide-laden

HLA molecules, amounting to about 100,000 to 300,000 class I or class II products of each of the HLA genes. Because each HLA molecule has one peptide bound to it, an uninfected cell displays hundreds of thousands of self peptides on its surface. Some of these peptides are present in the thousands, whereas others are represented by a few copies; most peptide species have 100 or so copies on the surface of each cell. Each cell thus displays a heterogeneous collection of peptides, and the surface of a cell resembles rows of well-stocked stalls at a bazaar, with bargain hunters looking over the stock. But if, in this metaphor, the vendors are the HLA molecules and the peptides the goods, who are the potential buyers? They are a group of lymphocytes reared in the thymus and then turned loose to roam the body—*the T cells* (Klein et al., 2000a; Klein et al., 2000b).

appendix (Figure 5-2). By 1968, lymphocytes had been divided into two classes: **lymphocytes called B cells** that are derived from and mature in bone marrow, and **lymphocytes called T cells** that are derived from bone marrow but travel to and mature in the thymus gland (Figure 5-3). T cells make up 70% to 80% of the lymphocytes circulating in the body. Circulating T cells are a heterogeneous group of cells with a wide range of different functions. When a T cell encounters another cell, it uses various probes or detecting devices on its surface—known as receptors—to examine the fragments displayed on an antigen-presenting cell's surface (Figure 5-1). The fragments displayed on the Antigen Presenting Cell (APC) disclose to the scanning T cell whether the APC being scanned is normal and to be left unharmed, or infected and to be destroyed. The protein fragments are cupped inside tiny holders called class II major histocompatibility complexes (class II MHCs). To be more specific, each individual T cell expresses a receptor (**T Cell antigen Receptor, TCR**), which recognizes a ligand (a compound that fits a particular receptor) composed of an antigenic peptide, 8–15 amino acids long, bound to a **self-major-histocompatibility-complex (MHC) molecule** (also **referred to as HLA-human leukocyte antigen system**) (see Point of Information 5.1). Thus, a T cell does not directly recognize a soluble antigen, but rather recognizes an antigen displayed on the surface of an **antigen-presenting cell (APC)** like a B cell or macrophage. There are about

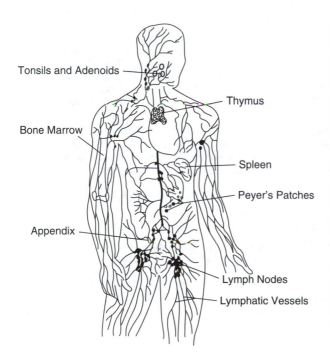

Tonsils and Adenoids

Bone Marrow

Appendix

Thymus

Spleen

Peyer's Patches

Lymph Nodes

Lymphatic Vessels

FIGURE 5-2 Organs of the Human Immune System. The organs of the immune system are positioned throughout the body. They are generally referred to as lymphoid organs because they are concerned with the development, growth, and dissemination of lymphocytes, or white cells, that populate the immune system. Lymphoid organs include the bone marrow, thymus, lymph nodes, spleen, tonsils, adenoids, appendix, and the clumps of lymphoid tissue in the small intestine called Peyer's patches. The blood and lymphatic fluids transport lymphocytes to and from all the immune system organs. Gut-associated lymphoid tissue contains 50% to 60% of the body's lymphocytes, and those lymphocytes, according to Peter Anton at UCLA, contain six times more CD4 receptors than do CD4+ or T4 cells circulating in the blood. Other lymphoid tissue contains about 98% of lymphocytes and blood contains about 2%. These data may mean that the gut is the preferred site of HIV replication in untreated patients.

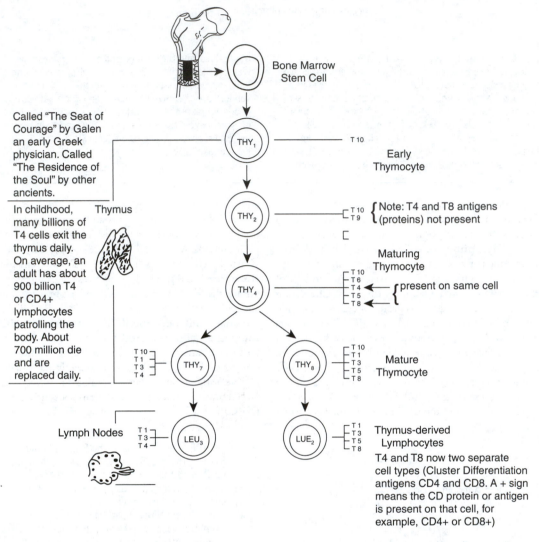

Bone Marrow
Stem Cell

Called "The Seat of
Courage" by Galen
an early Greek
physician. Called
"The Residence of
the Soul" by other
ancients.

In childhood,
many billions of
T4 cells exit the
thymus daily.
On average, an
adult has about
900 billion T4
or CD4+
lymphocytes
patrolling the
body. About
700 million die
and are
replaced daily.

Thymus

THY₁ — T 10

Early
Thymocyte

THY₂ — T 10 / T 9   Note: T4 and T8 antigens (proteins) not present

Maturing
Thymocyte

THY₄ — T 10 / T 6 / T 4 / T 5 / T 8   present on same cell

T 10 / T 1 / T 3 / T 4 — THY₇

THY₈ — T 10 / T 1 / T 3 / T 5 / T 8

Mature
Thymocyte

Lymph Nodes

T 1 / T 3 / T 4 — LEU₃

LUE₂ — T 1 / T 3 / T 5 / T 8

Thymus-derived
Lymphocytes

T4 and T8 now two separate
cell types (Cluster Differentiation
antigens CD4 and CD8. A + sign
means the CD protein or antigen
is present on that cell, for
example, CD4+ or CD8+)

FIGURE 5-3 T Lymphocyte **Cluster Differentiation (CD)** Antigen in Humans. The CD marker or antigen on a T cell tells something about what the cell does. For example the CD4 and CD8 T cells have different jobs to do. Stages of thymic differentiation (that is, the presence of the different antigens or proteins on their membrane surfaces) are defined on the basis of reactivity to monoclonal antibodies. Schematic pictures of cells represents thymocytes within specific stages of a defined phenotype: T1–T10.

10 billion APCs located in the lymphoid organs. The receptors of T cells are different from those of B cells because they are "trained" to recognize fragments of antigens that have been combined or complexed with HLA class II molecules. As T cells circulate through the body, they scan the surfaces of body cells for the presence of foreign antigens that have become associated with the HLA molecules. The antigen present on the APC signals to the T cell whether the APC should be left unharmed or whether the APC is

infected and should be destroyed. This function is sometimes called **immune surveillance.**

The Cytotoxic and Helper (T4 or CD4+) Lymphocytes

Two of the important kinds of T cells are **cytotoxic** or **killer T** lymphocytes, (CTL) and **helper T** lympho-cytes. Killer T cells carry the **CD8 protein antigen** and are called T8 or CD8+ cells. CD8 or T8 cells are suppressor cells that bring an end to an immune re-

BOX 5.1

HOW LARGE IS A TRILLION?

The human body is made up of many trillions of cells. For example, the human immune system contains at least a trillion lymphocytes dedicated to destroying foreign substances that endanger health. But, a trillion of anything is a very large number. Can we really appreciate just how large a trillion of something is? Perhaps the following will help.

1. A stack of 1 trillion one-dollar bills would reach a height of 69,000 miles.

2. It would take a person 11.5 days to count to 1 million and 31,688 years to count to 1 trillion—1, 2, 3, 4, 5 . . . !

3. A stack of 1 trillion HIV (Figure 5-4) would be over 62 miles high (diameter of HIV = 1000 angstroms: $(1 \times 10^{12})(1000)$
$(1 \times 10^{-10}) = 1 \times 10^5$ meters = 62.15 miles).

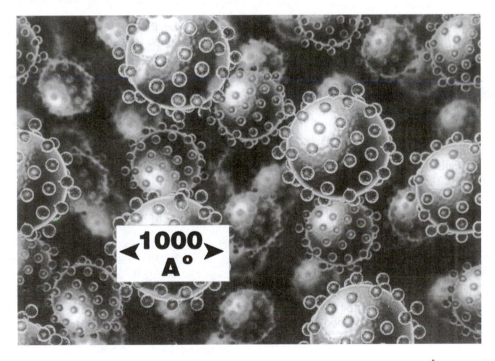

FIGURE 5-4 Dimensions of HIV in Angstroms. HIV has a diameter of 1000 angstroms (Å). It would take 254,000 HIV laid side by side to equal 1 inch in length. *(Illustration courtesy of the author)*

sponse that is no longer needed. Helper T cells carry the **CD4 protein antigen** and are called **T4** or **CD4+ cells.** The CD4 and CD8 proteins or antigens located on their respective T lymphocytes act similar to a bar code or number on a football jersey; the proteins or antigens identify the cell type. Killer or CTL T cells bind to cells carrying a foreign antigen and destroys them. But CD4+ or T4 cells do not kill cells directly; they interact with B cells and CTL cells and help them respond to foreign antigens. The CD4+ or T4 cell has the role of a quarterback in football; it calls the plays for the rest of the lymphocyte team.

The Loss of T4 or CD4+ Lymphocytes when compared to T8 or CD8+ Lymphocytes and Its Biological Impact

The ratio of CD4 cells to CD8 cells is often reported. This is calculated by dividing the CD4 value by the CD8 value. In healthy people, this ratio is between 0.9 and 1.9, meaning that there are about 1 to 2 CD4 cells for every CD8 cell. In people with HIV infection, this ratio drops dramatically, meaning that there are many times more CD8 cells than CD4 cells.

Ashley Haase, director of the University of Minnesota Microbiology Department, estimated that healthy young adults harbor approximately 200 billion mature CD4+ cells. In HIV-positive patients, this total number is halved by the time the CD4+ cell count falls to 200 cells/μL of blood. In the more advanced stage of HIV disease, the destruction of parenchymal lymphoid spaces is so extensive that a total body CD4+ cell count has not even been attempted (Haase, 1999).

It is believed that T4 cells recognize only those antigens of viruses, fungi, and other parasites; and trigger only those parts of the immune system necessary to act against these agents. Indeed, the viruses, fungi, and other parasites produce the majority of opportunistic infections when the T4 cells have been depleted by HIV.

It was unknown if B cells begin to malfunction soon after HIV infection. In late 2001, investigators at the National Institute of Allergy and Infectious Diseases (NIAID) reported that the presence of HIV in infected patients causes B cells (a) to produce excessive amounts of nonessential antibodies, (b) to fail to respond to physiological signals, and (c) to be at risk of becoming cancerous. Some of these changes can be reversed with the use of antiretroviral drugs (Moir et al., 2001).

In Summary

The two types of lymphocytes, B cells and T cells, play different roles in the immune response, though they

may act together and influence each another's functions. The part of the immune response that involves B cells is often called **humoral immunity** because it takes place in the body fluids. The part involving T cells is called cellular immunity because it takes place directly between the T cells, other cells, and their antigens. This distinction is misleading, however, because strictly speaking, all adaptive immune responses are cellular—that is, they are all initiated by cells (the lymphocytes) reacting to antigens. **B cells** may initiate an immune response, but the triggering antigens are actually eliminated by soluble products that the B cells release into the blood and other body fluids. These products are called **antibodies** and belong to a special group of blood proteins called **immunoglobins.** When a B cell is stimulated by an antigen that it encounters in the body fluids, it transforms, with the aid of T4 cells, into a larger cell, a blast cell. The blast cell begins to divide rapidly, forming a clone of identical cells. Some of these transform further into plasma cells—in essence, antibody-producing factories. These plasma cells produce a single type of antigen-specific antibody at a rate of about 2000 antibodies per second. The antibodies then circulate through the body fluids, attacking the triggering antigen.

What Happens to the Immune System after HIV Infection

HIV enters the body via infected body fluids: blood, semen, and vaginal secretions. Once inside, HIV specifically infects active T4 or CD4+ cell. However, while HIV devastates CD4 or T4 cells, most of the time it cannot infect them. Some 95% of these cells are in a resting state during which HIV cannot infect them. It is only when these cells become activated—rapidly multiplying to kill invading microorganisms—that HIV infects the cells, uses their genetic machinery to replicate, and eventually kills the cells. The resting CD4 cells' antiviral protection derives from the protein APOBEC3G, an enzyme that could have evolved in mammals as a natural antiviral defense. HIV has a protein, called VIF, that appears to disarm these cells by neutralizing APOBEC (see explanation in Chapter 3). APOBEC exists in lightweight and heavyweight versions. In resting cells, the lightweight APOBEC is lethal to HIV. But when T cells are activated, the free-floating, lightweight APOBEC proteins are gathered into the heavyweight complexes that are vulnerable to HIV.

The new CD4 cells direct the body's immune response against infection. As HIV takes over the T4 cells, it alters their growth and reproduction through a complicated process that leads to the T4 cells' destruction. The ratio of T4 cells to T8 cells then changes. In healthy people, the number of T4 cells is greater than the number of T8 cells. In HIV-infected individuals, a decline in the T4 count signals the progress of immune system deterioration. The results are debilitating: The T4 cells are not as responsive to antigen identification, macrophages become less responsive, and B cells produce fewer specific antibodies and lose their normal responsiveness. At this point, the immune system becomes dysfunctional and the host becomes vulnerable to attack from opportunistic infections. (Chapter 6 discusses the different opportunistic infections.)

Uses of the T4 or CD4+ Cell Count

Doctors use a test that counts the number of T4 or CD4+ cells in a cubic millimeter or μL (microliter) of blood. A normal count in a healthy, HIV-negative adult can vary but is usually between 600 and 1200 T4 cells/μL. About 2% of the body's T4 cells are in the blood; the rest are in tissues such as lymph nodes. Changes in your T4 cell count (which looks only at the blood) may reflect the movement of cells into and out of the blood, rather than changes in the total number of T4 cells in your body. The absolute CD4 count is obtained by multiplying the estimated percentage of CD4 cells in a blood sample by the total number of white blood cells in the body. It is the absolute CD4 count of about 350 that is used as the criterion to start ART.

A metaphor that can be used to describe the differences between percent and absolute CD4 counts is that the absolute count is like measuring the total number of red cars on the highway at any one time—if measured at rush hour, there would be more than at midnight. The real question, however, is how many red cars are there in the city (or CD4s in your body); presumably, the percentage of red cars remains the same at rush hour and at midnight. Percentage is a way to smooth over variations in the traffic or CD4 cells in multiple samples.

In some cases, in order to help understand changes in your absolute T4 count, a physician may determine what proportion of a blood sample's lymphocytes are T4+ cells. This is called the T4 or CD4+ percentage. In HIV-negative people a normal result is around 30%. This means that 30% of your lymphocytes are CD4+ cells. The normal range is between 20% to 40%. A T4 percentage which falls below about 15% is understood to reflect a risk of serious infections. Most people with HIV find that their T4 count falls over time. This often happens at a variable rate, so the count can still be quite stable for long periods. It is useful to have a T4 or CD4+ count measured regularly for two reasons: (1) to monitor one's immune system and help one decide whether and when to take anti-HIV drugs and treatments to prevent opportunistic infections (OI); and (2) to help monitor the effectiveness of any anti-HIV drugs being taken. If your T4 or CD4+ count is persistently below 350, your immune system is weakened and you are at a gradually increasing risk of OI the further it falls. If it drops below 200–250 you are at increased risk for serious OI. At less than 350 both European and U.S. treatment guidelines now recommend beginning ART. One effect of anti-HIV drugs is to improve the state of the immune system. This is crudely reflected in an increase in the T4 or CD4+ count. Evidence suggests that the cells' ability to fight OI is also improved. For example, people taking antiretroviral drugs, who find their T4 count rises and stays above 250 cells, may no longer need to take drugs that may have been prescribed to prevent *Pneumocystis* pneumonia (PCP) or other opportunistic infections. Monitoring the changes in your T4 count while you are taking antiretrovirals can help the doctor decide whether the treatment is working or whether it is time to try different options. A fall in T4 count would be a sign the treatment is not working and may need to be switched to a new regimen. However, the T4 count isn't the only consideration when making these decisions; viral load results, how well you feel, and which treatments have been used before are also considered.

Understanding the Results

Factors other than HIV can affect your T4 or CD4+ count including infections, time of day, smoking, stress, and which lab tests the blood sample. So it is very important to watch the trend in your CD4+ count over time, rather than to place too much emphasis on a single test that may be misleading. Doctors will normally suggest measuring the T4 or CD4+ count every three to six months if one has a relatively high count, no symptoms, and is not taking antiretroviral drugs. They may suggest more frequent counts if decisions have to be made such as starting treatments, the development of HIV-related symptoms, or if the decline in CD4+ cells appears to be increasing.

The Antibody

Antibodies are Y-shaped molecules that bind to specific foreign proteins, or pieces of protein, called antigens.

When antibodies on the surface of a B cell snag an undesirable or foreign protein, *both disappear inside the cell*. Eventually, as previously discussed, a bit of the foreign protein may reemerge, attached to a self recognizable protein molecule called a **class II protein** (Figure 5-1). The pair, the small piece of foreign protein attached to a self class II protein, acts as a red flag to T4 cells, which set off an aggressive immune response.

(For an excellent review of the concept of antigen processing and presentation, see Unanue, 1995; for class I and class II proteins, Strominger et al., 1995; for the concept of self, Zinkernagel, 1995; for cell-mediated immunity, Doherty, 1995).

B Cells Make Antibodies and Release Them into the Bloodstream

After an antibody and virus join, they are digested by macrophages or cleared from the blood by the liver and spleen. Some B cells and T cells become memory cells, which are stored by the immune system. Memory cells appear to recall their history and remember the antigen they have previously encountered. However, if the antigen, say a virus, has mutated (changed), as the flu virus does yearly, previous antibodies will not affect it. New antibodies must be created to neutralize or cancel out the new mutant virus. While this antibody production is taking place, the viral invader has time to multiply and infect new cells, and the infected person suffers the symptoms of the flu.

SIDEBAR 5.1

MEASURES AND COUNTERMEASURES: THE HUMAN IMMUNE SYSTEM VS. VIRUSES

A war has existed between humans and viruses that invade human cells and cause disease. Probably from the first encounter, prehuman to first humans, viruses became able to *hide* inside human cells. The immune system in turn adapted by developing a means of surveying and identifying cells containing a hidden virus. Viruses then adapted by deceiving the immune surveillance system; the immune system then evolved a better means to *mark* cells carrying the virus. This game of hide-and-seek between the virus and the immune system continues. Learning the means by which the virus attempts to trick the immune system carries over into the study of tumor cells. They must also escape the immune system's surveillance system and do so by using several of the same ploys used by the virus. From what microbiologists have learned so far, different viruses have evolved different ways of getting rid of expression of class I proteins, the flagpole of self proteins. But the mechanisms are amazingly different in different viruses. Examples are:

Cytomegalovirus (CMV)—A virus that may cause birth defects in the fetus and the rapid onset of blindness in people with AIDS. On entering a cell, CMV stops self-identity proteins from reaching the cell membrane. If the class I proteins can't reach the membrane neither will pieces of CMV. The immune system is blinded to the fact the CMV is inside the cells. The immune system counters with a natural killer cell that destroys all cells that do not contain a self protein on their surface! But CMV over time evolved a means to produce a fake self protein that passes for the real one. The natural killer cells are successfully fooled.

Adenovirus—The virus causing common colds. This virus can also stop self proteins from reaching the membrane carrying identifying pieces of virus. Further, this virus is able to make the cell divide so it can replicate itself. The cell then becomes cancerous (replication out of control), begins to destroy itself—but the virus has evolved a way to stop the cell's self-destruction, so the cell continues to divide. The process is similar to what happens in tumor cells.

HIV—This virus has the most deadly scheme of all. This virus infects cells of the immune system—most often the T4 cells that are essential to the initiation of the immune response. Similar to other viruses, HIV has to disable the self-alerting system. One of HIV's genes, call **nef**, makes a protein that attaches to the self proteins, just inside the cell's membrane. The other end of the nef protein carries an address label, readable by the cell's internal sorting system that directs proteins to their proper place. The message carried by the nef protein says, in the cell's sorting code, "Haul to garbage dump and recycle," tricking the infected cell into pulling down its self proteins and destroying them. The nef protein also tags the CD4 proteins for destruction in the same way. Like the self proteins, the CD4's stick up through the cell membrane. What does HIV gain from having the cell destroy CD4 proteins? That's the million-dollar question investigators are working on. The reason may be to prevent other viruses from entering the cell or because in latching onto the CD4 proteins, the nef protein dislodges and energizes another protein that is known to activate the T cells. The cell's activation to make more HIV may be the answer.

Can the Immune System Remember HIV Exposure?

The immune system works because it produces antibody against an antigen and in addition creates immune memory cells. But this does not appear to occur when the immune system is exposed to HIV. Yes, antibody is made, but when HIV disappears (is reduced to below measurable levels using antiretroviral therapy or HAART), so does the immune defense against it. There are few if any memory cells to protect should HIV rebound or break through drug suppression replication. In the mid-1990s, Francis Plummer and colleagues at the University of Nairobi stunned scientists when they announced the discovery of a group of Kenyan female prostitutes who appeared resistant to HIV infection, surviving infection for years despite more than six customers a week without condom protection in a society where upward of 20% of their customers were likely to be HIV positive. Vaccine researchers were ecstatic because the discovery offered evidence that people could successfully become immune to HIV—something some scientists had argued might be impossible. But at the Seventh Conference on Retroviral and Opportunistic Infections (2000) Plummer's group had distressing news: 10% of the apparently resistant prostitutes became HIV positive from 1996 to 1999. Their infections coincided with the women's decisions to **decrease their exposure** to HIV by having fewer customers or insisting that the men wear condoms. Kevin De Crock, an HIV investigator, said, "It suggests that HIV antigen stimulation is required for the maintenance of resistance." De Crock said it may be that the immune system is not capable of remembering without a constant presence of HIV (too few memory cells made?). This would appear to be an HIV catch 22—to control HIV it must be present, but the control will over the long run be insufficient to stop the progression to AIDS.

ANTIBODIES AND HIV DISEASE

Resistance to HIV does not seem to be the same as the more common examples of immunity. The body's protective countermeasures against measles and mumps are absolute. Years after exposure, there is no hint within the body of the foreign agents that cause those diseases. After children become immune to mumps, they can no longer infect other people. Immunity to these diseases occurs because the immune system makes neutralizing antibody, antibody that binds to and directly inhibits or neutralizes the function of infectious agents. Memory immune cells are able to produce neutralizing or cancelling antibody whenever these infecting agents enter the body. In contrast, it has been shown that although the immune systems of most people initially produce neutralizing HIV antibodies, the continued evolution of HIV in their bodies results in a series of mutant HIV that are not efficiently neutralized or cancelled via antibody response. Thus over time, the ratio of effective neutralizing antibody production to new virus production becomes disproportionate, that is, more virus exists than effective neutralizing antibody, and at this time the level of T4 or CD4+ cells begins to drop. T4 cells drop because antibodies to HIV reduce circulating HIV in the plasma (viral load) without affecting HIV replication or cell-to-cell spread of HIV. This means that the production of mutant HIV to existing antibody never ceases, resulting in continued T4 cell infection and loss. Eventually there are too few T4 cells to ward off opportunistic infections (see Chapter 7 for additional information on T4 cell replacement and HIV production).

The rapid production of HIV mutants without the same rapid production of a neutralizing or cancelling antibody against each mutant means that sometime after infection, much if not most of the antibody in some people may be nothing more than useless

---

POINT OF INFORMATION 5.2

THE BIG QUESTION

◆ How does HIV, which at first glance does not appear to be a highly formidable foe, persist in the body for such long periods of time and continue multiplying and progressively causing more and more damage until a fatal outcome is reached?

◆ Why does the immensely powerful immune system of the body, an organ system that has evolved over millennia of challenges from a wide variety of infectious and noninfectious invaders to become an exceedingly effective defender of the body against agents far more virulent than HIV, now appear to be powerless against it?

The answer: Because HIV, unlike other agents that enter the human body, (virus, bacteria, fungus, and protozoa) infects immune system cells, in particular **the T4 or CD4+ cell that governs the response of the entire immune system.** Without T4 cells the immune system cannot function—like a car without gas, all the parts are there but nothing happens.

---

antibody copy (antibody to the initial strain or strains of HIV). In these people, HIV disease would most likely progress more swiftly than in persons whose immune system can keep up with the production of somewhat useful antibody to match the formation of HIV mutants. This may be one important reason why some people progress to AIDS and death so rapidly when compared to other HIV-infected people.

Immune Activation: A Clue to AIDS Progression?

Recently, researchers have suggested that a natural process called **immune activation** may determine why infection with HIV progresses differently in different people.

Immune activation occurs whenever immune system cells detect foreign invaders and send out chemical signals to draw other cells into the fight. It occurs at the beginning of any infection and, in the case of HIV, seems to remain engaged throughout. Researchers speculate that HIV turns this normally beneficial response into a cellular malfunction.

Since the early days of HIV/AIDS, scientists have realized that a higher-than-normal proportion of immune cells become and stay activated in a person with HIV than in someone responding to another infection. Ironically, activation makes immune cells more vulnerable to the infection. That's because, when activated, immune cells begin allowing HIV to hijack their cellular machinery in order to copy its viral genes. Stephen Deeks, a well-known HIV/AIDS investigator, said, "The links between immune activation and AIDS seem to be solid. That's especially important because no drug therapy devised so far can wipe out an HIV infection, and a vaccine able to completely prevent it is unlikely. Understanding how HIV and a patient's immune system interact could lead to measures to help infected people live with the virus. Tracking immune activation might someday help doctors decide when to start, stop, and switch drug therapies."

Infection-Enhancing Antibodies

Ramu Subbramanian and colleagues at the University of Montreal (2002) reported that infection-enhancing antibodies (IEAs) make up most of the antibody humoral response to HIV infection. Their results show that the anti-HIV humoral immune response consists of a mixture of antibodies that may inhibit or enhance HIV infection and whose ratios may vary in different stages of the infection. Seventy percent of blood serums from HIV-infected persons contained IEAs. Such antibodies enhance HIV's ability to infect cells!

HIV Protected from Human Antibodies

Humans create antibodies against a number of HIV proteins, namely the envelope proteins (gp120), the transmembrane protein (gp41), and the proteins of HIV's core (gp24). But, *antibodies cannot enter cells*. The antibody can only attack HIV in the plasma. Plasma is the fluid part of the blood and does not include the blood cells. Once inside a host cell, *HIV is protected from antibodies*. Such cells, monocytes, and macrophage and dendritic cells carry HIV internally. All these cell types serve as **HIV reservoirs** in the body. In addition, these cells travel to all distant points within the body and deliver HIV. The self antiretroviral chemicals that these cells generate appear to be ineffective against their hidden traveling companion, HIV (Moir et al., 2000; Olinger et al., 2000).

Latency or Dormancy and Immunologic Memory

HIV latency or dormancy is a consequence of the normal physiology of CD4+ T lymphocytes. At any given time, most CD4+ T lymphocytes are in a resting state. Resting lymphocytes are profoundly quiescent or quiet cells with a low metabolic rate and a unique morphology characterized by a small cytoplasmic volume. In adults, about half of the resting cells are **naïve,** meaning they have yet to encounter an appropriate antigen. The remaining cells are memory cells that have previously responded to an antigen. Antigen-driven responses involve a burst of cellular division and differentiation, giving rise to **memory cells.** These cells have an altered pattern of gene expression enabling long-term survival and rapid responses to the same antigen, should they meet again in the future. With regard to HIV, the virus infects immunologic memory cells, creating a reservoir of HIV within the body. That is, within these memory cells HIV gene expression is largely or completely silenced. In the absence of HIV gene expression, latent cells differ from their uninfected memory cells only by the presence of HIV DNA integrated into the memory cells' DNA. It is difficult to envision any targeting mechanism that will allow specific elimination of this reservoir of HIV-infected dormant or silent memory cells because they cannot be distinguished from the uninfected memory cells.

Perhaps the most disturbing discovery concerning HIV reservoirs in 2001 is the work of Robert Siliciano at Johns Hopkins University. This discovery is disturbing because little is known about memory cells' life span and whether they can be eradicated. Memory cells are programmed to sit and wait for viruses to attack; their job is to keep a record of the germs that the body has previously encountered so that the immune system will be ready the next time it is confronted with those antigens. What HIV has done is tap into the most fundamental aspect of the immune system—a person's immunological memory. It's the perfect mechanism for the virus to ensure its survival. Because the cells are the immune system's memory, they must survive for a long time, creating a latent or dormantly infected reservoir of HIV in the body. This reservoir is the single biggest obstacle to getting rid of HIV. Anthony Fauci, director of the National Institute of Allergy and Infectious Diseases said, "We are not going to be eliminating this reservoir. Whether you can measure it or not doesn't seem to have a significant impact on the clinically relevant phenomenon of what happens when you stop taking the drug."

Once HIV gets inside these cell reservoirs as a **provirus,** it is likely to remain there for the rest of the cell's life (person's life) unless some other antiviral mechanism within the body or some chemical agent is able to destroy the provirus. To date, no such drug has been found to be effective against the HIV provirus.

UPDATE 2008—Pauline Chugh and colleagues (2008) reported on the steps HIV takes to hide out in macrophage cells (one of two major cell types that act as HIV reservoirs; the other is the memory T cells). The research team found that HIV produces a protein that turns on a particular cell survival pathway. After a multistep process, it activates an enzyme called **Akt** that in turn prevents cell suicide. They placed macrophage in laboratory dishes and added drugs known to block the **Akt** pathway. The drug miltefosine blocked the formation of the **Akt** protein, and those treated cells died. This drug is already known to be safe to humans as it is used to treat Leishmaniasis patients (an intestinal disease of humans and other animals caused by the protozoan Leishmania). The real problem is how many macrophages are infected. If too many are infected, how will their loss affect the body's immune system? Miltefosine may be a first and very meaningful step in eliminating one of the two main HIV reservoirs in the body.

CELLULAR MICRO-RNAS CONTRIBUTE TO HIV LATENCY IN RESTING PRIMARY CD4+ T CELLS

Seventeen years ago, no one had even heard of microRNAs. These small but abundant regulatory, noncoding RNAs—initially thought to be an oddity of nematode biology—appear to control gene expres-sion in all animals, as well as in plants, some viruses, and at least one unicellular alga. So far, scientists have tracked their activity in all major organ systems. Some animal microRNAs (miRNAs) are specific to a single tissue or cell type, while others are expressed across multiple organs, and each organ seems to have a unique miRNA profile or characteristic of expression among a set of miRNAs. These profiles change throughout development and during diseases such as cancer, suggesting that they may be useful as diagnostic tools. There's still a lot to learn. MiRNAs inhibit messenger RNA (mRNA) translation, but most miRNAs have not yet been matched with mRNA targets. Their significance, however, is unquestionable. Deepak Srivastava of the University of California, San Francisco, said, "Almost every important gene and pathway will be regulated at multiple levels by a variety of microRNAs. It's really an entirely new layer of biology."

In October 2007, Jialing Huang and colleagues may have found one important explanation as to how HIV can remain dormant or latent in resting CD4+ cells. They found that HIV recruits cellular miRNAs to control the translation of viral RNA into protein. The production of HIV protein is the last step in the creation of HIV antigens, which make the virus visible to the immune system. The research team showed that a cluster of miRNAs bind to a certain location in the viral RNA, which in turn blocks the creation of important proteins and HIV replication.

Resting CD4 cells, they found, are enriched with more than the normal amount of these miRNAs when compared to the activated T cells. When the researchers blocked miRNA-caused viral inhibition, they found that the HIV again was active and able to replicate—proving miRNA's critical role in maintaining latency. They suggest that using miRNA inhibitors might become a kind of therapeutic approach to get the virus out of hiding, making it visible and a target for the immune system.

IMMUNE SYSTEM DYSFUNCTION

When HIV first arrives in the body, there are no immune memory T cells that know how to deal with it. The body has never experienced HIV. As with any other first exposure to an infection, it is the job of **naïve** or **unexposed T cells** to respond (Figure 5-5). Returning to the scene in the lymph nodes, naïve T4 or CD4+ cells get recruited to fight HIV and in turn they become infected. As these infected T cells begin to

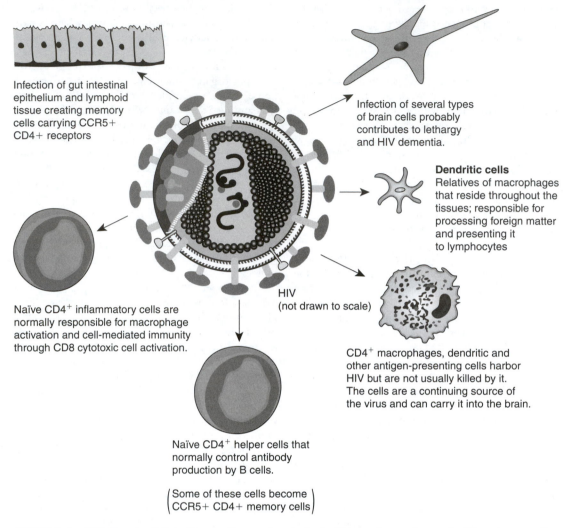

Infection of gut intestinal epithelium and lymphoid tissue creating memory cells carrying CCR5+ CD4+ receptors

Infection of several types of brain cells probably contributes to lethargy and HIV dementia.

Dendritic cells
Relatives of macrophages that reside throughout the tissues; responsible for processing foreign matter and presenting it to lymphocytes

Naïve CD4$^+$ inflammatory cells are normally responsible for macrophage activation and cell-mediated immunity through CD8 cytotoxic cell activation.

HIV
(not drawn to scale)

CD4$^+$ macrophages, dendritic and other antigen-presenting cells harbor HIV but are not usually killed by it. The cells are a continuing source of the virus and can carry it into the brain.

Naïve CD4$^+$ helper cells that normally control antibody production by B cells.

(Some of these cells become
CCR5+ CD4+ memory cells)

FIGURE 5-5 HIV's Favorite Cellular Targets. On entering the body, HIV attaches to those naive T lymphocyte cells carrying CD4+ CCR5+ receptors. Certain of the infected T cells revert back to a resting stage, becoming memory cells infected with HIV or silent reservoirs of HIV in the body. *(Adapted from Eugene Nester, Microbiology, McGraw-Hill Publishing Company)*

divide, HIV is able to replicate and release new viruses from each infected cell. Viral load counts in the blood will usually rise rapidly during this period called **primary** or **acute infection.** During the acute phase HIV also creates latent HIV reservoirs in lymphoid tissue. During this period, a small fraction of the T cells that are activated to fight HIV revert back to a resting, or memory, state. As the cells rest or become dormant, so do the viruses they harbor. In effect, HIV causes two

infections: an active infection that spreads via infected T4 cells to other parts of the body, including the brain; and a dormant, or latent infection that persists in lymphoid tissue to become HIV cell reservoirs.

If this process is allowed to continue unchecked, the large pool of naïve T cells becomes slowly drained. To understand why, think of the lake metaphor. The water flows out of the lake at a rate greater than the amount of water coming in, so if the siphoning isn't stopped, the lake eventually empties. Studies have shown that the naïve T cell pool does indeed dwindle in HIV infection. In fact, a recent study shows that the loss of newly produced naïve T4 cells is strongly linked to disease progression.

ORIGINAL ANTIGENIC SIN

Although there are many facets to immune system dysfunction that investigators have yet to understand, there is one phenomenon that may help us to understand why some diseases leave people with immunity against future attacks while other diseases, like dengue (ding-ee) fever, make people sicker the second time around. Or why some HIV-infected people fare better immunologically and live longer without antiretroviral drugs than others. The explanation for this phenomenon may have to do with **"original antigenic sin"** (OAS). OAS is defined or recognized by the manner in which the immune system responds to vaccination against a disease. In OAS, vaccination creates memory cell DNA sequences that **increase** susceptibility to future exposure to the same disease. For example, if the vaccine were to use "virus A" (HIV), the immune system would learn to recognize it and attack. Later, if a very similar but not identical form of the type A virus (or mutant HIV) were to show up, the body would mobilize against the original type A (HIV) and produce immune cells that might not be fully effective against the new invader, a changed or mutant type A or HIV. In second infections, the immune system does not make new antibodies that exactly fit the antigen but instead looks in its memory cells to see if any antibody messages already exist to do the job. Because the memory cells already know something about the attacking virus, in effect they are halfway round the track when the gun goes off. So the immune system goes on the attack (makes antibodies) directed at the "original" cause of the disease, type A virus or HIV. This is "Original Antigenic Sin." The advantage is that a response can be quickly mobilized. The disadvantage is that the response is shaped by previous antigen, and it may not be the best fit to the current form of that antigen. This idea was originally developed in studies of influenza, which is caused by a virus that changes or mutates so often that new vaccines have to be developed annually. OAS would mean that no new batch of flu vaccine will be 100% effective. How effective the vaccine will be depends on the effects of the OAS— how close the antibodies, now produced, fit the new

mutant flu virus or how structurally close these antibodies are to the originally formed antibodies. The more similar the antibodies, the less effective they will be against new mutant flu viruses or perhaps HIV.

For clarification, if a person's white blood cells or B cells are making four antibodies against four antigen sites that worked against one variety of the flu virus, and he or she contracts another variety of the flu virus that shares only two of those antigenic sites, then his or her immune system will be predisposed to make antibodies against only the two sites the different flu viruses have in common. That is, the immune system mounts an attack **directed at the original form of the virus.** Moreover, the immune system will never learn to recognize the two new antigenic sites that are present on the new flu strain, choosing instead to go with what worked in a prior case of infection. Over time, as the flu virus continues to mutate and has progressively less in common with the original "remembered" antigenic sites, the immune system becomes less prepared to recognize newer flu strains. In effect, the immune system forgoes whole classes of random combinations that might actually work against the new mutant flu virus in favor of tried-and-true varieties, carried in the memory bank, that will not.

How Invading HIV Gets to the T4 or CD4+ Cell: Dentritic Cells Just Doing Their Job!

Based on the recent investigations of American and Dutch scientists, it appears that HIV hijacks immune cells to enter the body's immune system.

Dendritic cells are the watchdogs of the immune system. They are located just below the skin surface and under moist mucosal tissue on surfaces like those of the mouth, gut, genital, and urinary tracts. When dendritic cells see a foreign invader such as a microorganism or virus, they capture it, shred it, and display pieces of proteins from the invading pathogen on their surfaces. These displayed proteins serve to alert other immune system cells such as T4 cells that the body is under attack. What recent investigations now show is that HIV attaches to dendritic cells and hitches a ride into the lymphoid tissues where it then infects T4 cells. The dendritic cell has finger-like projections that carry a protein receptor called **DC-SIGN** (dendritic cell-specific ICAM-3-grabbing nonintegrin). HIV adheres to DC-SIGN and is carried from the mucosal lining of the cervix or rectum to the lymph nodes where it transfers HIV to the T4 cells through their coreceptors CXCR4 (R-4) and CCR5 (R-5) (Steinman, 2000; Geijtenbeck et al., 2000). Thus, another puzzle piece is in place toward the complete understanding of how HIV successfully attacks the human immune system.

Dendritic Trojan Horses

According to Melissa Pope (2002), as capable as dendritic cells are of kicking off a multipronged immune response to any invading pathogen that crosses their paths, something goes terribly wrong when they are confronted with HIV. Herein lies the paradox. The very cells that should be activating the immune system against this pathogen end up facilitating the virus infection. It is now known that some dendritic cells can actually become infected with HIV and replicate the virus. It also appears that the R 5 receptor on immature dendritic cells permits infection and replication to occur.

How HIV Enters T4 or CD4+ Cells and Macrophages

HIV researchers have known since 1984 that human CD4 cell membrane receptors alone are sufficient for binding HIV to the T4 lymphocyte membrane but CD4 receptors are not sufficient for HIV envelope fusion with the T4 cell membrane or for HIV penetration or entry into the cell's interior. This knowledge has enticed many groups of AIDS researchers to search for additional receptors, coreceptors to CD4, that HIV uses to enter a cell after binding to it.

THE SEARCH FOR ADDITIONAL RECEPTORS (CORECEPTORS) TO CD4: FUSIN OR CXCKR-4 (R-4)

In May 1996, Ed Berger (Figure 5-6) and colleagues reported finding a receptor that allowed syncytium-inducing (SI) strains of HIV (HIV that causes T4 cells to form clusters—they attach to each other) to enter T4 cells. Strains of HIV that do not induce T4 cell syncytium formation (NSI) could not enter T4 cells. Berger and colleagues named this T4 cell receptor **FUSIN.** In August 1996 Conrad Bleul and colleagues identified a chemokine, **CXC stromal cell-derived factor-1 (SDF-1)** that binds to the FUSIN receptor and blocks HIV entry. They named this chemokine **R-4.** This coreceptor functions preferentially for T cell line-tropic HIV strains.

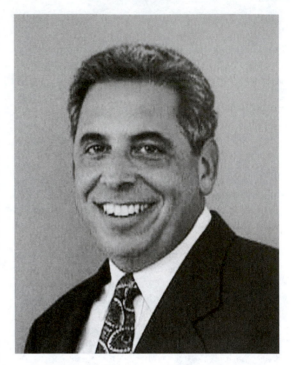

FIGURE 5-6   Edward A. Berger, Chief of the Molecular Structure Section, Laboratory of Viral Diseases at the National Institutes of Allergy and Infectious Diseases. In Spring 1996, he and colleagues discovered the first coreceptor **R-4** or FUSIN that HIV needs to complete its attachment and entry into T4 lymphocytes. In 2007 he received the Bernard Field's Memorial Lectureship award *(Photograph courtesy of National Institutes of Health)*

CCKR-5 (R-5) RECEPTOR

Within two months after the FUSIN receptor data were reported an additional coreceptor called CCKR-5 (R-5) was found. This coreceptor functions mainly in macrophage cells. Members of the research teams who have contributed to the discovery of the R-5 receptor believe that macrophage-tropic or M-tropic HIV strains occur in greatest number early on after HIV infection and then, sometime later during HIV disease the predominant HIV strain shifts to HIV strains that use the FUSIN receptor (R-4) on T4 cells. HIV, by shifting receptors, may be avoiding the suppressive activity of the chemokines that block the R-5 receptor. Figure 5-7 shows a diagram of this suggested **receptor swap** that occurs sometime during HIV disease progression. One of the great unsolved puzzles of HIV dis-

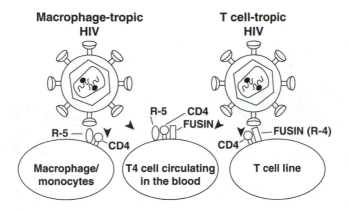

FIGURE 5-7 Coreceptors Required for HIV to Enter Human Cells. HIV can be broadly divided into two classes: those more suitable (tropic) to infecting macrophage, a major reservoir of HIV, and those that infect T4 cells in the lymph nodes or other tissues. HIV usually uses one of two coreceptors, R-5 or R-4 to enter the CD4+ lymphocyte. Macrophage-tropic HIV isolates infect macrophages but fail to infect HIV T cell lines, while T4 HIV strains fail to infect macrophage. But HIV of both classes efficiently infect T4 cells isolated from peripheral blood mononuclear cells (PBMC). Macrophage-tropic HIV appear to be preferentially transmitted by sexual contact and constitute the vast majority of HIV present in newly infected individuals (Zhu, 1993). The T-tropic viruses generally appear late in the course of infection during the so-called "phenotypic switch" that often precedes the onset of AIDS symptoms (Conner et al., 1994). The molecular basis of HIV-1 tropism appears to lie in the ability of envelopes of macrophage-tropic and T-tropic viruses to interact with different coreceptors located on macrophage or T4 cells. Macrophage-tropic viruses primarily use R-5 (80%), R-4 (20%) and less often R-3 and R-2, newly described chemokine receptors, while T-tropic HIV tend to use FUSIN (R-4) (Hill et al., 1996; Moore, 1997).

ease is *why*, during disease progression, does HIV lose its ability to infect macrophage and become T cell tropic? *Why* does HIV switch to other cell receptors?

Figure 5-8 represents the use of R-5 and/or R-4 as necessary HIV attachment sites in conjunction with CD4 to enter a T lymphocyte or macrophage. HIV coreceptor switching R5 to R4 occurs in about half of those in treatment.

EMERGENCE OF HIV STRAINS THAT VARY IN THEIR LETHAL ABILITIES

During the course of HIV disease, viral strains emerge in an infected person that differ widely in their ability to infect and kill different cell types, as well as in their rate of replication. Scientists are investigating why strains of HIV from people with advanced disease appear to be more virulent and infect more cell types than strains obtained earlier from the same person. Part of the explanation may be the expanded ability of the virus to use other coreceptors, such as R-4.

HIV is truly the Houdini virus of all viruses to date. This virus has the ability to change in response

to the human immune system. And not in any predictable pattern. HIV mutates into new forms and escapes—like Houdini, but from the immune system.

IN SEARCH OF GENETIC RESISTANCE TO HIV INFECTION

At this point in the HIV/AIDS pandemic it is believed that about 95% of HIV-exposed people are susceptible to HIV infection and HIV disease progression. This statement is made because it has long been known that some persons who have deliberately avoided safer sex practice and who have had unprotected sex with HIV-infected persons failed to become HIV-infected! The question that has continued to puzzle HIV investigators is, how can multiple HIV-exposed persons remain uninfected? Pieces of that puzzle began to fall into place when two gay males came forward who, despite repeated unprotected sex with companions who died from the disease, remained HIV negative. Neither quite understood why he was spared, but they pressed scientists to come up with the answer. HIV investigators Rong

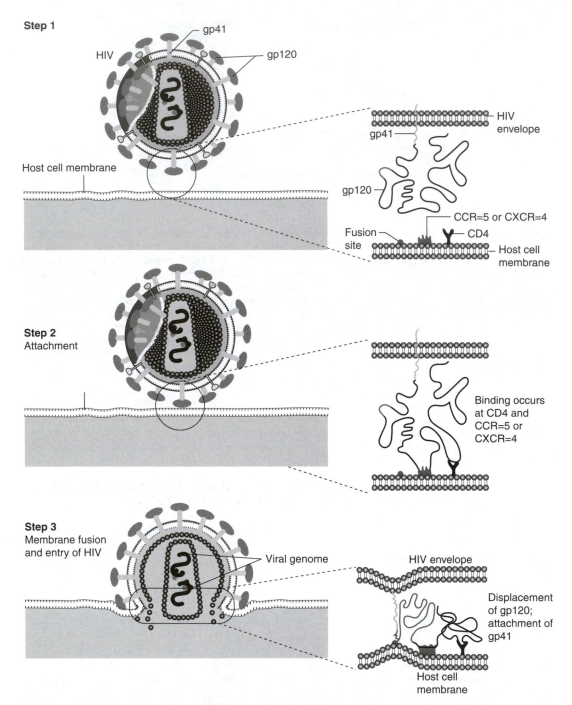

FIGURE 5-8 Attachment and Entry of HIV into a Host Cell, Schematic Representation of CD4 Receptor Binding Step 1: Virion in close proximity to the cell membrane; blowup showing gp120 protein and sites of reaction with host cell receptors. **Step 2:** Initial contact of gp120 is with CD4. Attachment to a chemokine receptor such as R-5 or R-4 must occur before membrane fusion and entry of the viral genome can take place. **Step 3:** Membrane fusion probably is mediated by gp41.

Liu and coworkers (1996) and Michel Samson and coworkers (1996) reported that repeated HIV-exposed but uninfected people have a 32-nucleotide deletion in the gene that produces the R-5 receptors on macrophage. The protein produced by this gene is severely damaged and does *not* reach the cell surface to act as an R-5 chemokine receptor. Without R-5 receptors, the envelope of HIV cannot fuse with the envelope of macrophage to gain entrance into the cell. Thus, people who carry both defective R-5 genes' **homozygotes** (they received one defective gene from each parent) are resistant to HIV infection. If one is **heterozygous** (that is, one carries one defective gene and one normal gene), one will produce the R-5 receptor that HIV needs to penetrate macrophage, but they are fewer in number. Thus, there are fewer R-5 receptors so there are fewer R-5 receptors available for HIV attachment. As a result, heterozygous people are *less* resistant to HIV infection than the homozygous mutant (receptorless) people, but are *more* resistant than people who have two normal genes (homozygous normal) who are the most susceptible to HIV infection. (O'Brien, 1998).

Michael Marmor and colleagues (2001) reported that white gay males who are heterogeneous were 70% less likely to become HIV-infected than those without the mutation. Survival analysis also shows that disease progression is slower in R-5 deletion heterozygotes than in individuals with the normal R-5 gene. Jesper Eugene-Olsen and colleagues (1997) reported that individuals who are heterozygous for the 32-base-pair deletion in the R-5 gene have a slower decrease in their T4 cell count and longer AIDS-free survival than individuals with the wild-type gene for up to 11 years of follow-up.

Sean Philpott and colleagues reported in 1999 that children who inherit the R-5 mutation are protected from vertical HIV infection (mother to newborn via breast milk).

Will the Mutant R-5 Gene Protect People from All Subtypes of HIV?

This genetic defect, the 32-nucleotide deletion, prevents infection only with the strain of HIV (Subtype B) that is transmitted sexually and is prevalent in the United States and Europe. It does not necessarily protect against other strains of HIV transmitted through intravenous drug use or blood transfusions, or strains prevalent in Africa.

Should Everyone Be Tested for the Presence of the R-5 Gene?

Researchers agree that getting tested for the gene would not be difficult, but it would not be of great value because the tested person could still be infected by other strains of HIV. It must be assumed that most people do not carry a pair of defective R-5 genes because 95% or more of HIV-exposed people become HIV-infected.

Who Carries the Defective R-5 Gene?

Perhaps most surprising, HIV investigators found that the homozygous genetic defect is common: **It is present in 1% of whites of European descent.** But it appears to be absent in people from Japan and Central Africa; about 20% of whites are heterozygous for this gene.

Recent studies conducted at Stellenbosch University show that the R-5 gene deletion is virtually absent in the South African black population. Most likely there are other genes involved in the complexity of susceptibility to infection.

Why Does This Gene Exist?

Scientists speculate that the mutant form of R-5 protected against some disease that afflicted Europeans but not Africans. The obvious candidates would be the Black Death of 1346, the plague and/or smallpox. Both lethal diseases are at least 700 years old, enough time for genetic selection to take place. Those without the mutant R-5 gene died, the survivors reproduced and the gene became dispersed within the surviving population. Stephen O'Brien said that the chance of this gene *randomly* reaching its current frequency in the white population is about zero. The idea that a mutant gene can confer protection against a specific infection is not new. The mutation that causes sickle cell anemia provides people carrying one copy of it with resistance (but not immunity) to malaria. There is some evidence that the cystic fibrosis mutation may protect against typhoid fever.

These ideas for why the R-5 gene exists remind us that we carry a genetic record of the diseases of the past and that, at least for some, those genes have once again come to the rescue. In contrast to mutant forms of genes being beneficial, is the report by He Weijing and colleagues (2008) that the mutant form of the Duffy Antigen Receptor for chemokines, which helps protect people living in sub-Saharan Africa from malaria common to the region, could make them more susceptible to HIV infection. The researchers estimated that this gene mutation could account for about 11 percent or 2.7 million HIV infections in Sub-Saharan Africa. This study does have its skeptics who say that the prevalence of HIV infection among those who carry the mutation versus those who do not is barely statistically significant.

T4 CELL DEPLETION AND IMMUNE SUPPRESSION

Means by Which T4 Cells May Be Lost

1. *Filling CD4 Receptor Sites*—There is evidence from in vitro studies that HIV can attack CD4 receptor sites in at least two ways. First, HIV can attach, via its gp160 "spikes," to CD4 receptor sites. Second, HIV is capable of releasing or freeing its exterior gp120 envelope glycoprotein, thereby generating a molecule that can actively bind to CD4-bearing cells (Gelderblom et al., 1985). As a result of filling the receptor sites on the T4 cells, the T4 cells lose their immune functions; that is, the T4 cell does not have to be infected with HIV to lose immune function. In addition, CD4-bearing cells that attach the free gp120 molecule then become targets for immune attack by antibody-mediated antibody-dependent cell cytotoxicity (ADCC) and non-antibody-mediated cytotoxic T cells. Both events can result in the destruction of uninfected CD4-bearing cells.

2. *Syncytia Formation*—The formation of syncytia involves fusion of the cell membrane of an infected cell with the cell membranes of uninfected CD4 cells, which results in giant multinucleated cells (Figure 3-8). A direct relation between the presence of syncytia and the degree of the cytopathic effect of the virus in individual cells has been demonstrated in vitro, and HIV isolated during the accelerated phase of infection in vivo has a greater capacity to induce syncytia in vitro.

3. *Apoptosis*—Programmed cell death, or apoptosis (a-po-toe-sis), is a normal mechanism of cell death that was originally described in the context of the response of immature thymocytes to cellular activation. It is a mechanism whereby the body eliminates autoreactive clones of T cells.

In a typical day, 60 billion to 70 billion cells die. Much of this normal cellular turnover involves **apoptosis.** When apoptotic pathways are defective, insufficient cell death can lead to cancers and autoimmune diseases, and excessive cell death can result in neurodegeneration or stroke. Accordingly, much work is being done to define key players in apoptosis.

4. *Cofactors May Help Deplete T4 Cells*—HIV-infected people who are asymptomatic show a wide variation in HIV disease time and progression to AIDS. It is believed that cofactors may be responsible for some of the time variation with regard to disease progression.

Many agents may act as cofactors to activate or increase HIV production. Although, in general, it is not believed that any cofactor is necessary for HIV infection, cofactors such as nutrition, stress, and infectious organisms have been considered as agents that might accelerate HIV expression after infection. Three new human herpes viruses (HHV-6, 7, and 8) may be cofactors and play a role in causing immune deficiency. They have been shown to infect HIV-infected T4 cells and activate the HIV provirus to increase HIV replication. Cytomegalovirus, Epstein-Barr virus, hepatitis B and C viruses, and tuberculosis have also been associated with increased HIV expression. Over time, investigators expect to find other sexually transmitted diseases that behave as cofactors associated with HIV infection and expression.

Drugs may also be cofactors in infection. Used by injection-drug users (IDUs), heroin and other morphine-based derivatives are known to reduce human resistance to infection and produce immunological suppression. *Pneumocystis* pneumonia is about twice as frequent in heroin users as in homosexuals. It is believed that the heroin has an immunosuppressive effect within the lungs.

Blood and blood products may also act as cofactors in infection because they are immunosuppressive. Because blood transfusions save lives, their long-range effects are generally overlooked. Transfusions in hemophiliacs, for example, result in lowered resistance to viruses such as cytomegalovirus (CMV), Epstein-Barr, and perhaps HIV. Seminal fluid (fluid bathing the sperm) may also act as a cofactor in infection because it also causes immunosuppression. One of its physiological functions is to immunosuppress the female genital tract so that the sperm is not immunologically rejected.

IMPACT OF T4 CELL DEPLETION

The overall impact of T4 cell depletion is multifaceted. HIV-induced T4 cell abnormalities alter the T4 cells' ability to produce a variety of inducer chemical stimulants such as the **interleukins** that are

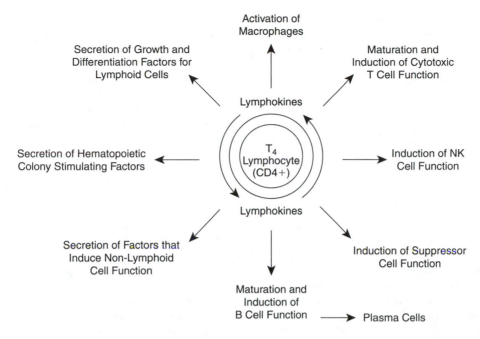

FIGURE 5-9 The T4 or CD4+ Cell Role in the Immune Response. T4 lymphocytes are responsible directly or indirectly for inducing a wide array of functions in cells that produce the immune response. *(Adapted from Fauci, 1995)*

necessary for the proper maturation of B cells into plasma cells and the maturation of a subset of T cells into cytotoxic cells (Figure 5-9). Thus the critical basis for the immunopathogenesis of HIV infection is the depletion of the **T4 lymphocytes,** which results in profound immunosuppression.

Presumably, with time, the number of HIV-infected T4 cells decrease to a point where, in terminal AIDS patients, *few normal T4 cells exist.*

Saha Kunal and colleagues reported on the isolation of CD8+ lymphocytes from HIV-infected patients who produced new HIV. The HIV produced by the CD8+ cells were able to infect both the CD4+ (T4) and CD8+ (T8) cells. CD4+ produced HIV-infected CD8+ cells without using the R-4 or R-5 coreceptors that HIV use to infect CD4+ cells. These data are additional evidence of HIV's ability to adapt to existing biology and to continue to replicate itself.

ROLE OF MONOCYTES AND MACROPHAGES IN HIV INFECTION

Some scientists now believe that T4 cell infection alone does not cause AIDS. They believe that equally important to T4 cell infection is **dendritic, monocyte,** and **macrophage** infection (Bakker et. al.,

1992). Monocytes change into various types of macrophages (given different names) in order to search and destroy foreign agents within tissues of the lungs, brain, and interstitial tissues, tissues that connect organs. Despite the name changes, all forms of macrophages basically work the same way: They ingest things. Some macrophages travel around within the body, others become attached to one spot, ingesting.

Macrophages, like dendritic cells, are often the first cells of the immune system to encounter invaders, particularly in the area of a cut or wound. After engulfing the invader, the macrophage makes copies of the invader's antigens and displays them on its own cell membrane. These copies of the invader antigens sit next to the self molecules. In effect, the macrophage makes a "wanted poster" of this new invader. The macrophage then travels about showing the wanted poster to T4 or CD4+ cells, which triggers the T4 cells into action. Macrophages also release chemicals that stimulate both T4 cell and macrophage production and draw macrophages and lymphocytes to the site of infection.

Macrophage: Trojan Horses

Macrophages may play an important role in spreading HIV infection in the body, both to other cells and to HIV's target organs. First, HIV enters a macrophage and spreads from macrophage to macrophage before the immune system is alerted. Second, macrophages, in their different forms, travel to the brain, the lungs, the bone marrow, and to various immune organs, carrying HIV to these organs.

HIV's ability to infect brain tissue is particularly important. The brain and cerebrospinal fluid (CSF) are specially protected sites. CSF cushions the brain and the spinal cord from sudden and jarring movements. The blood-brain barrier, a chemical phenomenon, normally stops foreign substances from entering the brain and the CSF. But HIV-infected monocytes can pass through this barrier. For HIV, monocyte-macrophages are Trojan horses, enabling HIV to enter the immune-protected domain of the central nervous system—the brain, the spine, the rest of the nervous system.

HIV isolates taken from macrophages appear to grow better in macrophages than in lymphocytes. In human cell culture experiments, HIV isolates taken from lymphocytes appear to grow better in lymphocytes than in macrophages. These peculiarities of replication rates may be evidence of separate tissue-oriented HIV strains.

HIV-infected macrophages have proven to be a major problem in efforts to control and stop HIV infection. Some become reservoir cells protecting HIV from immune destruction.

WHERE DO T4 OR CD4+ CELLS BECOME HIV INFECTED?

The Human Gut-Associated Lymphatic Tissue (GALT)—Despite 25 years (1983–2007) of research on HIV, debates continue about the path from infection to immunological mayhem and failure. There is abundant evidence that HIV preferentially infects and decimates T4 or CD4+ lymphocytes, and some researchers have long argued that direct killing alone causes the profound CD4+ loss that is the hallmark of AIDS. That prompted David Ho to once wear a button saying, "It's the virus, stupid." Another camp contends that HIV infects a relatively small number of CD4+ cells and indirectly causes the massive death of uninfected CD4+ cells by activating them, a process that leads to their premature death.

The studies of Daniel Douek and colleagues (2004–2005) indicated there was both a direct and indirect killing of CD4+ cells beginning with the primary infection of CD4+ cells in **gut-associated lymphatic tissue (GALT)**. Douek and colleagues present fascinating and galvanizing evidence on how HIV blazes through CD4+ cells starting in the lymphatic tissue of the gut (Figure 5-10), then moving into lymph nodes and the blood. Regardless of how HIV enters the body at infection, HIV attaches to CD4+ cells that have surface receptors known as CCR5 (R-5). The vast majority of CD4+/R-5+ cells reside in the gut. The investigators provide a startling photograph taken during colonoscopies. Whereas the uninfected person's ileum had mounds of lymphoid tissue that contained CD4+/R-5+ (Figure 5-10a), the landscape of the ileum of a person recently infected by HIV was scraped clean (Figure 5-10b). The investigators noted that, "You have absolutely no GALT at all—it's completely wiped out." This is absolute evidence that direct killing caused this loss. These investigators provide compelling evidence for a rapid and profound depletion of R-5+ CD4+ cells in the GALT of patients in the first several weeks of HIV infection. GALT is the major reservoir for activated CD4+ cells in the body. Thus, about 50% of the body's memory CD4+ cells are lost within about two weeks after infection by the direct effects of HIV. Interestingly, while there is a significant increase in peripheral blood CD4 cell counts after 6 months on antiretroviral therapy, there is no increase in GALT CD4 cell counts. Thus CD4 depletion in GALT may not be reversible. This may explain treatment failure in some patients. As the diseases progresses to a chronic infection, indirect killing—which takes place, to a large degree, in the lymph nodes—creates additional CD4+ cell loss. The investigators propose that when HIV destroys GALT immunity, other pathogens flourish, which in turn overactivates the lymph production of CD4+ cells, many of which will soon die even though they are uninfected. "Just as the inflammation caused by hepatitis destroys the liver, chronic inflammation of the lymph nodes or immunitis destroys their architecture, leading to massive buildup of collagen, causing fibrosis."

The investigators showed that the greater the amount of collagen in lymph nodes, the less able infected people were to respond to antiretroviral drugs. This may mean that the differences in individual collagen levels may determine their response to drug therapy. The most important ramifications of this improved understanding of how HIV causes disease could be in vaccine research. A vaccine that triggers immune responses in the GALT may best prevent the initial HIV infection.

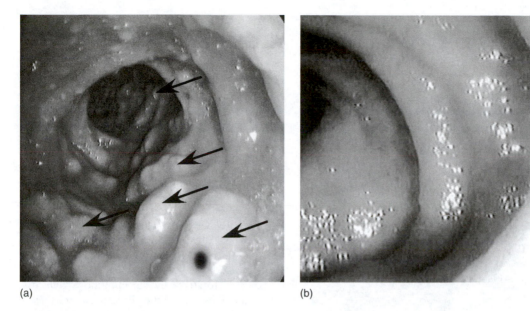

(a)   (b)

FIGURE 5-10 Gastrointestinal Tract Endoscopy: Before and After. (a) The interior lining of the gut of an uninfected person showing numerous lymph node patches. (b) The gut lining stripped of lymph node patches in an HIV-infected person. *(Photographs from Brenchley et al.,* Journal of Experimental Medicine, *2004, Vol. 200, pp. 749–759 by copyright permission of The Rochefeller University Press.)*

A separate study on GALT, by Moraima Guadalupe and colleagues (2006), and Liliana Belmonte and colleagues (2007) showed that even when blood tests show that viral load is undetectable and CD4+ or T4 cell counts are responding well to HIV treatment, there is likely ongoing viral replication and immune system damage occurring in the gut. In other words, HIV replication in the gut is not influenced by HIV drugs. These investigators explained that GALT accounts for 70% of the body's immune system, and restoring GALT function is crucial to ridding the body of HIV. They concluded that blood measurements of viral load and CD4+ cell counts do not provide an accurate analysis of what is happening in GALT.

The Human Lymph Nodes—The **lymph nodes,** which are pea-sized capsules that trap foreign invaders and produce immune cells, are all over the body and are connected by vessels much like those that transport blood (Figure 5-2). Deep within the lymph nodes researchers have found millions of viruses. Based on those data, Fox suggested that HIV uses the lymph nodes as places to meet up with immune cells. Infected T4 cells leave the lymph nodes and new un-

infected cells arrive to become infected. Years later, when enough GALT and lymph node immune cells have been killed, the patient's defenses become so impaired that he or she is vulnerable to any one of a wide array of opportunistic infections—AIDS has arrived.

Anthony Fauci (Figure 5-11), the head of the National Institute of Allergy and Infectious Diseases (NI-AID), and Sonya Heath and colleagues (1995) agree that there are many more HIVs in the lymph nodes than in the blood. Studies in Fauci's laboratory have shown that there are many millions of HIV particles stuck to what are known as **follicular dendritic cells (FDC)** located in hotspots of immune activity in the lymph tissue called germinal centers of an infected individual.

The follicular dendritic cells, which have thousands of long feathery squid-like tentacles emanating from them and whose normal function is to filter and, acting like fly paper, trap antigens for presentation to antibody-producing B lymphocytes, serve as highly effective collection centers for extracellular HIV particles. Virtually every lymphocyte in a lymph node is enmeshed in the processes of these cells. Follicular dendritic cells themselves are susceptible to HIV infection, and appear to place huge numbers of virus

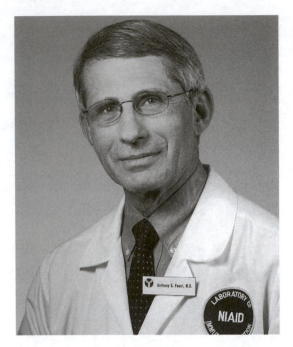

FIGURE 5-11 Anthony S. Fauci, M.D, Director, National Institute of Allergy and Infectious Diseases, National Institutes of Health, Associate Director of NIH for AIDS Research. He received the 2001 Annunzio Humanitarian Award for his impact on the understanding and treatment of infectious diseases/AIDS. In 2007 he received the Mary Woodard Lasker Public Service Award, The Kober Medal—the highest honor of the Association of American Physicians—and the National Medal of Science, bestowed by the president of the United States (Photograph courtesy of National Institute of Allergy and Infectious Diseases)

particles into intimate contact with other cells that are susceptible to HIV infection (Haase et al., 1996; Knight, 1996). FDC also serve as latent reservoirs for HIV.

During the clinically latent phase, the lymph nodes of an infected individual are slowly destroyed.

In the final phase of an infection, the follicular dendritic network completely dissolves and the architecture of the lymph node collapses to produce what Fauci called a "burnt-out lymph node," or Douek's equivalent of collagen causing lymph node fibrosis. With regard to HIV-caused CD4+ cell death, Douek states that with the initial infection of CD4+ cells, rapid renewal of lost CD4+ cells essentially means there will be more cells for HIV to infect! "Unlike any other viruses that we

know of, unlike any other diseases, HIV is a virus that generates its own targets." With this collapse, large amounts of HIV are released into the circulatory system and an ever-increasing number of peripheral cells are infected with HIV (Edgington, 1993).

Implications of a High HIV Replication Rate

Based on Ho and colleagues' kinetic studies of viral replication, it can be estimated that the population of HIV undergoes between 3000 and 5000 replication cycles **(generations)** over the course of 10 years, producing a minimum of 10^{12} (1 trillion) HIV in an HIV-infected person. This creates a lot of opportunity for HIV RNA evolution because genetic mutations occur most commonly during replication. Some mutations will weaken HIV in such a way as to expose it to attack by the immune system. But other mutations will aid the virus, speeding its replication and increasing the chances it can evade the immune system. Because HIV gets so many chances to replicate, it evolves and mutates, and those strains with the greatest replication efficiency gradually win out. This is Darwinian evolution going on in one patient.

In 1996 the hope was that HAART could wipe out HIV. This hope was based on two ideas, both later proved to be wrong: that the drugs would completely stop the virus from reproducing, and that there were no reservoirs where the HIV could hide. But HIV has the uncanny ability to reestablish itself in a variety of cell types. Even the most rigorous attempts to reduce or eliminate HIV from these reservoirs have failed. Scientists had vastly underestimated the extent of virus activity in an HIV-infected person, particularly during the asymptomatic or clinically latent phase. These and other recent studies should satisfy the major unanswered question concerning HIV disease/AIDS, which was, "Where is the virus?" During the 1980s, it was difficult to find medium to high levels of HIV in persons with HIV disease or even in those persons in the later stages of AIDS. We now know that there are large amounts of HIV present early on in the gut and lymph nodes of HIV-diseased people and in viral reservoirs. Perhaps the most troubled group of researchers now may be those currently developing AIDS vaccines. (See Chapter 9 for a discussion about possible HIV vaccines.)

Summary

After a healthy person is HIV-infected, he or she makes antibodies against those viruses that are in the bloodstream, but not against those that have become integrated as HIV proviruses in the host immune cell DNA. Over time the immune system cells that are involved in antibody production are destroyed. Evidence is accumulating that cofactors such as nutrition, stress, and previous exposure to other sexually transmitted diseases that increase HIV expression are associated with HIV infection and HIV disease. Agents that suppress the immune system may also play a significant role in establishing HIV infection. In short, HIV infection is permanent. HIV attaches to CD4-bearing cells and enters those cells using one or more of at least four chemokine receptors **R-2, R-3, R-4 (FUSIN),** and **R-5.** These coreceptors allow HIV to fuse with the cell membrane, and enter the cell after HIV attachment to the CD4 receptor. As seen in Chapter 3, HIV undergoes rapid genetic change, and, as far as is known, attacks only human cells—mostly of the human immune system. It is also known that the body's natural immune response against HIV is inadequate in containing or controlling the virus. Indeed, since the discovery of HIV, there has never been a documented case in which an individual's immune system has ever completely eradicated the virus following established infection. It has recently become quite clear that large amounts of the virus are produced within weeks after HIV infection. The virus remains, for the most part, in the gut and lymph nodes until very late in the disease process.

Review Questions

(Answers to the Review Questions are on page 426.)

1. Which cell type is believed to be the main target for HIV infection? Explain the biological impact of this particular infection.

2. What is CD4, where is it found, and what is its role in the HIV infection process?

3. Is there a period of latency after HIV infection— a time when few or no new HIV are being produced?

4. True or False: HIV is the cause of AIDS.

5. True or False: HIV primarily affects red blood cells.

6. True or False: Lymphocytes have a major role in the immune response to antigens.

7. True or False: All T and B lymphocytes inhibit or destroy foreign antigens.

8. True or False: CD4 and CD8 molecules are antibodies.

9. True or False: HIV belongs to the family of retroviruses.

10. True or False: Cytotoxic and suppressor T lymphocytes are the main targets of HIV.

11. True or False: The latent period is that time between initial infection with HIV and the onset of AIDS.

12. True or False: HIV can spread to infect new cells after it buds out of infected cells.

13. True or False: HIV causes the gradual destruction of cells bearing the CD4 molecule.

14. The most effective use of T4 cell counts in the clinical management of patients with HIV infection is for:

    A. determining when to initiate therapy.
    B. assessing risk of disease progression.
    C. deciding on prophylaxis for opportunistic infections.
    D. measuring the antiretroviral effect of initial therapy.

15. What cells of the immune system are the prime targets of HIV?

6

Opportunistic Infections and Cancers Associated with HIV Disease/AIDS

CHAPTER CONCEPTS

- Suppression of the immune system allows harmless agents to become harmful opportunistic infections (OIs).
- OIs respond well to Highly Active Antiretroviral Therapy (HAART).
- OIs in AIDS patients are caused by viruses, bacteria, fungi, and protozoa.
- In the United States, about 95% of the HIV infected are coinfected with herpes 1 and/or 2. About 40% are coinfected with hepatitis C, and 36% are coinfected with tuberculosis.
- Annually, March 24 is recognized as World Tuberculosis (TB) Day.
- Nearly one-third of the world's population is infected with Mycobacterium tuberculosis.
- Between 700,000 and 800,000 people with tuberculosis are coinfected with HIV.
- Human Herpes Virus-8 is believed to be the cause of Kaposi's sarcoma.
- The cost of treating OIs can be very high.
- There are two types of Kaposi's sarcoma (KS): classic and AIDS-associated.
- Cancers associated with HIV/AIDS are presented.
- KS is rarely found in hemophiliacs, injection drug users, and women with AIDS.
- The clinical presentation of OIs has been impacted by the use of protease inhibitors.

WHAT IS AN OPPORTUNISTIC DISEASE?

Humans evolved in the presence of a wide range of parasites—viruses, bacteria, fungi, and protozoa that do not cause disease in people with an intact immune system. But these organisms can cause a disease in someone with a weakened immune system, such as an individual with HIV disease. The infections they cause are known as **opportunistic infections** (OIs). Thus, OIs occur after a disease-causing virus or microorganism, normally held in check by a functioning immune system, gets the opportunity to multiply and invade host tissue after the immune system has been compromised. For most of medical history, OIs were rare and almost always appeared in patients whose immunity was impaired by either cancer or genetic disease.

With improved medical technology, a steadily growing number of patients become severely immunosuppressed because of medications and radiation used in bone marrow or organ transplantation and cancer chemotherapy. HIV disease also sup-

presses the immune system. Perhaps as a corollary to their increased prevalence, or because of heightened physician awareness, OIs seem to be occurring more frequently in the elderly, who may be rendered vulnerable by age-related declines in immunity. New OIs are now being diagnosed because the pool of people who can get them is so much larger, and, in addition, new techniques for identifying the causative organisms have been developed. However, most of the infections considered opportunistic are not reportable to state or federal governments which interferes with a clear-cut count of their growing numbers.

Although OIs are still not commonplace, they are no longer considered rare—they occur in tens of thousands of HIV/AIDS patients. But despite this increase, physicians and their patients have reasons to be optimistic about their ability to contain these infections. The reasons are: (1) In a massive federal effort, driven by the HIV/AIDS epidemic, researchers are finding drugs that can prevent or treat many of the OIs; and (2) various anti-HIV drug therapies have shown promise for warding off OIs by boosting patients' immune systems.

THE PREVALENCE OF OPPORTUNISTIC DISEASES

The prevalence of OIs in the United States is very high. There are some 500,000 HIV-seropositive individuals with T4 or CD4+ cell counts below 200/μL of blood. Worldwide, there are between 12 and 18 million HIV infected with a T4 or CD4+ cell count of 200 or less. More than 100 microorganisms—bacteria, viruses, fungi, and protozoa—can cause disease in such individuals, even though only a fraction of these (17) are included in the current surveillance definition for clinical AIDS. In a large survey from the Centers for Disease Control and Prevention (CDC), such OIs were diagnosed in 33% of individuals at one year and in 58% at two years after documentation of a T4 cell count below 200/μL. In late 2008 the CDC presented its latest guidelines for prevention and treatment of OIs in HIV-infected persons. The new treatments for OIs have extended the survival of AIDS patients, but they have also opened new issues. With the growing proportion of longer-term AIDS survivors, new OIs have become prominent, together with concerns about cost, compliance, drug interactions, and quality of life (Laurence, 1995; *MMWR*, 1995b). The six most common AIDS-related OIs are bacterial pneumonia, candidal esophagitis, pulmonary/disseminated TB, mycobacterium avium complex disease, herpes simplex reinfection, and *Pneumocystis* pneumonia or PCP. The year 1997 marked the first time, since the AIDS pandemic began in the United States, that the incidence of AIDS-defining OIs among HIV-infected persons fell in number from the previous year's total. The reason: the use of antiretroviral drugs.

OPPORTUNISTIC INFECTIONS IN HIV-INFECTED PEOPLE

AIDS is a devastating human tragedy. It appears to be killing about 95% of those who demonstrate the symptoms. One well-known American surgeon said, "I would rather die of any form of cancer rather than die of AIDS." This statement was not made because of the social stigma attached to AIDS or because it is lethal. It was made in recognition of the slow, demor-

alizing, debilitating, painful, disfiguring, helpless, and unending struggle to stay alive.

Because of a suppressed and weakened immune system, viruses, bacteria, fungi, and protozoa that commonly and harmlessly inhabit the body become pathogenic (Figure 6-1). Prior to 1998, about 90% of deaths related to HIV infection and AIDS were caused by OIs, compared with 7% due to cancer and 3% due to other causes. Now, with the use of antiretroviral drugs, OIs cause about 50% of deaths. Liver and kidney organ failure, heart disease, and various cancers are on the increase as the cause of death in AIDS patients.

HIV-Related Opportunistic Infections Vary Worldwide

The course of HIV infection tends to be similar for most patients: Infection with the virus is followed by seroconversion (HIV test changes from negative to positive) and progressive destruction of T4 or CD4+ cells. Yet the opportunistic infections and malignancies that largely define the symptomatic or clinical history of HIV disease vary geographically. People with HIV and their physicians in different regions confront distinct problems, mainly because of differences in exposure, in access to diagnosis and care, and in general health.

Comparisons between the data about opportunistic infections in different countries must be made with care. But most developing nations lack the facilities and trained personnel to identify opportunistic infections correctly; consequently, their prevalence may be underreported. Clinicians in developed countries can order sophisticated laboratory analyses to identify pathogens. Those in developing countries must rely on signs and symptoms to make their diagnoses. Oral candidiasis and herpes zoster are easy to diagnose without laboratory backup because the lesions are visible. While some pneumonias and types of diarrhea can be specified, others, such as extrapulmonary tuberculosis, cytomegalovirus infections, cryptococcal meningitis, and systemic infections such as histoplasmosis, toxoplasmosis, microsporidiosis, and nocardiosis, go underreported due to the lack of laboratory facilities.

Socioeconomic Factors

Geography explains much about the varying patterns of opportunistic infections, but a decisive factor is often financial capacity. On the most fundamental

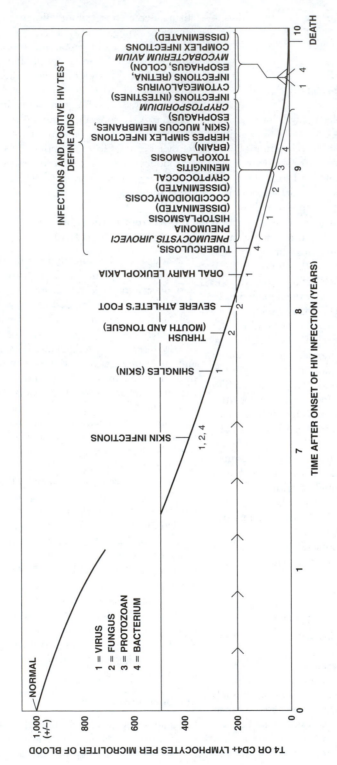

FIGURE 6–1 General Progression of Opportunistic Infections in Untreated Adolescent/Adults After HIV Infection. Normal T4 or CD4+ cell count in adolescent/adults is, on average, about 1000/μL of blood. There is a relationship between the drop in T4 lymphocytes and the onset of opportunistic infections (OIs). The first sign of an OI begins under 500 T4 cells/μL. As the T4 or CD4+ cell count continues to drop, the chance of OI infection increases. Note the variety of OIs found in AIDS patients with 200 or less T4 cells/μL.

THE CHANGING SPECTRUM OF OPPORTUNISTIC INFECTIONS

Fourteen years ago there was hardly any standardized use of protective agents to block the infectious complications or opportunistic infections (OIs) associated with HIV-induced immunodeficiency. Now there is an array of drugs that can be used in strategies to prevent or delay nearly all the major OIs. With this advancement has come the need to weigh the pros and cons of the various strategies. Cost, antimicrobial resistance, drug interactions, and pill overload are all important considerations.

EFFECT OF ANTI-HIV THERAPY ON OPPORTUNISTIC INFECTIONS

As presented in Chapter 4, the use of anti-HIV combination drug therapy has produced a number of unexpected results in patient response to those drugs. Soon after combination therapy began, physicians witnessed a rather confusing or unusual presentation of OIs. In some cases certain OIs improved, in others the situation deteriorated. Such changes in OI expression are occurring now, at a time when hundreds of thousands of HIV-infected Americans are on Highly Active Antiretroviral Therapy (HAART).

TREATMENT IN THE HAART ERA

HAART therapy appears to help the human immune system. When HIV patients take retroviral medicines that control HIV replication, their immune systems begin to recuperate in ways that are puzzling and controversial. For example, patients recover immunity to some deadly opportunistic infections but appear unable to fight diseases for which they were vaccinated as children, for example, tetanus, or to target HIV itself. Collectively, such observations indicate HAART patients can only raise successful immune responses against pathogens they see regularly. For example, cytomegalovirus is an organism found in almost everybody's blood, so the immune systems of HAART patients see the pathogen constantly and generate cells and antibodies that attack it. But tetanus is something people rarely encounter, so HAART patients, unlike their HIV-negative counterparts, fail to raise immune responses against it. The ultimate irony is

that HAART, when successful, destroys all but a few million HIVs that are forced into hiding.

Recent studies suggest that the incidence of esophageal candidiasis and, by inference, other forms of *Candida* infection has fallen by 60% to 70% in patients treated with HAART. The use of HAART dramatically changed the epidemiology of opportunistic infections and is clearly associated with gradual recovery of the immune system (Powderly et al., 1998; Ledergerber et al., 1999).

This information aside, when HIV is controlled with the antiretroviral drugs, immunity to infections—other than HIV—usually starts to return. As a result, some opportunistic infections go away without specific treatment; and sometimes patients can stop prophylactic treatment for certain opportunistic diseases. However, entering year 2009, it is still unclear who can stop prophylaxis safely, and who cannot.

Studies from 1998 through 2008 using protease inhibitor drugs in HAART have shown that virtually no patient whose T4 level rose to and stayed over 200 to 300 per microliter of blood (μL) developed an OI. This is the strongest evidence to date that immune reconstruction is occurring with antiretroviral drug therapy, and suggests that it occurs early and with quite modest improvements in T4 cell levels. The implication is that the search for immunorestorative therapy other than with the current antiretroviral is somewhat less urgent than previously believed, though still a clear priority.

VIRAL LOAD RELATED TO OPPORTUNISTIC INFECTIONS

HIV clinicians have recently looked at the predictive value of plasma HIV RNA for the development of three OIs: PCP, CMV, and MAC. Using a database of patients participating in AIDS Clinical Trial Groups (ACTG), for every 1-log increase in plasma HIV RNA level, the risk of developing one of these OIs was increased two- to threefold. Plasma HIV RNA level was predictive of an increased risk of an OI independent of T4 cell count, which also predicted OI risk. This information confirms that maintaining control of viral replication may be a critical component of preventing OIs in HIV-infected patients.

level, money is needed to create an infrastructure that limits exposure to pathogens. Thus, while few people with HIV in wealthy countries develop certain bacterial or protozoal infections, they are a major

cause of death in poor areas that cannot provide clean water and adequate food storage facilities.

Financial resources also affect clinicians' abilities to diagnose AIDS and, when appropriate, to provide the proper medicine. AIDS patients in Africa often die of severe bacterial infections because they don't have the antibiotics or the clinical care they need. They don't survive long enough to develop diseases such as PCP.

United States, Europe, and Africa—The United States and Europe on one end, and Africa on the other, represent the global extremes of financial resources for health care. The most common opportunistic infections each region faces reflect the overall quality of health care, sanitation, and diet. For example, Thailand and Mexico belong to the large group of nations that have intermediate incomes and correspondingly intermediate patterns of HIV complications (Harvard AIDS Institute, 1994).

AIDS patients rarely have just one infection (Table 6-1). The mix of OIs may depend on lifestyle and where the HIV/AIDS patient lives or has lived. Thus, a knowledge of the person's origins and travels may be diagnostically helpful. (Note: a number of the symptoms listed in the CDC definition of HIV/AIDS can be found associated with certain of the OIs presented.)

Fungal Diseases

In general, healthy people have a high degree of innate resistance to fungi. But a different situation prevails with opportunistic fungal infections, which often present themselves as acute, life-threatening diseases in a compromised host (Medoff et al., 1991).

Because treatment seldom results in the eradication of fungal infections in AIDS patients, there is a high probability of recurrence after treatment (DeWit et al., 1991).

Fungal diseases are among the more devastating of the OIs and are most often regional in association. AIDS patients from the Ohio River Basin, the Midwest, or Puerto Rico have a higher-than-normal risk of histoplasmosis (his-to-plaz-mo-sis) infection. In the Southwest, there is increased risk for coccidioidomycosis (kok-sid-e-o-do-mi-ko-sis).

In the southern Gulf states, the risk is for blastomycosis. Other important OI fungi such as ***Pneumocystis jiroveci***-(nu-mo-sis-tis yer-row-vet-see), ***Candida albicans*** (kan-di-dah al-be-cans), and ***Cryptococcus neoformans*** (krip-to-kok-us knee-o-for-mans) are found everywhere in equal numbers. Because of their importance as OIs in AIDS patients, a brief description of histoplasmosis, candidiasis, *Pneumocystis carinii* pneumonia, and cryptococcosis are presented.

Histoplasmosis (**Histoplasma capsulatum**)—Spores are inhaled and germinate in or on the body (Figure 6-2). This fungal pathogen is endemic in the Mississippi and Ohio River Valleys. Signs of histoplasmosis include prolonged influenza-like symptoms, shortness of breath, and possible complaints of night sweats and shaking chills. Histoplasmosis in an HIV-positive person is considered diagnostic of AIDS. In about two-thirds of AIDS patients with histoplasmosis, it is the initial OI. Over 90% of cases have occurred in patients with T4 cell counts below $100/\mu L$ (Wheat, 1992).

Candidiasis or Thrush (**Candida albicans**)—This fungus is usually associated with vaginal yeast infections. It is a fungus quite common to the body and in particular inhabits the alimentary tract. It is normally kept in check by the presence of bacteria that live on the linings of the alimentary tract. However, in immunocompromised patients, especially those who have received broad spectrum antibiotics, candida multiplies rapidly. Because of its location in the upper reaches of the alimentary tract, if unchecked, it may cause mucocutaneous candidiasis or **thrush,** an overgrowth of candida in the esophagus and in the oral cavity (Figure 6-3). Mucosal candidiasis has been associated with AIDS patients from the very beginning of the AIDS pandemic (Powderly et al., 1992). In women, overgrowth of candidiasis also occurs in the vaginal area.

Oral or esophageal candidiasis causes thick white patches on the mucosal surface and may be the first manifestation of AIDS. Because other diseases can cause similar symptoms, candidiasis by itself is not sufficient for a diagnosis of AIDS.

A New Name for *Pneumocystis Carinii* Is *Pneumocystis Jiroveci* (yee-row-vet-see)

In September 2002, James Stringer and colleagues, based on DNA evidence, reported that *Pneumocystis carinii* is the species that infects rats and that *Pneumocystis jiroveci* infects humans. Given the compelling evidence that the human form of *Pneumocystis* is a separate species, the most important objection to designating it as such has been the problem that this name change could create in the medical literature, where the disease caused by *P. jiroveci* is widely known as *Pneumocystis carinii* pneumonia. This problem can be avoided by taking the species name out of the disease name. Under this system, PCP would refer to

Table 6-1   Some Common Opportunistic Diseases Associated with HIV Infection

Organism/Virus	Clinical Manifestation
Protozoa	
Cryptosporidium muris	Gastroenteritis (inflammation of stomach–intestine membranes)
Isospora belli	Gastroenteritis
Taxoplasma gondii	Encephalitis (brain abscess), retinitis, disseminated
Fungi	
Candida sp.	Stomatitis (thrush), proctitis, vaginitis, esophagitis
Coccidioides immitis	Meningitis, dissemination
Cryptococcus neoformans	Meningitis (membrane inflammation of spinal cord and brain), pneumonia, encephalitis, dissemination (widespread)
Histoplasma capsulatum	Pneumonia, dissemination
Pneumocystis jiroveci	Pneumocystic pneumonia
Bacteria	
Mycobacterium avium complex (MAC)	Dissemination, pneumonia, diarrhea, weight loss, lymphadenopathy, severe gastrointestinal disease
Mycobacterium tuberculosis (TB)	Pneumonia (tuberculosis), meningitis, dissemination
Viruses	
Cytomegalovirus (CMV)	Fever, hepatitis, encephalitis, retinitis, pneumonia, colitis, esophagitis
Epstein-Barr	Oral hairy leukoplakia, B cell lymphoma
Hepatitis C (HCV)	Liver cirrhosis or cancer (major reason for liver transplants)
Herpes simplex	Mucocutaneous (mouth, genital, rectal) blisters and/or ulcers, pneumonia, esophagitis, encephalitis
Papovavirus J-C	Progressive multifocal leukoencephalopathy
Varicella-zoster	Dermatomal skin lesions (shingles), encephalitis
Cancers	
Kaposi's sarcoma	Disseminated mucocutaneous lesions often involving skin, lymph nodes, visceral organs (especially lungs and GI tract)
Primary lymphoma of the brain	Headache, palsies, seizures, hemiparesis, mental status, or personality changes
Systemic lymphomas	Fever, night sweats, weight loss, enlarged lymph nodes

Patients with compromised immune systems are at increased risk for all known cancers and infections (including bacterial, viral, and protozoal). Most infectious diseases in HIV-infected patients are the result of proliferation of organisms already present in the patient's body. Most of these opportunistic infections are not contagious to others. The notable exception to this is tuberculosis.

Disclaimer: This table was developed to provide general information only. It is not meant to be diagnostic nor to direct treatment.

(Adapted from Mountain-Plains Regional Education and Training Center HIV/AIDS Curriculum, 4th ed., 1992 updated, 1997; and from MMWR 2002.)

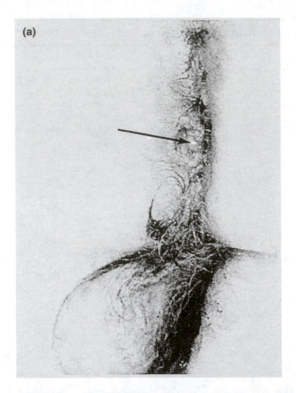

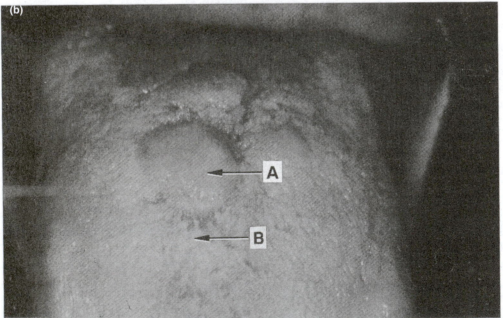

FIGURE 6–2 (a) Anal Histoplasmosis. Histoplasmosis is caused by *Histoplasma capsulatum* and causes infection in immunocompromised patients. (b) AIDS patient's tongue showing multiple shiny, firm *Histoplasma* erythematous nodules (see arrow A) and thrush (see arrow B). (*A, Courtesy of the Centers for Disease Control and Prevention, Atlanta; B, Courtesy of Marc E. Grossman, New York*)

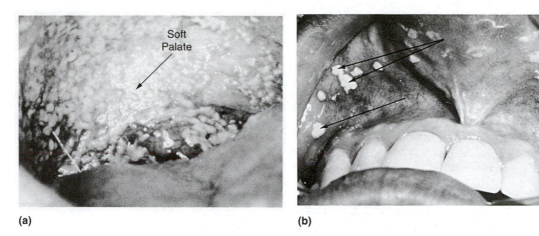

(a) **(b)**

FIGURE 6-3 Thrush **(a)** An overgrowth of *Candida albicans* on the soft palate in the oral cavity of an AIDS patient. **(b)** Creamy patches of candida that can be scraped off, leaving a red and sometimes bleeding mucosa. (**A,** *Courtesy of the Centers for Disease Control and Prevention, Atlanta;* **B,** *Schiodt, Greenspan, and Greenspan 1989. American Review of Respiratory Disease, 1989, 10:91–109. Official Journal of the American Thoracic Society* © *American Lung Association*)

Pneumocystis pneumonia. This simple modification accommodates the name change pertaining to the *Pneumocystis* species that infects humans. Furthermore, adopting this change makes the acronym appropriate for describing the disease in every host species, none of which, except rats, is infected by *P. carinii*. In summary, the acronym PCP will be retained in the literature. But the causative agent will be referred to as *Pneumocystis jiroveci* or Pj pneumonia where necessary. **From this point forward in the book, PCP will be used with the understanding that it is caused in humans by *Pneumocystis jiroveci*.**

Virtually everyone in the United States by age 30 to 40 has been exposed to *P. jiroveci*. It lies dormant in the lungs, held in check by the immune system. Prior to the AIDS epidemic, PCP pneumonia was seen in children and adults who had a suppressed immune system as in leukemia or Hodgkin's disease and were receiving chemotherapy. In the AIDS patient, the onset of PCP pneumonia is insidious—patients may notice some shortness of breath and they cannot run as far. It causes extensive damage within the alveoli of the lungs.

Prior to 1981, fewer than 100 cases of PCP infection were reported annually in the United States; yet 80% of AIDS patients develop PCP pneumonia at some time during their illness. This is one of the few AIDS-related conditions for which there is a choice of relatively effective drugs. The first of these to be

made available was the intravenous and aerosolized versions of pentamidine. There are frequent recurrences of this infection. PCP accounted for a diagnosis of AIDS in over 65% of AIDS cases in 1990. In 1994 it had fallen to 20% due to available therapy (Ernst, 1990; Murphy, 1994). The triad of symptoms that almost always indicates the onset of PCP during HIV disease is fever, dry cough, and shortness of breath (Grossman et al., 1989). PCP pneumonia is unlikely to develop in people with HIV disease unless their T4 cell count drops below 200 (Phair et al., 1990).

Viral Diseases

Hepatitis C—Hepatitis means an inflammation or swelling of the liver. Viruses can cause hepatitis. Alcohol, drugs (including prescription medications) or poisons can also cause hepatitis. In late 1999, **hepatitis C** caused by the hepatitic C virus **(HCV)** was classified as an OI because the relative risk for liver-associated death is increased sevenfold in HIV-positive patients compared to non-HIV-infected individuals. It is estimated that 200 million people worldwide are infected with the hepatitis C virus. Over 4 million of the infected live in America.

HIV/HCV Means Double Trouble

The hepatitis C virus (HCV) is now at least four times as widespread in America as HIV. It kills between

10,000 and 15,000 each year and is predicted to kill 30,000 a year by 2010. Its transmission is similar to that of HIV. About 30% of people living with HIV infection in America, about 250,000 people, are believed to be coinfected with the HCV. Among some groups, primarily HIV-positive current and former intravenous-drug users, the coinfection rate is thought to be about 90%. According to the National Hemophilia Foundation, the coinfection rate among HIV-positive hemophiliacs is equally high. For those who become infected with HCV, the virus produces no symptoms for 10–30 years. Then symptoms like fatigue, joint and abdominal pain, nausea, and lapses in concentration begin to set in. Because doctors have not traditionally screened patients for the virus, many people do not even know they are infected until their livers show signs of serious damage. Studies now indicate that HIV can greatly speed the progression of hepatitis C. That means that many with HIV may suffer advanced liver disease (cirrhosis of the liver) after just 5 or 10 years, even as the antiretroviral drugs boost their life expectancies. Studies on HCV's effects on AIDS patients have been contradictory, but the coinfection has been associated with a higher risk of progression to HIV disease and AIDS. The antiretroviral drugs used to fight HIV, particularly the protease inhibitors, place a great strain on the liver, the organ whose function is to metabolize them. Over the last nine years (2000–2008), hepatitis C coinfections have been and will most likely continue to be the leading cause of liver failure and death in AIDS patients. Some patients infected with both viruses find that their bodies have great difficulty tolerating many HIV/AIDS and HCV drugs. At present, there is no national policy for dealing with this virus.

Herpes Viruses

Because of a depleted T4 or CD4+ cellular component of the immune system, AIDS patients are at particularly high risk for the herpes family of viral infections: cytomegalovirus, herpes simplex virus types 1 and 2, varicella-zoster virus, and Epstein-Barr virus.

Cytomegalovirus (CMV)—This virus is a member of the human herpes virus group of viruses. CMV is the perfect parasite. It infects most people asymptomatically. When illness does occur, it is mild and nonspecific. There have been no epidemics to call attention to the virus. Yet CMV is now considered the most common infectious cause of mental

retardation and congenital deafness in the United States. It is also the most common viral pathogen found in immunocompromised people (Balfour, 1995).

The virus is very unstable and survives only a few hours outside a human host. It can be found in saliva, tears, blood, stool, cervical secretions, and in especially high levels in urine and semen. Transmission occurs primarily by intimate or close contact with infected secretions. The incidence of CMV infection prior to the beginning of HAART therapy in 1996 varied from between 30% and 80% depending on the geographical community tested. In the 1980s, over 90% of homosexual males tested positive for CMV (Jacobson et al., 1988).

CMV infection of AIDS patients usually results in prolonged fever, anemia (too few red blood cells), leukopenia (too few white blood cells), and abnormal liver function. **CMV also causes severe diarrhea and HIV-associated retinitis resulting in eventual blindness** (*Emergency Medicine,* 1989; Lynch, 1989).

Prior to HAART therapy, 75% of AIDS patients had an eye disease, with the retina the most common site (Russell, 1990). The retina, which is a light-sensitive membrane lining the inside of the back of the eye, is also part of the brain and is nourished by blood vessels. AIDS-related damage to these vessels produces tiny retinal hemorrhages and small cotton wool spots—early indicators of disease that are often detected during a routine eye examination (Figure 6-4). Since the beginning of HAART therapy, CMV retinitis has fallen to about 5% in AIDS patients.

In unusual circumstances, the virus can produce dramatic symptoms, such as loss of vision within 72 hours. Without treatment, CMV can destroy the entire retina in three to six months after infection.

Herpes Viruses Types 1 and 2 (HSV-1 and -2)—The name *herpes* comes from the Greek *herpein*—"to creep." Members of the *Herpesviridae* family have been identified in a variety of animals, and they all share certain features, including an ability to establish latency following primary infection, as well as a potential to reactivate and cause further disease. Herpes infections are among the most commonly diagnosed infections among the HIV/ AIDS population. Almost all HIV-infected individuals (95%) are coinfected with HSV-1 and/or HSV-2. Both viruses cause *severe* and progressive eruptions of the mucous membranes.

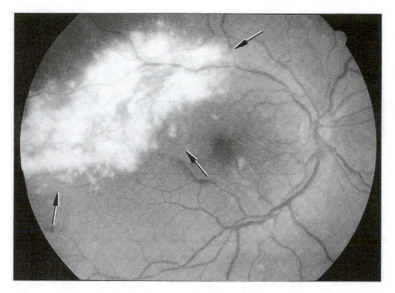

FIGURE 6-4 Cytomegalovirus Retinitis. The disease, as seen in this photograph, involves the posterior pole of the right eye. Fluffy white infiltrate (**cotton wool spots**) with a small amount of retinal hemorrhage can be seen in the distribution of the superior vascular arcade. (*Courtesy of Scott M. Whitcup, M.D., National Eye Institute, National Institutes of Health, Bethesda, Md.*)

HSV 1 affects the membranes of the nose and mouth. Also, when herpetic lesions involve the lips or throat, 80% to 90% of the time they either precede or occur simultaneously with **herpes-caused pneumonia** (Gottlieb et al., 1987). Bacterial or fungal super-infections occur in more than 50% of herpes-caused pneumonia cases and are a major contributory cause of death in AIDS patients.

Mortality from HSV pneumonia exceeds 80% (Lynch, 1989). Herpes may also cause blindness in AIDS patients. The following is from Paul Monette's *Borrowed Time:*

> I woke up shortly thereafter, and Roger told me—without a sense of panic, almost puzzled—that his vision seemed to be losing light and detail. I called Dell Stead-man and made an emergency appointment, and I remember driving down the freeway, grilling Roger about what he could see. It seemed to be less and less by the minute. He could barely see the cars going by in the adjacent lanes. Twenty minutes later we were in Dell's office, and with all the urgent haste to get there we didn't really reconnoiter till we were sitting in the examining room. I asked the same question—what could he see?—and now Roger was getting more and more upset the more his vision darkened. I picked up the phone to call Jamiee, and by the time she answered the phone in Chicago he was blind. **Total blackness, in just two hours!**
>
> The retina had detached. (An operation on retinal attachment was successful and sight was restored. The cause of the retinal detachment was a herpes infection of the eyes.)

HSV-2 affects the membranes of the vagina, penis, and anus, causing severe ulcers in and on these organs.

Herpes of the skin can generally be managed with oral **acyclovir** (Zovirax), Foscavir, or Famvir.

Herpes Zoster Virus (HZV)—Like herpes simplex, this virus has the potential to cause a rapid onset of pneumonia in AIDS patients. Untreated HZV pneumonia has a mortality rate of 15% to 35%. HZV is now monitored as an early indicator that HIV-positive people are progressing toward AIDS.

Protozoal Diseases

An increasing number of infections that have not been observed in immunocompromised patients are being found in AIDS patients. Two such infections are caused by the protozoans *Toxoplasma gondii,* and *Cryptosporidium muris.*

Toxoplasma gondii—*T. gondii* is a small intracel-lular protozoan parasite that lives in vacuoles inside host macrophages and other nucleated cells. It appears that during and after entry, *T. gondii* pro-duces secretory products that modify vacuole mem-branes so that the normal *fusion* of cell vacuoles with lysosomes containing digestive enzymes is blocked. Having blocked vacuole-lysosome fusion, *T. gondii* can successfully reproduce and cause a disease called **toxoplasmosis** (Joiner et al., 1990). It can infect any warm-blooded animal, invading and multiply-ing within the cytoplasm of host cells. As host immunity develops, multiplication slows and tissue cysts are formed. Sexual multiplication occurs in the intestinal cells of cats (and apparently only cats); oocysts form and are shed in the stool (Sibley, 1992). Transmission may occur transplacentally, by ingestion of raw or undercooked meat and eggs containing tissue cysts or by exposure to oocysts in cat feces (Wallace et al., 1993).

In the United States, 10% to 40% of adults are chronically infected but most are asymptomatic. *T. gondii* can enter and infect the human brain causing **encephalitis** (inflammation of the brain). Toxoplasmic encephalitis develops in over 30% of AIDS patients at some point in their illness (Figure 6-5). The signs and symptoms of cerebral toxoplasmosis in AIDS patients may include fever, headache, confusion, sleepiness, weakness or numbness in one part of the body, seizure activity, and changes in vision. These symptoms can get worse and progress to coma and death unless toxoplasmosis is promptly diagnosed and treated. Thus, for most AIDS patients, it is believed that *T. gondii* is latent within their bodies and is reactivated by the loss of immune competence.

Cryptosporidium—*Cryptosporidium* is the cause of cryptosporidiosis, and is a member of the family of organisms that includes *Toxoplasma gondii* and *Isospora*. Its life cycle is similar to that of other organisms in the class Sporozoa. Oocysts are shed in the feces of infected animals and are immediately infectious to others. In humans, the organisms can be found throughout the GI tract. *Cryptosporidium* causes **profuse watery diarrhea** of 6 to 26 bowel movements per day with a loss of 1 to 17 liters of fluid (a liter is about 1 quart). It is an infrequent infection in AIDS patients, usually occurring late in the course of disease as immunological deterioration progresses.

Studies of transmission patterns have shown infection within families, nursery schools, and from person to person, probably by the fecal-oral route. The infection is particularly common in homosexual men, perhaps as a consequence of anilingus (oral-anal sex). About 15% of people with HIV/AIDS are infected with this parasite.

Bacterial Diseases

There is a long list of bacteria that cause infections in AIDS patients. These are the bacteria that normally cause infection or illness after the ingestion of contaminated food, such as species of *Salmonella*. Others, such as *Streptococci, Haemophilus,* and *Staphylococci* are common in advanced HIV disease. A number of other bacteria-caused sexually transmitted diseases such as syphilis, chancroid, gonorrhea, and chlamydial diseases are also associated with HIV disease.

One difference between AIDS and non-AIDS individuals is that bacterial diseases in AIDS patients are of greater severity and more difficult to treat. Two bacterial species, *Mycobacterium avium intracellulare* and *Mycobacterium tuberculosis* are of particular importance as agents of infection in AIDS patients (Table 6-2).

Mycobacterium avium intracellulare (MAI)—Over the past 40 years, MAI has gone from a rare, reportable infection to something that is common in most large American communities. Unlike tuberculosis, which is almost exclusively spread person to person, MAI is, in most instances, environmentally acquired. MAI exists in food, animals, water supplies, and soil, and enters people's lungs as an aerosol when they take showers.

MAI occurs in about 25% of people with HIV disease and has been implicated as the cause of a non-specific **wasting syndrome.** AIDS patients demonstrate **anorexia** (inability to eat), weight loss, weakness, night sweats, diarrhea, and fever. Some patients also experience abdominal pain, enlarged liver or spleen, and malabsorption. In contrast to viral infections, this bacterium rarely causes pulmonary or lung problems in AIDS patients. Among persons with AIDS, the risk of developing disseminated MAI increases progressively with time. AIDS patients surviving for 30 months had a 50% risk of developing disseminated MAI. It appears most HIV-infected per-

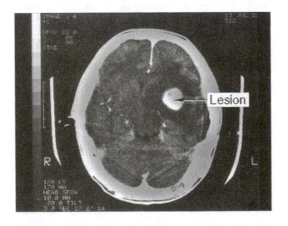

FIGURE 6–5 *Toxoplasma gondii* Lesions in the Brain. Radiographic imaging shows a deep ring-enhancing lesion located in the basal ganglia. *(Courtesy of Carmelita U. Tuazon, George Washington University)*

Table 6-2 Categories of Organism and Viral Involvement in Opportunistic Diseases

Symptoms	Causative Agent	Symptoms	Causative Agent
Generally Present		Proctocolitisa[1]	*Entamoeba histolytica*
Fever, weight	*Pneumocystis jiroveci*	(diarrhea,	Campylobacter
loss, fatigue,	Cytomegalovirus	abdominal pain,	Shigella
malaise	Epstein-Barr virus	rectal pain)	Salmonella
	Mycobacterium avium intracellulare		*Chlamydia trachomatis*
	Candida albicans		Cytomegalovirus
		Proctitisa[1]	*Neisseria gonorrhoeae*
Diffuse Pneumonia		(pain during	Herpes simplex
Dyspnea, chest	*Pneumocystis jiroveci*	defecation,	*Chlamydia trachomatis*
pain, hypoxemia,	Cytomegalovirus	diarrhea, itching,	*Treponema pollidum*
abnormal chest	*Mycobacterium tuberculosis*	and perianal	
X-ray	*Mycobacterium avium intracellulare*	ulcerations)	
	Candida albicans		
	Cryptococcus neoformans	**Neurological Involvement**	
	Toxoplasma gondii	Meningitis,	Cytomegalovirus
		encephalitis,	Herpes simplex
Gastrointestinal Involvement		headaches,	*Toxoplasma gondii*
Esophagitis	*Candida albicans*	seizures, dementia	*Cryptococcus neoformans*
(sore throat,	Herpes simplex		Papovavirus
dysphagia)	Cytomegalovirus (suspected)		*Mycobacterium tuberculosis*
Enteritis	*Giardia lamblia*	Retinitis	Cytomegalovirus
(diarrhea,	*Entamoeba histolytica*	(diminished	*Toxoplasma gondii*
abdominal pain,	*Isospora belli*	vision)	*Candida albicans*
weight loss)	Cryptosporidium		
	Strongyloides stercoralis		
	Mycobacterium avium intracellulare		

[1] Especially in those persons practicing anal sex.

Adapted from Amin, 1987.

For Sexual Exposures—People should use male latex condoms during every act of sexual intercourse to reduce the risk of exposure to cytomegalovirus, herpes simplex virus, and human papillomavirus, as well as to all other sexually transmitted pathogens. Use of latex condoms will help prevent the transmission of HIV to others. Avoid sexual practices that may result in oral exposure to feces (oral-anal contact) to reduce the risk of intestinal infections such as cryptosporidiosis, shigellosis, campylobacteriosis, amebiasis, giardiasis, and hepatitis A and B.

sons will develop disseminated MAI if they do not first die from other OIs (Chin, 1992).

World Tuberculosis (TB) Day

World TB Day is observed on March 24 each year and commemorates the date in 1882 when Dr. Robert Koch announced the discovery of *Mycobacterium tuberculosis,* the bacterium that causes tuberculosis (TB). Worldwide, TB remains one of the leading causes of death from infectious disease. An estimated two billion persons (i.e., one-third of the world's population) are infected with *M. tuberculosis.* Each year, approximately nine million persons become ill from TB; of these, nearly two million die from the disease. World TB Day provides an opportunity for TB programs, nongovernmental organizations, and other partners to describe problems and solutions re-

lated to the TB pandemic and to support worldwide TB control activities.

Tuberculosis dates back to at least 4000 B.C. and was present in ancient Egypt, Greece, Rome, and India. Known as consumption, it was responsible for one in five deaths in 17th century London.

Tuberculosis (TB) is now the leading cause of illness and death in people infected with HIV. TB is spread almost exclusively by airborne transmission. TB has been observed in elephants, cattle, mice, and other animal species.

The disease can affect any site in the body, but most often affects the lungs. When persons with pulmonary TB cough, they produce tiny droplet nuclei that contain TB bacteria, which can remain suspended in the air for prolonged periods of time. (With respect to transmission, the cough to TB is like sex to HIV.) Anyone who breathes air that contains these droplet nuclei can become infected with TB. It has been suggested that there is a minimal chance of inhaling HIV in blood-tinged TB sputum (Harris, 1993).

An estimated 10 to 15 million Americans are infected with TB bacteria. About 10% of otherwise healthy persons who have latent tuberculosis infection will become ill with active TB at some time during their lives. With HIV disease, the risk is 10% per year. It has been estimated that through year 2008, 14 million HIV-infected people worldwide will be coinfected with TB. No two diseases are more inextricably linked. HIV infection severely weakens the immune system, allowing TB to become active. A person with an HIV infection is 50 times more likely to express the symptoms of TB than a non HIV-infected person. HIV accelerates the disease! Were it not for HIV, global TB infections would be declining. Without effective drug therapy for TB, millions of coinfected (HIV/TB) Africans will die of TB over the coming years.

Tuberculosis is not generally considered to be an OI because people with healthy immune systems contract TB. After infection with *M. tuberculosis* about 5% of immunocompetent individuals will develop TB (Daley, 1992).

Drug Resistant TB

In 2005, an outbreak of extremely drug resistant TB (XDR-TB) occurred in Kwazulu-Natal province in South Africa. This strain of TB received national attention at the 2006 International AIDS meeting in Toronto, Canada. XDR-TB strains are resistant to at least seven of the most important drugs used to treat TB. The two most important first-line anti-tuberculosis drugs are isoniazid and vifampin, the two second-line drugs are of the fluorquinolone class, and the three other very useful drugs are third-line drugs. About 30,000 cases of XDR-TB occur each year and are present throughout South Africa!

TB AND HIV

According to the World Health Organization, TB worldwide is the leading cause of death in HIV-infected people. TB has killed at least 200 million people since 1882, the date of the discovery of the bacterium that causes TB. Millions more die from TB each year. Globally, TB was estimated to account for 30% of AIDS-related deaths each year from 2000 through 2008. In the United States, 14% of HIV/AIDS patients are also coinfected with TB.

Other Opportunistic Infections

Other opportunistic infectious organisms and viruses and the diseases they cause and possible therapies are listed in Table 6-1. Table 6-2 separates OIs into the body parts most affected by a particular organism or virus.

From diagnosis until death, the AIDS battle is *not* just against its cause, HIV, but against those organisms and viruses that cause OIs. Opportunistic infections are severe, tend to be disseminated (spread throughout the body), and are characterized by multiplicity. Fungal, viral, protozoal, and bacterial infections may be controlled for some time but are rarely curable.

CANCER OR MALIGNANCY IN HIV/AIDS PATIENTS

Common sense tells us that viruses should be cleared from our bodies just like any other invading pathogen. However, many are not cleared entirely and are able to persist by establishing latent or dormant infection. In many cases, virus-host interactions have evolved over the millennia such that viruses reproduce, remain viable, and are transmitted. During this time, host immune systems contain these viral infections and prevent severe illness or death. Examples of such viruses include herpesviruses and papillomaviruses. Herpesviruses that can establish latent and long-term infection in host humans include cytomegalovirus (CMV) or human herpesvirus 5 (HHV-5), Kaposi's sarcoma-associated herpesvirus (KSHV) or human herpesvirus 8 (HHV-8), and Epstein-Barr virus (EBV). Many of the viruses that become latent in the body—for example, HPV, CMV, and EVB—are quite common in the human population but do not always lead to the development of a cancer. It is now known that infection with HIV changes the playing field, and the environment of immunosuppression may eventually tip the scale in favor of these viruses, leading to an increased risk of cancer.

Malignancy

The word "malignancy" means a cancer. Specifically, cancer is an abnormal growth of cells that divide uncontrollably and may spread to other parts of the body. There are many kinds of cancer, which can involve just about any part of the body.

HIV infection carries with it a high susceptibility to certain cancers. Because of the severe and progressive impairment of the immune system, host defense mechanisms that normally protect against certain types of cancer are lost.

Cancer is a significant cause of mortality and morbidity in people infected with HIV; in fact, 30% to 40% will develop a malignancy or cancer during their lifetime. The majority of cancers affecting HIV-positive people are those established as **AIDS-defining** Kaposi's sarcoma (KS), non-Hodgkin's lymphoma, invasive cervical cancer, and progressive multifocal leukoencephalopathy (oral and anal). However, other types of cancer, **non-AIDS defining** but AIDS associated or opportunistic, also appear to be more common among those infected with HIV. While not classified as AIDS-defining, these malignancies are rising in the HIV/AIDS community (Table 6-3). The introduction of highly active antiretroviral therapy (HAART) has since 1996 resulted in decreased mortality and morbidity in cases of AIDS-defining cancers. The majority of people in developed countries infected with HIV are now living with only mild to moderate immunosuppression because of wide access to antiretroviral therapy. The widespread use of antiretroviral drugs has altered the incidence of cancer by increasing the prevalence of some types of cancer in the HIV-infected population.

Of the four types of AIDS-associated cancers, KS occurs with the greatest frequency and is discussed in some detail. The other three cancer conditions are briefly described. (For a review of HIV/AIDS-related cancers read Hessol, 1998; Grulich 2000; Newcomb-Fernandez, 2003.)

Table 6-3 Some Non–AIDS-Defining Cancers with Increased Incidence in the HIV-Infected Population

Leukemia	Esophagus	Kidney
Multiple myeloma	Lip	Colorectal
Skin cancer	Tongue	Brain and CNS
Penile	Stomach	Heart
Vulva/Vagina	Larynx	Angiosarcoma
Leiomyosarcoma	Hodgkin's disease	Squamous cell
Burkitt's lymphoma	Pancreas	carcinoma
Pharynx	Liver	

Note: The four most frequent non-AIDS cancer-related deaths are lung cancer, cancer of the gastrointestinal tract, including liver cancer, blood-related cancers, such as leukemia and Hodgkin's disease, and anal cancer. Considering that HIV-positive patients are living longer due to the use of antiretroviral therapy, researchers believe that death rates due to non–AIDS-related cancers will likely continue to overshadow death rates associated with classic AIDS-related cancers. (Adapted from Jennifer Newcomb-Fernandez in *RITA* 9:5–10, 2003; Hessol et. al., 2007 and Patel et. al. 2008)

Kaposi's Sarcoma (cap-o-seas sar-com-a)

No other HIV/AIDS-related opportunistic disease attacks and singles out one segment of the population as KS does with HIV-positive gay men. Men with KS outnumber women approximately 19 to 1; HIV-positive homosexual men with KS outnumber heterosexual men almost as significantly. KS is extremely rare in hemophiliacs with HIV.

HIV infection represents an overwhelming risk factor for the development of KS, which was rare in the United States (incidence less than 1/100,000/year) before the HIV epidemic. It is an aggressive disease, with involvement of the gut, lung, pleura, lymph nodes and the hard and soft palates.

In the United States, Kaposi's sarcoma is at least 300 times more common in people with HIV/AIDS than in the general population.

KS was first described by Moritz Kaposi in 1877 as a cancer of the muscle and skin. Characteristic signs of early KS were bruises and birthmark-like lesions on the skin, especially on the lower extremities. KS was described as a slow-growing tumor found primarily in elderly Mediterranean men, Ashkenazi Jews, and equatorial Africans.

Kaposi's sarcoma as described by Moritz Kaposi is called classic KS and it differs markedly from the KS that occurs in AIDS patients (Figure 6-6). Classic KS has a variable prognosis (forecast), is usually slow to develop, and causes little pain **(indolent).** Symptoms of classic KS are ulcerative skin lesions, swelling **(edema)** of the legs, and secondary infection of the skin lesions.

Kaposi's Sarcoma and AIDS

The HIV/AIDS epidemic has brought a more virulent and progressive form of KS marked by painless, flat to raised, pink to purplish plaques on the skin and mucosal surfaces that may spread to the lungs, liver, spleen, lymph nodes, digestive tract, and other internal organs. In its advanced stages it may affect any area from the skull to the feet (Figure 6-7). In the mouth, the hard palate is the most common site of KS (Figure 6-8) but it may also occur on the gum line, tongue, or tonsils.

The prevalence of KS among gay men in 1981 was 77%; by 1987, it had fallen to 26% and by 2004 to less than 5% in gay men on HAART.

Human Herpes Virus Is the Kaposi's Virus—Most HIV/AIDS researchers now believe that HIV is not the primary pathological agent for Kaposi's sarcoma; rather, they believe a herpes virus is the primary cause.

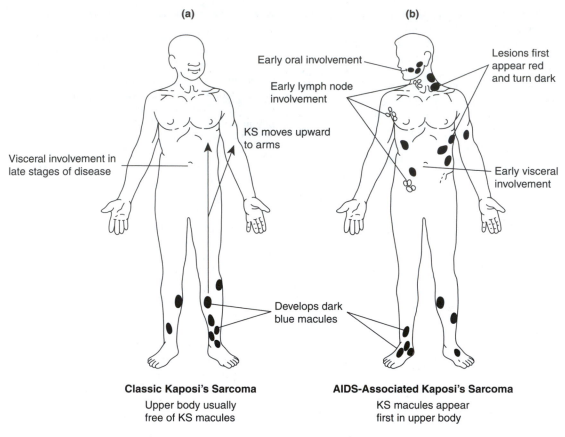

(a)

Early oral involvement

Early lymph node involvement

KS moves upward to arms

Visceral involvement in late stages of disease

(b)

Lesions first appear red and turn dark

Early visceral involvement

Develops dark blue macules

Classic Kaposi's Sarcoma
Upper body usually
free of KS macules

AIDS-Associated Kaposi's Sarcoma
KS macules appear
first in upper body

FIGURE 6-6 Classic and AIDS-Associated Kaposi's Sarcoma. **(a)** Patients with classic KS (non-AIDS-related) demonstrate violet to dark blue bruises, spots, or macules on their lower legs. Gradually, the lesions enlarge into tumors and begin to form ulcers. KS lesions may, with time, spread upward to the trunk and arms. The movement of KS appears to follow the veins and involves the lymph system. In the late stages of the disease, visceral organs may become involved. **(b)** For AIDS patients, initial lesions appear in greater number and are smaller than in classic KS. They first appear on the upper body (head and neck) and arms. The lesions first appear as pink or red oval bruises or macules that, with time, become dark blue and spread to the oral cavity and lower body, the legs, and feet. Visceral organs may be involved early on and the disease is aggressive. However, death is not caused by KS.

In December 1994, Yuan Chang and colleagues reported that they found DNA sequences that appear to represent a **new human herpes virus (HHV-8)** in KS tissue. Evidence continues to accumulate indicating that HHV-8 is the infectious agent responsible for KS (Kledal et al., 1997; Said et al., 1997).

Many research papers on whether herpes virus 8 causes KS have been published in recognized scientific/medical journals. It appears there is a cause-and-effect relationship; HHV-8/KS.

The work of Charles Rinaldo and colleagues (2001) reveals that healthy non HIV-infected people who carry HHV-8 have a healthy immune response and control the virus. HIV-infected persons who carry HHV-8 have

a poor immune response to the virus, which then becomes a precursor for the expression of KS.

The Kaposi's virus may have entered the same population in which HIV is endemic, which would explain why the two are often transmitted together. HIV may produce the right conditions for Kaposi's development by causing growth factor production, and possibly by suppressing the body's immune defenses against cancer.

Lymphoma (lim-fo-mah): Cancer of the Lymph Glands

Lymphomas are the second most common cancer in HIV and are now the seventh most common cause

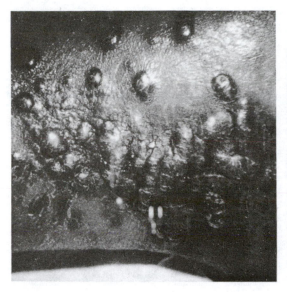

FIGURE 6-7 Kaposi's Sarcoma on Lower Leg of an AIDS Patient. (*Courtesy of Nicholas J. Fiumara, M.D., Boston*)

of death for people with AIDS. A lymphoma is a neoplastic disorder (cancer) of the lymphoid tissue (Figure 6-9). B cell lymphoma occurs in about 1% of HIV-infected people, but makes up about 90% to 95% of all lymphomas found in people with HIV disease (Herndier et al., 1994; Scadden, 2002). Although it occurs most often in those demonstrating persistent generalized lymphadenopathy (swollen lymph glands), the usual site of lymphoma growth is in the brain, the

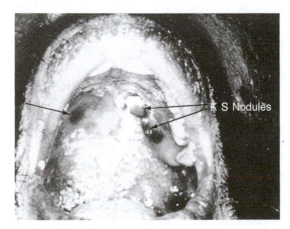

FIGURE 6-8 Oral Kaposi's Sarcoma. KS can be seen on the hard palate and down the sides of the oral cavity. (*Courtesy of Nicholas J. Fiumara, M.D., Boston*)

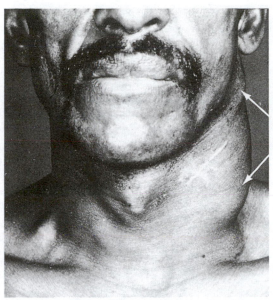

FIGURE 6-9 HIV/AIDS Patient Demonstrating a Lymphoma of the Neck. (*Courtesy of the Centers for Disease Control and Prevention, Atlanta*)

heart, or the anorectal area. The most common signs and symptoms are confusion, lethargy, and memory loss. Lymphomas are increasing in incidence primarily due to the extension of the life span of AIDS patients because of medical therapy (Tables 6-1 and 6-3).

AIDS-Related Lymphomas (ARL)

AIDS-related lymphomas (ARL) are a heterogeneous group of aggressive non-Hodgkin's lymphomas occurring 60-fold more frequently in HIV-infected individuals than in the non–HIV-infected population. ARL shortens life more than any other commonly occurring cancer in HIV infection. Some changes in the distribution and outcome of ARL have been documented since the advent of HAART. These changes vary among the various forms of ARL. While the incidence of ARL in HIV infection has decreased overall since the beginning of HAART in 1995, there has been no change within any patient grouping defined by CD4+ T cell counts.

Non-Hodgkin's Lymphoma

The risk of non-Hodgkin's lymphoma (NHL, also referred to as AIDS-related lymphoma) is substantially increased in the HIV-infected population, with risks ranging from about 100 to 200 times that of the general population. Many agree that the risk of developing NHL increases with lower CD4 T cell counts and further progression of HIV infection. Moreover, NHL is more prevalent in HIV-positive women than in high-risk HIV-negative women, indicating that immunosuppression, rather than other risk factors, is associated with the increased incidence of NHL in the HIV-positive community. No definitive conclusions can be drawn regarding the effect of HAART on the incidence of NHL, although it continues to be one of the most common malignancies afflicting those with HIV infection.

Progressive Multifocal Leucoencephalopathy (leuco means white; encephalo means brain; pathy means disease)

Progressive multifocal leucoencephalopathy (PML) is an opportunistic infection caused by a papovavirus [Jamestown Canyon virus (JCV)] affecting about 5% of AIDS patients. It is usually fatal within an average of 3.5 months and there is no treatment. In a few patients spontaneous improvement and prolonged survival have been reported. Some observations have indicated that cytosine arabinoside, a potent antiviral, may reverse the symptoms of PML. Symptoms of PML include altered mental status, speech and visual disturbances, gait difficulty, and limb incoordination (Guarino et al., 1995).

Invasive Cervical Cancer

Though invasive cervical cancer (ICC) is considered an AIDS-defining condition, the association between HIV and cervical cancer is somewhat inconsistent. Some analyses report no increase in incidence that is coincident with the AIDS epidemic, and no correlation between immunosuppression and increased risk of developing the cancer. Indeed, HIV-positive women with ICC tend to have higher CD4 T cell counts than HIV-positive patients with other malignancies. Still, other studies report that HIV-positive women are approximately five to nine times more likely to have ICC than are seronegative women, and this cancer accounts for 55% of AIDS-related malignancies in some settings. Moreover, the clinical course becomes even more aggressive when CD4 T cell count is low. Decreased CD4+ cell counts are associated with an increased risk of becoming infected with the human papillomavirus (HPV). HPV is associated with almost all cases of cervical cancer, and women who are HIV infected are even more likely to be coinfected with HPV. The use of HAART does not appear to affect the incidence of ICC.

Human Papillomavirus (HPV)

There are over 100 viruses known as human papillomavirus (HPV). They are common. One study found HPV in 77% of HIV-positive women. HPV is transmitted easily during sexual activity. It is estimated that 75% of all sexually active people between ages 15 and 49 get at least one type of HPV infection. Some types of HPV cause common warts of the hands or feet. Several types of HPV cause genital warts on the penis, vagina, and rectum. Those with HIV can get worse sores in the rectum and cervical areas. HPV can also cause problems in the mouth or on the tongue or lips. Other types of HPV can cause abnormal cell growth known as dysplasia. Dysplasia can develop into anal cancer in men and women, or cervical cancer, or cancer of the penis.

Can HPV Infection Be Prevented?

There is no easy way to tell if someone is infected with an HPV. People who don't have any signs or symptoms of HIV infection can transmit the infection. And condoms do not totally prevent the transmission of HPVs. HPVs can be transmitted by direct contact with infected areas that aren't covered by a condom. A vaccine called Gardasil was approved in 2006. However, it has not been tested in or approved for people already infected with HPV.

Summary for HIV and Cancers

The cancer prognosis for people infected with HIV tends to be worse compared to seronegative cancer patients regardless of the type of cancer (Table 6-3). Perhaps because of a suppressed immune system and impaired immune surveillance, cancers take a more aggressive clinical course in those infected with HIV. HIV-positive patients typically present with more advanced cancer at the time of diagnosis, and the average age of diagnosis is usually younger in HIV-positive patients compared to seronegative patients; this is particularly true with lung and testicular cancers.

The Impact of HAART

Preliminary data suggest that with the exception of KS, HAART has not had a significant impact on cancer incidence in the HIV-positive population, though it may be premature to draw any definitive conclusions at this time. Widespread availability of HAART has only occurred within the last dozen years, and many of the cancers discussed require years to develop.

While the goal of antiretroviral therapy is the suppression of HIV replication, failure to accomplish this objective is common in clinical practice. Also, data suggest that the continuing efficacy of present antiretroviral therapy may allow more HIV-infected patients to survive with long-term mild to moderate immunosuppression, thereby placing such patients at risk for the development of lymphoproliferative disorders such as Hodgkin's and non-Hodgkin's lymphomas. Indeed, recent data suggest that 23% to 50% of patients receiving HAART developed Hodgkin's and non-Hodgkin's lymphomas despite effective HIV suppression and high CD4 T cell counts. These results substantiate the idea that the development of lymphomas in HIV-infected individuals is a complex process.

HIV Provirus: A Cancer Connection

In early 1994 AIDS investigators reported that HIV, on entering lymph cell DNA, activated nearby cancer-causing genes (oncogenes). The evidence suggests that HIV itself may trigger cancer in an otherwise normal cell.

These findings may mean that a variety of retroviruses that infect humans may also cause cancer (McGrath et al., 1994). Such findings raise concerns for developing an HIV vaccine. Using a weakened strain of HIV to make the vaccine may, when used, increase the incidence of lymphoma and other cancers.

DISCLAIMER

This chapter is designed to present information on opportunistic infections in HIV/AIDS patients. The author does not accept any responsibility for the accuracy of the information or the consequences arising from the application, use, or misuse of any of the information contained herein, including any injury and/or damage to any person or property as a matter of product liability, negligence, or otherwise. No warranty, expressed or implied, is made in regard to the contents of this material. This material is not intended as a guide to self-medication. The reader is advised to discuss the information provided here with a doctor, pharmacist, nurse, or other authorized healthcare practitioner and to check product information (including package inserts) regarding dosage, precautions, warnings, interactions, and contraindications before administering any drug, herb, or supplement discussed herein.

Summary

One of the gravest consequences of HIV infection is the immunosuppression caused by the depletion of the T4 or CD4+ helper cell population; suppressed immune systems allow for the expression of opportunistic diseases and cancers. The OI, end organ failures, and cancers kill AIDS patients, not HIV per se. It is the cumulative effect of several OIs that creates the chills, night sweats, fever, weight loss, anorexia, pain, and neurological problems.

KS is characterized as a cancer that can spread to all parts of an AIDS patient's body. About 20% of AIDS patients, mostly gay men, have KS. It is not usually found in hemophiliacs, injection-drug users, or female AIDS patients.

Review Questions

(Answers to the Review Questions are on pages 426–427.)

1. Define opportunistic infection (OI).

2. Which OI organism expresses itself in 80% of AIDS patients? Where is it located and what does it cause?

3. Which of the protozoal OI organisms causes weight loss, watery diarrhea, and severe abdominal pain?

4. Which of the bacterial OIs causes "wasting syndrome," night sweats, anorexia, and fever?

5. True or False: Kaposi's sarcoma (KS) is caused by HIV. Explain.

6. Name the two kinds of KS.

7. True or False: KS affects all AIDS patients equally. Explain.

8. True or False: Candidiasis and ulceration may be present in patients with HIV infection.

9. True or False: Oral candidiasis occurs frequently with HIV infection.

10. True or False: The use of combination anti-HIV drug therapy, especially those combinations containing a protease inhibitor, have substantially decreased the severity and number of OIs in AIDS patients.

A Profile of Biological Indicators for HIV Disease and Progression to AIDS

CHAPTER CONCEPTS

- Why all the fuss about HIV/AIDS?
- Clinical signs and symptoms of HIV infection and AIDS are presented.
- Stages of HIV disease vary substantially.
- HIV replication is rapid and continuous in HIV-infected lymphoid cells.
- AIDS Dementia Complex presents as mental impairment.
- Viral load indicates current viral activity.
- T4 or CD4+ cell counts indicate degree of immunologic destruction.
- Information on long-term survival is presented.
- Serological changes after HIV infection are presented.
- The rate of clinical HIV disease progression is variable among individuals infected with HIV.
- The development of AIDS over time is discussed.
- Elite controllers and long-term survivors, with and without drug therapy.
- Classification of HIV/AIDS progression is presented.
- Clinical indicators to track HIV disease progression are listed.
- Diarrhea is the most common gastrointestinal sign and symptom of HIV/AIDS infection.
- Humanized mice may become a model animal system in which to study the pathology of HIV/AIDS.
- Clues to pediatric AIDS diagnosis are presented.

HIV has the vexing capacity to do the right thing for itself and the wrong thing for those it infects.

SNAPSHOT 7.1

HIV/AIDS UNITED STATES: ESTIMATED KEY DATA 2009

1. New HIV Infections Annually over 56,000
2. People Living with HIV/AIDS—1.2 million
3. People with HIV/AIDS Not in Care—about 50%
4. People Who Don't Know They Are HIV Infected—about 27%

HIV DISEASE DEFINED

The diagnosis of AIDS in the 1980s was most often associated with a quick death. Mortality came quickly and was inevitable within a few months of the diagnosis. It was at the time, and still is, one of the few terminal diseases that elicits the questions, **"How did you get it?"**

By the mid-1980s the CDC had learned enough about HIV infection to call it a disease. That made sense, as the vast majority of those who became infected became ill. HIV infection leads to the loss of T4 or CD4+ cells, which in turn produces a variety of signs and symptoms of a **nonspecific disease** with initial acute fever-associated illness or mononucleosis-like symptoms that may last up to four weeks or longer. After the initial symptoms, most individuals enter a clinically asymptomatic phase (see Case in Point 7.1). This means the infected person feels well while his or her immune system is slowly compromised. It has been shown that long-lasting symptomatic **primary** HIV infection predicts an increased risk of rapid development of HIV-related symptoms and AIDS, but it is not known whether the different responses to HIV infection are caused by viral factors, host factors, or both. Virulent (extremely infectious) strains of HIV have

WHY ALL THE FUSS ABOUT HIV/AIDS?

Why has the U.S. federal government spent over $238 billion over the past 22 years (1987–2008) on just this one disease? More money has been spent on HIV/AIDS in its relatively short history than on any other human disease in our history. In addition, the public/private sector has spent a sum equal to or greater than the government over the same time period. (See Chapter 14 for a breakdown of the billions spent on this disease.)

First, over the past years, AIDS has been killing about 2.5 million people each year worldwide. Through 2009, an estimated 24 million people will have died of AIDS worldwide. Malaria, TB, heart disease, cancer—no other disease is spreading or growing at this rate. In spite of HIV/AIDS campaigns in most countries, there is little evidence so far of any slowdown in the spread of the epidemic. By the end of 2009, about 59 million people are expected to have been infected by HIV.

Second, this virus is mainly transmitted during sexual intercourse. Since few human societies talk openly and honestly about sex, this makes this disease difficult to discuss; and since sex is a very private activity, it makes the transmission of HIV very difficult to control.

Third, it has an extraordinary capacity for change and rapid global spread.

Fourth, there is a long asymptomatic period between infection and illness. On average, it takes about 10 to 12 years for someone infected with HIV to develop AIDS. During this time, the HIV infected will show few if any recognizable symptoms, but they will be able to infect other people. This long asymptomatic period is rare in human infectious disease. People dying today represent those infected 10 to 20 years ago; the results of anything we do now to reduce transmission will not be apparent for years.

Fifth, HIV/AIDS is more serious than many more common diseases because of the age groups it attacks. Some diseases—measles and diarrhea, for example—affect mainly infants and children; others, such as heart disease and cancer, affect mainly the old. But because HIV is predominantly transmitted

sexually, AIDS mainly kills people in their twenties through forties. A major increase in deaths among these age groups, society's most productive groups, has a much greater impact socially and economically than deaths that occur among children or old people would have.

Sixth, in the past, plagues were often marked by their lack of discrimination, by the way in which they killed large numbers of people with little regard for race, wealth, sex, or religion. But AIDS was different from the beginning. It immediately presented a political as much as a public health problem. Homosexuals, who until the pandemic had been mostly closeted in the United States, were suddenly at the heart of a health crisis as profound as any in modern American history.

Seventh, with respect to therapy, HIV disease/AIDS requires the use of some of the most expensive and toxic drugs in medical history.

Eighth, it is a disease that has severely stigmatized those who have it.

Ninth, it is a disease that has parents burying their children.

Tenth, and lastly, this virus means there are other viruses in waiting. This has awakened our most primal fear; dying a horrible death by an unknown agent. Examples include the West Nile encephalitis virus that struck the New York City metropolitan area in the summer and fall of 1999, the SARS virus that struck in 2003, and the avian flu virus that began its global spread in 2005.

So why all the fuss about HIV/AIDS? It is caused by a unique virus that changes itself faster than a rumor making the gossip column of a tabloid. It is lethal, it is transmitted, most often sexually, it affects people in their reproductive and most productive years, it is exceptionally expensive to treat, it defies our best scientists who are working to create a vaccine for preventing infection and transmission, and it is a disease that has severely stigmatized those who have it.

HIV has one requirement to continue its presence on earth: a human host!

been characterized by their rapid replication, **syncytium-inducing (SI sin-sish-e-um)** capacity, and tropism (attraction) for various types of T cells. It is known that the biological properties of HIV strains in asymptomatic HIV-infected individuals with normal T4 or CD4+ cell counts may predict the subsequent development of HIV-related disease, and that patients who harbor SI isolates develop immune deficiency more rapidly. It is not clear whether the appearance of more virulent strains during the symptomatic phase of the infection is a cause or an effect of progressive immune deficiency (Nielson et al., 1993). Several studies have demonstrated that a long period of fever around the time of **seroconversion** (the presence of detectable HIV antibody in the serum) is associated with more rapid development of immune deficiency (Pedersen et al., 1989).

Spectrum of HIV Disease

Because the immune system slowly falters, HIV disease is really a spectrum of disease (Figure 7-1). At one end of the spectrum are those infected with HIV who look, feel, and are perfectly healthy. At the opposite end are those with advanced HIV disease **(symptomatic AIDS)** who are visibly sick and require significant medical and psychosocial support (Figure 7-2). Between these two extremes, HIV-infected people may develop illnesses that range from mild to serious. Symptoms can include persistent fevers, chronic fatigue, diarrhea, swollen lymph nodes, night sweats, skin rashes, significant weight loss, visual problems, chest pain, and fungal infections

of the mouth, throat, and vagina. Illness from these conditions can be severe and disabling, and some people may die without ever being diagnosed with AIDS. Also, people with HIV disease may develop neurologic disorders, which can cause forgetfulness, memory loss, loss of coordination and balance, partial paralysis, leg weakness, mood changes, and dementia. These symptoms may occur in the absence of any other symptoms. The interval between initial HIV infection and the presence of signs and symptoms that characterize AIDS is variable and may range, in those who have not used antiretroviral drugs, from several months to a median duration of about 11 years (Figure 7-3).

Defining Incubation and Latency

Because of the long delay in determining what happened after HIV infection and progression to AIDS,

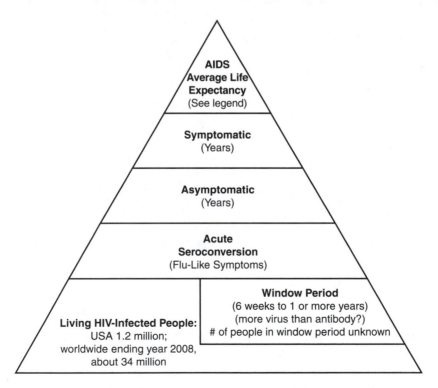

FIGURE 7-1 (a) The HIV/AIDS Pyramid. This figure demonstrates that current AIDS cases are coming from an existing pool of HIV-infected persons. In the United States, of those infected, about 25% to 30% do not yet know they are HIV positive. Although both the asymptomatic and symptomatic periods may last for years, once a person is diagnosed with AIDS, the average life expectancy without AIDS drug cocktails is two to three years. Life expectancy for those now on combination drug cocktails depends on the state of the individual's immune system and response to antiretroviral therapy.

VARIATION OF INITIAL SYMPTOMS AFTER HIV INFECTION

Case I: Male, Age 35, Los Angeles, California

One evening, for no apparent reason, John began sweating profusely. Soon after, a red rash began on his arms, face, and legs and then covered his body. Simultaneously, breathing became difficult and he was rushed to an emergency room. By then he was shaking violently. After medication and a battery of tests his problem could not be defined. This brief illness passed, but some years later, during a blood screen for insurance purposes he came up HIV positive. He immediately reflected back on his earlier illness and its cause.

Case II: Male, Age 29, Los Angeles, California

This case is in marked contrast to Case I. Feeling the pinch of a sore throat, this male went to his physician for an antibiotic. On examination, he had a yeast infection that appeared far back in his throat. This raised suspicion and he agreed to an HIV test. It came back positive. He had no other illness. He was treated, the sore throat vanished, and he is thriving in a long asymptomatic period.

the terms **incubation** and **latency** are used, in many cases interchangeably, causing some confusion. In this chapter, the two terms are used with respect to **clinical** observations as follows: **Clinical incubation** is that period after infection through the window period or when anti-HIV antibody production is measurable. **Clinical latency** is the time period from detectable anti-HIV antibody production (sero-conversion—the person now tests HIV-antibody positive) through the asymptomatic period—a time prior to the expression of opportunistic diseases. This time period, being asymptomatic, may last from 1 to 30 years—the average being about 11 years. The beginning and end of these periods will vary from person to person and their susceptibility and expression of HIV disease and whether they are on drug therapy.

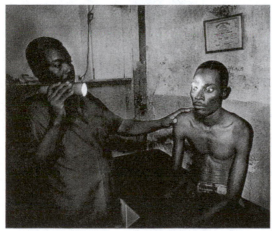

(a)

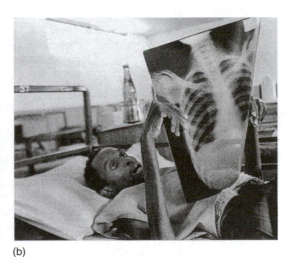

(b)

FIGURE 7-2 HIV/AIDS: The Beginning and the End. (a) Because he has no electricity in his office in Cite Soleil, Haiti, this physician uses a flashlight to examine an HIV-positive patient who is in the first stages of the infection. This physician sees, on average, one new HIV-infected person each day. (b) At age 28, Jean David looks at his X-ray, which, along with his medical history, according to his physician, indicates his impending death from AIDS. Jean David died soon after this picture was taken. He left an HIV-infected wife and HIV-infected 14-month-old daughter. (*Photos by Mike Stocker/South Florida Sun-Sentinel*)

Adult/Adolescent HIV Disease Continuum to AIDS

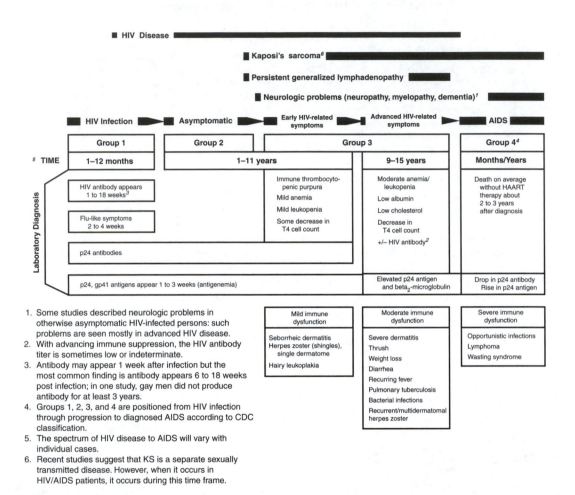

FIGURE 7-3 Spectrum of HIV Infection, Disease, and the Expression of AIDS, no therapy involved. Seroconversion means that HIV antibodies are measurably present in the person's serum. With continued depletion of T4 or CD4+ cells, signs and symptoms appear, announcing the progression of HIV disease to AIDS. Although HIV antibodies have been found as early as 1 week after exposure, **most often seroconversion occurs between weeks 6 and 18; 95% within 3 months, 99% within 6 months** (see Figure 7-5). The level of an individual's infectiousness is believed to be greatest within the first months after infection and again when the T4 cell count drops below 200. However, people who are HIV-infected can transmit HIV at any time.

STAGES OF HIV DISEASE (WITHOUT DRUG THERAPY)

The course of the disease in the infected individual varies substantially. At the extremes are individuals who show either little evidence of progression (loss in T4 cells) 10 to 30 years following infection (about 3%) or extremely rapid progression and death within less than two to three years. In general, HIV-infected adults experience a variety of conditions, categorized into four stages: **acute infection, asymptomatic, chronic symptomatic,** and **AIDS.**

HLABISA, AN AIDS-RAVAGED TOWN IN KWAZULU NATAL PROVINCE

In 1994, 10% of adults in Hlabisa (Sha-BEE-sa) were HIV infected. By 2004, over 30% or 75,000 people were HIV positive.

In the desperately crowded clinics and hospital wards, the scale of the epidemic is clear enough. This district of 250,000 people sits amid the hills of KwaZulu Natal, which has the highest adult rate of HIV infection of any province in South Africa. It is one of the few communities in South Africa in which government researchers have kept statistics on HIV infection rates for over decade. Its story offers a rare and intimate look at one community ravaged by the plague. It marks the faces of young widows who trudge the road in somber capes and skirts, traditional mourning garb. It inspires the medicine makers who brew slivers of tree bark and bundles of dried leaves into elixirs sold in used Coca-Cola bottles. "Two spoons in the morning, two spoons in the afternoon," advises a herbalist who charges $1.25 a bottle. Chilled bodies that are often stacked one on top of another swamp the morgue.

FEAR, DENIAL, AND GUILT

Professional men in Hlabisa boast over beers about extramarital affairs and the pleasures of unprotected sex. Some church leaders burn condoms and assail people with the virus as sinners. Prominent community members die in silence because the disease is considered so shameful. The disease is so deadly and so frightening that many hospital employees are reluctant to call it by name. They say a patient is immune compromised, or that he suffers from "that disease." Others simply say, "You know what he's got." It is as if uttering the word might infect the tongue.

HEALTHCARE CHOICE: HOSPITAL OR HEALER?

Hospitals

On any given day there are more patients than available beds. In the male ward, 80% of men are HIV positive and about half the nursing positions are vacant. The first event in morning rounds is to count those who died of AIDS or a combination of HIV infection and tuberculosis. Of those who die, about half are under age 30! In the first six months of 2001, of 500 people who took HIV tests, 63% tested positive. One of the staff nurses has six

children, four daughters and two sons. She leaves boxes of condoms on their bedroom dressers. The two things that give her the greatest sense of peace are taking her pills and watching those boxes empty. The children do not comment—she watches and replenishes the condom supply as needed.

Healers or Sangomas

In Southern Africa, a sangoma undergoes a long apprenticeship studying plant lore and making diagnoses that can include playing a guessing game with the patient, dancing into a trance, reading cast banes or waiting for the answer to come in a dream. In Hlabisa, physicians believe that virtually all their patients first visit a sangoma—a traditional healer. Donald McNeil describes the residence of one of the preeminent sangomas in Hlabisa. She is 57-years-old. The walls of her home are covered with dried birds, the python skins she stabbed herself, and a crocodile her husband speared—from which, she says, she can make a lotion that renders a man's skin bulletproof. The floor is covered with hundreds of medicine containers, as humble as a Yum Yum peanut butter jar and as ornate as a set of gourds covered with beadwork. But there is also a box of latex gloves, which she wears when inspecting sores. When she injects a patient with a porcupine quill tipped with brown gunk from the Yum Yum jar, she makes a point of wiping the quill afterward with alcohol. Asked about those precautions, she proudly displayed the framed certificate from a 1998 workshop on "The Traditional Healer's Role in AIDS: Sexually Transmitted Diseases and Primary Health Care" offered at Hlabisa Hospital. One of the sangoma's patients said that her illness was sent to her from her ancestors as a test. She also has a goat's bladder tied into her hair to remind her ancestors that she had sacrificed a goat to them.

Traditional Therapy

Because traditional Zulu medicine focuses chiefly on digestion, bile, and mucus, sangomas often give emetics or enemas. Some are simply dishwashing liquid or toothpaste. But others contain powerful herbs that can cause serious drug interactions. Enemas are used for anything from constipation to hysterical crying. However, enemas can rapidly dehydrate patients and send them into kidney or liver failure. For those who receive herbs causing them to throw up (emetics), it defeats the use of antiretroviral drugs.

Primary HIV Infection or the Acute Disease Stage

The clinical syndrome of primary HIV infection was recognized and documented in 1985, about two years after the initial identification of the causative agent of AIDS. By 1991 it was known that this symptomatic period is associated with an explosive replication of the virus, which is then partially controlled as the illness resolves spontaneously. Reports in 1993 further showed the population of HIV during this early period of infection to be quite homogeneous, in distinct contrast to the diverse quasispecies that are typically found in chronically infected persons. The course and time frame of the infection are illustrated graphically in Figure 7-3. The course of Primary

HIV Infection (PHI) is limited to a few weeks or months, whereas the entire course of HIV infection can span many years. Specifically, PHI is the period after infection with HIV but before the development of detectable antibodies or seroconversion (see Figure 7-4).

The acute stage usually develops in two to eight weeks during PHI. Up to 70% of infected individuals develop a self-limited (brief) illness similar to influenza or mononucleosis: high spiking fever, sore throat, headaches, and swollen lymph nodes. Some may develop a rash, vomiting, diarrhea, and thrush (yeast infection in the mouth). This is referred to as the **acute retroviral syndrome.** The symptoms generally last about one to four weeks and resolve spontaneously (Table 7-1). The acute stage can be over quickly and easily missed. The acute phase is marked by high levels of HIV production, of 1 to 10 million copies per milliliter of blood. During this phase, large numbers of HIV spread throughout the body, seeding themselves in various organs, particularly lymphoid tissues such as the lymph nodes, spleen, tonsils, and adenoids (Figure 7-4). During this time frame, HIV infects monocytes, macrophage, T4 or CD4+ cells, and follicular dendritic cells. Within these safe havens, HIV can persist for years despite Highly Active Antiretroviral Therapy (HAART). This pool of latently infected cells is established very early after HIV enters the body—even if the person takes drug therapy immediately after exposure to HIV.

During acute primary infection, patients have extremely high levels of viral replication but a variable antibody immune response. The level of cytotoxic T lymphocytes (CTLs) targeted against HIV appears to increase significantly, an attempt by the cellular part of the immune system to contain the high rate of HIV replication. It is now believed that the increase in the presence of CTLs and chemical factors they produce bring about a milder illness and a reduction in HIV to a **lower set point**—a steady state of viral load. The higher this set point the more rapidly HIV disease progresses to AIDS. (The presence of CTLs and long-term survival is presented in Box 7.3.) At this time in HIV infection and in some cases for weeks or months, neutralizing antibodies to HIV are not measurable—thus antibody testing, whether at clinical labs or using a home testing kit, is negative. This period of high viral replication in the absence of detectable antibody is called the **window of infectivity before**

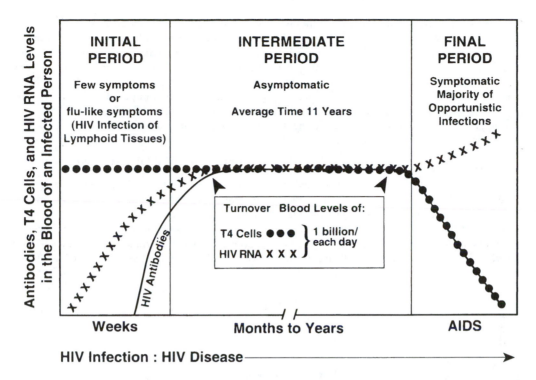

FIGURE 7-4   Relationship of T4 or CD4+ cells, HIV Antibodies, and HIV RNA Levels (Viral Load) Beginning with HIV Infection Through AIDs. Within a week to weeks after HIV infection, HIV becomes seeded throughout the body's blood and lymph system. HIV reproduction (infection of T4 cells) begins almost immediately in the lymph system. The T4 cell population also begins rapid reproduction to replace T4 cell loss. This is why the T4 graph line stays at the same level through the **asymptomatic** period. The immune system begins to turn out HIV antibodies, in general 6 to 18 weeks later (window period, see Figure 7-5). Note that during the asymptomatic period T4 cell and HIV replication and antibody production keep pace. With time, however, T4 cells fail to replace losses, HIV continues to replicate, antibody levels drop due to loss of T4 signals to B cells to produce antibodies, and opportunistic infections begin—the **symptomatic** period. Without therapy this period lasts on average about two to three years. For people using HAART, the average number of years one can survive in the symptomatic period is when on drug therapy now between 8 and 16 years.

seroconversion or window period. During this period, patients may be highly infectious, about 10 times more infectious than in the asymptomatic stage. The viral burden in genital secretion is particularly high during this time. Mathematical models suggest that 56% to 92% of all HIV infections may be transmitted during this period of acute infection (Quinn, 1997; Wainberg, 2007).

Table 7-1   Primary HIV Infection: Signs and Symptoms (Department of Health and Human Services [DHHS] Guidelines [*Ann Intern Med* 2002; 137:381])

Fever—96%	Myalgias—54%	Hepatosplenomegaly—14%
Adenopathy—74%	Diarrhea—32%	Weight loss—13%
Pharyngitis—70%	Headache—32%	Thrush—12%
Rash[1]—70%	Nausea & vomiting—27%	Neurologic symptoms[2]—12%

1. Rash—erythematous maculopapular rash on face and trunk, sometimes extremities, including palms and soles. Some have mucocutaneous ulceration involving mouth, esophagus, or genitals.

2. Aseptic meningitis, meningoencephalitis, peripheral neuropathy, facial palsy. Guillain-Barre syndrome, brachial neuritis, cognitive impairment, or psychosis.

A true state of **biological latency,** according to the work of Xiping Wei and coworkers (1995) and David Ho and coworkers (1995), does not exist in the lymph nodes at any time during the course of HIV infection. The Wei and Ho investigations show that from the time of infection HIV replication is rapid and continuous, and within two to four weeks the infecting HIV strain is replaced by drug-resistant mutants. Each day over 1 billion HIV are produced and mostly destroyed and millions of T4 cells are infected, dying, and replaced. Over time the immune system fails to destroy HIV and replace its T4 cell losses and HIV disease progresses. Also, over time, many T4 cells in the lymphoid organs probably are activated by the increased secretion of certain cytokines such as tumor necrosis factor–alpha and interleukin-6. T4 or CD4+ cell activation allows uninfected cells to be more easily infected and causes increased replication of HIV in infected cells. Other components of the immune system are also chronically activated, with negative consequences that may include the suicide of cells by a process known as programmed cell death or apoptosis and an inability of the immune system to respond to other invaders.

Asymptomatic HIV Disease Stage

Following acute illness, an untreated infected adult can remain free of symptoms from 6 months to a median time of about 11 years. During the asymptomatic period, measurable HIV in the blood drops to a lower level but it continues to replicate and to destroy T4 cells within the lymph nodes while the body

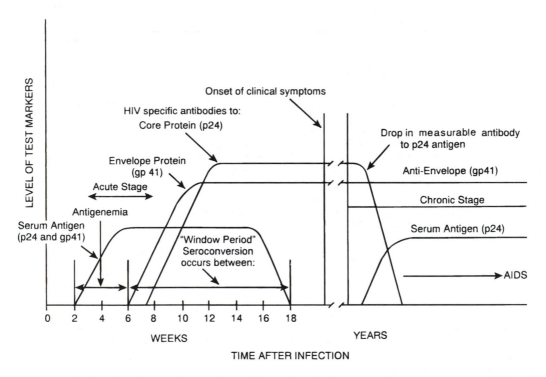

FIGURE 7-5 Profile of Serological Changes After HIV Infection. The dynamics of antibody response to HIV infection were determined by enzyme immunoassays (EIA). Note that during antigenemia, specific HIV proteins (antigens) can be detected before seroconversion occurs. Perhaps other HIV proteins will allow even earlier detection of HIV infection. Once antibodies appear, some antigens like p24 and gp41 disappear only to show up again later on. Note also that although antibody production is a sign that the immune system is working, in HIV-infected people it is not working well enough. Although envelope and core protein antibodies are being produced as clinical illness begins, as the p24 antibody drops, the illness becomes more serious. (*Adapted from Coulis et al., 1987*)

continues to produce new T4 cells and antibodies to fight the virus (Figure 7-5). An asymptomatic individual appears to be healthy and performs normal activities of daily living.

Symptomatic HIV Disease Stage

The symptomatic phase can last for months or years before a diagnosis of AIDS occurs. During this phase, as viral replication continues, T4 or CD4+ cells drop significantly. As the number of immune system cells decline, the individual develops a variety of symptoms such as fever, weight loss, malaise, pain, fatigue, loss of appetite, abdominal discomfort, diarrhea, night sweats, headaches, and swollen lymph glands. Ultimately, HIV overwhelms the lymphoid organs. The follicular dendritic cell networks break down in late-chronic-stage disease and virus trapping is impaired, allowing spillover of large quantities of virus into the bloodstream. The destruction of the lymph node structure seen late in HIV disease may stop a successful immune response against HIV and other pathogens as well. Individuals at this stage, with a T4 cell count of 500 or less/μL of blood, often develop thrush, oral lesions, and other fungal, bacterial, and/or viral infections. The duration of these symptoms varies, but it is common for HIV-infected individuals to have them for months at a time. Of those persons in the symptomatic stage and not using HIV drug therapy, about 30% developed AIDS-associated infections within five years.

Response to HAART

The CD4+ count typically begins to increase at four to eight weeks after viral suppression with HAART and then increases an additional 50–100 cells/mm^3/year in some patients. Normal CD4+ cell counts range between 600 and 1200 cell/mm.^{3}

AIDS: Advanced HIV Disease Stage

The diagnosis of AIDS is a marker, not an end in itself. Currently, most people recover from their first, second, and third AIDS-defining illnesses. People with AIDS are a very heterogeneous group—some feel well and continue working for several years, others are chronically ill, and some die rather quickly.

Patients with AIDS became an even more diverse group after the 1993 expansion of the Centers for Disease Control and Prevention's definition of AIDS. People in excellent health are diagnosed with AIDS if they test HIV positive and their T4 or CD4+ cell count is less than 200/μL of blood.

The final stage of HIV infection is called AIDS. During this time there is continued rapid viral replication that finally upsets the delicate balance of HIV production/T4 cell infection to T4 cell replacement. The virus largely depletes the cells of the immune system. It has been suggested that during the AIDS stage, serious immunodeficiency occurs when HIV diversity exceeds some threshold beyond which the immune system is unable to control HIV replication (Nowak et al., 1990; Wei et al., 1995; Cohen, 1995).

Finally the Question—How Long Can an HIV-Infected Person Live?

SLOW DANCE

Have you ever watched kids on a merry-go-round,
or listened to rain slapping the ground?

Ever followed a butterfly's erratic flight,
or gazed at the sun fading into the night?

You better slow down, don't dance so fast,
time is short, the music won't last.

Do you run through each day on the fly,
when you ask, "How are you?" do you hear the reply?

When the day is done, do you lie in your bed,
with the next hundred chores running through your head?

You better slow down, don't dance so fast,
time is short, the music won't last.

Ever told your child, we'll do it tomorrow,
and in your haste, not see his sorrow?

Ever lost touch, let a friendship die,
'cause you never had time to call and say hi?

You better slow down, don't dance so fast,
time is short, the music won't last.

When you run so fast to get somewhere,
You miss half the fun of getting there.

When you worry and hurry through your day,
It's like an unopened gift thrown away.

Life isn't a race, so take it slower,
Hear the music before your song is over.

—David L. Weatherford

The average time someone survives from the moment of HIV infection until death continues to increase. At the beginning of the epidemic, the average time was about 10 years. Many people confuse the date of diagnosis with the date of actual infection. The latter date is most often not known. Many years may separate the dates of infection and diagnosis. For the U.S., it currently is estimated at least 25% of persons infected with HIV today, utilizing drugs and treatments available, will survive on average for about 30 years. According to the Antiretroviral Therapy Cohort Collaboration 2008 report, if one lives in a high-income country, is currently age 20 and on effective drug therapy one can expect to live, on average, to age 70. In contrast, an HIV-negative 20-year-old can expect to live, on average, to age 80. But averages are exactly that—averages. More precise estimates for individuals depend on current and past HIV RNA levels, current and past T4 or CD4+

cell counts, number of antiretroviral regimens used, adherence to therapy, response to therapy, and current health status. About 5% of HIV-infected persons are estimated to be long-term nonprogressors. That is, in the absence of therapy, these individuals maintain a T4 or CD4+ cell count of about 450 cells per microliter of blood and typically have HIV RNA levels of less than 5000 copies/mL of blood. It is not clear what immunologic features distinguish these individuals from the other 95% of HIV-infected persons (see Boxes 7.2 and 7.3).

Symptoms and Impairment

In the symptomatic stages of HIV disease, an individual's ability to carry on the activities of daily living is impaired. The degree of impairment varies considerably from day to day and week to week. Many individuals are debilitated to the point that it becomes difficult to hold steady employment, shop for food, or do household chores. It is also quite common for people with AIDS to experience phases of intense life-threatening illness, followed by phases of seemingly normal functioning, all in a matter of weeks. For a good review on the mechanisms of HIV disease, read *The Immunopathogenesis of HIV Infection* by Giuseppe Pantaleo et al. (1993), Bucy (1999), and Yu (2000).

HIV Can Be Transmitted During All Four Stages

A person who is HIV-infected, even while feeling healthy, may unknowingly infect others. *The greatest risk of HIV transmission occurs within the acute period, the first several months after infection, and again when the T4 cell count drops below 200.*

HIV DISEASE WITHOUT SYMPTOMS, WITH SYMPTOMS, AND AIDS

Michael is a 31-year-old Hispanic male who complains of fatigue, headache, muscle aches, sore throat, and nausea. Physical assessment demonstrates a skin rash on his trunk and swollen lymph glands. His temperature is 98°F (37°C); other vital signs are within normal limits. Laboratory findings including white blood cell count, platelet count, and blood chemistry are normal. Michael states that his symptoms began one week ago. Subsequent laboratory testing will confirm that Michael has acute retroviral

---

SIDEBAR 7.2

WHAT IS MEANT BY THE TERM *WASTING* DURING HIV DISEASE

Body wasting during HIV disease is sometimes referred to as AIDS WASTING. Wasting is not well understood, but it involves the involuntary loss of more than 10% of body weight, plus more than 30 days of either diarrhea or weakness and fever. Wasting is linked to disease progression and death. Part of the weight lost during wasting is fat. More important is the loss of muscle mass. This is also called lean body mass, or body cell mass. Lean body mass can be measured by bioelectrical impedance analysis (BIA). This is a simple, painless office procedure. AIDS wasting together with lipodystrophy can cause serious body shape changes. Wasting is the loss of muscle. Lipodystrophy is a loss of fat from one area and the accumulation of fat in another area of the body (see Figures 4–11 and 4–12).

UPDATE 2008—With the use of ART beginning in 1995 came a slow but constant weight gain in those persons on ART. AIDS researchers and advocacy groups say the waistlines of HIV patients are growing right along with the girths of uninfected Americans as the disease shifts from a death sentence to a chronic condition. Although exact numbers are hard to obtain, new research suggests that nearly two-thirds of the HIV population may be overweight or obese, mirroring the U.S. population. It appears that today, for those who respond to ART, their problem is no longer "wasting" but obesity.

syndrome that accompanies primary HIV infection (PHI). But the odds are high that in almost every emergency room or physician's office in the country, Michael will be misdiagnosed. He is likely to be told that he has a viral infection, probably the flu, and sent home with instructions for supportive care.

A person may have no symptoms **(asymptomatic)** but test HIV positive. This means that the virus is present in the body. Although he or she has not developed any of the illnesses associated with HIV disease, it is possible to transmit the virus.

In time, most people with HIV disease progress to AIDS. A person has AIDS when the defect in his or her immune system caused by HIV disease has progressed to such a degree that an unusual infection or tumor is present or when the T4 or CD4+ cell count has fallen below 200/μL of blood. In AIDS patients, a number of diseases are known to take advantage of the damaged immune system. These include opportunistic infections and tumors such as Kaposi's sarcoma or lymphoma, a malignancy of the lymph glands. The presence of one of the opportunistic diseases or a T4 cell count of less than 200, along with a positive HIV test, establishes the medical diagnosis of AIDS. Thus the disease we call AIDS is actually the end stage of HIV disease. It is important to remember that AIDS itself is not transmitted—the virus is. AIDS is the most severe clinical form of HIV disease.

The term "full-blown AIDS" is often used on TV and in the press but not in this textbook. Terms such as advanced HIV disease or advanced AIDS are not only more accurate but also more meaningful.

PRODUCTION OF HIV-SPECIFIC ANTIBODIES

During the 25 years (1983–2008) since the discovery of HIV, scientists have constructed a serological or antibody graph of HIV infection and HIV disease. The graph reveals how soon the body produces HIV-specific antibodies after infection and about when the virus begins its reproduction. Different parts of the graph (Figure 7-5) have been filled in by Paul Coulis and colleagues (1987), Dani Bolognesi (1989), and Susan Stramer and colleagues (1989). The history of the HIV antibody is not yet complete, but the order of appearance and disappearance of antibodies specific for the serologically important antigens over the course of HIV disease has been described.

Note that Figure 7-5 shows that HIV plasma viremia (the presence of virus in blood plasma) and antigenemia (an-ti-je-ne-mi-ah—the persistence of antigen in the blood) can be detected as early as two weeks after infection. This demonstrates that viremia and antigenemia occur prior to seroconversion. Using HIV proteins produced by recombinant DNA methods (making synthetic copies of the viral proteins), antibodies specific for gp41 (a subunit of glycoprotein 160) are detectable prior to those specific for p24 (a core protein) and persist throughout the course of infection. Levels of antibody specific for p24 rise to detectable levels between six and eight weeks after HIV infection but may disappear abruptly. The drop in p24 antibody has been shown to occur at the same time as a rise in p24 antigen in the serum. This strange phenomenon is thought to be due to the loss of available p24 antibody in immune complexes—too little p24 antibody is being made to handle the new virus being produced. It is believed that this imbalance is one of the important factors that moves the patient toward AIDS. A sudden decrease in anti-p24 is considered by many scientists to be a prognostic indicator that people with HIV disease are moving toward AIDS.

Some AIDS researchers and healthcare professionals believe that 90% to 95% of those persons infected with HIV will eventually develop AIDS. Without antiretroviral drugs, approximately 50% of people with HIV disease will progress to AIDS within 8 years after infection. At 10 years 70% will have developed AIDS. After that, an additional 25% to 45% of the remainder will develop AIDS.

Classification of HIV/AIDS Progression

There are several classifications that spell out the progression of signs and symptoms from HIV infection to the diagnosis of AIDS. The classifications were developed to provide a framework for the medical management of patients from the time of infection through the expression of AIDS. All classification systems are fundamentally the same—they group patients according to their stage of infection, based on signs that indicate a failing immune system (Royce et al., 1991).

The most widely accepted classification because of its greater clinical applicability, comes from the CDC. The CDC classification uses four mutually exclusive groupings (Figure 7-7). The groupings are based on the presence or absence of signs and symptoms of disease, and clinical and/or laboratory findings and the

BOX 7.1

EVOLUTION OF HIV DURING HIV DISEASE PROGRESSION

HIV is a unique retrovirus. For example, mitosis, a form of cell division, is a requirement for the nuclear entry of most retroviral nucleic acids. In contrast, mitosis does not appear to be required for nuclear entry of HIV nucleic acids, particularly in terminally differentiated cells (for example, macrophages and dendritic cells) (Freed et al., 1994). Second, HIV lacks any mechanism to correct errors that occur as its genetic material is being duplicated, so a few days or weeks after initial infection, there may be a large population of closely related, but not identical, viruses replicating in an infected individual. In the **quasi**-steady-state condition, there are successive generations of viral progeny, with each generation following the next by about 2.6 days. Approximately 140 generations of virus are produced over the course of a year and 1400 generations over the course of 10 years, allowing production of an extraordinary number of genetic variants. Some variants can provide preexisting drug-resistant forms or enable rapid development of resistance under drug pressure, and some enable the viral population to escape immune activity.

VIRAL POOL

The viral pool in an HIV-infected person is estimated to be about 10 billion viruses and each is genetically different from all other HIV in the pool. It is known from experimental data that about 1 in 1000 particles is infectious, so the infectious viral pool may be on the order of 10 million viruses. With a genome of approximately 10^4 nucleotides, and from 1 to 10 billion HIV variants made daily, mutations most likely occur at every nucleotide position on a daily basis (Ho, 1996). This creates an enormous potential for viral evolution. On average, the HIV that is transmitted to another individual will be over 1000 generations removed from the initial HIV infection. This extent of replication per transmitted infection (transmission cycle) is probably without equal among viral and perhaps bacterial infections (Coffin, 1995). Regardless of the underlying mechanism of immunodeficiency, it is becoming apparent that the force that is driving the disease is the constant repeated cycles of HIV replication.

LIFE SPAN OF HIV

Alan Perelson and colleagues (1996) reported data collected from five HIV-infected people after administering ritonavir through 7 days. Each person responded with a similar pattern of decline in plasma HIV RNA. Their results: Infected T4 cells had an average life span of 2.2 days. Plasma HIV RNA had an average life span of 0.3 days. The results also suggest that the minimum duration of the HIV life cycle in human T4 cells is 1.2 days on average and that the average HIV generation time—defined as the time from release of a virus until it infects another cell and causes the release of a new generation of HIV—is 2.6 days. The lifetime of HIV in resting or latent T4 cells may range from 6 months to perhaps an infinite amount of time. Such cells can produce HIV when activated.

TREATMENT FAILURE

Virologic Failure

Failure to reduce the viral load to an undetectable level *or*
Failure to reduce the viral load by at least 2 to 2.5 $\log_{10}$ *or*
A persistent increase in viral load following a period of adequate suppression

Immunologic Failure

Failure to restore the T4 or CD4+ cell count to more than 200 cells/mm^3 *or*
Failure to significantly increase T4 cell count *or*
A persistent decline in T4 cell count after a period of immune reconstitution

Clinical Failure

Development of new opportunistic infections (OIs) *or*
Failure to resolve pretreatment OI, wasting, or dementia

(Adopted from Soloway et al., 2000)

With new techniques for quantitating plasma HIV RNA, infected individuals can be evaluated for response to antiretroviral therapy.

MUTANT HIV OVERWHELM THE IMMUNE SYSTEM

As HIV multiplies and mutant forms are produced, the immune system responds to these new forms. But ultimately the sheer number of *different* viruses to which the immune system must respond becomes overwhelming. It's a bit like the juggler who tries to keep too many balls in the air: The result is disastrous. Once the immune system is overwhelmed, the latest escape mutant—which may not necessarily be the most pathogenic one to come along—will predominate and immune deficiency will progress.

A University Student's Message To Her Classmates

"People want to know that you care before they care what you know...."

James F. Hind

Worried about how she could make a difference in her generation's reaching out to help the HIV infected, this student felt that she could help her classmates become involved by raising a sensitive issue and asking them to think deeply about what she had to say. She said, "I asked myself how can I get your attention in a meaningful way? For example, if I were given an assignment to write a message so that all of you would feel differently about this pandemic once I shared it with you, what would I say?" She then went on to tell her classmates that "In writing this message, I would tell people our age to imagine their best friend coming to them and telling them they are HIV positive. Imagine your best friend has just told you that he or she is infected with HIV, that he or she will ultimately progress to AIDS and die. Suddenly, the person who you have grown up with, and who you confide in for everything will over time become terminally ill with a condition that will cause him or her to visibly suffer. You watch your best friend wither away, in pain, and there will be nothing you can do to help. Eventually, you will be at the funeral, and the cause of death will be AIDS. If your friend had only been cautious that ONE time, he or she would still be here today. Will you be careful? Will you help stop the spread of HIV?" (see Figure 7-6.)

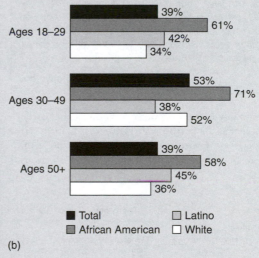

Ages 18–29
- 39% (Total)
- 61% (African American)
- 42% (Latino)
- 34% (White)

Ages 30–49
- 53% (Total)
- 71% (African American)
- 38% (Latino)
- 52% (White)

Ages 50+
- 39% (Total)
- 58% (African American)
- 45% (Latino)
- 36% (White)

■ Total   ☐ Latino
▨ African American   ☐ White

(b)

FIGURE 7-6 (b)   Percent who say they personally know someone who now has AIDS, has died from AIDS, or has tested positive for HIV. "Kaiser Family Foundation *Survey of Americans on HIV/AIDS,* Part Three—Experiences and Opinions by Race/Ethnicity and Age," (#7140), The Henry J. Kaiser Family Foundation, August 2004. The information was reprinted with permission from the Henry J. Kaiser Family Foundation. The Kaiser Family Foundation, based in Menlo Park, California, is a non-profit, independent national healthcare philanthropy and is not associated with Kaiser Permanente or Kaiser Industries.

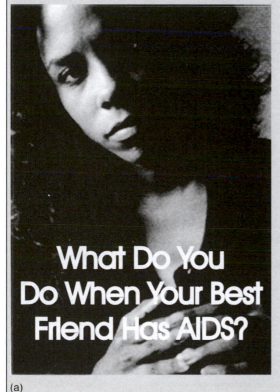

What Do You Do When Your Best Friend Has AIDS?

(a)

FIGURE 7-6 (a)   The Photograph Presents Its Own Message. *(Courtesy of the Centers for Disease Control and Prevention, Atlanta)* but lacks HIV antibodies and signs and symptoms of HIV disease.

The majority of people in Group 1 remain asymptomatic. Some may experience flu- or mononucleosis-like symptoms that generally disappear in a few weeks. In relatively few cases the patient moves rapidly from mild symptoms into severe opportunistic infections and is diagnosed with AIDS.

In Group 2, antibodies are present but most patients remain free of HIV disease symptoms. Regardless of the lack of outward clinical symptoms, 90% of those who are asymptomatic experience some form of immunological deterioration within five years (Fauci, 1988).

In Group 3, asymptomatic people from Groups 1 and 2 become symptomatic and demonstrate lymphadenopathy in the neck, armpit, and groin areas. Although a number of other diseases may cause the lymph nodes to swell, most swelling declines as the other symptoms of illness fade. However, with HIV infection, the lymph nodes remain swollen for months, with no other signs of a related infectious disease. Consequently, lymphadenopathy is sometimes called **persistent generalized lymphadenopathy** (PGL). People with PGL may experience night sweats, weight loss, fever, on-and-off diarrhea, fatigue, and the onset of oral candidiasis or thrush (see Figure 6-3). Such signs and symptoms are prodromal (symptoms leading to) for AIDS. Studies have shown that people in Group 3 appear to become more infectious as the disease progresses.

chronology of their occurrence. Group 1, acute infection, means the person is **viremic** (that is, many virus particles are present in his or her blood or serum). There are *no measurable antibodies;* one is HIV positive

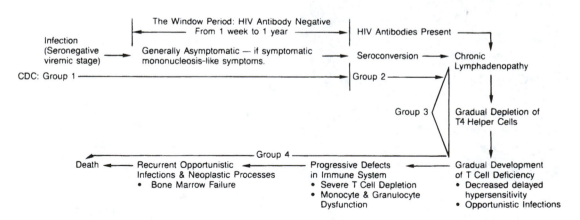

FIGURE 7-7 Clinical History of HIV Infection According to Centers for Disease Control and Prevention Groupings. Seroconversion means that HIV antibodies are measurably present in the person's serum. With continued depletion of T4 cells, various signs and symptoms appear announcing the progression of HIV disease into AIDS. Although HIV antibodies have been found as early as 1 week after exposure, most often seroconversion occurs between weeks 6 and 18 but may not occur for up to 1 year or more.

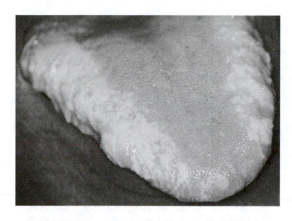

FIGURE 7-8 Oral Hairy Leukoplakia of the Tongue. An early manifestation, it is virtually diagnostic of AIDS. The white shaggy-appearing or corrugated "hairy" patches typically occur on the lateral borders of the tongue and are caused by the Epstein-Barr virus (EBV). These white plaques cannot be removed. *(Courtesy of Stuart Fischman, D. M. D.)*

People in Group 4 have been diagnosed with AIDS. They fit the 1987 CDC criteria for AIDS diagnosis. (The CDC AIDS diagnostic criteria are listed in Table 1-1.) Hairy leukoplakia (Figure 7-8) is virtually diagnostic of AIDS in Group 4 patients. Statistics show that about 30% of all the newly HIV infected will progress to Group 4 (AIDS) every 5 years, so that about 90% will have been diagnosed with AIDS within 15 years. Not all the opportunistic infections (OIs) or cancers will appear in any one AIDS patient. But some OIs, like *Pneumocystis* pneumonia, occur in some 80% of AIDS patients prior to their deaths.

PROGNOSTIC BIOLOGICAL MARKERS RELATED TO AIDS PROGRESSION

The ideal marker would be able to predict HIV disease progression, be responsive to antiretroviral therapy, and explain the variance in clinical outcome due to therapy. It is, however, unlikely that any one marker will be able to fulfill all these criteria in HIV infection. Therefore, individual markers used to track HIV infection to AIDS are presented.

p24 Antigen Levels

p24 is a specific protein located in the core or inner layer of HIV. Because the immune system produces antibody against foreign protein, antibody is made against p24. A positive test for p24 antigen in the blood means that HIV production is so rapid that it overcomes the available antibody (Figure 7-5). This raised p24 antigen level condition occurs at least twice: once shortly after infection and again during the AIDS period when the immune system is rapidly deteriorating and unable to produce sufficient antibody to deal with newly produced HIV.

Those who, during the early stage of HIV infection, test p24 antigen positive are likely to progress to AIDS earlier than those who test p24 negative. Thus, a positive p24 test is an early and serious warning sign for HIV-infected people (Escaich et al., 1991; Phillips et al., 1991a).

p24 Antibody Levels

High levels of p24 antibody indicate that the immune system is functioning well and clearing the body of free HIVs. High antibody levels appear to slow the progression toward AIDS. Typically, p24 antibody levels are high during a person's asymptomatic or latent stage (Figure 7-4). However, antibody levels begin to decrease and p24 antigen levels rise, indicating a loss of immune function.

Other Markers

Beta-2 microglobulin (B-2M) is a low molecular weight protein that is present on the surface of almost all nucleated cells. As cells die, this compound is released into body fluids. Thus there is always some B-2M in the blood because of normal cell degeneration and replacement. However, in a chronic illness with increased cell destruction, as in HIV infection, B-2M increases beyond normal levels.

To date, a B-2M level of 5 mg/L or higher is the best available indicator of progression to AIDS within three years. Levels below 2.6 are considered normal. B-2M protein increases dramatically shortly after infection occurs, then declines, and finally rises again with AIDS. B-2M can be used with T4 counts to foretell which HIV-positive individuals face the greatest immediate risk of progressing to AIDS.

T4 and T8 Lymphocyte Levels

The most extensive use of data for AIDS progression risk identification involves the number of T4 or CD4+ and T8 or CD8+ cells circulating in the blood (Anderson et al., 1991; Burcham et al., 1991; Phillips et al., 1991b).

BOX 7.2

DEVELOPMENT OF AIDS OVER TIME

HIV-INFECTED AND THEIR PROGRESSION TO AIDS WITHOUT ANTIRETROVIRAL THERAPY

A spectrum of clinical expression of disease can occur after HIV infection. Approximately 10% of HIV-infected subjects progress to AIDS within the first 2 to 3 years of HIV infection (rapid progressors). People with greater than 50,000 HIV RNA copies/mL at 6 months after infection are the most likely to be rapid progressors. About 60% of adults/adolescents will progress to AIDS within 12 to 13 years after HIV infection (slow progressors). Approximately 5% to 10% of HIV-infected subjects are clinically asymptomatic after 20 to 30 years. They have stable peripheral blood T4 cell levels of greater than 500 (long-term nonprogressors or LTNPs) People with AIDS having low T4 cell counts who have survived for 5 years or more without therapy are usually described as long-term survivors (LTS). Some 6% of persons diagnosed with clinical AIDS are long-term survivors.

THE ELITE AND VIREMIC CONTROLLERS

Some HIV positive people do not need ART. They are considered elite.

Elite controllers, as defined by Steve Deeks, University of California at San Francisco, are HIV-positive people who have their viral load at nondetectable levels or ess than 50 copies of HIV RNA per mL for at least two years without using antiretroviral drugs. Is it possible that some of the elite controllers have eradicated HIV? Studies on this question are in progress. But, it's hard to prove a negative. Viremic controllers are HIV-positive people whose immune systems have kept the virus under 2000 for at least one year without antiretrovirals. Neither group progresses to AIDS. Researchers believe it is unlikely that elite or viremic controllers can transmit the virus. Bruce Walker, director of Partners AIDS Research Center at Massachusetts General Hospital, and colleagues have enrolled 200 elite controllers in a study, and the researchers in the next six months plan to enroll 1000 more elite and 1000 viremic controllers. If the true frequency of elite and viremic controllers is one in 300, there should be about 4000 of them to be recognized (found). The researchers plan to compare genetic sequences of HIV in the elite controllers to other HIV-positive people, as well as HIV-negative people, to determine whether there are genetic variations that can explain why elite and viremic controllers can suppress the virus. Researchers need to enroll at least 1000 elite controllers so that their genetic findings can have significance.

POSSIBLE EXPLANATION FOR ELITE CONTROLLERS?

One possibility is that these "HIV resistant" people have been infected with a heavily compromised, mutated strain of HIV. For example, they may carry HIV with a mutant or non-functional nef gene. In this case, nef minus HIV would not be able to activate CD4 lymphocytes. A few cases of nef-depleted HIV were discovered in blood-transfused people in the early 1980s. These people, some 29 years later, are still without the symptoms of HIV/AIDS. However, the R5 nucleotide mutation (discussed in Chapter 5), which confers some resistance to HIV infection, is found in only a few elite controllers. For example, neither Robert Massie (infected in 1978 and currently thriving) nor Rob Rosenthal (infected in 1986 and currently thriving) carry the R5 mutation (see Box 7-3). It is possible that elite controllers inherited a unique set of HLA (human leukocyte antigen) molecules that sit on the surface of the T cells and identify the virus to the immune system, which then can kill the virus and the cell. Even in elite controllers, however, protective HLA types are found in only a very small percentage of patients. Perhaps it is the neutralizing antibody responses. They are lower in patients with acute infections than in patients with chronic infections, and titers (level of antibody) are especially high in long-term nonprogressors.

These elite and viremic controllers all have one thing in common, a functional squad of memory T4 or CD4+ cells that respond to HIV infection. Such people have an immune system that remembers HIV and controls it over time, or else they are infected with defective HIV that cannot promote their pathological condition.

The elite and viremic controllers (LTNPs or LTS) are a very important group to study as they control infection without antiretroviral drug intervention and thus should provide valuable information on disease progression and how it is influenced by immunological, virological, and genetic factors.

Cytokines

An important chemical signal (or cytokine) used by cells is interleukin 10 (IL-10). When produced in large amounts by cells, IL-10 can weaken the immune re-

BOX 7.2   (*continued*)

sponse against viruses, bacteria, and fungi. Some researchers think HIV may trick the immune system into producing large amounts of IL-10, weakening the body's ability to fight the virus. Researchers at Mt. Sinai Hospital in Toronto reported at the Eighth Conference on Retroviruses and Opportunistic Infections that T lymphocyte cells taken from nonprogressors and healthy HIV-negative people produced relatively low levels of IL-10. But such cells taken from people with AIDS produced between two and five times more IL-10. The researchers found that those who took highly active antiretroviral therapy (HAART) were able to significantly reduce their levels of IL-10.

One thing is clear from the studies of nonprogressors thus far: Not all are the same. Some show distinct features not shared by others, yet somehow all experience nonprogression. The reasons behind this phenomenon may be virologic, immunologic, or both. However, no common genetic correlate has yet been identified to explain long-term nonprogression.

AIDS: LONG–TERM SURVIVORS WITH DRUG THERAPY

Current and continued use of AIDS drug cocktails containing at least one protease inhibitor has increased the number of long-term survivors. Survival after the onset of AIDS, without HAART, has been increasing in industrialized countries from an average of less than 1 year to over 5 years at present. With therapy, on average, survival time has been increased by 5 to 30 years, depending on the case and

therapy. Survival time with AIDS in developing countries remains short and is estimated to be, on average, less than 2 years. Longer survival appears to be directly related to routine treatment with antiretroviral drugs, the use of drugs for opportunistic infections, and a better overall quality of health care.

The majority of AIDS cases occurs before age 35, and over 90% of all AIDS deaths occur in people under the age of 50 worldwide.

Philip Rosenberg and colleagues (1994) reported that the length of incubation and progression from HIV infection to AIDS, without treatment, varied according to the age at the time of infection. Younger ages were associated with a slower progression to AIDS. The estimated median treatment-free clinical incubation period was about 11 years for those infected at age 20, 9.9 years for infection at age 30, and 8.1 years for infection at age 40.

LONG–TERM UNDETECTABLE

The goal for antiretroviral drug therapy is to get the viral load or number of HIV to undetectable levels in the blood—that is, maintaining a viral load of less than 50 copies of HIV RNA per milliliter of blood. Using the new antiretroviral combination once- and twice-a-day drugs like Kaletra, Combivir, Truvada, and Trizivir has kept HIV at undetectable levels in some patients for five years and counting (see Table 4-1).

T4 cells and the ratio of T4 cells to T8 cells found in the blood have, since 1997, been widely used as prognostic indicators for AIDS progression. T4 cell counts, however, are not ironclad predictors of HIV disease progression. In some cases persons with HIV disease and very low (less than 50 or 100) T4 counts remain healthy; conversely, some HIV-diseased persons have relatively high counts (over 400) and are quite ill. *T4 counts are notoriously fickle*—their counts can vary widely between labs or because of a person's age, the time of day a measurement is taken, and even whether the person smokes (Sax et al., 1995).

Lymph Nodes, the T Cell Zones, T4 or CD4+ Cell Production, and HIV Infection

The T cell zone in the lymph nodes is involved with 98% of the body's T4 or CD4+ cells. It is also where 99% of HIV production occurs. As HIV replication continues it causes inflammation, scarring, and eventual destruction of the T cell zone. Newly produced T4 cells have little room in the scarred T cell zone to divide. If they divide there is a high probability they will become infected. With this new knowledge reported in 2003, researchers now believe they understand why

BOX 7.3

ARE THERE LONG-TERM ADULT HIV INFECTED NONPROGRESSORS—YES!—WHY?

HIV infected long-term nonprogressors (LTNP) in the absence of HIV drug therapy are defined as those persons who are still alive 10 or more years after they tested HIV positive, with seroconversion documented by history or stored serum samples, absence of symptoms, and normal and stable T4 cell counts (at least 500 T4 cells/microliter of blood). Studies through 2008 suggest that 12% to 15% of HIV-infected people remain asymptomatic with near normal T4 cell counts for about 8 to 12 years (Conant, 1995; Levy, 1995; updated). At least three people are known to be asymptomatic now, 30 years after HIV infection! The question is: How does their immune system differ from those who do not live as long?

SOME MALE, LONG–TERM NONPROGRESSORS (LTNP)

One of the longest long-term nonprogressors is Robert Massie. He was infected in 1978. By the end of 2009, he will have lived for 31 years with his HIV infection. Massie is the current executive director of Ceres, a coalition of environmental, investor, and advocacy groups. In 1994, he went to the Massachusetts General Hospital, urging doctors to study him. He told them that he was infected with HIV, had never been treated, and that his immune system was fine. Massie first learned he was infected in 1984, when he had an HIV test as part of a research study. He was not surprised by the result, he explained, because he is a hemophiliac, and, like virtually every other American with this genetic disease who was alive in the early 1980s, he was repeatedly exposed to HIV through the blood clotting factors made from the pooled blood of donors (see Chapter 8). Massie kept waiting to become ill. "I would read a report saying it could be as long as five years before you come down with symptoms of AIDS and die, then it could be as long as seven years, then as long as ten years, then twelve years. I always thought I was at the limit." When Massie's doctors looked back at his blood samples, which they had stored in hemophilia research projects, they found antibodies to HIV as early as 1979. They suspect that he was infected in November 1978 when he became gravely ill. Massie said, "One day I was sitting at my desk and I suddenly felt overwhelmingly tired, incapable of talking, I was so tired." He had a fever and symptoms that led doctors, at that time, to suggest pneumonia, tuberculosis, a cerebral hemorrhage, and a seizure disorder. So, in 1994, when Massie arrived at Massachusetts General

Hospital, he had been infected with HIV for 16 years. Now age 55, he has been infected for more than half his life. Since then, Massie has been meeting with Bruce Walker, an infectious disease specialist in HIV infection. The first question for Walker was what was Massie's T4 or CD4+ cell count? He found Massie had near-normal levels of T4 cells. Walker said, "This was the first evidence that HIV followed the rules that other viruses follow." It meant that his body's immune system could control HIV.

A similar documented case of a long-term nonprogressor to date is that of Kai Brothers, a gay male who was also infected about 31 years ago. His T4 count remains normal. Brothers is a patient of HIV/AIDS investigator Jay Levy, director of the University of California Laboratory for Tumor and AIDS Research. He is 47 years old and believes he was infected in 1978. Brothers, like Massie, has never taken antiretroviral drug therapy. Levy believes that about 5% of the HIV infected will remain capable of living successfully with the infection. Anthony Fauci, director of the National Institute of Allergy and Infectious Diseases, believes the number of such LTN make up less than 1% of this population. Regardless of the percentage of such people, they are very hard to locate, but they make up an essential part of HIV/AIDS research subjects.

OTHER CASES OF LTNP

In 1983, at age 71, a man became HIV positive. He received a contaminated blood transfusion while undergoing colon surgery. He suffered no symptoms and no loss of immune function. He celebrated his 81st birthday before dying of natural causes. He is one of five patients who came to the attention of an AIDS researcher as he was preparing a routine update on transfusion-related HIV infections. All five people were infected by the same donor. And 10 to 15 years later, none of the remaining four had suffered any effects.

The blood donor was a gay male who had contracted the virus during the late 1970s or early 1980s and gave blood at least 26 times before learning he was infected. After locating the donor researchers found that the man was just as healthy as the people who got his blood.

A 41-year-old San Francisco artist has beaten the odds by living with the virus that causes AIDS for 25 years. He has only routine medical complaints: the stuffiness of an occasional head cold or the aches and pains of a flu. He has never taken an anti-HIV

BOX 7.3   *(continued)*

drug. His own immune system seems to have held the virus at bay.

Susan Buchbinder and colleagues (1992, 1994) reviewed 588 HIV-infected gay men. Thirty-one percent were still AIDS-free 15 years after infection. They attempted to determine why these men lived while others died of HIV/AIDS. Some long-term survivors have low T4 cell counts, some have never taken antiviral therapy, and some have high T4 cell counts. If it can be determined why or how their bodies have delayed the progression of HIV disease, then perhaps new approaches to treating all HIV-infected persons will follow.

Buchbinder and colleagues have found that three aspects of the healthy survivors' immune system appear to delay HIV disease progression: Survivors have strong cytotoxic lymphocyte activity, or T8 cell activity, and have higher levels of antibodies against certain HIV proteins.

Stephen Migueles and colleagues (2002) examined a group of 15 nonprogressors who have controlled HIV for up to 20 years without antiretroviral therapy. They found no significant difference in the number of T8 or CD8+ cells between nonprogressors and the others. Instead, they found that the nonprogressors' CD8+ cells were better able to divide and proliferate when called into action and they also produced higher levels of a molecule called perforin, which helps kill off cells infected with HIV. This study represents the first time scientists have observed a difference in the HIV-specific CD8+ T cell response of nonprogressors and suggests a mechanism whereby the CD8+ T cells of nonprogressors control HIV while those of most HIV-infected individuals do not.

SOME FEMALE, LONG-TERM NONPROGRESSORS

For years, some 18 women have intrigued AIDS investigators because they have remained HIV-free despite having frequent, unprotected sex with an infected partner. Researchers at the University of Medicine and Dentistry of New Jersey found that in most of the women, key immune cells worked in various ways to block HIV from multiplying in their bodies. During the study, only one became infected with HIV, and that took nine years of frequent, unprotected sex. The 17 uninfected women had unprotected sex with their HIV-positive partners for periods ranging from 1 year to 11 years dating as far back as the mid-1980s. Tests on their blood focused on two types of immune cells, cytotoxic or CD8+ and T4 or CD4+ cells, which kill invading organisms and rev up the rest of the

immune system. The CD8+ cells and the CD4+ cells separately were mixed with HIV proteins in laboratory dishes mimicking how they would interact in a person's body and researchers watched for reactions. In many samples, the CD4+ cells rapidly reproduced, as if stimulating the rest of the immune system and the CD8+ cells. Also, they produced two different substances that stopped the virus from reproducing. The research team expected to find one immune response protecting the women from HIV infection, but instead found different types of immune responses spread among the 17 women (Skurnick et al., 2002).

In the Pumwani district of Nairobi, a group of 100 women have become well known to HIV researchers around the world by offering evidence that the immune system can, in rare cases, fight off HIV. The evidence derives from a group of women sex workers (prostitutes) established in 1984 by Elizabeth Ngugi and colleagues from the University of Nairobi and the University of Manitoba. Despite an estimated 60 or more unprotected exposures to HIV every year, one of the highest documented exposure rates in the world, 100 of the 2000 women enrolled in the study have tested negative for HIV infection for at least five years, and for some women up to 22 years. Studies of these highly exposed persistently seronegative (HEPS), also referred to as exposed seronegative (ESN), women convinced many skeptics that immunological resistance to HIV is possible, and by extension so is an HIV vaccine.

More recently, 98 prostitutes of Maniper, India, who routinely have had unprotected sex with their clients for years have remained HIV negative, and 54 of these women during the interim have had HIV-negative babies. Again, why they remain HIV negative despite repeated exposure to HIV is unknown.

A 2008 report by Tada Hirbod and colleagues on 113 Kenyan sex workers repeatedly exposed to HIV showed that 89 remained HIV negative and 24 became HIV positive. Studying cervicovaginal secretions in both groups of women, they found that highly exposed, persistently negative (HEPS) women were far more likely to have vaginal secretions containing a type of antibody called immunoglobulin A (IgA) that was active against HIV. These women were also more likely to have evidence of HIV-specific CD4 cell proliferation in their cervicovaginal tracts than were those who had become infected with HIV. This study is the first to show an association between reduced HIV transmission and prior detection of both genital HIV-neutralizing IgA and HIV-specific CD4 proliferation. (Hirbod et al., 2008.)

BOX 7.3   (continued)

Heterosexual Men Exposed to HIV Remain HIV Negative

In a study by Mario Clerici and colleagues (2003), 14 HIV-negative men remained HIV negative after repeated exposure to HIV from HIV-infected female partners after four years of unprotected sex. On average, the 14 couples said they had sex 14 times a year. Why they remain HIV negative is unknown.

Current evidence suggests that between 5% and 10% of HIV-infected people will live up to 20 or more years. It should be mentioned that if the average time from infection to AIDS is 11 years, statistically speaking, survivors at 20+ years are expected to occur. Time will tell. For other accounts of long-term survivors, see the articles by Cao (1995), Pantaleo (1995), Kirchhoff et al., (1995), Baltimore (1995), Gegny (2000), and Migueles (2000).

IMMUNE CELL RECEPTORS, MOLECULES THAT BIND TO THESE RECEPTORS (LIGANDS), AND T4 OR CD4+ AND CTL CELL INFLUENCE ON SURVIVAL

Chemokine Receptors: An Association of Coreceptors to Progression to AIDS

As discussed in Chapters 4 and 5, the **chemokine receptors** [the four most familiar are CCKR-5 (R-5), CXCKR-4 (R-4), CCKR-3 (R-3), and CCKR-2 (R-2)] reside on immune system cell membranes. The receptors act as host sites for a variety of chemokines that need entry into such cells. But scientists recently learned that these chemokine receptors also act as **coreceptors** to the CD4 receptor, the receptor to which HIV first attaches. That is, HIV anchors to the cell's CD4 receptor, but it also needs to bind with a coreceptor, one of the chemokine receptors, in order to complete its entry into the cell. **Genetic mutations** that inhibit given chemokine receptor formation and/or reduce the numbers of such receptors on the immune cell membrane offer such cells a complete or partial resistance to HIV infection. A double or homozygous mutation at R-5 makes some people resistant to HIV infection, but the R-2 mutation only slows the progression of HIV disease to AIDS. Such mutations contribute to some people's long-term survival. Both CCKR-5 and CCKR-2 receptor mutations offer this protection (Balter, 1998; Collman, 1997; Cocchi et al., 1995; Feng et al., 1996). Exciting research published in 1998 reports that the genetic mutation that interferes with the X-4 receptor actually interferes with the *production* of the specific chemokine that attaches to the R-4 receptor. It appears that this mutation causes the overproduction of a chemokine called Stromal Derived Factor-1 (SDF-1). With an excess in the environment, SDF-1 fills available R-4 receptor sites, blocking HIV attachment. So, those persons carrying an SDF-1 mutation, although HIV infected, progress through HIV disease at a much slower pace, delaying the onset of AIDS as much as 7 to 10 years later than average (Winkler et al., 1998; Balter, 1998). Thus it appears that, in some people, the progression rate to AIDS is linked to the types of coreceptors people carry on their T4 cells and macrophages (Reynes et al., 2001).

CHILDREN

Micheline Mishrahi and colleagues (1998) reported that children carrying one copy (heterozygous) of the mutant R-5 gene demonstrate a substantial reduction in progression of HIV disease to AIDS.

---

some people respond well to antiretroviral drug therapy and have their T4 cell counts increase while others on drug therapy do not experience T4 cell increase. They believe the increase of T4 cells or lack of it is associated with the amount of T cell zone destruction.

Performing T4 or CD4+ Cell Counts in HIV-Infected People Continues to Be Essential

A major player in the body's immune system is the T4 or CD4+ cell. By binding with CD4+ cells, HIV can kill them and stop the associated production of antibodies, leaving the immune system weakened and vulnerable to opportunistic disease. Doctors gauge the health of the immune system by counting T4 or CD4+ cells. A healthy, HIV-negative adult has between 600 and 1200 CD4+ cells per cubic millimeter of blood. If the count falls below 350, the immune system has become weakened. Further loss leads to immune suppression and the onset of opportunistic diseases.

Thus, accurate and reliable measures of T4 or CD4+ lymphocytes are essential to the assessment of the immune system of HIV-infected persons. The progression to AIDS is largely attributable to the decrease in T4 lymphocytes. Consequently, the Public Health Service (PHS) has recommended that T4 lymphocyte levels be monitored every three to six months in all HIV-infected persons. The measurement of T4 cell levels has been used to establish de-

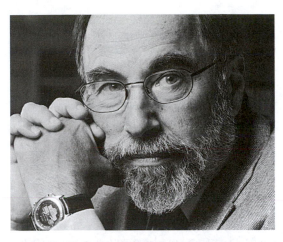

FIGURE 7-9 David Baltimore, 1975, Nobel Prize Molecular Biologist and President of the California Institutes of Technology. (*Photograph © David Baltimore*)

cision points for initiating prophylaxis for a variety of opportunistic infections. Moreover, T4 lymphocyte levels are a **criterion** for categorizing HIV-related clinical conditions by CDC's classification system for HIV infection and surveillance case definition for AIDS among adults and adolescents (*MMWR*, 1997).

Levels of HIV RNA in the Blood: Viral Load

David Baltimore (Figure 7-9), the Nobel Prize-winning retrovirologist, and coworkers have found a useful clinical predictor of HIV disease progressors, *levels of HIV RNA in the blood. More RNA means more HIV,* and that makes patients get sicker sooner. HIV RNA is a more sensitive measure of HIV than other antibody type assays and may detect the virus earlier than it would be seen otherwise.

Since the reported work of Baltimore and others on the levels of HIV RNA in the blood, Denis Henrard and coworkers (1995) have concluded that the stability of HIV RNA levels suggests that an equilibrium between HIV replication rate and efficacy of immunologic response, **a set point,** is established shortly after infection and persists throughout the asymptomatic period of the disease (Figure 7-5). Thus, a defect in immunologic control of HIV infection may be as important as the viral replication rate for determining AIDS-free survival. Because individual steady-state levels of HIV RNA are established soon after infection, HIV RNA levels can, as Baltimore suggests, be useful markers for predicting clinical outcome.

Viral load measurements indicate the amount of current HIV activity. T4 cell counts indicate the degree of immunologic destruction. Thus, the best monitor of disease progression is the use of both the T4 cell count and viral load (Merigan et al., 1996; Katzenstein et al., 1996; Voelker, 1995; Goldschmidt et al., 1997).

No current viral or immunological markers adequately reflect drug toxicities caused by therapy.

HIV INFECTION OF THE CENTRAL NERVOUS SYSTEM (CNS)

The nervous system has two parts. The brain and the spinal cord are the central nervous system (CNS). The nerves and muscles are the peripheral nervous system. Peripheral means around the outside. A wide variety of CNS abnormalities occur during the course of HIV infection. They result not only from the opportunistic infections and malignancies in the immunodeficient individual, but also from direct HIV infection of the CNS. It was believed that because some brain cells contain CD4-like receptors they were receptive to HIV infection. In addition, other brain cells contain a glycolipid that allows for HIV infection (Ranki et al., 1995). However, more recent research shows that after HIV-infected monocytes migrate to the brain, become tissue macrophage, and release HIV, the virus *does not* infect brain cells; rather HIV resides in brain spaces, in the cerebrospinal fluid. In 2004, Yan Xu and colleagues reported that it is the molecular products of HIV and not the virus itself that cause nerve cell death which leads to neurodegeneration and associated cognitive and motor dysfunctions. HIV investigators believe that HIV may invade the brain within a few weeks to months after HIV infection.

The CNS and Antiretroviral Therapy

HIV infection of the CNS has to be treated with antiviral drugs. Yet, the blood-brain barrier keeps many drugs out of the central nervous system. The barrier is a tight network of blood vessels that protects the brain and spinal cord from most infectious agents or poisons in the bloodstream. Several anti-HIV drugs do get through the blood-brain barriers. A special concern is that people with CNS problems may need extra help remembering to take their medications.

Genetic analysis and clinical studies have revealed that HIV in the cerebrospinal fluid (CSF) of some people with AIDS-related dementia evolves *independently* of the HIV in their blood, leading to at least two genetically distinct forms of the virus. This finding poses a new challenge for treatment of these patients, suggesting that drugs effective against HIV in their blood may not do the job in the central nervous system, and vice-versa. Why HIV evolves independently in the CSF of the demented patients is not clear. It may reflect a separate viral subpopulation thriving in their central nervous system, or maybe those with dementia have progressed further in immunodeficiency that may allow HIV to become more virulent. Scientists at Gladstone Institute of Virology and Immunology also found preliminary evidence that in some AIDS dementia patients HIV in the CSF compartment is more resistant to antiretroviral drugs than is HIV in the blood. This can cause a rebound of virus levels in the CSF while the viral load in the blood is suppressed. Ongoing studies of resistant mutations should clarify this pattern (Haas et al., 2000).

AIDS Dementia Complex

HIV/AIDS associated dementia or AIDS Dementia Complex (ADC) is a progressive brain disorder that causes confusion, memory loss, difficulty with thinking and speaking, and balance problems. ADC is characterized by severe changes in four areas: a person's ability to understand, process, and remember information (cognition); behavior; ability to coordinate muscles and movement (motor coordination); or emotions (mood). These changes are called ADC when they're believed to be related to HIV itself rather than to other factors that might cause them, such as other brain infections or drug side effects.

Different Neurological Problems Affecting People with HIV in the Era of HAART

Currently, about 10% to 15% of people on highly active antiretroviral therapy (HAART) experience severe AIDS Dementia Complex (ADC). The spectrum of problems affecting people with HIV on HAART is changing. For example, neurocognitive disorders are now fewer and milder than those found, say, ten years ago. HAART is having a profound effect on reducing the symptoms associated with ADC.

How Does HIV Cause ADC?

While it is clear that HIV can cause serious nervous system disease, how it causes ADC is unclear. In general, nervous system and mental disorders are caused by the death of nerve cells. While HIV does not directly

infect nerve cells, it's thought that HIV can somehow kill them indirectly. Macrophages—white cells that are prevalent in the brain and act as large reservoirs for HIV—appear to be HIV's first target in the central nervous system. HIV-infected macrophages can carry HIV into the brain from the bloodstream.

In 2005, Paul Thompson and colleagues published a report saying that HIV is selective in how it attacks the brain and that drug therapy does not appear to slow HIV-associated brain damage. The brain provides a sanctuary for HIV where most drugs cannot follow. Using 3D imagery they found that AIDS patients had 10% to 15% thinner-than-normal brain tissues in regions that control movement, language and feeling. The tissue loss shown in the brain imaging of the AIDS patients correlated with motor and cognitive defects that the patients showed in multiple brain function tests.

A progressive dementia (mental deterioration) due to HIV infection of the central nervous system develops in about half of AIDS patients (depending on their life span, Figure 7-10). Pathological changes in the CNS are observed in up to 80% of those autopsied (McGuire, 1993). But the mystery remains as to why some HIV-infected people develop dementia while others do not. Some people with high viral loads were not demented, while others with low viral loads had dementia.

NEUROPATHIES IN HIV DISEASE/AIDS PATIENTS

Soon after it enters the body HIV colonizes in the brain and other nerve tissues. Within the compartment of the nervous system, the virus remains, often at high concentrations and with time can lead to a spectrum of problems spanning from localized disease of the brain to distal peripheral neuropathy.

Neuropathies are functional changes in the peripheral nervous system; therefore, any part of the body may be affected. Although neuropathies are not OIs, they may result from the presence of certain OIs. **Peripheral neuropathy** is caused by nerve damage and is usually characterized by a sensation of pins and needles, burning, stiffness, or numbness in the hands, feet, legs, and toes. It is a common, sometimes painful, condition in HIV-positive patients, affecting up to 30% of people with AIDS. At autopsy, two-thirds of AIDS patients have neuropathies. Neuropathy has been a continuous problem for patients throughout

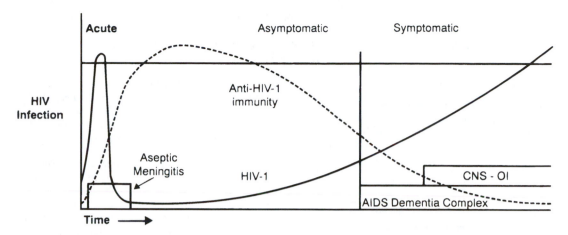

FIGURE 7-10 Central Nervous System Events After HIV Infection. Note that aseptic meningitis (an inflammation of the membrane of the brain and spinal cord in the absence of viral or bacterial infection), when it occurs, occurs early after HIV infection. Although usually apparent later, AIDS dementia complex may begin during the early-late phase. The late phase represents the period during which major AIDS-defining opportunistic infections occur. The headings acute, latent, early-late, and late refer to periods after HIV infection. It appears that opportunistic infection of the brain occurs after the onset of ADC. (*Adapted from Price, 1988*)

the HIV/AIDS epidemic. It is most common in people with a history of multiple opportunistic infections and low T4 or CD4+ cell counts. There is a wide range of expression among patients with neuropathy, from a minor nuisance to a disabling weakness. The kinds of neuropathies occurring in people with HIV/AIDS are numerous and must be identified before appropriate treatment can be prescribed. The underlying cause of the most common type of peripheral neuropathy remains elusive. What was a common complaint early in HIV infection of severe neuropathy—usually, burning feet, causing patients to walk on their heels—has diminished. The decrease in such complaints may be attributable to the antiviral effects of the drug ZDV. On the other hand, new varieties of drug-induced nerve damage (neuropathies) have been recognized with the use of nucleoside, non-nucleoside reverse transcriptase inhibitors, and protease inhibitor antivirals.

PEDIATRIC CLINICAL SIGNS AND SYMPTOMS

Currently over 90% of pediatric AIDS cases are newborns and infants who received HIV from mothers who were injection-drug users or were the sexual partners of IDUs. For those who become HIV-infected during gestation, clinical symptoms usually develop within six months after birth. Few children infected as fetuses live beyond two years, and survival past three years used to be rare; but with the use of anti-HIV drugs and therapy for opportunistic diseases, some children born with HIV are still alive at age 28 and some are raising their own children!

The clinical course of rapid HIV disease progression in infants diagnosed with AIDS is marked by failure to thrive, persistent lymphadenopathy, chronic or recurrent oral candidiasis, persistent diarrhea, enlarged liver and spleen (hepatosplenomegaly), and chronic pneumonia (interstitial pneumonitis). Bacterial infections are common and can be life-threatening. Bacterial infection and **septicemia** (the presence of a variety of bacterial species in the bloodstream) is a leading cause of death.

Less than 25% of AIDS children express the kinds of OIs found in adult AIDS patients. Kaposi's sarcoma occurs in about 4% of them. Young AIDS children experience delayed development and poor motor function. Older AIDS children experience speech and perception problems (See Chapter 11 for more on the effects of HIV on children.)

BOX 7.4

SCIENTISTS NEED A SMALL ANIMAL MODEL IN WHICH TO STUDY HIV DISEASE—
WHY ISN'T THERE ONE?

WHY THE NEED FOR A SMALL ANIMAL MODEL

HIV/AIDS researchers typically describe HIV as a wily, stealthy, and clever killer. But researchers who have been struggling for over two decades to get HIV to infect small animals have another adjective for the virus: impotent. HIV causes AIDS only in humans. If it could be coaxed to infect mice and rats—and, better yet, make them sick—the payoff could be enormous. Robert Gallo, head of the Institute of Human Virology in Baltimore, said, "Instead of five animals in an experiment, we'd have 500. Instead of waiting two years to get results, you'd wait two months. It would greatly catapult the field forward." But until recently, attempts to develop a rodent model for AIDS have been frustrating. HIV, it seems, is just too picky.

To date, scientists do not really know how HIV kills cells that carry the CD4 protein on their outer membranes—mostly those cells of the human immune system, the T lymphocytes. But that is not all that is unknown about how this unique virus attacks, inserts itself into human DNA, replicates, and exits the cell. To learn more about the devastation HIV brings to humans after cellular infection, replication, and release into the bloodstream, scientists must use chimpanzees and rhesus macaque monkeys. Yet HIV does not cause AIDS in these animals. HIV evolved in humans and to date, only causes AIDS in humans. But there are no other animals that are closer to the human system in which to study the infection and disease process. So scientists have routinely infected these primates with an HIV/SIV (human/simian or monkey virus/hybrid virus called SHIV). This hybrid virus will cause AIDS-like symptoms in these primates. But these primates are scarce and expensive. Chimpanzees cost up to $50,000 each. Rhesus macaque monkeys, more abundant than chimpanzees, but still short in supply, cost up to $5000 each. Breeding of either species takes years.

Scientists in a number of laboratories have, for years, been trying to develop specific strains of mice and rats to use as animal models to study HIV. In early 2008, Shifeng Sun and colleagues reported on creating and infecting a humanized immune system in mice with HIV. The mice were born with no immune system of their own; a human immune system developed after the transplantation of human fetal liver and thymus tissue and immune cells. After HIV particles were introduced into the rectums of the mice, six of seven showed evidence of HIV infection. Three of four mice produced antibodies to HIV, as humans do. On autopsy, HIV production was noted in the lymph nodes, spleen, other immune tissues, lungs, intestines, and male and female reproductive tracts. That the mice's bodies produced an immune response suggests they could be used to test HIV vaccine candidates. They might also represent an important advancement in the search for protective microbicides that could be applied in the rectum or vagina. Also, in early 2008, Paul Denton and colleagues prevented vaginal HIV infection in five humanized mice using Truvada-a combination of tenofovir and emtricitabine. The mice received Truvada for seven days before exposure to HIV. By contrast, 7 out of 8 mice not treated and exposed to HIV became infected.

Summary

The clinical signs and symptoms of HIV infection and AIDS have been addressed in the previous chapters. However, there are two major classification systems used to diagnose patients as they progress from HIV infection to AIDS. The first is the Walter Reed System. It recognizes six stages of signs and symptoms that a person passes through to AIDS. The CDC uses four groupings to identify the stage of illness from infection to AIDS. Both systems revolve around the recognition of a failing immune system, persistent swollen lymph nodes, and opportunistic infections. Mysteries still to be resolved are exactly why and how HIV kills cells, and why some people stabilize after the initial symptoms of HIV infection while others move directly on to AIDS.

One disorder that was not immediately recognized in AIDS patients is AIDS Dementia Complex (ADC), a progressive mental deterioration due to HIV infection of the central nervous system. ADC develops in over 50% of adult AIDS patients prior to death. Research has shown that some of the symptoms of this dementia can be reversed with the use of the drug zidovudine.

Review Questions

(Answers to the Review Questions are on page 427.)

1. Name the two major AIDS classification systems used in the United States.

2. What percent of HIV-infected individuals will progress to AIDS in 5 years; in 15 years?

3. What is the neurological set of behavioral changes in AIDS patients called?

4. Name three body organs and their associated AIDS-related diseases.

5. True or False: Currently the single most important laboratory parameter that is followed to monitor the progress of HIV infection is the T4 cell count.

6. True or False: The average time from infection to sero-conversion is two weeks. Explain.

7. True or False: Being infected with HIV and being diagnosed with AIDS are the same thing. Explain.

8. True or False: The average length of time from infection with HIV to an AIDS diagnosis is approximately two years.

9. Write a brief essay on: (a) In general, about how long HIV can reside in the body before one shows signs of HIV infection. (b) In general, about how long it takes the body to generate antibodies to HIV after infection.

10. The general signs and symptoms associated with HIV/AIDS include:

    A. recurrent fever

    B. weight loss for no apparent reason

    C. white spots in the mouth

    D. night sweats

    E. all of the above

11. If you were infected with HIV, you might show symptoms . . .

    A. within a few weeks

    B. within a year

    C. in 10 or more years

    D. any of the above

12. All of the following symptoms are chracteristic of AIDS, except

    A. fever

    B. fatigue

    C. diarrhea

    D. blindness

    E. weight loss

13. Which of the following is a cause of T_4 cell death in HIV disease?

    A. Replication of HIV lyses the cell.

    B. Infected cells are destroyed by cytotoxic T cells (T_C).

    C. Infected cells are attacked by natural killer cells.

    D. Cells are killed by fusion and syncytium formation.

    E. All of the above.

Epidemiology and Transmission of the Human Immunodeficiency Virus

---

CHAPTER CONCEPTS

- First evidence of HIV-1, 1959, Central Africa.
- In 1985, HIV-2 was isolated in West Africa.
- Transmission of HIV into the United States may have been via Haiti.
- Behavior is associated with HIV transmission.
- HIV is not casually transmitted.
- HIV is not transmitted to humans by insects. Only people transmit HIV!
- HIV transmission is being reported from 194 countries and among all ages and ethnic groups.
- The four basic mechanisms of HIV transmission are: sexual contact, needles and syringes, mother to child, and blood transfusions. All involve an exchange of body fluids.
- HIV enters the body through the mucosal lining of the vagina, vulva, penis, rectum, or mouth during sex.
- A single copy of HIV causes an HIV infection.
- One new route of HIV transmission has been discovered in the last 27 years: prechewed food!
- First documented case of HIV transmission via deep kissing is presented.
- Highest frequency of HIV transmission in the United States is among homosexual and bisexual males and among injection-drug users.
- High-risk activities of gay males presented.
- Serosorting is preferentially picking sexual partners of the same HIV status.
- It has been found that most HIV-infected people do not infect others.
- Male circumcision prevents HIV transmission into males but does not affect women's HIV risk.
- Sperm washing: an effective means of providing HIV free fertilizations.
- Swiss experts say HIV positive people with undetectable viral load and no sexually transmittable diseases **do not** transmit HIV.
- Other countries, HIV infection, and injection-drug use.
- HIV/AIDS in the Caribbean.
- Worldwide, highest frequency of HIV transmission is among heterosexuals.
- Blood banks in several countries knowingly allowed the distribution of HIV-contaminated blood.
- HIV-infected athletes want to compete.
- Death due to HIV infection is placed in perspective.
- Interactions between HIV and sexually transmitted diseases are discussed.
- Prenatal HIV transmission generally occurs after the 12th to 16th week of gestation, most often during childbirth and breast-feeding.
- Zidovudine (ZDU or AZT) and nevirapine decrease perinatal HIV transmission.
- National HIV/AIDS resources phone numbers are listed.
- Play the game—see if you can tell who is HIV positive or not.

When a population becomes infected with a contagious disease, an epidemic results. **Epidemic** is derived from Greek and means "in one place among the people." To understand how an infectious disease can spread or remain established in a population, investigators must consider the relationship between an infectious disease agent and its host population. The study of diseases in populations is an area of medicine known as **epidemiology (ep-i-de-mi-ol-o-gy).**

Complacency and HIV Infection

The danger of complacency has been learned from earlier epidemics. Complacency about HIV infection is especially dangerous because the infection can remain hidden for years. Because many infected people remain symptom-free for years, it is hard to be sure just who is infected with the virus. The more sexual partners, the greater the chances of encountering one who is infected and subsequently becoming infected.

With regard to HIV infection, it is your behavior that counts. The transmission of HIV can be prevented. HIV is relatively hard to contract and with exceptions, can be avoided.

The presence of HIV/AIDS is not isolated—the transmissibility of HIV between individuals and across borders and populations is what drives this global pandemic and makes it imperative that nations work together to prevent the continued transmission of HIV. On an individual level, IT IS NOT IMPORTANT HOW YOU GOT HIV, WHAT IS IMPORTANT IS HOW YOU LIVE YOUR LIFE WITH THE VIRUS.

How HIV Enters the Body

In all cases, HIV is transmitted in one of two ways: first, as the virus itself, or second, within an HIV-infected cell. The virus is held within the white blood cells of the immune system and is carried Trojan horse-style within the fluid of one person into the body of another.

HIV and Sexual Transmission

Epidemiological data suggest that sexual transmission, in general, is relatively inefficient, in that exposure to HIV often does not produce infection. HIV is transmitted more efficiently intravenously than through sexual routes. However, worldwide the predominant mode of transmission of HIV is through exposure of mucosal surfaces of the vagina, vulva, penis, rectum, or mouth to infected sexual fluids (semen, cervical/vaginal, rectal) and during birth. Sexual transmission of HIV now accounts for about 90% of infections worldwide.

Factors Driving Sexual Transmission

There is evidence from around the world that many factors play a role in initiating a sexually transmitted HIV epidemic or driving it to higher levels. Among the **behavioral** and **social factors** are (a) condom use, (b) proportion of the adult population with multiple partners, (c) overlapping (as opposed to serial) sexual partnerships—individuals are highly infectious when they first acquire HIV and thus are more likely to infect any concurrent partners, (d) sexual networks (often seen in individuals who move back and forth between home and a far-off workplace), (e) age mixing, typically between older men and young women and children, and (f) poverty and in particular women's economic dependence on marriage or prostitution, robbing them of control over the circumstances or safety of sex.

Biological factors include (a) high rates of sexually transmitted infections, especially those causing genital ulcers, (b) low rates of male circumcision, and (c) high viral load HIV levels in the bloodstream that are typically highest when a person is first infected and again in the late stages of illness.

While all these factors help spread the virus, it is not known exactly how much each of them contributes and to what extent they need to be combined in order to spread the epidemic. The issue of male circumcision is a good example. Many countries in which all boys are circumcised before puberty have very limited epidemics, and even in some countries with wider epidemics, circumcised men have lower HIV rates than uncircumcised men (see discussion on the benefits of male circumcision later in this chapter).

HIV: Other Routes of Transmission?

People do not "catch" HIV in the same way that they "catch" the cold or a flu virus. Unlike colds and flu viruses, HIV *is* **not,** according to the CDC, spread by tears, sweat, coughing, or sneezing. The virus *is* **not** transmitted via an infected person's clothes, phone, or toilet seat. HIV *is* **not** passed on by eating utensils, drinking glasses, or other objects that HIV-infected people have used that are free of their blood.

HIV *is* **not** transmitted through daily contact with infected people, whether at work, home, or school. Insects **do not** transmit the virus. Kissing is also considered very low risk: There is only one documented case to prove that HIV is transmitted by kissing. Paul Holmstrom and colleagues (1992) report that salivary HIV antibodies are detected regularly in HIV seropositive subjects. The route of HIV into saliva is not fully understood. Both salivary glands and salivary leukocytes have been shown to harbor HIV. Gingival fluid (fluid seeping out of the gums) has been regarded as the main source of salivary HIV antibodies and infectious HIV.

In its 1990 supplemental guidelines for cardiopulmonary resuscitation (CPR) training and rescue, the Emergency Cardiac Care Committee of the American Heart Association (AHA) noted that there is an extremely small theoretical risk of HIV or hepatitis B virus (HBV) transmission via cardiopulmonary resuscitation (CPR). To date no known case of seroconversion for HIV or HBV has occurred in these circumstances.

WE MUST STOP HIV TRANSMISSION NOW!

Education and advocacy for risk reduction remain important tools for preventing HIV infection. Used alone however, they will never accomplish the objective of slowing the speed and extent of the virus's spread. This can only be achieved by combining educational and early intervention efforts with specific measures guiding those resources to the people who need them most: those who are already infected and to their sex and drug partners.

Ending year 2009, there will be over 1.2 million AIDS cases in the United States. Figure 8-1 breaks this number down according to means of HIV infection—sexual behavior, drug use, medical exigencies, and undetermined causes. Figure 8-2 gives a breakdown by transmission category for 40,000 AIDS estimated cases for 2009.

EPIDEMIOLOGY OF HIV INFECTION

The first scientific evidence of human HIV infection came from the detection of HIV antibodies in preserved serum samples collected in Central Africa in 1959. The first AIDS cases appeared there in the 1960s. By the mid-1970s HIV was being spread throughout the rest of the world. The earliest places to experience the arrival of HIV were Central Europe and Haiti. Transmission into the United States may have been by tourists who had vacationed in the area of Port-au-Prince, Haiti (Swenson, 1988).

On entry into the United States the virus first spread among the homosexual populations of large cities such as New York and San Francisco. The first **recorded** AIDS cases in the United States occurred in 1979 in New York. The first **CDC-reported** AIDS cases were in New York, Los Angeles, and San Francisco in 1981. In all cases, the diagnosis of AIDS was based on clinical descriptions.

According to the CDC's first clinical AIDS definition, at least one case of AIDS occurred in New York City in 1952 and another in 1959. Both males demonstrated opportunistic infections and *Pneumocystis jiroveci* pneumonia, a hallmark of HIV infection. This early evidence of AIDS suggests that the virus might have been in the United States, Europe, and Africa at about the same time (Katner et al., 1987). If HIV has been present

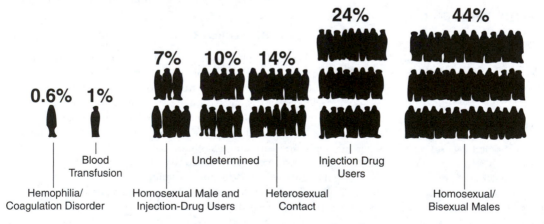

FIGURE 8-1 Cumulative AIDS Cases by Route of Transmission. At the end of 2009, there will be about 1.2 million AIDS cases in the United States. This diagram gives the percentage of adults and adolescents in each group. Groupings are according to sexual preference, drug use, medical conditions, and others not associated with any of these. *(Courtesy of CDC, Atlanta—updated)*

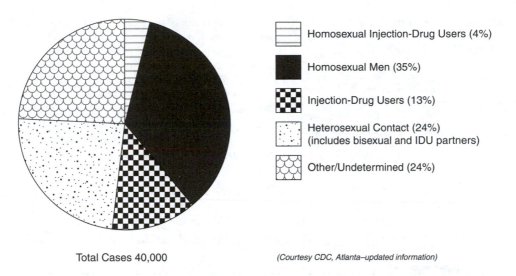

Homosexual Injection-Drug Users (4%)

Homosexual Men (35%)

Injection-Drug Users (13%)

Heterosexual Contact (24%)
(includes bisexual and IDU partners)

Other/Undetermined (24%)

Total Cases 40,000   (Courtesy CDC, Atlanta–updated information)

FIGURE 8-2   Adult/Adolescent AIDS Cases by Transmission Category Estimated for 2009, United States.

for decades as suggested, its failure to spread may reflect a recent HIV mutation, a major change in social behaviors conducive to HIV transmission, or both. For example, the sexual revolution and the widespread use of birth control pills, which began in the 1960s, and the subsequent decrease in the use of condoms may have contributed to the transmission of HIV.

TRANSMISSION OF TWO STRAINS OF HIV (HIV-1/HIV-2)

The spread of HIV-1 is global. The clinical presentation of AIDS caused by HIV-1 is similar regardless of geographical area.

HIV-2 is a genetically distinct strain. HIV-2 was first discovered in 1985 in West Africa. It is believed to have been present in West Africa as early as the 1960s. Clinical data demonstrate that HIV-2 has a reduced virulence compared to HIV-1 (Marlink et al., 1994).

It appears that HIV-2, like HIV-1, may spread worldwide. HIV-2 has already spread from West Africa to other parts of Africa, Europe, and the Americas. Both HIV-1 and HIV-2 are transmitted or acquired through the same kinds of exposure.

Because over 99% of global AIDS cases are caused by the transmission of HIV-1, only data that pertain to HIV-1 (HIV) will be presented unless otherwise stated.

IS HIV TRANSMITTED BY INSECTS?

In spite of convincing evidence of the ways in which HIV can be transmitted, it remains difficult for the general public to believe that a virus that appears to spread as rapidly as HIV is not either highly contagious or transmitted by an environmental agent. After all, there are many viral and bacterial diseases that are highly contagious and transmitted by insects. The question was asked: Is this virus being transmitted by insects?

Necessary data to resolve the question is available. Epidemiological data from Africa and the United States suggest that HIV is not transmitted by insect bites. If it were, many more cases would be expected among school-age children and elderly people, groups that are proportionally underrepresented among AIDS patients. In one study of the household contacts of AIDS patients in Kinshasa, Zaire, where insect bites are common, not a single child over the age of 1 year had been infected with HIV, while more than 60% of spouses had become infected.

In 1987, the Office of Technology Assessment (OTA) published a detailed paper on the question of whether blood-sucking insects such as biting flies, mosquitoes, and bedbugs transmit HIV (Miike, 1987). The conclusion was that the conditions necessary for successful transmission of HIV through insect bites and the probability of their occurring rule out the possibility of insect transmission as a virus has to overcome many obstacles. It must avoid digestion in the gut of the insect, recognize receptors on the external surface of the gut, penetrate the gut, replicate in insect tissue, recognize and penetrate the insect salivary glands, and subsequently escape into the lumen of the salivary duct. Webb and colleagues (1989) inoculated bedbugs intraabdominally (belly) and mosquitoes intrathoracically (chest) with HIV to enable the virus to bypass gut barriers. HIV failed to replicate in either.

significant factor in the spread of AIDS. Jerome Goddard reported (1997) that blood-sucking arthropods (for example, mosquitoes and bedbugs) for good biological reasons, **cannot** transmit HIV. The

HIV TRANSMISSION

If most HIV-exposed people can become HIV infected, can most infected people *transmit* HIV to

---

SNAPSHOT 8.1

TOP 14 MYTHS ABOUT HIV/AIDS

Beginning with the least believable at number 14 If you do not recognize these statements as myth, you will by the time you complete this chapter/book.

14. Gambian President Yahya Jammeh claims he can cure AIDS in three days.
13. Teenagers aren't really at risk.
12. Mostly gay men and drug users get it.
11. There is a cure, but only rich people like Magic Johnson can afford it.
10. You only need to get tested if you don't know your sex partner that well.
9. You can tell someone has AIDS just by looking at them.
8. Heterosexual women are not at risk.
7. You shouldn't kiss, hug, or share a meal or drink with someone who is HIV positive or has AIDS.
6. Wearing the Red Ribbon is the only way to help fight the AIDS pandemic.
5. It's really only bad in developing, third-world countries.
4. You don't hear so much about it anymore, so it must not be that bad.
3. The U.S. government has the secret to cure HIV/AIDS locked away and only the rich and powerful receive this cure.
2. The U.S. government developed HIV/AIDS to reduce the black population (Ross et. al 2007).
1. In 2003, Jeremiah Wright, former long-time pastor to Senator Barack Obama, the 2008 presidential candidate, said that the U.S. government had "lied" about inventing HIV as a means of perpetrating black genocide. And in April 2008 he said that he believes the U.S. government is "capable" of having invented HIV as a means of committing genocide against people of color (CNS News.com 4/28/08).

Other Rumors and Hoaxes Going Around

1. I received an e-mail warning that a man who was believed to be HIV positive was recently caught placing blood in the ketchup dispenser at a fast food restaurant. Because of the risk of HIV transmission, the e-mail recommended that only individually wrapped packets of ketchup be used.
2. A child in Florida tested HIV positive after being stuck by a used needle found on a playground.
3. HIV can easily be transmitted through contact with unused feminine (sanitary) pads.
4. The CDC has discovered a mutated version of HIV that is transmitted through the air.
5. Many people are getting stuck by HIV blood-containing needles in phone booth coin returns, movie theater seats, gas pump handles, and other places.

NOTATION: HIV IS ONLY CARRIED BY PEOPLE—ONLY PEOPLE CAN TRANSMIT HIV!

others? This is a difficult question to answer. Infection with HIV appears to depend on a large number of variables that involve the donor, recipient, and portal of entry. The most important variables are mode of transmission, viral load, which subtype and variant of HIV is present, and the recipient's genetic resistance.

Global Patterns of HIV Transmission

Worldwide there are now three types or patterns of HIV epidemics unfolding. The first pattern is occurring in wealthy countries, such as the United States, where the epidemics are heterogeneous but dominantly involve **male-to-male** sexual transmission. After a long period of decline, those epidemics are now showing troubling signs of resurgence, largely due to unsafe sexual practices among gay men.

The second pattern is seen in sub-Saharan Africa and Latin America, driven by **heterosexual** transmission. Africa continues to have the largest numbers of people living with HIV and dying of AIDS.

The third pattern and labeled as explosive by UNAIDS has almost nothing to do with sex. It is driven by **needles shared among people who inject narcotics.** All over the world the narcotics-driven HIV pandemic seems to begin, unnoticed by government officials, in isolated communities of injection-drug users, spreads like wildfire, and then suddenly takes on national significance. The most disturbing examples

---

BOX 8.1

A NEIGHBOR'S STORY: PUBLIC IMAGE, PUBLIC FEAR

We have over the last 27 years witnessed educated people offering misrepresentation and fantasy about HIV infection and AIDS. We have listened to them distort the truth by presenting false perceptions rather than facts. If education is to become a major player in prevention of the spread of HIV, the mix of myth and fantasy must be replaced by reality—and this can be done by giving the proper respect to a new disease in our lifetime.

THE NEIGHBOR

Some neighbors were having a garage sale. Their friend came over and asked them a question about AIDS. They mentioned that he should talk to the professor next door and he came over to the house. He said, "I'm looking for the truth about who is, and who isn't HIV infected and how I can tell people that are HIV infected from those who are not." I asked if he cared to share the reason for the questions and he immediately told me that he divorced three years ago and has been so frightened by the information he has seen on TV, heard on the radio, and read in the paper that he has remained celibate for three years and that it has truly affected his quality of life. He said, "I'm afraid to have sex with any woman I date because I believe almost every woman in Jacksonville and elsewhere carries HIV. It's driving me insane. My male friends are still having sex. Are they crazy or am I the fool?" I took the second question first. I assured him that his worst fears were correct. You can't tell the HIV positive from the HIV negative just by their appearance. Infected and noninfected all look alike—

at least in the early and middle stages of the disease. For the second question of who is and who is not HIV infected, I gave him some details relating to people's behavior, the particular behavioral risk groups and I said that if he did not belong to such groups or did not have a blood transfusion before 1985–1986, and that if he had some information about his sexual partner and did not change sexual partners too frequently and always used a condom, he could feel as safe as one can. The expression on his face went from concern to relief. He shook my hand repeatedly. He thanked me profusely and he said, "I feel like the media, the government, the gays, and everyone else has cheated me out of three years of my life. I can never get that back." I said, "Yes, to some degree that is true, but here you stand after three years still HIV negative. Would you like to exchange three years of free-wheeling sexual encounters for an HIV infection?" He agreed that he would not, but we both understand his point. We all need to understand his point. Misinformation—data skewed by ignorance or lack of education causes fear. And failure to give an accurate representation of a disease, from both the medical and social vantage points, can cause a great deal of harm—in ways that most of us would not begin to contemplate. Did I give him the right advice? No, because I did not give him advice at all. I simply attempted to put things in their proper perspective. He did not leave me less afraid of dying of AIDS. He left me with the idea that he could have his sex life restored without dying from AIDS, provided he maintains his low-risk behavior.

—The Author

---

of this phenomenon are the epidemics of Eastern Europe and Asia, which regionally are in the midst of an HIV explosion that was predicted some years ago. Injection-drug use-associated HIV infections are out of control in Russia, China, and Indonesia.

Across the globe, depending on the developing nation, IDU is associated with the highest incidence of HIV transmission; in other countries it may be via men having sex with men, or heterosexual sex among males and females.

HIV TRANSMISSION IN FAMILY/HOUSEHOLD SETTINGS

Several studies of the family members of AIDS patients have failed to demonstrate the spread of HIV through household contact. The only cases in which family members have become infected involved the sexual partners of AIDS patients or children born to mothers who were already infected with the virus. Even individuals who bathed, diapered, or slept in the same bed with AIDS patients have not become infected. In one study, family members shared toothbrushes with the infected person and no one became infected.

Perhaps the best evidence *against* casual HIV transmission comes from studies of household members living with blood-transfused AIDS patients (Peterman et al., 1988). Transfusion infection cases are unique because their dates of infection are known retrospectively. Prior to the onset of AIDS symptoms, the families were unaware that they were living with HIV-infected individuals. Family life was not altered in any way, yet family members remained uninfected. In some cases, the transfusion patients were hemophiliacs who received weekly or monthly injections of blood products and became HIV infected. From the combined studies of these households, only the sexual partners of infected hemophiliacs became infected.

Although contact with blood and other body substances can occur in households, transmission of HIV is rare in this setting. Through 2008, at least 11 reports have described household transmission of HIV not associated with sexual contact, injection-drug use, or breast-feeding. Of these 11 reports, 7 were associated with documented or probable blood contact. In one report, HIV infection was diagnosed in a boy after his younger brother had died as the result of AIDS; however, a specific mechanism of transmission was not determined.

NONCASUAL TRANSMISSION

The routes of HIV transmission were established *before* the virus was identified. The appearance of AIDS in the United States occurred first in specific groups of people: homosexual men and injection-drug users. The transmission of the disease within the two groups appeared to be closely associated with sexual behavior and the sharing of IV needles. By 1982, hemophiliacs receiving blood products, as well as the newborns of injection-drug users, began demonstrating AIDS. By 1983, heterosexual female partners of AIDS patients demonstrated AIDS. **Twenty-seven years** of continued surveillance of the general population has failed to reveal other categories of people contracting HIV/AIDS (Table 8-1). It became apparent that the infectious agent was being transmitted within specific groups of people, who by their behavior were at increased risk for acquiring and transmitting it (Table 8-2). Clearly, an exchange of body fluids was involved in the transmission of HIV, even in the three cases of HIV being transmitted via prechewed food reported on by the CDC in 2008.

Bodily Fluids

With the announcement that a new virus had been discovered, further research showed that this virus was present in a number of body fluids. Thus, even before there was a test to detect this virus, the public was told that it was transmitted through body fluids exchanged during intimate sexual contact, contaminated hypodermic needles, contaminated blood or blood products, and from mother to fetus. In addition it was concluded that the widespread dissemination of the virus was most likely the result of multiple or repeated viral exposure because the data from transfusion-infected individuals indicated that they did not necessarily infect their sexual partners. In other words, it was concluded early on and later confirmed that this virus was not transmitted as easily as other blood-borne viral diseases such as hepatitis B, or viral and bacterial sexually transmitted diseases. Table 8-3 lists the means of HIV transmission worldwide. Table 8-4 lists the means of HIV transmission in the United States.

Mobility and the Spread of HIV/AIDS

Mobility is an important epidemiological factor in the spread of communicable diseases. This becomes particularly obvious when a new disease enters the

Table 8-1 HIV Transmission and Infection[1]

CHAIN OF HIV INFECTION

Agent causing the disease	HIV
Major reservoirs (source of HIV in the body)	Lymph nodes, intestines, blood, genitals
Replication site of HIV	Mostly inside T4+ or CD4–bearing lymphocytes
Portal of exit (how does HIV leave the body)	Mucosal openings, skin breaks, bleeding, or expulsion of body fluids
Transfer or transmission of HIV (from one human to another)	Via body fluids
Portal of entry (how does HIV enter the body)	Mucosal openings, skin breaks, areas of bleeding, injection, prechewed food.

TRANSMISSION ROUTES

Blood Inoculation

Transfusion of HIV-infected blood and blood products
Needle sharing among injection-drug users
Needle sticks, open cuts, and mucous membrane exposure in healthcare workers
Use of HIV-contaminated skin-piercing instruments (ears, acupuncture, tattoos)
Injection with unsterilized syringe and needle (mostly in undeveloped countries)

Sexual Contact: Exchange of semen, vaginal fluids, or blood

Homosexual, between men
Lesbian, between women
Heterosexual, from men to women and women to men
Bisexual men and women

Perinatal

Intrauterine
Peripartum (during birth)
Breast-feeding

[1]To reduce the risk of spreading HIV, use condoms during sexual activity. Do not share drug injection equipment. If you are HIV infected and pregnant, talk with your doctor about taking anti-HIV drugs. If you are an HIV-infected woman, talk with your doctor about breast-feeding. Protect cuts, open sores, and your eyes and mouth from contact with blood and other bodily fluids. If you think you've been exposed to HIV, get tested and ask your doctor about taking anti-HIV medications.

Table 8-2 Adult/Adolescent AIDS Cases by Sex and Exposure Categories, Estimated Through 2008, United States[a]

Male Exposure Category (77%)	Total No.
1. Men who have sex with men	360,591
2. Injecting drug use	223,223
3. Men who have sex with men and inject drugs	55,805
4. Hemophilia/coagulation disorder	8,585
5. Heterosexual contact:	120,197
a. Sex with injecting–drug user	44,473
b. Sex with person with hemophilia	240
c. Sex with transfusion recipient with HIV infection	952
d. Sex with HIV-infected person, risk not specified	74,532
6. Receipt of blood transfusion, blood components, or tissue	4,293
7. Other/undetermined	85,855
Total male AIDS cases	858,550

Female Exposure Category (23%)	
1. Injecting drug use	117,967
2. Hemophilia/coagulation disorder	–
3. Heterosexual contact:	125,660
a. Sex with injecting–drug user	50,264
b. Sex with bisexual male	6,786
c. Sex with person with hemophilia	879
d. Sex with transfusion recipient with HIV infection	1,131
e. Sex with HIV-infected person, risk not specified	66,600
4. Receipt of blood transfusion, blood components, or tissue	2,565
5. Other/undetermined	10,258
Total Female AIDS cases	256,450
Total male/female cases	1,115,000

[a]Pediatric cases, 9800. These calculations only give a general idea of risk. They can tell you which activities carry a higher or lower risk. They cannot tell you if you have been infected. If, for example, the risk is 1 in 100, it doesn't mean that you can engage in that activity 99 times without any risk of becoming infected. You might become infected with HIV after a single exposure. That can happen the first time you engage in a risky activity.

scene. In the early stage of the HIV/AIDS epidemic, for example, the route of the virus could be associated with mobility.

The first HIV-infected people in some Latin American and European countries reported a history of foreign travel. In some African countries, spread of the virus could be traced along international roads. Today, increasing numbers of HIV infections have been observed to be associated with the relaxation of travel restrictions in Central and Eastern Europe.

Table 8-3 How HIV Is Transmitted Worldwide, 2008

Exposure	Efficiency, %	% of Total
Blood transfusion/ blood products	>90	3
Perinatal	20–40	9
Sexual intercourse[a]	0.1–1.0	80
Injection-drug use	0.5–1.0	8

[a]Heterosexual intercourse over 70%
(Source: WHO/Global Programme on AIDS and UNAIDS, updated 2006)

Table 8-4 An Approximation of How an Estimated 1,800,000 Americans Became Infected with HIV, through 2008

180	—healthcare workers got infected from the blood or body fluids of patients;
24,120	—children infected through their mothers;
38,700	—people got HIV from infected blood or blood products;
126,000	—people did not know how they were infected, did not report their risk, or died before anyone could find out;
117,000	—people were infected who had both unprotected sex and shared needles;
450,000	—people were infected who shared needles;
1,044,000	—people were infected through unprotected sex.

(Based on data from HIV/AIDS Surveillance Report, CDC, Year-End Edition, 2006, updated)

Few countries are unaffected by HIV/AIDS. This has made it clear that restrictive measures such as refusal of entry to people living with HIV/AIDS and compulsory testing of mobile populations are ineffective measures to stop the spread of the virus. In times of increasing international interdependency, it is an illusion to think that the disease can be stopped at any border.

Number of HIVs Required for Infection

A recent article by George Shaw of the University of Alabama at Birmingham and colleagues (2008) revealed that most HIV infections can be traced back to the transmission of a *single* HIV that penetrates the body's defenses.

For the study, Shaw and colleagues analyzed blood samples from 102 people who had recently become HIV infected. The investigators genetically analyzed the samples and were able to count generations of HIV.

They found that the HIV in 76% of the infected people could be traced back to a single copy of the virus! The remaining 24% of infections were traced back to between two and five viruses. In the majority of cases, the single virus crossed the sexual mucosa and infected a single cell. Shaw said, "That cell makes a lot of viruses; you have a firestorm of HIV replication over the next couple of weeks. Very quickly the person is populated by millions of viruses." Shaw and his colleagues believe that these findings help explain why it usually takes several exposures to HIV to become infected, why the transmission of HIV is so inefficient, and why condoms help prevent HIV transmission. The investigators believe the findings are significant because they indicate that if researchers are trying to develop a vaccine or microbicide to prevent HIV infection, the only thing it has to prevent is the transmission of a single virus, in most cases. In addition, the investigators believe these findings help to clarify our understanding of the acute and early stages of HIV transmission.

In striking contrast to a single copy of HIV crossing the sexual mucosa, it is known that for other sexually transmitted infectious agents like bacteria and spirochetes, many copies of these agents cross the mucosa to cause infection.

Shaw said, "The findings are crystal clear; they will stand up to scientific study."

Body Fluid Transmission

High levels of HIV have been isolated from blood, semen, vaginal fluids, serum, and breast milk. Lower levels of HIV are found in saliva, tears, urine, lung fluid, and cerebrospinal fluid.

Cases of low levels of HIV in cell-free body fluids and within the cells of these fluids does not mean that HIV cannot be transmitted via these fluids or cells—it can, but the dose (number of viruses) is so small that the risk of infection is minimal. Also, no one has been identified as becoming infected with HIV due to contact with a body fluid on an environmental surface. CDC studies show that high concentrations of HIV in a drying fluid became 90% to 99% less infectious over several hours; thus the reason for the low number of healthcare workers contracting HIV infection after touching, being splashed by, or needle sticking themselves with blood containing HIV.

Highest Concentration of HIV in The Body

HIV is found in greatest numbers within T4 or CD4+ cells, macrophages, monocytes and dendriditic cells, and in blood, vaginal fluids and semen. Laboratory findings, along with overwhelming empirical observations, support the scientific conclusion that the major route of HIV transmission is through human blood and sexual activities involving exchange of semen and vaginal fluids. Semen carries significantly larger numbers of HIV than vaginal fluid. It appears that of all body fluids, these three contain the largest number of infected lymphocytes (Figure 8-3), which provide the largest HIV concentration in a given area at a given time.

Presence of HIV-Infected Cells in Body Fluids

Blood—Red blood cells do not contain nuclei; therefore, they have no DNA for HIV to use to replicate itself. Recent observations indicate that both latent and HIV-producing cells are present throughout the course of infection in the blood. Thus it is probable that HIV-infected people harbor substantial numbers of HIV-infected CD4 macrophage and monocyte cells in their blood from soon after the initial infection through the terminal stage of the disease.

Semen—A single specimen of ejaculate contains between 1 million and 10 million nonspermatozoal

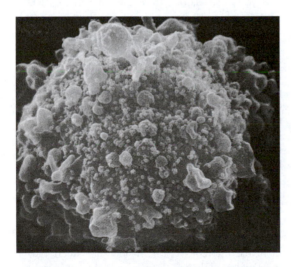

FIGURE 8-3 Electron Micrograph of an HIV-Infected T4 Lymphocyte. The T4 or CD4+ cell has produced a large number of HIVs that are located over the entire lymphocyte. Each HIV leaves a hole in the cell membrane. The photograph shows part of the convoluted surface of the lymphocyte magnified 20,000 times. (*Courtesy of The National Biological Standards Board, South Mimms, U.K.*)

cells, and many leukocytes including T4 cells, macrophage, and monocyte cells. But the number and type of cells in the semen of a healthy man differs considerably from day to day.

Reducing the numbers of lymphocytes and macrophages in semen could decrease the chances of infection. Christopher Pilcher and colleagues (2007) reported that HIV in semen reached its peak at four weeks after infection, and HIV shedding was almost completely contained by week 10, reflecting perhaps the host immune response. Lee Harrison and colleagues (2000) reported on 93 HIV-positive men on antiretroviral drugs. Before drug treatment, 74% had detectable levels of HIV in their semen. After six months on therapy 33% had detectable HIV in their semen.

Sperm—HIV is present in seminal fluid and white blood cells but not in sperm. Through washing and the use of centrifugal force, sperm can be separated from the other components of semen and then injected into the woman's body or used for in vitro fertilization. In studies issued over the past decade, some 4500 fertilizations using treated sperm from HIV-positive men have been conducted worldwide without any infection of either mother or child, according to Deborah Cohan, an obstetrician and gynecologist at the University of California at San Diego. While the sperm washing is relatively cheap—roughly $200—fertility treatments can be expensive. Uterine insemination, the so-called turkey baster method, costs approximately $1,000 while in vitro fertilization, in which the egg is fertilized outside the body, can cost between $10,000 and $15,000.

Saliva—Saliva contains few CD4, macrophage or monocyte cells. There continues to be some concern over the presence of HIV in saliva because of the exchange of saliva during deep kissing, the saliva residue left on eating utensils, and saliva on instruments handled by healthcare workers, especially in dentistry. Results of studies on hundreds of dental workers, many of whom have cared for AIDS patients, have shown no evidence of HIV infection (Friedland et al., 1987 updated). Also, in a CDC study, none of 48 healthcare workers became infected after parenteral (IV) or mucous membrane exposure to the saliva of HIV-infected patients (Curran et al., 1988). Studies by Fox (1991), Archibald (1990), and Pourtois (1991) showed that human saliva contains factors that inhibit HIV infectivity.

First Documented Kissing Transmission Case

Although about 59 million people around the world will have been HIV-infected by the end of 2009 there are remarkably few reports of its spread by kissing, dental treatment, biting, or coughing. Even among those people whose bodies are actively shedding HIV, their saliva usually contains only noninfectious components of the virus.

In July 1997, the first documented case of HIV transmission via deep kissing was reported by the CDC. In this *one* case, the man was HIV positive, via IDU in 1988. Both he and his female partner had serious gum (periodontal) disease. His gums routinely bled with brushing or flossing. Investigators at the CDC believe that the HIV was transmitted via blood within the man's oral cavity due to oral lesions onto the mucus membrane of the woman (*MMWR*, 1997).

Breast-Feeding: Mother's Milk—Breast milk contains CD4, macrophage and monocyte cells. Several studies have shown that HIV can be transmitted by breast-feeding. Van de Perre and coworkers (1993 updated) found that infection of babies via breast milk was most strongly correlated with the presence of HIV-infected cells in the milk, suggesting that infection might be cell-mediated. However, infection was also correlated with low levels of antibodies to HIV, suggesting that infection may be initiated by cell-free virus.

Prechewed Food—Aditya Gaur and colleagues (2008) reported that after ruling out other routes of transmission, such as breastfeeding, sexual abuse, blood transfusion, or needle stick injury, the investigators looked at caregivers and discovered that in two cases, HIV-positive mothers were in the habit of giving prechewed food to their infants. In one case, the child died of AIDS before the route of transmission was discovered, but the other child is receiving antiretroviral treatment. In the third case, a child was diagnosed with HIV at the age of 15 months in 1993. The infant's mother was HIV negative, and the strain of HIV carried by her HIV-positive partner was genetically dissimilar to the infant's strain, prompting the investigators to look elsewhere. They subsequently discovered that the child's great aunt had often looked after the child between the ages of 9 and 14 months and had given it prechewed food. The aunt died of AIDS in 1993.

They also discovered that in two of three cases, medical records showed evidence of bleeding gums and mouth sores during the period they were giving prechewed food to the infants. In the third case, no information was available on the caregiver's oral health for the period prior to the child's infection, but the virus found in the child was closely related, and no other explanation could be found for the child's HIV infection. The CDC believes that in developing countries prechewed food may be more common due to the lack of prepared baby foods, so it may pose a greater risk in settings where HIV prevalence is high and oral health poor.

Notation—This is essentially a newly discovered route of HIV infection!

Dentist with AIDS Infects Patient During Tooth Extraction?

In July 1990, the CDC reported on the possible transmission of HIV from a dentist with AIDS to a female patient (*MMWR*, 1990a). This case, like no other before it, sent chills through many. But why this case? Because the vast majority of people go to dentists! They don't inject drugs and are not gay. This case, however, is difficult to resolve. For example, two years had elapsed from the time of the dental work to when the patient, Kimberly Bergalis, was diagnosed with AIDS. Both patient and dentist, David J. Acer of Stuart, Fla., were uncertain of exactly what happened. Some of the pertinent factors in this case are (1) review of dental records and radiographs suggest that the two tooth extractions were uncomplicated; (2) interviews with Bergalis and the dentist did not identify other risk factors for HIV infection. Bergalis, age 22, stated over national TV in 1990 that she was still a virgin. This point was disputed on June 19, 1994, during the TV program *60 Minutes* (with Mike Wallace). Yes, she did engage in sexual foreplay, but not intercourse. Yes, she was infected with the human papilloma virus, which can be sexually transmitted, but this is not at all uncommon in immune-suppressed AIDS patients with no history of sexual intercourse; (3) nucleotide sequence data indicated a high degree of similarity between the HIV strains infecting her and the dentist; and (4) the time between the dental procedure and the development of AIDS was short (24 months), and Bergalis developed oral candidiasis 17 months after infection. At this time, only 1% of infected homosexual/bisexual men and 5% of infected transfusion recipients develop AIDS within two years of infection.

Who Was David Acer?—David Acer, a bisexual, was diagnosed with symptomatic HIV infection in 1986 and with AIDS in 1987. He died on September 3, 1990. Since then, 1100 of his 2500 patients were contacted for HIV testing. In January 1991, the test results of 591 of these patients revealed that five were HIV positive: a 68-year-old retired school teacher, a middle-aged father of two, a 37-year-old carnival worker, an unemployed drifter, and a 19-year-old student. As with Bergalis, infection in these patients may have come from some other source. All six patients denied having sexual contact with the dentist or with one another (*MMWR*, 1991a). If an absolute case can be made that Acer transmitted the virus to Bergalis, this will be the first documented case of a healthcare professional infecting a patient.

Bergalis died of AIDS on December 8, 1991. She was 23 years old and weighed 48 pounds.

How Did David Acer Infect His Patients?—There is no shortage of ideas as to how Acer might have infected his patients. For example, he could have used the same dental instruments on himself or his sexual partners that he used on his patients without sterilizing them.

The actual route of HIV transmission in the Acer-Bergalis case will most likely never be known. There have been suggestions that the dentist did not wish to die alone and chose certain people to infect. It was suggested that he may have attempted to infect still others, but was unsuccessful. A friend of the dentist said that he believed that Acer intentionally infected his patients to call attention to the HIV/AIDS problem in the United States. Acer felt that mainstream America was ignoring the problem.

A CDC estimate put the theoretical risk of HIV transmission from an HIV-infected dentist to a patient during a procedure with potential blood exposure at 1 chance in 260,000 to 1 chance in 2.6 million (Friedland, 1991).

(Read Denis Breo (1993). The dental AIDS cases—murder or an unsolved mystery? *JAMA*, 270: 2732–2734.)

Conclusion—Beginning 2009, two of the six, Lisa Shoemaker and Sherry Johnson, believed to have been infected by Acer have progressed to AIDS but are still alive; Kimberly Bergalis, Richard Driskill, John Yecs, and Barbara Webb have died. To date, the six people have received $10 million from Acer's insurance company.

In 2005, Madrid, Spain—A Spanish woman, who tested HIV negative, was infected with HIV by her obstetrician during a cesarean section. The case is reported in the January 9 edition of *AIDS*. It is believed that the infection occurred as a result of a needle stick injury by the doctor, who was homosexual and did not know he was infected with HIV at the time. Genetic analysis of the obstetrician's and the patient's HIV indicated that the doctor was the likely source of the infection.

Since this case, investigations have been completed involving over 22,000 patients of 63 HIV-infected physicians, surgeons, and dentists, and no other cases of this type of transmission have been identified in the United States.

Sexual Transmission of HIV: The AIDS Pandemic Signals the End of the Sexual Revolution in the United States

The predominant mode of global HIV transmission is through sexual contact. Not all sexual practices are equally likely to result in HIV transmission (Table 8-5). HIV usually gains access to the immune system at mucosal or membrane lining surfaces. Such surfaces include the oropharynx (throat area), rectum, and genital mucosa. Mucosal surfaces are rich in Langerhans cells, dendritic cells that trap antigens and virus particles. In addition, lymphoid aggregates are found throughout the tissue immediately below the mucosal surface.

Sexual Behavior and Risk of HIV Infection

Sexual transmission of HIV occurs when infected blood, semen, or vaginal secretions from an infected person enter the bloodstream of a partner. This can happen during anal, vaginal, or oral penetration, in descending order of risk. Unprotected anal sex by a male or female appears to be the most dangerous, since the rectal wall is very thin. Masturbation or self sex is the safest. In general, a person's risk of acquiring HIV infection through sexual contact depends on (1) the number of different partners, (2) the likelihood (prevalence) of HIV infection in these partners, and (3) the probability of virus transmission during sexual contact with an infected partner. Virus transmission, in turn, may be affected by biological factors, such as concurrent sexually transmitted disease (STD) infections in either partner. Behavioral factors, such as type of sex practice and use of condoms, or varying levels of infectivity in the source partner (for example

Table 8–5 Sexual Activity According to Degree of Risk for Transmitting HIV

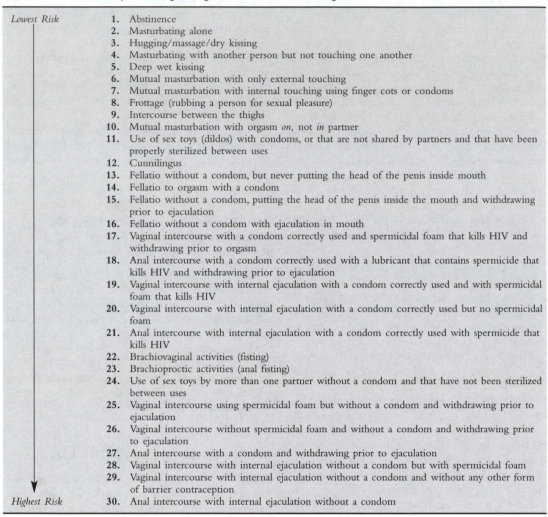

Lowest Risk

1. Abstinence
2. Masturbating alone
3. Hugging/massage/dry kissing
4. Masturbating with another person but not touching one another
5. Deep wet kissing
6. Mutual masturbation with only external touching
7. Mutual masturbation with internal touching using finger cots or condoms
8. Frottage (rubbing a person for sexual pleasure)
9. Intercourse between the thighs
10. Mutual masturbation with orgasm *on,* not *in* partner
11. Use of sex toys (dildos) with condoms, or that are not shared by partners and that have been properly sterilized between uses
12. Cunnilingus
13. Fellatio without a condom, but never putting the head of the penis inside mouth
14. Fellatio to orgasm with a condom
15. Fellatio without a condom, putting the head of the penis inside the mouth and withdrawing prior to ejaculation
16. Fellatio without a condom with ejaculation in mouth
17. Vaginal intercourse with a condom correctly used and spermicidal foam that kills HIV and withdrawing prior to orgasm
18. Anal intercourse with a condom correctly used with a lubricant that contains spermicide that kills HIV and withdrawing prior to ejaculation
19. Vaginal intercourse with internal ejaculation with a condom correctly used and with spermicidal foam that kills HIV
20. Vaginal intercourse with internal ejaculation with a condom correctly used but no spermicidal foam
21. Anal intercourse with internal ejaculation with a condom correctly used with spermicide that kills HIV
22. Brachiovaginal activities (fisting)
23. Brachioproctic activities (anal fisting)
24. Use of sex toys by more than one partner without a condom and that have not been sterilized between uses
25. Vaginal intercourse using spermicidal foam but without a condom and withdrawing prior to ejaculation
26. Vaginal intercourse without spermicidal foam and without a condom and withdrawing prior to ejaculation
27. Anal intercourse with a condom and withdrawing prior to ejaculation
28. Vaginal intercourse with internal ejaculation without a condom but with spermicidal foam
29. Vaginal intercourse with internal ejaculation without a condom and without any other form of barrier contraception

Highest Risk

30. Anal intercourse with internal ejaculation without a condom

(Source: Shernoff, 1988 Journal of Contemporary Social Work)

viral load) related to clinical stage of disease also increase the risk of HIV transmission/infection. Based on these factors, the risk for HIV infection is highest for an uninfected partner of an HIV-infected person practicing unsafe sex. In February 2001 researchers at the University of North Carolina, Chapel Hill reported that HIV could be transmitted via unprotected sex between 5 and 13 days after infection. Persons who have sex partners with risk factors for HIV infection or who themselves have multiple partners with high rates of injection-drug, "crack"

cocaine, and methamphetamine use, prostitution, and other STDs are also at increased risk.

Circumcision and HIV Transmission

As summarized in an editorial authored by Daniel Halperin of the University of California, San Francisco, and Robert Bailey of the University of Illinois at Chicago in a recent issue of *The Lancet,* the highly vascularized foreskin (fold of skin covering the end of the penis) contains a higher density of Langerhans cells—the primary target cells for sexual transmission of HIV—than cervical, vaginal, or rectal mucosa (Helperin, 1999). They also note the foreskin is more susceptible to traumatic epithelial disruptions (tears) during intercourse, which allows additional vulnerability to blood, ulcerative STDs and HIV.

A summary on the Technical Meeting on Male Circumcision–Global held in Washington, D.C., in September 2002 states that a synthesis of 28 studies shows that circumcised men are 50% less likely to be infected by HIV than noncircumcised men.

It is estimated that if male circumcision became routine across sub-Saharan Africa, 6 million new HIV infections and 3 million deaths could be prevented over the next 20 years. Currently, the results of the three randomized controlled trials conducted in Kenya, South Africa, and Uganda showed that circumcision does protect males from HIV infection. The three studies showed that circumcision reduced the risk of HIV infection by 60% (Gray et al., 2007; Wawer et al., 2007).

Male Circumcision Doesn't Affect Women's HIV Risk

In two recent reports on the effect of male circumcision as it relates to HIV infection in women of HIV-positive circumcised partners, there did not appear to be any benefit to the women. These studies were conducted in Uganda and Zimbabwe (Turner et al., 2007; Wawer et al., 2008; Tobian et al.,2008).

The World Health Organization (WHO) and the UNAIDS Secretariat convened an international expert consultation to determine whether male circumcision should be recommended for the prevention of HIV infection. Based on the evidence presented, which was considered to be compelling, experts attending the consultation recommended that male circumcision now be recognized as an additional important intervention to reduce the risk of heterosexually acquired HIV infection in men. Currently, it is estimated that 665 million men or about 30% of men worldwide have been circumcised. In the U.S. about 70% of the current male population has been circumcised.

Warnings—The UN agencies emphasize that male circumcision does not provide complete protection against HIV infection. It should never replace other known effective prevention methods and should always be considered to be part of a comprehensive prevention package, which includes correct and con-sistent use of male or female condoms, reduction in the number of sexual partners, delaying the onset of sexual relations, and HIV testing and counseling. In other words, although circumcision is effective, people cannot circumcise their way out of this pandemic.

Problems—The circumcision operations in the studies were done in state-of-the-art clinics and they were done well, but real-world application may be different. There can be complications. And there are a finite number of those complications. The operation takes about 20 to 30 minutes with moderate to severe side effects. In most cases it takes up to 30 days to heal, and the aftereffects of the operation can be very painful. Add to this the cultural and religious aspects of having this operation.

Lastly, extrapolating the African needs to the U.S. epidemic is difficult. While the African trials dealt with heterosexual men, in the U.S. the highest risk groups are men who have sex with men (MSM), drug injectors who share needles, and women who have sex with high-risk men. The U.S. AIDS epidemic, unlike the one in Africa, is not generalized. So far, there has been no rush of U.S. men seeking circumcision.

Danger of HIV Infection via Artificial Insemination

By early year 2009, 15 women were reported to have been HIV infected through the use of anonymous donor sperm to initiate pregnancy: one in Germany, two in Italy, four in Australia, two in Canada, and six in the United States. Thirty recipients of semen from HIV-infected donors refused to be HIV tested (Guinan, 1995 updated). All cases except Germany occurred *before* the availability of HIV antibody testing. But 28 years into the AIDS epidemic, the increasingly popular fertility business remains largely unregulated and unmonitored, even though it traffics in semen, long known to be one of the two main HIV transmission routes.

Only a few states (New York, California, Ohio, Illinois, and Michigan) require HIV testing of semen donors. There are no federal regulations.

In 2007, Louis Bujan and colleagues reported on the current effectiveness of sperm washing to eliminate HIV. The retrospective study involved eight European clinics. The study involved 1036 couples in which the man was HIV positive and the woman HIV negative. These couples had over 3000 cycles of assisted reproduction using washed sperm. Not a single case of HIV transmission occurred in 463 live births! On the basis of this finding, the investigators write, "It is neither ethically nor legally justifiable to exclude individuals from infertility services on the basis of male HIV infection."

CONCLUSION: Sperm washing is a safe option for HIV-discordant couples.

Personal Choice—Personal Risks

Ray Bradbury wrote that "living at risk is jumping off a cliff, and building your wings on the way down." About 90% of the HIV infections that occur within the heterosexual noninjection-drug use population occur through one or more sexual activities. Some 90% of the HIV infections that occur among gay males occur through anal intercourse (Kingsley et al., 1990). In any sexual activity, HIV is transmitted via a body fluid (see Figures 8-4 and 8-5).

Eighty Percent of New HIV Infections Come from Risky Behavior by Just 20 Percent of Infected People. Stop Them and We Stop HIV Transmission?

The 80/20 Rule—The fact that specific high-risk behavioral groups sustain the current HIV infection rate in the United States has led scientists to name this phenomenon the 80/20 Rule: 80% of the new infections are caused by 20% of the HIV-infected population.

David Holtgrave (2004) of Emory University's Rollins School of Public Health analyzed HIV transmission rates between 1978 and 2000. Holtgrave found that transmission rates dropped during the 1980s from essentially 100% to about 5.49%. The rate fell again slightly at the beginning of the 1990s, then remained relatively stable at 4.0–4.34%. Holtgrave believes this rate is surprisingly low. The drop indicates a real success of HIV prevention programs.

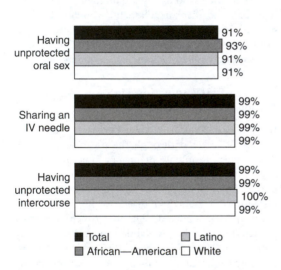

FIGURE 8-4   Knowledge About HIV Transmission: Percent who say that HIV can be transmitted in the following ways . . . (Correct answers) National random sample of 2,902 respondents age 18 and older. "Kaiser Family Foundation *Survey of Americans on HIV/AIDS,* Part Three—Experiences and Opinions by Race/Ethnicity and Age," (#7140), The Henry J. Kaiser Family Foundation, August 2004. The information was reprinted with permission from the Henry J. Kaiser Family Foundation. The Kaiser Family Foundation, based in Menlo Park, California, is a nonprofit, independent national healthcare philanthropy and is not associated with Kaiser Permanente or Kaiser Industries. These data were updated, August 2006 by Kaiser public opinion spotlights.

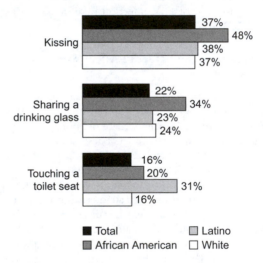

FIGURE 8-5   Misconceptions About HIV Transmission: Percent who say that HIV can be transmitted in the following ways, or say they don't know . . . (Incorrect answers) National random sample of 2,902 respondents age 18 and older. "Kaiser Family Foundation Survey of Americans on HIV/AIDS, Part Three—Experiences and Opinions by Race/Ethnicity and Age," (#7140), The Henry J. Kaiser Family Foundation, August 2004. The information was reprinted with permission from the Henry J. Kaiser Family Foundation. The Kaiser Family Foundation, based in Menlo Park, California, is a nonprofit, independent national health care philanthropy and is not associated with Kaiser Permanente or Kaiser Industries. These data were updated, August 2006 by Kaiser public opinion spotlights.

Following Holtgrave's findings, it means that in the mid-1980s virtually everyone who became HIV positive infected in turn someone else during any given year. With greater education and counseling, by the late 1990s the annual odds of someone passing his or her virus fell to 4.0 to 4.34%. And this would mean that at least 95% of persons living with HIV didn't transmit the disease to another person during any given year through 2008.

HIV/AIDS investigators have developed estimates of the risk of transmission of HIV. These estimates can give you a general idea of which activities are more or less risky. They cannot tell you that any activity is safe, or how many times you can do them without getting infected.

Following is a presentation of the different behavioral groups and how they put themselves at risk for HIV infection and transmission.

Heterosexual HIV Transmission: Key Factors

Heterosexual HIV transmission means that the virus was transmitted during heterosexual sexual activities. As such, the proportion of HIV infection and AIDS cases among the heterosexual population in the United States is now increasing at a greater rate than the proportion of HIV infections and AIDS cases among homosexuals or IDUs. The key factors for persons at highest risk for heterosexually transmitted HIV infection include adolescents and adults with multiple sex partners, those with sexually transmitted diseases (STDs), and heterosexually active persons residing in areas with a high prevalence of HIV infection among IDUs. In 1985, fewer than 2% of HIV infections were in the heterosexual population. In 2008, about 37% of new HIV infections were in the heterosexual population, with 64% of these occurring in women!

Heterosexual HIV Transmission: Africa and Asia— Heterosexual intercourse is the most common mode of transmission of HIV in developing countries.

Africa: In Africa, over 80% of infections are acquired heterosexually, while mother to child transmission, gay men, injection-drugs use and transfusion of contaminated blood account for the remaining infections.

Asia and Latin America: Heterosexual contact and injection drug use are the main modes of HIV transmission in South and Southeast Asia. Studies in Haiti and other Caribbean and Third World countries indicate that HIV transmission is most prevalent among the heterosexual population. Globally, hetero-

---

BOX 8.2

HIV/AIDS ROULETTE

CASE I: THE WOMAN EXECUTIVE

I am a successful executive woman. A year ago I applied for life insurance. I was required to take an HIV antibody test. It came back positive.

I am not a prostitute or promiscuous. I am not and have never been an injection-drug user. I am not a member of a minority group, indigent nor homeless, and I have not slept with a bisexual male (?).

I don't fit any of the stereotypes that people have designated for those infected with HIV. I got HIV from a man I love and have been seeing for five years. He is not homosexual or bisexual. He has never used injection drugs. He had no idea he was carrying the virus. He believes he may have been infected about six years ago by a woman with whom he had a brief, meaningless relationship. For that one indiscretion we will both pay the ultimate price.

CASE II: THE HIV-INFECTED MALE

A 21-year-old man walked into a sexually transmitted disease clinic and told the doctor he had "the clap," or gonorrhea, but he carried HIV.

When a counselor inquired about his sex partners, he told them about several, including a 12-year-old girl. The girl had gone elsewhere to be treated for gonorrhea and tested positive for HIV.

The man admitted to sleeping with 27 women, including 13 teenagers. Ten of the partners couldn't be found. Of the 17 others, 12 tested positive for HIV.

The man has since died, and the clinic has not been able to track all of his sexual partners.

There is a message to be found in these two cases: People with HIV are much more dangerous to a community than someone with AIDS. On average, the HIV infected are asymptomatic for 11 years. Those with AIDS and not treated, are usually symptomatic. They are losing weight. They are sick. They have little or no sexual appetite. Those with HIV are healthy and vigorous. That's where the sexual roulette begins.

---

sexual transmission now accounts for over 90% of HIV/AIDS cases.

Vaginal and Anal Intercourse—Among routes of HIV transmission, there is overwhelming evidence that HIV can be transmitted via anal intercourse. In vaginal intercourse, male-to-female transmission is much more efficient than the reverse. This is believed to be due to (1) a consistently higher concentration of HIV in semen than in vaginal secretions, and (2) abrasions in the vaginal mucosa (lining or membrane). Such abrasions in the tissue allow HIV to enter the vascular system in larger numbers than would occur otherwise, and perhaps at a single entry point.

That same reasoning explains why the **receptive** rather than the **insertive** homosexual partner is more likely to become HIV-infected during anal intercourse. It appears that the membranous linings of the rectum, rich in blood vessels, are more easily torn than are those of the vagina. In addition, recent studies indicate the presence of receptors for HIV in rectal mucosal tissue.

Homosexual Anal Intercourse—As of 2008, about 27% of homosexual men in San Francisco were/are HIV infected, probably the highest density of infection anywhere in the developed world. "It colors everything we do out here," said a gay activist. "The gay community, to a large extent, is about addressing AIDS. It has to be, because it's literally a war: Your entire community is under siege."

In a single year, 1982, 21% of the uninfected gay male population became infected, and for some reason not yet known, many of those infected early, died early. "Soon everyone, and I mean everyone, had a friend who was dying" (Science in California, 1993). During 1995 through mid-1997, three gay men died of AIDS each day. From mid-1997 through 2008, using aggressive anti-HIV drug therapy, daily deaths from AIDS has dropped to less than two per week (Conant, 1995 updated).

It appears that of all sexual activities, anal intercourse is the most efficient way to transmit HIV (DeVincenzi et al., 1989). Major risk factors identified with regard to HIV transmission among gay males include anal intercourse (both receptive and insertive), active oral-anal contact, number of partners, and length of homosexual lifestyle (Kingsley et al., 1990).

POINT TO PONDER 8.1

SWISS EXPERTS SAY INDIVIDUALS WITH AN UNDETECTABLE VIRAL LOAD AND NO SEXUALLY TRANSMITTABLE DISEASES (STDS) WILL NOT TRANSMIT HIV DURING SEX

Swiss HIV experts have produced the first-ever consensus statement to say that HIV-positive individuals on effective antiretroviral therapy and without sexually transmitted infections are sexually noninfectious (Vernazza et al., 2008).

The statement says that "after review of the medical literature and extensive discussion," the Swiss Federal Commission for HIV/AIDS resolves that, "an HIV infected person on antiretroviral therapy with completely suppressed viraemia (effective ART) is not sexually infectious, i.e., cannot transmit HIV through sexual contact." However, the Commission said, "it realizes that medical and biologic data available today do not permit proof that HIV infection during effective antiretroviral therapy is impossible, because the non-occurrence of an improbable event cannot be proven." The statement also discusses the implications of the consensus findings for doctors, for HIV-positive people, for HIV prevention, and for the legal system.

Seth Kalichman and colleagues (2008) reviewed 19 studies examining the relationship between the viral load found in blood versus that in semen. The bottom line of their review as it relates to the Swiss study is that semen that has an undetectable viral load is still potentially infectious and that cells in semen can contain HIV proviral DNA (HIV DNA embedded in the host-cell DNA) and can act as vehicles for the sexual transmission of HIV.

Comments from the American Center for Disease Control and Prevention

With the publication of the Swiss study, the CDC immediately released the following statement:

An article recently published by Switzerland's Federal Commission for HIV/AIDS states that HIV positive individuals on effective antiretroviral therapy are not at risk for transmitting HIV to their sexual partners under certain circumstances. The Commission acknowledges that there are no scientific data that the risk of transmission in these circumstances is zero. The Centers for Disease Control and Prevention (CDC) underscores its recommendation that people living with HIV, who are sexually active, use condoms consistently and correctly with all sex partners. (February 2008)

The CDC statement was followed by similar statements from the WHO and UNAIDS.

GAY MEN PUTTING THEMSELVES AT HIGH RISK FOR HIV INFECTION

Experts believe one reason risky behavior continues among the young is that they have not yet seen their friends die of the disease.

Another is simply the kind of risk-taking common among the young—the same impulse that prompts teenagers to drive fast or take up smoking. In three large American cities, 66% of gay men surveyed had **unprotected sex** in the last 18 months. **One in five** gay men in San Francisco and New York City said they had **unprotected sex** with an HIV-negative partner or with a partner whose HIV status was unknown. Linda Valleroy and colleagues at the CDC reported at the Eighth Conference on Retroviruses, February 2001, on testing and interview results of 2400 gay men ages 23 through 29. The men were from Baltimore, Dallas, New York, Los Angeles, Miami, and Seattle. Over 12% or 293 of the men were new HIV positives. **Twenty-nine percent** knew they were HIV positive before testing! Forty-six percent said they had unprotected oral sex during the previous six months. These data shocked the researchers.

On January 29, 1999, the *San Francisco Chronicle* carried a story about an $8 admission for a night of communal sex—the rules: no clothes, no condoms, no discussion of HIV. The article also covers an Internet link offering gay men the **extreme sex party** where becoming infected or HIV-infecting another is the erotic allure of the party. Still another twist is the **Russian Roulette Party** where three noninfected men have sex with five others, one of the five being HIV positive!

Exit the Condom

During a health inspection of a gay sex club, the inspector felt something crunch underfoot. It was an empty blister pack of **Viagra.** The inspector, San Francisco's director of sexually transmitted disease prevention, began to wonder whether Pfizer's impotence drug was contributing to unsafe sexual behavior and fueling an increase in HIV and other diseases. As a result of follow-up studies, he believes he has his answer. In the first three months of 2003, 43 new cases of syphilis and 14 new HIV infections have been diagnosed in Viagra users in San Francisco. Together these data imply that gay men are reverting to unsafe sex. And all this comes after the state and federal government has spent millions of dollars on AIDS education and prevention.

Effect of Highly Active Antiretroviral Therapy (HAART) on Sexual Behavior and HIV Transmission

Recent studies on HIV-infected gay males in San Francisco revealed that the use of HAART reduced HIV transmission by 60%. However, the increase in unprotected anal sex rose from about 8% in 2000 to 25% in 2003 during the same time period. This behavioral change, going from protected to unprotected anal sex has offset the beneficial effects of HAART. In addition to these data, John McGowan and colleagues (2004) reported that of those diagnosed with HIV in New York, 41% of men and women continued to have unprotected sex. Their reasons were trading sex for money or drugs and the availability of HAART. For those who need it, being on HAART has taken away much of their fear, and the uninfected at-risk population no longer sees the pallid face of death in public places as in the past—they never developed the fears of yesterday, the days before HAART. For many with HIV/AIDS the time of disbelief and terror evolved into burnout and despair, which in turn has now become a time of recuperation and salvation. The newly infected mostly see salvation through HAART. They see magazine ads that show hot muscular men living life to the fullest thanks to HAART. Other ads show couples holding hands, sending messages that the road to true love and happiness is being HIV positive. Unlike the photos of buff men in the ads, most who are on drug cocktails are not having the time of their lives. They spend mornings in the bathroom throwing up or suffering from diarrhea. They spend afternoons at doctor's appointments, clinics and pharmacies. And they spend endless evenings planning their estates and trying to make ends meet because they are not well enough to support themselves and HAART. **The reality is, AIDS is not fun. It's not sexy or manageable. AIDS is a debilitating, deforming, terminal and incurable disease. And the drugs used can bring on heart, kidney, and liver disease, cancer, and a host of daily discomforts, like never being too far from the nearest toilet.**

The Use of Methamphetamine (Crystal or Tina)

"Whenever I want sex, I want meth and whenever I am high on meth, I want sex." The use of crystal meth by gay and heterosexual men is not new, it is the sudden accelerated use of the drug among gay men that is of major concern.

BOX 8.3

ONCE, WHEN WE WERE HEROES
BY MARK KING, JUNE 2006

My brother Richard smiles a lot. He has an easy laugh. But there was a time, years ago, when he held a poisonous drink in his hands and begged his dying lover not to swallow it. A time when Richard held the concoction they had prepared together and wept.

Emil couldn't wait. He took the drink from Richard quickly because the release it offered was something more rapturous than the appeals of his lover of thirteen years. It was Emil's wish to die on his own terms if living became unbearable, a promise one to the other. When that time arrived, however, Richard wanted another moment, just a little more time to say, "I love you, Emil," over and over again before the drink would close Emil's eyes and quietly kill him.

Richard has a charming store in my hometown today where he sells collectibles and does theater in his free time. Emil consumed the drink twenty years ago.

There were people who displayed remarkable courage then. People who lived and died by their promises and shared the intimacy of death and then the world moved forward and grief subsided and lives moved on. But make no mistake, there are heroes among us right now. There is a shy, friendly man at my gym with silver hair and a handsome face. There was a time when his sick roommate deliberately overdosed after his father told him that people with unspeakable disease will suffer in hell. My gym friend performed CPR for an hour before help arrived but the body never heard a loving word again.

There is courage among us, astonishing courage and we summoned it and survived. And then years passed. We got new jobs and changed gyms. There was a time when old friends called to say goodbye, and by goodbye they meant forever. When all of us had a file folder marked "Memorial" that outlined how we wanted our service to be conducted. When people shot themselves and jumped off bridges after getting their test results. There is profound, shocking sadness here, right here among us, but years went by and medicine got better and we found other lives to lead. Our sadness is a distant, dark dream.

My best friend Stephen just bought a new condo. He's having a ball picking out furniture. But there was a time when he knew all the intensive care nurses by name. When a phone call late at night always meant someone had died. And just who, exactly, was anyone's guess. Stephen tested positive in the 1980s, shortly after I did. A few months after the devastating news, he agreed to facilitate a support group with me. We regularly saw men join the group, get sick and die, often within weeks. Watching them disintegrate felt like a preview of coming attractions. But Stephen was remarkable, a reassuring presence to everyone and worked with the group for more than a year despite the emotional toll and the high body count.

There is bravery here, still, living all around us. But the bravest time was many years ago and times change and the yard needs landscaping and there's a brunch tomorrow. There was a time when I sat beside friends in their very last minutes of life, and I helped them relax, perhaps surrender, and told them comforting stories. And lied to them. Jeremy lost his mind weeks before he died. Sometimes he had moments of sanity when we could have a coherent conversation before his dementia engulfed him again. It was a time when you were given masks and gloves to visit friends in the hospital. He was agitated with the business of dying and told me he couldn't bear to miss what might happen after he'd gone. I had an idea. "I tell you what," I offered. "I'm from the future and I can tell you anything you would like to know." "OK then, what happens to my parents," he asked. I thought it might be a distracting game but Jeremy's confused mind took it very seriously. "They went to Hollywood and won big on a game show so they never did need your support in their old age," I answered. He looked relieved at the thought. "What about Streisand and Bette," he smiled. "They are canonized as saints, of course. And they raise totally hot gay sons that run for office and win." He barely took the time to enjoy this thought before his hand grabbed my wrist tightly, almost frantically. He pulled me closer. "When..." he began, and a mournful sob swelled inside him in an instant, his eyes begging for relief. "When does this end?" There was an awful, helpless silence. His eyes beckoned for a truth he could die believing. "It does end," I finally managed, although nothing suggested it would. "It ends, Jeremy, but not for a really long time." He digested each word like a revelation, and slowly relaxed into sleep. Two days later fluid filled his lungs and Jeremy drowned.

There is compassion here enough for all the world's deities and saints acting in concert. Infinite compassion for men who lived in fear and checked every spot when they showered for Kaposi sarcoma, and for disowned sons wasting away in the guest

BOX 8.3   *(continued)*

room of whoever had the space. But we get older and friends don't ask us to hold their hand when they stop breathing and the fear fades and I bought new leather loafers and the White Party is coming. The truth is simply this, and no one will convince me otherwise, my most courageous self, the best man that I'll ever be lived two decades ago during the first years of a horrific plague. He worked relentlessly alongside a million others who had no choice but to act. He secretly prayed to survive even above the lives of others and his horrible prayer was answered with the death of nearly everyone close to him. To say I miss that brutal decade would only be partially true. I miss the man I was forced to become when an entire community abandoned tea dances for town hall meetings, when I learned to offer help to those facing what terrified me most. Today, the lives of those of us who witnessed the horror have become relatively normal again perhaps mundane. We prefer it. We have new lives in a world that isn't choking in disease. But once, there was a time when we were heroes.

Mark King is a longtime activist and writer living in Fort Lauderdale. He can be reached at marksking@aol.com

Meth use and attendant HIV transmission has become such a concern across the nation that in New York City, Gay Men's Health Crisis, one of the nation's largest gay AIDS/HIV groups, has launched a major education campaign. The organization is putting up billboards, sending out mailings, sponsoring workshops and dispatching counselors into the community to talk about meth abuse and HIV. Meth, a psychostimulant that excites pleasure centers in the brain, makes users feel euphoric for hours. The drug impairs judgment, lowers inhibitions, keeps people awake for days and can increase sexual arousal. They go from feeling like wallflowers to feeling like supermen, and safer sex messages are just forgotten. This drug has become almost normalized in the gay community. One gay male said, "It gives people a way to have sex for hours and hours and hours. It's the greatest euphoria you can ever feel."

Party and Play

Meth is so linked with this subculture of gay men engaging in anonymous sex with strangers that men advertise either that they have the drug or want it during sex in personal ads and on the Internet. Their notices carry the phrase "PnP" for "party and play," a euphemism for crystal methamphetamine and sex. For one gay male, his friends introduced him to crystal meth on a Thursday evening and he stopped using it on Monday morning. He lost count over the weekend when he hit having sex with 12 men. About a month later he developed a flu-like syndrome, got tested and he was HIV positive. In his mind he was thinking this was just one weekend. One weekend and it will impact him for the rest of his life.

Circuit Parties—Circuit parties got their name from those who travel to various cities—the circuit—to attend several parties each year. The parties, which began in 1986, essentially are the gay version of raves, parties that are popular among some young people. There are two or three circuit party weekends a month. Among the cities where they are held: Montreal, San Francisco, Atlanta, Palm Springs, Miami, and Washington. The parties are not universally popular among gay men, although many say they have attended one. The parties generally attract professionals ages 21 to 35. The parties began with the intention of fund raising and community building. But somewhere along the way, the original intent of the party has become diluted. Now, circuit parties have become weekend bashes. They attract thousands of mostly young gay men who dance until dawn and whose admission fees raise millions of dollars for AIDS prevention groups and gay charities. But, according to Ronald Johnson, an official of the circuit party organization, "It (circuit parties) became a social phenomenon above and beyond what (we) intended and beyond what (we) could control." Health officials say the parties have become a reflection of the risky behavior that is contributing to rising rates of HIV infection among gay men. Drugs are so prevalent at the parties that organizers often hire medical teams to treat overdoses. Troy Masters, publisher of a gay newspaper in New York, who now opposes these parties said, "You wouldn't find the American Cancer Society throwing a smoking party." Gay Men's Health Crisis, which was founded in 1981 and serves 11,000 clients annually in the New York area, stopped holding its party in 1998 after it became known for drug use and sex. Two Philadelphia couples said they attend up to eight parties a year and usually take Ecstasy pills with a liquid shot of GHB or some ketamine, which can be liquid or powder. They agreed that "if you don't do drugs, you're not going to enjoy it as much."

Barebacking: Chasing The Bug—Intentionally Seeking HIV Infection

Bug chasing sounds like a group of children running around chasing crickets, butterflies, or grasshoppers. Enter Robert, age 30. He routinely hooks up with three to four men each week for unprotected sex—he hopes they are all HIV positive! For Robert, bug chasing is mostly about the excitement of doing something that everyone sees as crazy and wrong. Keeping this part of his life secret is part of the turn-on. That forbidden aspect makes HIV infection incredibly exciting for him, so much so that he seeks out sex exclusively with HIV-positive men. "This is something that no one knows about me, it's mine. It's my dirty little secret." He compares bug chasing to the thrill you get by "screwing your boyfriend in your parents' house," or having sex on your boss's desk. You are not supposed to do it, and that's exactly what makes it so much fun. When asked why he wants to become infected, his eyes light up as he says that the actual moment of transmission, the instant he gets HIV will be the "most erotic thing I can imagine." When asked whether he is prepared to live with HIV after that "erotic" moment, he dismisses living with HIV as a minor annoyance. Like most bug chasers, he has the impression that the virus isn't such a big deal anymore. "It's like living with diabetes. You take a few pills and get on with your life."

It has recently been observed that a minority of both HIV-positive and negative men have begun to consciously, willfully, and proudly engage in unprotected anal sex. The new phenomenon is referred to as raw, skin-to-skin, or bareback sex. Such behavior in this group leads to the intentional transmission and reception of HIV! This form of barebacking is referred to as **"bug chasing" or "chasing the bug."** These HIV-negative gay men seek to become HIV infected.

Brotherhood of the Infected: Bug Chasers and Gift Givers

According to Yvonne Abraham of the *Boston Globe Online,* and DeAnn Gauthier (1999), health professionals are seeing something unexpected in the gay community: a small group of men who want to contract HIV in the belief that it offers community and kinship. Increasing numbers of chat rooms and websites approach the subject of men who want to convert from HIV negative to positive. Marshall Forstein, medical director of mental health at Fenway Community Health Center in Boston, says some of the men feel lonely or shunned and believe that HIV will bring them attention from friends and caregivers. One California activist who stopped using condoms and later contracted HIV also noted, "When I was entering the gay community at the height [of the epidemic], I felt like I'd joined the war. And that somehow transformed HIV into this rite of passage as opposed to something to be reviled and avoided." Some websites even discuss conversion parties, where uninfected men can have unprotected sex with HIV-positive men to try to contract the virus. The groups refer to HIV infection as a rebirth and a way to bond with a new family. According to Gauthier, bug chasing as a form of bareback sex actually involves two categories of participants. There are the HIV-negative men who seek to become infected with the virus (bug chasers), and there are the **gift givers,** HIV-positive men who seek to share their gift of HIV to others. Chasers typically advertise for partners with statements such as: "Will let you _____ me raw only if you promise to give me all your diseases like AIDS/herpes, etc. Let's do it." Gift givers, on the other hand, typically make comments such as: "Attention neg men! Why stay locked in a boring world of sterile sex when you can join the ranks of the AIDS Freedom Fighters? Let me give you my gift and set you free." Becoming "bug brothers" may occur one-on-one but is just as likely to result at special marathon group sex parties that are held for the purpose of seroconverting as many HIV-negative participants as possible. That individuals would knowingly participate in such events is shocking not only to some members of the gay community, but also the community at large (Gauthier, 1999).

The story of chasing HIV until infected is presented in a film, *The Gift.* It became available in 2003 and was shown nationally on the Sundance TV network on February 2, 2004. It is a powerful presentation of gay men in search of **The Gift,** HIV.

The High Rate of HIV Infection Among Gay Men on South Beach, Miami

Miami's South Beach—Hot music, hot spots, hot sun, hot bodies. The once sagging tip of Miami Beach has been turned into the playground of the beautiful, the rich, and the chic. South Beach is also a growing mecca for young gay men. In a world

RACIAL GAP SEEN IN HOMOSEXUAL HIV RATES AMONG MEN HAVING SEX WITH MEN (MSM): ON THE DOWN LOW

In 2005, Frangiscos Sifakis, from Johns Hopkins Bloomberg School of Public Health in Baltimore, and colleagues with the National HIV Behavioral Surveillance system tested 1767 MSMs at venues where they normally congregated, such as bars, clubs, and social organizations, in five different cities. Overall, 25% tested positive for HIV. However, the infection rate differed by race—46% among blacks, 21% among whites, and 17% among Hispanics. About half of those who tested positive were unaware of their HIV infection. Of those with unrecognized HIV infections, 64% were black, 18% were Hispanics, and 11% were white. Although most had undergone testing in the past, the researchers found that 58% with unrecognized infections had not been tested during the previous year. Stephanie Behel from the CDC in Atlanta said, "We know that persons who are aware of their HIV status take measures to seek treatment and reduce risk behaviors, which underscores the importance of annual HIV testing for MSM, particularly among black-American MSM."

FEAR, HATE, SECRETS, AND LIES: THE CLIMATE WHICH KEEPS HIV TRANSMISSION GOING: ON THE DOWN LOW

The highest rate of HIV infection in the United States occurs among bisexual black men. And that has implications for black women, who are 19 times more likely to be infected than white women. That's because many black men have unprotected sex with other men but then conceal that fact and have unprotected sex with women. This behavior is called **On The Down Low.** These men are bisexual. They do not identify themselves as gay or homosexual. There are, of course, white bisexual men who pose the same threat to white women. For example, the outing of former New Jersey Governor James McGreevey in 2004 makes the point that some closeted gay white men can or may expose their wives and girlfriends to HIV. Some sociologists believe that gay or bisexual black men are more afraid to come out of the closet than whites because they already face racial discrimination and are reluctant to take on the added burden of homophobia.

Though AIDS researchers have suspected for years that a culture of clandestine gay sex was helping to fuel the HIV epidemic, the "down low" syndrome has only recently become widely known. In 2005, J.L. King wrote a book, *On the Down Low: A Journey Into the Lives of "Straight" Black Men Who Sleep with Men,* about his secret life, and he appeared on the Oprah Winfrey TV show to discuss his sexual lifestyle, on The Down Low.

In 2006, Preeti Pathela and colleagues reported on a survey of 4193 men ages 18 and older in New York City. Four percent said they were homosexual, 91.7% said they were heterosexual, and 5% said they were bisexual. The study found that about 10% of the men who said they were heterosexual had slept with a man but not a woman in the previous year, and that such men were less likely to have had an HIV test than men who said they were homosexual. The study also found that 22% of men who had sex with men but who described themselves as heterosexual used condoms, compared with 55% of men who considered themselves gay. According to the researchers, the findings imply that physicians should not depend on a man's self-described sexual orientation when assessing his risk for contracting HIV or other sexually transmitted infections.

---

where homosexuality is often confined to the closet, it is a place to be out and to be open. But behind the perfect tans, there is dark reality. According to a new study one in every six gay men between the ages of 18 and 29 in South Beach has tested HIV positive.

William Darrow, AIDS researcher who surveyed 87 gay men ages 18 to 29 and 70 gay men age 30 and older, said, "People seem to think they're on a holiday there from everything—including AIDS." Darrow's survey showed that about 75% of gay men in both age groups had unprotected anal sex.

Gay Men Serosorting to Prevent HIV Infection

Many people living with HIV have based sexual and romantic choices on serostatus since the beginning of the epidemic. In recent years, an official term for this behavior was coined by prevention experts and is frequently used in the scientific literature: **serosorting.**

Serosorting is defined as "the practice of preferentially choosing sex partners, or deciding not to use condoms with selected partners based on their disclosed concordant (agreed with) HIV status." Matt Golden (2006) of the University of Washington,

Seattle Center for AIDS and STDs (sexually transmitted diseases) looked at serosorting as a prevention activity adopted by gay men. Data from Golden's clinic found that HIV-positive patients were particularly likely to serosort. Forty percent and 49% of his HIV-positive patients, respectively, had unprotected receptive and insertive sex with HIV-positive partners but only 3% and 6%, respectively, with HIV-negative partners.

In November 2006, the San Francisco Department of Public Health began a highly visual print and web campaign featuring silhouettes of naked men embracing in erotic poses with their HIV status branded on their shoulders, with a caption reading, "Sero-Sorting is a Prevention Strategy."

PROBLEM

According to David Butler and colleagues (2007), in certain high-risk populations and settings, there may be a significant percentage of people who believe they are negative but are instead in the early throes of HIV infection. Harold Jaffe and colleagues (2007) stated that 10% to 15% of 15- to 29-year-old men who have sex with men (MSM) are HIV infected, but about 67% of these do not know they are infected, and 60% of these men thought they were at **low** risk! Butler says that, "the effectiveness of serosorting on the basis of mutual disclosure of perceived HIV status is a flawed strategy for reducing sexual transmission of HIV when it does not consider the prevalence of recent HIV infections in specific populations.

Heterosexual Anal Intercourse—A number of sexuality-oriented surveys of the heterosexual population indicate that between one in five and one in ten heterosexual couples have tried or regularly practice anal intercourse. Bolling (1989) reported that 70% to 80% of women may have tried anal intercourse and that 10% to 25% of these women enjoyed anal sex on a regular basis. He also reported that 58% of women with multiple sex partners participated in anal sex. James Segars (1989) reported that the highest rates of anal sex occur among teenagers who use drugs and older married couples who are broadening their sexual experiences.

Although it may increase the risk of HIV infection, it must be emphasized that anal intercourse is not necessary for HIV transmission among heterosexuals. In fact, most HIV-infected heterosexuals say they have never practiced anal intercourse.

Risk of HIV Infection; Number of Sexual Encounters—The risk of HIV infection to a susceptible person after one or more sexual encounters is very difficult to determine. In some cases, people claim to have become infected after a single sexual encounter.

In some reported transfusion-associated HIV infections, the female partners of infected males remained HIV negative after five or more years of unprotected sexual intercourse. Television star **Paul Michael Glaser** said that he had unprotected sexual relations with his wife Elizabeth for five years prior to her being diagnosed as HIV-infected. He was not HIV-infected. She received HIV during a blood transfusion, but was not diagnosed until after their firstborn child was diagnosed with HIV. In other studies of heterosexual HIV transmission, many couples had unprotected sexual intercourse over prolonged periods of time with no more than 50% of the partners becoming HIV infected. There are many instances of heterosexuals and homosexuals who remained HIV negative after having repeated sexual intercourse with HIV-infected partners.

The Biological Factor

The fact that not all who are repeatedly exposed become infected suggests that biological factors may play as large a role in HIV infection as behavioral factors. For biological reasons, some people may be more efficient transmitters of HIV; while others are more susceptible to HIV infection, that is, require a smaller HIV infective dose. Some people carry genes that may make them resistant to HIV infection (see "Mutant R-2 and R-5 Genes" in Chapter 5).

Number of Sexual Partners and Types of Activity—One relatively large risk factor for HIV infection in both homosexuals and heterosexuals is believed to be the number of sexual partners. The greater the number of sexual partners, the greater the probability that one of the partners is HIV positive.

The scale of multiple-partnering during the late twentieth century and continuing into the twenty-first century is unprecedented. With over 6 billion people on earth, an ever-increasing percentage of whom are urban residents; with air travel and mass transit available to allow people from all over the world to go to the cities of their choice; with mass youth movements advocating, among other things, sexual freedom; with a feminist spirit alive in much of the industrialized world, promoting female sexual freedom; and with 47% of the world's population made up of people between the ages of 15 and 44—there can be no doubt that the amount of worldwide urban sexual energy is unparalleled.

Knowing Your Sexual Partner—The amount of protection one actually obtains from limiting one's number of partners depends mainly on who those partners are. Having one partner who is in a high-risk group may be more dangerous than having many partners who are not. An example of this is seen in prostitutes, who may be more likely to be infected by their regular injection-drug-using partners than by customers who are not in a high-risk group. The risk status of a person who remains faithful to a single sexual partner depends on that partner's behavior: If the partner becomes infected, often without knowing it, the monogamous individual is likely to become infected (Cohen et al., 1989).

The Effects of Sexual Partner Reduction in Uganda—In the mid-1980s Uganda had a 30% rate of HIV infection. Today it is less than 6%. A miracle? No, the bottom line was sexual partner reduction.

In 1986, the Uganda Ministry of Health started a vigorous HIV prevention campaign in which the slogans "Love Carefully," "Love Faithfully," and "Zero Grazing" (Uganda slang for don't have sexual partners outside the home) were posted on public buildings, broadcast on radio and in speeches by government officials, teachers, and AIDS prevention workers across the country. Religious leaders scoured the Bible and the Koran for quotations about infidelity. Also, newspapers, theaters, singing groups, and ordinary people spread the message of abstinence. In short, Uganda promoted their A, B, C approach to lowering the HIV infection rates—**A** for abstinence, **B** for be faithful (stay with one sexual partner), and **C** if you fail A and B, use a condom. As a result of these two prevention methods, in addition to sexual partner notification, the frequency of casual sex fell by 60% between 1989 and 1995. HIV-associated pregnancy rates fell by 50%. And there was a drop in the rate of HIV infection across Uganda. All of this was occurring at a time when condoms were not widely available. Some researchers have attributed Uganda's HIV prevention success to increased sexual abstinence among teenage girls, but statistics suggest that partner reduction, especially on the part of men, was far more important. Partner reduction has been an important factor in HIV prevention elsewhere as well. In Thailand, HIV infection rates declined steeply during the 1990s. Visits by men to sex workers also

fell by 60%. Among gays in America, HIV rates fell sharply during the 1980s. A significant part of this decline was attributable to the increased use of condoms, serosorting, and a reduction in sexual partners. In Zambia and northern Tanzania, where churches promoted faithfulness, HIV rates also declined. Meanwhile, in such countries as Botswana, South Africa, and Zimbabwe, condoms have been emphasized as the main method of prevention, and HIV rates have remained high.

Sexual Activities—In addition to a high-risk partner or a number of sexual partners, the types of sexual activities that occur are also significant (Table 8-5). Any sexual activity that produces skin, anal, or vaginal membrane abrasions (tear) prior to or during intercourse increases the risk of infection.

Orogenital Sex—Historically, it has been very difficult to establish the contribution oral genital sex makes to overall HIV transmission since few people engage solely in oral sex. Instead, many people also have vaginal or anal sex, which are recognized routes of HIV transmission. Though there have been a number of cases of apparent HIV transmission via oral genital sex, health professionals have tended to prioritize HIV prevention efforts in the areas of greatest risk. This strategy may have inadvertently downplayed the risks attached to oral genital sex, and left some individuals confused over risk reduction options.

How Risky Is Orogenital Sex?—Orogenital sex may be a greater risk factor for becoming HIV infected than previously thought. The risk of transmission is related to the presence of HIV at the sexual sites (oral, vaginal, penile, and anal), the amount of HIV present, and whether there are physical openings such as tissue tears or open sores (Rothenberg et al., 1998; Kahn et al., 1998).

After reviewing over 100 research reports Sara Edwards and colleagues (1998) concluded that HIV can be transmitted through oral sex. In a very rigorous study, Beth Dillon and colleagues (2000) appear to have clearly pinpointed oral transmission in approximately 7% of primary infection cases. By mid-2000, strong evidence for at least 30 cases of oral HIV infection were reported in the United States (Dillon, 2000). In Britain, Barry Evans, director of Public Health Laboratory Service, reported that oral sex may account for up to 8% of HIV infections among gay men. He said that oral sex leads to 30 to 50 new HIV infections annually in the

United Kingdom. Evans states that the risk of HIV infection via oral sex is greater than previously thought.

Susan Buchbinder and colleagues in 2001 calculated that the odds of acquiring HIV from any single act of oral sex with an infected partner are roughly 4 in 10,000 (1 in 2500) compared with odds of 4 in 1000 (1 in 250) for anal sex with a condom.

It should also be recognized that one can get other sexually transmitted diseases from oral sex, such as gonorrhea, syphilis, chlamydia, and herpes.

Prostitution (Sex Worker): United States

Sex Workers and Their Clients—A smartly dressed couple check into a four-star city hotel armed with a bottle of champagne and condoms. In a building across the street, a couple who has just met is putting on a condom. In a parking lot of the local high school, in the backseat of a car, two young people, high on dope, are removing one after finishing sex. Out in the suburbs, a man puts one on before he has sex with his regular partner at his home. In a bathroom of a public transportation system, another man is performing oral sex on his male partner. No, these are not couples engaged in affairs. They are not people who have just met at a bar, nor teenagers after the school dance. They are certainly not long-time lovers. They are all people who are part of the sex industry, sex workers and their clients (Figure 11-6).

Do Sex Workers Account for a Significant Transmission of HIV in the U.S.A.?—There is little if any evidence that prostitutes in the United States and most other developed nations play a large role in heterosexual HIV transmission (Cohen et al., 1989 updated).

A consequence of the attention prostitutes or sex workers have attracted in relation to AIDS in the United States and other developed countries is that

IF YOU DON'T TAKE A JOB AS A PROSTITUTE, WE CAN STOP YOUR BENEFITS

Because of the large unemployment rate in Germany, welfare reforms were instituted. One reform was the legalization of prostitution on the grounds that this would combat trafficking in women and cut links to organized crime. However, now that prostitution is no longer considered, by the law, to be immoral, there is really nothing but the goodwill of the job centers to stop them from pushing women into jobs they don't want to do, like prostitution! For example, a 25-year-old waitress who turned down a job providing sexual services at a brothel in Berlin faces possible cuts to her unemployment benefit under the new welfare reform laws introduced in 2005. Under Germany's welfare reforms, any woman under 55 who has been out of work for more than a year can be forced to take an available job, including one in the sex industry, or lose her unemployment benefits. The government had considered making brothels an exception on moral grounds, but decided that it would be too difficult to distinguish them from bars. As a result, job centers must treat employers looking for a prostitute in the same way as those looking for a dental nurse.

When the waitress looked into suing the job center, she found out that it had not broken the law. Job centers that refuse to penalize people who turn down a job by cutting their benefits face legal action from the potential employer. A lawyer from Hamburg who specializes in such cases said, "There is now nothing in the law to stop women from being sent into the sex industry. The new regulations say that working in the sex industry is not immoral any more, so jobs cannot be turned down without a risk to benefits."

One woman who had worked in call centers had been offered jobs on telephone sex lines. At one job center in the city of Gotha, a 23-year-old woman was told that she had to attend an interview as a nude model, and should report back on the meeting. Employers in the sex industry can also advertise in job centers. A job center that refuses to accept the advertisement can be sued. One woman who owns a brothel in central Berlin has been searching the online database of her local job center for recruits. She said, "Why shouldn't I look for employees through the job center when I pay my taxes just like everybody else."

For every sex worker who is HIV positive there is, somewhere, the partner from whom she or he contracted HIV. Given the fact that the chance of contracting HIV during a single act of unprotected sex is not high, infection in a sex worker is likely to mean that she or he has been repeatedly exposed to HIV by clients who did not or would not wear condoms. The more accurate way of reading the statistics of HIV infection in prostitutes or sex workers is to view them as an indication of how strong a foothold the epidemic has gotten within a community.

Prostitution (Sex Worker): Developing Countries

Do Sex Workers Account for a Significant Transmission of HIV in Developing Countries? The answer is YES—In a garbage-strewn alley in the city's red-light district, a 24-year-old prostitute slumps on a string bed, weak from tuberculosis and diarrhea. She knows she has AIDS but she has never heard of the multidrug cocktail that curbs the progress of the disease. Even if she had, she could never afford to buy it. Nobody wants the girls once they get sick, explains a health counselor who visits the alley each week. She says prostitutes with AIDS are shunned by many hospital doctors, brothel operators, and their own families. "We feel helpless; all we can do is comfort them and find them a place where they can go to die." This true vignette is happening in small towns, the suburbs, and in every large city in every country in developing nations. Many of the prostitutes are housewives out to make the difference between starvation and existence for their families. Many women knowingly risk exposure to HIV to economize the number of times they have to have sex with a stranger. They could make, say, the equivalent of $10 for one act of unprotected sex with one man, or they could make $10 for five acts of protected sex with five men. It is, for them, all about the money—a conscious choice, their only means of survival. The prostitutes sell their bodies for money or drugs to anyone who can afford their services. In some towns in Africa, Vietnam, and India between 50% and 90% of the prostitutes are HIV positive. Prostitution in developing countries is a large contributing factor to the spread of HIV/AIDS (Figure 11-6).

India—In Chennai, India, mobile brothels manned by cell-phone toting operators are proving profitable. For those in the trade, running a mobile unit makes sound business sense as it cuts down on operational

they tend to be seen as responsible for the spread of HIV—an attitude reflected in descriptions of prostitutes as reservoirs of infection or high-frequency transmitters. But, the sex worker is only the most visible side of a transaction that involves two people:

costs of renting a building and paying bribes. As for the client, it promises "pick and drop" sex workers at a place of his choice. More than 17 mobile units operate in the city, according to Chennai-based NGO Indian Community Welfare Organization (ICWO), which works with Commercial Sex Workers (CSWs). According to estimates, there are 6300 women sex workers operating throughout the city. Thirty percent said they couldn't use condoms with regular clients. Another 30% said, at times, they would forget to have their clients wear condoms and 10% felt that condom usage would prolong sexual activity. Another 10% said some clients would object to it. As for reasons why they chose to be sex workers, 31% respondents said they entered the profession due to family debts and 29% said their husbands deserted them. About 29% said their lovers had ditched them.

Risk Estimates for HIV Infection During Sexual Intercourse in the Heterosexual Population— Estimates of the risk of HIV infection from a single heterosexual encounter depend on the following: (1) the probability that the sexual partner carries the virus; (2) if one of the sexual partners is HIV positive, the size of their viral load (suppression of viral load reduces the risk of HIV transmission); and (3) the reduction in risk by using condoms and spermicides.

Choosing a partner who is not in a high-risk group provides almost 5000-fold protection compared with choosing a partner in the highest-risk category (Figure 8-6).

In 2005 Perry Halkitis, director of the Center for Health Identity, Behavior and Prevention Studies, New York University, reviewed the literature on HIV transmission. From the data collected, he calculated the odds of HIV infection during sex in the absence of a condom (see Table 8-6).

Sexual connections as seen here are sometimes referred to as sexual networks. Such networks may involve (a) **serial monogamists**—persons who go from one relationship to another, one at a time, and (b) those involved in **concurrent relationships**— persons involved with more than one sexual partner in a given period and going back and forth between them. Both behaviors increase the possibility of infection/transmission because earlier sexual partners can be infected by later sexual partners.

Condoms are estimated to provide about 10-fold protection.

The implication of this analysis is clear: *Choose sex partners carefully and use condoms.*

Other Studies on Heterosexual HIV Transmission

Nancy Padian and colleagues (1991) reported that women are 17.5 times more likely to become HIV infected from an infected male than men are to contract the disease from an infected female.

Viral Load and Heterosexual Transmission

Recent data from two separate HIV investigations shed light on the issue of gender transmission. Thomas Quinn and colleagues (2000) reported that the lower the level of HIV in the blood, the less likely HIV-infected persons will transmit the virus to their heterosexual sexual partner. This research team studied 400 heterosexual couples over 2.5 years. In each couple, only one person was HIV positive. No one with less than 1500 copies of HIV/milliliter of blood infected his or her partner. In those cases where one partner became infected, 80% of the time the viral load of the other partner was over 10,000. Such data confirm the benefit of lowering HIV levels in the blood via antiretroviral therapy.

INJECTION-DRUG USERS AND HIV TRANSMISSION

While a number of drugs are ancient, their injection is relatively recent. Injecting oneself is mainly a twentieth century innovation because that is when (after 1960) cheap and disposable syringes became available. Experience from IDU transmission of HIV indicates that once HIV enters an injection-drug use population, that country can expect a large and substantial HIV epidemic. IDU is a very efficient way of transmitting HIV, three times more efficient than through sexual intercourse.

HIV entered injection users during the mid-1970s and spread rapidly through 1983 largely unrecognized and unidentified. HIV transmission via IDU is the second most frequent risk behavior among adults/adolescents for becoming HIV infected in the developed world. Illicit drug injection occurs in at least 121 countries and HIV infection has been reported in IDUs in nearly all of these countries. Ending year 2009, of 1.2 million cases of AIDS that will be reported to CDC, 410,000 (36%) were directly or indirectly associated with injecting-drug use. Injecting-drug-user-associated AIDS cases include persons who are IDUs $n=352,600$, their heterosexual sex partners

DISTRIBUTION OF HIV-CONTAMINATED BLOOD:
FRANCE, GERMANY, THE UNITED STATES, AND OTHER COUNTRIES

Near the end he could not bring himself to visit his youngest brother, to see him dying of AIDS. He too was dying of AIDS. Their deaths would close out a family of four HIV-infected hemophiliac brothers, all diagnosed with AIDS. The first died at age 24, the second committed suicide at age 33, the last two brothers died in 1993. The four brothers became HIV infected about 1985 from using HIV-contaminated blood-clotting factor.

Blood banks, centers for blood transfusions, and companies involved in the creation and distribution of blood clotting factor VIII used to save the lives of hemophiliacs. Now they have been sued for selling blood and blood products that they should have known were contaminated with HIV. The use of these HIV-contaminated products by hemophiliacs became a worldwide tragedy. Many thousands of hemophiliacs have died prematurely because of these products. In France, over 4000 have been infected and over 1000 have died. French ministers were charged with collusion in poisoning people who used the contaminated blood products. In Germany, authorities closed blood plasma centers with charges of fraud, greed, and negligent bodily harm. The owners of the different plasma centers were charged with 5837 counts of attempted murder—corresponding to the number of blood products distributed.

In the United States, about 10,000 hemophiliacs became HIV infected after using blood products that either were not tested for HIV or if tested were distributed regardless. About 4,000 of them are still alive. France and Germany did the same thing. The evidence showed that the heads of the companies did not wish to discard large batches of blood products because it meant large financial losses! Other countries involved in similar HIV-contaminated blood distribution scandals are: Canada, Switzerland, Japan, India, Iran, Ireland, Pakistan, Russia, and China. Although each country's distribution of HIV-contaminated blood and blood products is scandalous, China may be the most scandalous of all.

China

In October 1996, China's Ministry of Public Health ordered thousands of state-run medical institutions to stop using a certain brand of serum albumin, a common blood product produced by a military-run factory.

Two years after Chinese journalists in Hong Kong and the United States first published reports that the blood product was contaminated with HIV, China's Foreign Ministry acknowledged that tests of some samples of the blood product indicated the presence of HIV. But, at the Department of Medicine Administration and Control, a Mr. Liu said: "No, no, it has never happened.

Some people outside China and some foreign journalists just made their reports on the basis of rumors."

In October 1998, in an effort to reduce the spread of HIV, the Chinese government created a law requiring that all blood products come from volunteers. Many countries banned the practice of payment for blood donation long ago, since there were concerns that the people who would be most likely to be strapped for money—such as drug users—would also be at high risk for blood-borne diseases. However, in China it can be hard to get donors because there is a cultural aversion to blood donation. Traditionally, the donation of blood is considered disrespectful to ancestors and parents; the culture also equates blood levels with health. Because China has a chronic blood shortage, many experts believe it will take several years for the illegal blood trade to die down. The government is trying to confront this problem by actively encouraging officials, students, and soldiers to donate blood.

Chinese health officials now believe that 50% of HIV-positive Chinese contracted HIV through the blood trade.

The Secret of China's Henan Province, 2001

Hints of a secret AIDS epidemic in China's countryside first began to surface in 2000. The depth of the tragedy and the unusually high incidence and impact of HIV/AIDS on villages in the Henan Province are now emerging, as disparate, dying farmers have begun to tell their stories of illness and death. All their stories begin with their willingness to sell their blood for needed money. The blood donors earned between $12 and $15 per donation. Some farmers reported donating blood 50 times in two months. Because of the plasma collection methods routinely used at the time throughout China, even those who donated only a few times ran a high risk of becoming ill. Blood from dozens of sellers was pooled and put into a huge centrifuge where it was spun at a speed sufficient to separate out the desired plasma. The remaining fraction, mainly red cells, was divided up and transfused back into the sellers, who felt the process to be healthful because it limited the blood loss.

The process was highly unsanitary. The result was once one blood seller in a village was infected with HIV or hepatitis, the rest were quick to become ill because the viruses from other people's bodies rode along with the red cells back into their veins. Because the sellers did not lose enough red cells with any donation to result in anemia, using this method meant that people could sell their blood frequently—raising their chance of infection.

In the village of Donghu, population 4500, every family has one or more members who suffer from fevers, chronic diarrhea, mouth sores, unbearable headaches, weight loss, racking coughs, and boils that do not heal. Residents estimate that more than 80% of adults carry HIV and more than 60% are already suffering debilitating symptoms. That would give this village, and the others like it in the province, localized rates that are the highest in the world.

Physicians who have worked in the Henan Province said more than a million people had probably contracted the virus from selling their blood. They add that while the sale of blood has stopped in the most severely affected villages, it continues elsewhere to a lesser extent, both in Henan and other provinces.

Repeats of the Henan tragedy also occurred in the provinces of Qinghai and Shaanxi.

Beginning 2009, China continues to downplay the effect of returning blood cells to paid donors in the Henan province. Officials have stopped villagers from traveling outside of Henan province or from speaking to the media. The epidemic in Henan province is still shrouded in silence because local officials were often involved in the profitable blood business. So while the authorities in Beijing held a big international conference in November 2001 and aired television dramas on the subject, repression and some concealment continues. Beginning in 2008, every batch of blood products nationwide was to be screened for HIV. This may be accomplished in 2009.

THE SECRET OF SHYMKENT (SHIM-KENT)—2007

In the industrial city of Shymkent near Uzbekistan (ooz-bek-a-stan), 118 children became HIV positive from blood transfusions in the summer of 2006. By mid-2007, 10 had died. All of the children were treated by 21 different healthcare workers; all received blood transfusions as ordered by these doctors. The doctors have been accused of medical malpractice. And many of the children's families were forced to move after experiencing HIV/AIDS-related discrimination. At trial, it became clear why the doctors prescribed the blood transfusions to treat these children. The doctors

charged patients $20 for 14 ounces or 467 milliliters of blood. The local blood bank received $10 and the doctors 10. A considerable amount of money in a country where doctors' salaries begin at $175 a month. The deputy chief physician at the Shymkent Infectious Diseases Hospital said, "Doctors' low wages force them to search for ways to generate additional revenue."

DUMB MEDICINE

Western doctors say that while pervasive corruption encourages many unnecessary transfusions, patients frequently demand transfusions. Doctors and patients in Russia and Eastern Europe, Central Asia, and parts of China and India truly believe that fresh infusions of blood can fortify a healthy body and remedy diseases that are not blood-related. One result, Western health officials say, is that throughout Central Asia and much of the developing world, local doctors prescribe tens of millions of unnecessary transfusions, putting people at heightened risk of contracting HIV/AIDS and other diseases transmitted by blood.

All of the factors listed above seem to have converged on the children of Shymkent. One 8-month-old boy received 25 unnecessary blood transfusions, according to court documents. The boy's transfusion regimen was halted only when he was found to have HIV. Michael O. Favorov, an epidemiologist and Central Asia program director of the Centers for Disease Control and Prevention, based in Atlanta, headed an extensive medical investigation by the agency that identified the transfusions of tainted blood as the source of the Shymkent outbreak. He said, "It's insane, this kid needed no blood." Kazakhstan's government has responded to the HIV outbreak by firing the health minister and four doctors and started construction on a pediatric HIV/AIDS facility in downtown Shymkent. Government health officials also have hired a Russian-speaking pediatric HIV/AIDS specialist from Israel to oversee treatment of the HIV-positive children. In addition, officials have conducted HIV tests among 8800 children nationwide who are on record for recently receiving blood transfusions. They found no new HIV cases.

RESULTS OF THE TRIAL

On July 28, 2007, 17 of the 21 healthcare workers were given jail sentences ranging from a few months to eight years. Four senior health officials received suspended sentences. The case is now under appeal.

SUMMARY

The issues in these blood scandals were delays in institution of donor screening, delays in screening donated blood with HIV antibody testing, and failure to withdraw contaminated factor from use and replace it with heat-treated factor for economic reasons—after it was known that these actions would protect individuals from infection.

According to the World Health Organization (WHO), the majority of nations are using unsafe blood with regard to HIV and hepatitis. The use of unsafe blood is most common in developing countries, home to 80% of the world's population, or some 4.8 billion people. Because of the high cost of blood testing, between $40 to $50 per unit, more than 13 million pints of blood annually are not checked for transmissible infections including HIV, malaria, and syphilis. Globally, transfusions of contaminated blood are thought to have caused up to 10% of AIDS infections. Moreover, unsafe transfusions and injection practices are estimated to cause up to 160,000 new HIV infections, 16 million new cases of hepatitis B,

and 4.7 million new hepatitis C infections each year. In response to these findings, the WHO, in cooperation with the International Federation of Red Cross and Red Crescent Societies, launched a global campaign to promote blood safety.

For the United States, the CDC states that over the past 24 years of blood screening for HIV (1985–2008) 52 adults and four children have developed AIDS after receiving an HIV-"negative" blood transfusion. This blood was taken in the window period before antibodies were made against HIV (Klein, 2000 updated). The majority of over 9000 HIV-contaminated blood transfusions occurred prior to 1985, the year when HIV blood screening began. It is estimated that about 50 new HIV-contaminated blood transfusions continue to occur each year in America. For additional information on blood scandals, read *Blood Feuds: AIDS, Blood and the Politics of Medical Disaster*, edited by Eric Feldman and Ronald Bayer, Oxford University Press, 1999.

Risk Group Activities May Place You in the Middle
of HIV Being Distributed Among Sexual Partners.

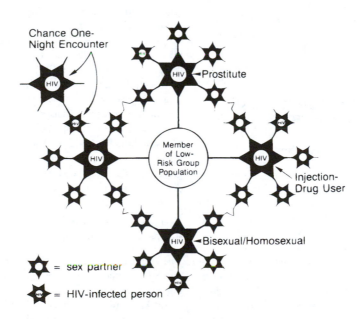

FIGURE 8-6 Risk Transmission of HIV. Sexual transmission can occur among homosexuals or heterosexuals. Prostitutes can be either male or female. The diagram shows possible bridges for transmission of HIV from high-risk groups into low-risk groups. To be safe, *you* must not become part of the chain.

Table 8-6 The Odds of Infecting Your Sexual Partner

If you're HIV positive and not using condoms and you are the:	Risk of your partner becoming infected:
Receptive partner of gay anal sex	1 in 1,250
Insertive partner of gay anal sex	1 in 122
Receptive partner of straight vaginal sex	1 in 1,000,000
Insertive partner of straight vaginal sex	1 in 111,111
Receiver of penile oral sex	1 in 1,250
Performer of penile oral sex	Negligible[1]
Receiver of vaginal oral sex	Negligible
Performer of vaginal oral sex	Negligible

Source: Jennifer Gong. POZ, November 2005, copyright 2005 CM Publishing LLC.

[1]Although the last three categories appear to be low risk, there are no guarantees.

n=51,250 and children n=8,200 whose mothers were IDUs or sex partners of IDUs. About half the females and about one-third of the heterosexual males who were diagnosed with AIDS had a sex partner who was an IDU (*HIV/AIDS Surveillance Report,* 1998 updated). It is estimated that half the estimated 56,000 new HIV infections in the United States, or 76 people per day through the year 2009, will be associated with IDUs. The epidemic among injection-drug users in New York City is an example of a very large, high-seroprevalence HIV epidemic. More than 100,000 injection-drug users have been infected with HIV, and over 50,000 cases of AIDS are reported among injection-drug users, their sexual partners, and their children in New York City (DesJarlais et al., 2000).

UNITED STATES: HETEROSEXUAL INJECTION-DRUG USE (IDU)

Women and Injection Drug Use

Over 90% of injection-drug users in the United States are heterosexuals. Thirty percent are women, of whom 90% are in their childbearing years. From 1988 to the beginning of 2009, female IDUs made up about 40% of all AIDS cases in women. Of the 41% of women infected by heterosexual contact, 38% were infected by having sex with a male IDU. During this same period about 8000 new cases of AIDS in children occurred—37% were from IDU mothers and 18% were from mothers whose sex partners were IDUs (*MMWR,* 1992; *HIV/AIDS Surveillance Report,* 2001 updated). Women IDUs and sexual partners of male IDUs represent the largest part (61%) of

the estimated 100,000 HIV-infected women of childbearing age. Thus, there is a direct correlation between HIV perinatal transmission and pediatric AIDS cases and injection-drug use.

Injection-Drug Use and HIV Infections in Other Countries

Worldwide there are about 16 million injection-drug users. Eighty percent of IDUs are men. An estimated 3 to 4 million past and current injecting-drug users are living with HIV/AIDS. Accordingly, in many countries, IDUs represent a significant proportion of those individuals who are in need of antiretroviral drugs. The dual epidemic of injection-drug use and HIV particularly affect resource-poor countries where there is limited access to HIV prevention measures such as needle and syringe exchange programs.

It appears that IDU is the major mode of HIV transmission in Kazakhstan, Malaysia, Vietnam, China, North America, Eastern Europe, The Newly Independent States, and the Middle East. Additionally, it is becoming more of an issue in West Africa and Latin America. The greatest problem has been seen in the Newly Independent States, in Eastern Europe, and in China.

Eastern Europe and the Former Soviet Union

The countries of Eastern Europe, countries of the former Soviet Union, and Russia are currently experiencing the most rapid spread of HIV anywhere in the world. Previously characterized by very low prevalence rates, the region now faces an extremely steep increase in the number of new HIV infections, up from 200,000 ending 1999 to about 1 million beginning 2009.

BOX 8.4

SPORTS AND HIV/AIDS: EARVIN "MAGIC" JOHNSON AND OTHER ATHLETES

HIV-INFECTED ATHLETES AND COMPETITION

The question regarding whether HIV-infected athletes should be allowed to compete has two facets:

1. Should these athletes be banned from competition to avoid the risk of spreading HIV infection?
2. Does the exercise that is demanded in competition accelerate the progression of HIV disease?

There is no hard, fast, scientifically supported answer to either question. However, as of the beginning of 2008, there has not been a single reported case of HIV transmission in any sporting event worldwide (Drotman, 1996 updated).

Magic Johnson: Professional Basketball Player, Los Angeles Lakers, HIV Positive

The first well-known HIV/AIDS-related name people became aware of in the United States was Rock Hudson, the famous movie star. He announced he had AIDS in July 1985 and died in October 1985. Rock Hudson's death from AIDS received international attention and was a major wake-up call to all Americans. The second well-known and respected personality to announce he was HIV infected was Magic Johnson, the National Basketball Association star. His announcement in 1991 came six years after Rock Hudson's. This shock was also felt around the world, especially in the United States and particularly in the African-American community. Now the U.S. community was forcefully aware of HIV/AIDs!

Earvin "Magic" Johnson said, "I thought the hardest thing I would ever have to do in life was try to beat fellow basketball greats Larry Bird and Michael Jordan on the basketball court. Instead the hardest thing was driving home from the doctor's office to tell my wife Cookie that I was HIV positive."

On November 7, 1991, Magic Johnson, age 32, appeared at a nationally televised press conference and said, "Because of the HIV virus I have obtained, I will have to announce my retirement from the Lakers today." He admitted having been "naïve" about AIDS and added, "Here I am saying *it can happen to anybody,* even me, Magic Johnson." He also assured the world that his wife, Cookie Kelly, two-months pregnant, had tested negative for the virus.

Some Events Since Magic's Announced Retirement

June 4, 1992—Earvin III is born *without* antibody to HIV. As of August 14, 2008, Magic is age 50. His wife, age 50 and son, age 18, are HIV negative.

In January 2003, Magic Johnson reached an agreement with Glaxo-Smith Kline (GSK), a leading antiretroviral drug manufacturer to use his image in promoting Combivir for HIV drug therapy among the urban black population. Newspaper, billboard, and subway posters include photos of a robust-looking Johnson and feature messages such as, "Staying healthy is about a few basic things: A positive attitude, partnering with my doctor, taking my medicine everyday."

His September 2007 checkup confirms he's still asymptomatic after 16 years.

In December 2006, through a partnership with the drug maker Abbott Laboratories, the I Stand With Magic initiative held HIV testing drives in 10 to 13 cities each year for the next five years; sponsored education and marketing drives, supported grassroots advocacy programs, and provided scholarships for doctors who staff HIV/AIDS programs in the black community. The $60 million campaign is to cut HIV/AIDS rates among black Americans by 50%.

Other Sports, Other Athletes—Basketball players are not the only athletes whose behavior may place them at risk for HIV infection. In 2007 there were 7131 professional athletes in the United States involved in boxing (4065), National Football League (1854), National Hockey League (784), and the National Basketball Association (428). Of these professionals, the CDC estimated 35 to be HIV positive.

John Elson (1991) wrote a revealing article for *Time* magazine just after Magic Johnson revealed his HIV status. Elson tells of groupies that follow athletes in all sports. They are usually college-age or older. Mainly they seek money, attention, and the glamour of associating with celebrated and highly visible "hard bodies." According to a 31-year-old who has had affairs with athletes in two sports, "For women, many of whom don't have meaningful work, the only way to identify themselves is to say whom they have slept with. A woman who sleeps around is called a whore. But a woman who has slept with Magic Johnson is a woman who has slept with Magic Johnson. It's almost as if it gives her legitimacy."

The Girls—Baseball players call them "Annies." To riders on the rodeo circuit, they are "buckle bunnies." To most other athletes, they are "wannabes" or just "the girls." They can be found hanging out anywhere they

BOX 8.4 (*continued*)

might catch an off-duty sports hero's eye and fancy, or in the lobbies of hotels where teams on the road check in. To the athletes who care to indulge them—and many do—these readily available groupies offer pro sport's ultimate perk: free and easy recreational sex, no questions asked. Recently, an HIV-infected female stated publicly that she had had sex with at least 50 Canadian ice hockey players. She could not recall their names. The sex may be free, but now there is a price for the lifestyle—HIV/AIDS.

Sports/Injuries/Blood—Concerns over the transmission of HIV are shared throughout sports, particularly those sports that cause blood-letting injuries—football, hockey, and boxing. In football Jerry Smith, a former Washington Redskin, died of AIDS in 1986; in December 2003, Roy Simmons, an offensive lineman for the New York Giants and Washington Redskins, revealed that he is HIV positive. He tested HIV positive in 1997 and has a homosexual lifestyle.

In 2005, according to the *New York Times,* Trevis Smith, a seven-season veteran of the Canadian Football League's Saskatchewan Roughriders, was arrested on October 28 and charged with aggravated sexual assault. The police disclosed Smith's HIV-positive status to the public saying such a warning was necessary. Team officials said they had been aware of Smith's status for about a year but privacy laws had prevented them from disclosing the information to his teammates. At a November 2 hearing, Smith was ordered by a judge to use condoms, disclose to his sexual partners that he is HIV positive, and give up his passport. The judge did not provide conditions on Smith's eligibility to continue playing in the CFL.

In 1996, the National Football League officials estimated that there was the *possibility* of one HIV transmission from body fluid exchange in 85 million football games played.

Boxing—In boxing, Esteban Dejesus, WBC lightweight champion, died of AIDS in 1989. Four other boxers are known to be HIV positive.

Tommy Morrison—In February 1996 Tommy Morrison, age 27, a heavyweight boxing title contender said, on announcing that he was HIV positive, "I honestly believed I had a better chance of winning the lottery than contracting this disease. I've never been so wrong in my life. I'm here to tell you I thought that I was bulletproof, and I'm not."

Morrison had his sperm washed free of HIV and fathered a boy in late 2003.

ATTENTION: In March 2007 Tommy Morrison took a repeated series of HIV tests and was found to be HIV negative! He said, "I was kicked to the curb and lost more than ten years of my career because of a false positive. I was using steroids at the time. I believe that's why the test came back the way it did. But I've taken five or six different tests in the last three or four months, and I passed them all." It is believed that the initial tests were either improperly run, his blood vial was mixed up in the laboratory, or the results were improperly interpreted. If someone truly tests HIV positive, they stay that way for life.

Ice Skating—In professional ice skating, the *Calgary Herald* and others reported, that by 2007, at least 45 top U.S. and Canadian male skaters and coaches had died from AIDS (among them Rob McCall, Brian Pockar, Dennis Coi, Shawn-McGill, Rudy Galindo, and Nicole Lesh).

Swimming—In February 1995, Greg Louganis, the greatest diver in Olympic history, announced that he had AIDS.

Tennis—Arthur Ashe died in 1993.

Baseball—Glenn Burke, outfielder, Los Angeles Dodgers/Oakland Athletics, died in 1995.

Race Car Drivers—It was reported in 1996 that Tim Richmond, race car driver, age 34, had died of AIDS. He won 13 Winston Cup races on the NASCAR racing circuit. One report states that Richmond may have infected up to 30 women (Knight-Tribune Service, March 27, 1996, A-1). His physician estimated that he was HIV positive for at least eight years. During this time, according to accounts of friends, he was sexually promiscuous. (Richmond actually died in 1989 but his story was kept silent until 1996.)

Ice Hockey—Bill Goldsworthy, five-time NHL All-Star, age 51, died of AIDS. He played 14 seasons in the NHL. He was diagnosed with AIDS in 1994. Goldsworthy said his health problem was caused by drinking and sexual promiscuity.

Injection-Drug Use in Russia

Russian health officials estimate there may be as many as 4 million IDUs. About half are HIV infected. They say up to 60% of IDUs are between ages 18 and 30 with precollege teenagers accounting for another 20%. Vadim Pokrovsky, head of the official AIDS prevention center, told a news conference broadcast on internet site www.presscentr.ru. that, "We are currently going through the peak of an epidemic among drug users. Currently about 90% of HIV infections are associated with IDU. In two or three years there will be another upsurge from sexual transmission of the disease."

Moscow—Change of Scene, Same Results

The hotbed of the disease had moved from the tiny Baltic enclave of Kaliningrad to Moscow and its suburbs. In some parts of Moscow, up to 5% of the young people are already HIV positive. If counted as a percentage of the population, Russia will reach U.S. levels. About 80% of the infected are aged 15 to 25. They will be lost in 10 years, just after they have finished their education. It means one gets infected at 20, graduates at 30, starts working, and dies. Murray Feshbach, a specialist in Russian demographic trends,

estimates that 5 to 10 million people will die of AIDS in Russia after year 2015.

Current estimates are that 36,000 adults/adolescents and 6600 babies are becoming HIV infected each year in Russia. The Russian federal government allocated $289 million in 2007 for its HIV/AIDS programs.

Epidemic in the Ukraine

The Ukraine's HIV/AIDS epidemic, the worst of all the former Soviet Union nations, is causing alarm among Ukrainian physicians and other neighboring countries. In a nation of 50 million people, about 250,000 (5%) are HIV positive, and the level of infection continues to rise.

Figure 8-7 presents the estimated new HIV infections for 2008 across the globe.

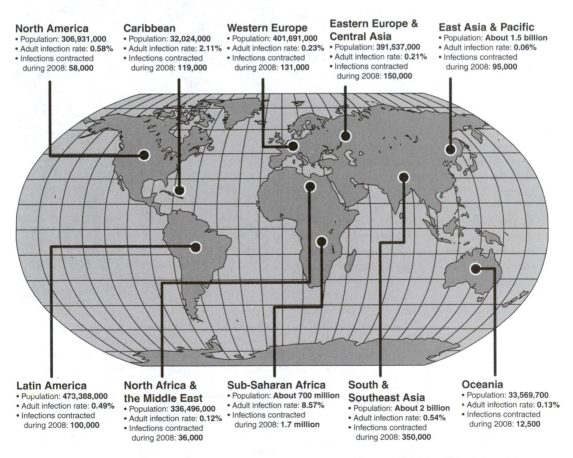

North America
- Population: **306,931,000**
- Adult infection rate: **0.58%**
- Infections contracted during 2008: **58,000**

Caribbean
- Population: **32,024,000**
- Adult infection rate: **2.11%**
- Infections contracted during 2008: **119,000**

Western Europe
- Population: **401,691,000**
- Adult infection rate: **0.23%**
- Infections contracted during 2008: **131,000**

Eastern Europe & Central Asia
- Population: **391,537,000**
- Adult infection rate: **0.21%**
- Infections contracted during 2008: **150,000**

East Asia & Pacific
- Population: **About 1.5 billion**
- Adult infection rate: **0.06%**
- Infections contracted during 2008: **95,000**

Latin America
- Population: **473,388,000**
- Adult infection rate: **0.49%**
- Infections contracted during 2008: **100,000**

North Africa & the Middle East
- Population: **336,496,000**
- Adult infection rate: **0.12%**
- Infections contracted during 2008: **36,000**

Sub-Saharan Africa
- Population: **About 700 million**
- Adult infection rate: **8.57%**
- Infections contracted during 2008: **1.7 million**

South & Southeast Asia
- Population: **About 2 billion**
- Adult infection rate: **0.54%**
- Infections contracted during 2008: **350,000**

Oceania
- Population: **33,569,700**
- Adult infection rate: **0.13%**
- Infections contracted during 2008: **12,500**

FIGURE 8-7   Global Impact of HIV/AIDS. About 35 million adults and children worldwide will be living with HIV/AIDS by the end of 2009, according to UNAIDS estimates. Estimated new infections for 2008, 2.5 million. (*UNAIDS; World Health Organization; U.S. Centers for Disease Control and Prevention; updated*)

China

The lifting of a ban on AIDS-related reporting in 2000 in the state-run media appears to have fed a public panic through alarmist reports that China is on the verge of an epidemic. The government recently projected that the number of people infected with HIV could rise to 10 million by 2015 from an estimated 1 million now if preventive measures are not enforced. The current estimate provided by the Chinese health officials is believed, by the WHO and UNAIDS, to be several times that high. By 2001 HIV infections were found in every province with prevalence rates of 77% among injection-drug users, ages 20 to 29, and 11% among prostitutes.

Caribbean HIV/AIDS: Big Problems Among Small Islands

In the Caribbean, an estimated 35,000 people die annually and 60,000 adults and children become infected. The total number of infected is about one million. The Caribbean has the highest rate of HIV infection in the world after sub-Saharan Africa, and AIDS is already the single greatest cause of death among young men and women in this region. The rate of HIV infection in the Caribbean is about four times that of North America, Latin America, and South and Southeast Asia. The rate is 35 times that found in East Asia and the Pacific and almost 10 times the rate in Western Europe (Figure 8-7). According to UNAIDS, if left unchecked HIV/AIDS will, by year 2020, cause 75% of deaths in the Caribbean. Such a scenario mimics what is happening in some parts of Africa. The disease has spread over the African continent through mobility. Long-haul truck drivers having sex with prostitutes along their routes have brought it home to wives and girlfriends. Likewise, throughout the Caribbean, tourists, truck drivers, shipmates, and soldiers have been important male agents of the spread of HIV, as is the use of injection drugs. In Puerto Rico, for example, over half of 30,000 plus AIDS cases were/are associated with IDU. Between 35% and 50% of injection-drug users are HIV infected. According to the CDC, Puerto Rico has the fourth-highest HIV infection rate of American states and territories, behind Washington D.C., New York City, and the U.S. Virgin Islands. Puerto Rico plays a special role as a global border town in the transmission of AIDS because it is a central transportation and commerce hub for the Caribbean. It is a favorite location for both trafficking drugs and smuggling people, especially from the Dominican Republic.

The Sex Trade, Women and Children: Two Examples, the Caribbean and Southeast Asia

Overall, in the Caribbean, the majority of HIV infection is sexually transmitted (Figure 8-8). According to a 2000 UNAIDS report, the spread of HIV is partly driven by older men who have numerous sex partners, and who seek out young women for sex and infect them. They in turn pass the virus on. If Caribbean women in general refuse unsafe sex and insist on the use of a condom, they often risk spousal

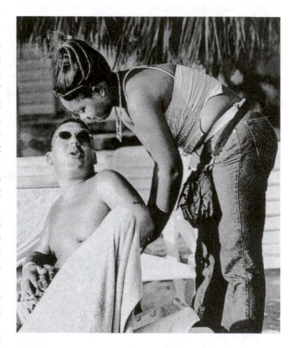

FIGURE 8-8 A Sex Worker Solicits a Tourist In Boca Chica, a Well-known Beach for Prostitution About 20 Minutes from Santo Domingo. About 100,000 women in the Dominican Republic are engaged in sex work. Most sex workers will tell you they will not have sex without a condom, but sometimes clients think that insistence on using a condom is a bargaining tactic based on economics. Since its first appearance in the Caribbean, AIDS has been a mobile epidemic closely linked to the region's underground sex trade and has altered the economy in many regions of the Caribbean and Latin America. *(Photo by Hilda M. Perez/South Florida Sun-Sentinel)*

abuse because it creates a suspicion of infidelity. Ten years ago there were seven times more infected men than women in the Caribbean. By 2003 that ratio had changed to 2 to 1.

Southeast Asia, The Golden Triangle

There are no reliable statistics on the number of children working in the sex industry worldwide, but the lowest figure cited is 1 million. The United Nations Children's Fund estimates that one-third of sex workers in Southeast Asia are 12 to 17-years-old. The smuggling of vast quantities of heroin and amphetamines from Myanmar and China through Thailand has given the region its infamous tag, "The Golden Triangle," but it's the explosion in the recruitment of girls into the lucrative Thai sex industry that has put this border town on the map. Every year, hundreds of young girls from Mae Sai, a town of 80,000 inhabitants on Thailand's northernmost border with Burma, are spirited away to brothels in Bangkok where they feed the insatiable appetite of the $20 billion commercial sex industry.

SNAPSHOT 8.4

HATE CRIMES AND VIOLENCE: A LOOK AT JAMAICA'S HIV/AIDS SCENARIO

On June 9, 2004, Jamaica's leading gay rights activist was murdered in his home, his body mutilated by multiple knife wounds. Within an hour after his body was discovered, a Human Rights Watch researcher witnessed a crowd gathered outside the crime scene. A smiling man called out, "Battyman (homosexual) he get killed!" Many others celebrated this murder, laughing and calling out, "Let's get them one at a time," "That's what you get for sin," "Let's kill all of them." Some sang "boom bye bye," a line from a popular Jamaican song about killing and burning gay men.

Jamaica's growing HIV/AIDS epidemic is unfolding in the context of widespread violence and discrimination against people living with and at high risk of HIV/AIDS, especially men who have sex with men. Myths about HIV/AIDS persist. Many Jamaicans believe that HIV/AIDS is a disease of homosexuals and sex workers whose moral impurity makes them vulnerable to it, or that HIV is transmitted by casual contact. Pervasive and violent homophobia, coupled with fear of the disease, impedes access to HIV prevention information, condoms, and health care.

Drugs and Daughters

Mae Sai has two main trades, drugs and daughters. A nongovernmental organization in Mae Sai that works with local girls who are at risk of being sold, estimates that of the village of Pa Tek's 800 families, 7 in every 10 have sold at least one daughter into the trade.

When a Burmese migrant in Pa Tek sold his 13-year-old daughter into prostitution for $114, his wife had one regret—they didn't get a good price for her. She said, "I should have asked for $228. He robbed us." The mother earns about $100 a year selling bamboo bowls in the local market and lives in a thatched hut in Pa Tek village on the outskirts of Mae Sai. With prices varying from $114 to $913 per daughter, the latter figure is equal to almost six years' wages for most families. Parental bonds in impoverished households are easily broken. In fact, child prostitution is so established that many brothel agents live in the village, and are often friends or relatives of the family from whom they buy the children. The director of the Child Protection and Rights Center in Mae Sai said, "Agents will come to the village with orders to fill so people in Bangkok, Thai men, and foreigners, mostly Europeans, can order girls like they order pizza. If they want a girl with thin hips and big breasts, the agents will come here and find her. They always deliver."

Caribbean Connection to America: South Florida

Five nations in the Caribbean with the highest infection rates have HIV infections in all segments of their populations. During the last 27 years about 300,000 Haitians have died of AIDS. UNAIDS estimates that Haiti, with 10% of the urban and 5% of the rural population infected (about 400,000; population 8.5 million), has the highest rate of HIV infection and 90% of all AIDS cases in the Caribbean. Next is the Bahamas at about 4% and 3% for Barbados. Guyana and the Dominican Republic are each at 2% with about 8% of their pregnant women HIV infected. (For data on Cuba, see Chapter 9.) The third National Caribbean American HIV/AIDS Awareness Day was celebrated June 8, 2008.

The Connection

The cruise ships and planes that leave and return to Fort Lauderdale and Miami weekly depend on the allure of tropical beaches, exotic ports, and lusty streets in the islands. Discount department stores depend on shirts sewn in Haitian textile plants, and increasingly, much of the low- and high-tech workforce essential to South Florida comes from Haiti, the Dominican Republic, and other Caribbean countries. In short, there is no way that South Florida can be spared the effects of the AIDS calamity in the Caribbean. The region is so tightly linked through culture, race, ethnicity, and economics that any public health crisis in the islands is felt here. In a highly mobile, global age, there are few boundaries that cannot be crossed. The disease, carried unknowingly among tourists and workers every day throughout the region, respects no borders.

Other Means of HIV Transmission

Other means of HIV infection have been documented. There has been a reported case of HIV transmission via **acupuncture.** It is believed that HIV-infected body fluids contaminated the acupuncture needles (Vittecoq et al., 1989). Unlicensed and unregulated **tattoo** establishments may also present an unrecognized risk for HIV infection to patrons. If the operator does not use new needles or needles that have been autoclaved (steam sterilized), the possibility exists that infection with HIV or a number of other blood-borne pathogens may take place. In addition, single-service or individual containers of dye or ink should be used for each client.

Organ/Tissue Transplants

On any given day, about 20,000 Americans are waiting for a transplant. There is a small but present risk of receiving HIV along with the transplant tissue. A CDC report revealed that a bone transplant recipient became HIV-infected from an HIV-infected donor. HIV transmission has also occurred in the transplantation of kidneys, liver, heart, pancreas, and skin (*MMWR,* 1988). In May 1991, the CDC reported on 56 transplant patients who received organs and tissues from an HIV-infected donor in 1985. A transplantation service company supplied tissues to 30 hospitals in 16 states. All tissues came from a single young male who was shot to death during a robbery. He twice tested HIV negative before his heart, kidneys, liver, pancreas, cornea, and other tissues were removed for transplant. By mid-1991, three recipients of these tissues had died of AIDS and six others were HIV positive. As of mid-1991, 32 other recipients had been located, 11 of whom tested HIV negative. It is unknown whether the others have ever been tested.

In May 1994, the CDC published guidelines for preventing HIV transmission through transplantation of human tissue (*MMWR,* 1994b).

In January 2007, four transplant recipients received HIV- and HCV- (hepatitis C virus) contaminated organs in three Chicago hospitals. By November 2007, all four were HIV and HCV positive. The CDC is investigating whether the four people may, in turn, have transmitted those viruses to others before they learned they were infected. The organ donor, via a screening questionnaire, was known to have engaged in high-risk activity, but pre-transplant tests were HIV negative, probably because the infections were too recent to generate antibodies. When organs are transplanted from such donors, the CDC recommends that the recipients be tested three months after their surgeries.

According to CDC guidelines, "High risk patients should be excluded from organ and tissue donation unless the risk to the recipient of not performing the transplant is deemed greater than the risk of HIV transmission and disease." In other words, this is a risk-versus-benefits calculation.

Since May 1994, at least 92 liver and kidney transplant cases have involved the use of human organs that were HIV positive. Of the 92 transplant cases, 70 of the patients were HIV negative prior to transplant and received organs that contained HIV. All became HIV positive. The average time for progression to AIDS was 32 months. The 22 people who were HIV positive prior to receiving an HIV-positive organ progressed to AIDS, on average, within 17 months (Horn, 2001). (See SIDEBAR 8.1.)

AIDS Patients and Organ Transplants

According to published reports, Larry Kramer, age 68, who cofounded the Gay Men's Health Crisis in 1981 and the AIDS Coalition to Unleash Power (ACT UP), suffered from end stage liver disease. Kramer said his situation was similar to that of a growing number of patients who live long enough with HIV to suffer from a second infection. After being rejected by other health centers, Kramer received a new liver at the Thomas E. Starzl Transplantation Institute in Pittsburgh on December 21, 2001. As of December 2002, Kramer's liver transplant has cost Medicare over $500,000 and Empire Blue Cross over $100,000 for the medications he must take, including $10,000 a month for Hepatitis B Immune Globulin, which he will receive for the rest of his life. Art Kaplan, director of the Center of Bioethics said that the medical community has yet to debate the ethics of transplanting organs into people with HIV/AIDS. This is largely because centers like Starlz are just beginning to create possibilities. Beginning 2009, over 60 HIV-positive people have received liver transplants, one heart, and one kidney transplant in the United States.

DISCUSSION QUESTION: Debate the ethics of giving an HIV-positive person an organ transplant in light of the fact that thousands of young and old noninfected people die each year while waiting for a transplant.

Influence of Sexually Transmitted Diseases on HIV Transmission and Vice-Versa

Sexual intercourse occurs more than 100 million times daily around the world. Results: 910,000 conceptions and over 600,000 cases of sexually transmitted disease. In the United States, according to the CDC, about 19 million new cases of sexually transmitted diseases occur each year. Nine million of these cases occur in 15- to 24- year-olds. By age 21, about one in five peo-

---

SIDEBAR 8.1

HIV/AIDS TRANSPLANT ERROR

MEXICO

MEXICAN DOCTORS TRANSPLANT HIV-INFECTED KIDNEYS

In February 1999, Mexican health officials fired five physicians and warned two others for transplanting HIV-infected kidneys into two patients. One of the two patients has since tested HIV positive. According to the regional director of the state-run hospital, the physicians did not wait for the results of the HIV test on the kidney donor before making the transplant.

In April 2002, the unofficial estimate was that 150,000 Mexicans required access to HIV/AIDS care and treatment. The epidemic in Mexico is centered among gay men ages 15 to 44. The number of HIV-infected women is rapidly rising.

ITALY

In February 2007, a 40-year-old woman died of a brain hemorrhage. With family consent, her organs were harvested and three of those organs, both kidneys and the liver, were separated and transplanted into three individuals. After the fact, it was found that the donor was HIV positive. All three organ recipients are on antiretroviral therapy.

---

ple has received treatment for an STD. At current rates at least one American in four will contract an STD at some point in his or her life. Over 50 organisms that can cause an STD are transmitted through sexual activity (Hooker, 1996). Regardless of these facts, data from the CDC in 2001 revealed that one in four physicians do not screen their patients for STDs. In addition, a GayHealth.com online survey conducted in May 2001 found 4 in 10 gay and lesbian patients have physicians who don't ask about their sexual practices. Over 40% of the men surveyed said they have not been vaccinated against either hepatitis A or B, potentially fatal viral liver infections spread through sexual activity. Men who have sex with men are at higher risk than the general population for these diseases. The annual cost of STDs in the United States is in excess of $10 billion. The latest U.S. government information on STDs and their treatment can be found in the updated STD Treatment Guidelines published by the CDC.

Association of STDs and HIV Infection: U.S.A.

STD researchers have long recognized that the behaviors that place individuals at risk for other STDs also increase their risk of becoming infected with HIV.

STDs are associated in several ways with HIV. Because STDs and HIV are spread by similar types of sexual activity, people who engage in behaviors that transmit HIV are also more likely to contract STDs, and vice-versa. Epidemiological evidence shows that populations and geographical regions in the United States with the highest STD rates also tend to have the highest rates of HIV. According to the CDC, "The geographic distribution of heterosexual HIV transmission closely parallels that of other STDs." In the past decade, high HIV incidence rates have shifted toward women infected through heterosexual activity, young adults, Black Americans, and people living in the southeastern United States, all populations with disproportionately high rates of STDs.

Tissues Most Often Infected with an STD

Infection by sexually transmitted diseases usually occurs through the mucosal (membrane) surfaces of the male and female genital tracts and rectum. The mucosal route also accounts for a large percentage of heterosexual and homosexual transmission of HIV. It is known that STDs increase the number of T4 or CD4+ cells (HIV target cells) in cervical secretions, thereby increasing the chance of HIV infection in women.

BOX 8.5

ASSAULT WITH HIV

Every state and territory has generic criminal statutes that could apply to conduct that exposed others to HIV. However, there is a growing frustration and fear about persons not revealing their HIV-positive status when they should (see the examples that follow).

Legislators around the country are passing an increasing number of laws intended to protect the public. This latest wave of legislation shifts the focus from earlier laws that protected the civil liberties of HIV-infected people to laws that seek to identify, notify, and in some cases punish people who intentionally place others at risk of contracting the virus. At least 32 states now make it a crime to knowingly transmit or expose others to HIV, with a third of those states enacting laws within the last five years.

According to Richard Lacayo (1997), Darnell McGee, age 28, through 1995 and 1996, had sex with at least 61 women ranging in age from 12 to 29. According to a Missouri public health report in February 1998, McGee had sex with at least 101 females, including four whose ages were 13 or 14. It is reported that McGee infected 18 women but Missouri officials believe he infected 30 women.

McGee knew what he was doing. According to the *St. Louis Post-Dispatch,* which broke the story, state records show that he tested positive in 1992 and was told the results.

On January 15, 1997, he was shot and killed, assailant unknown.

Darnell "Bossman" McGee is just one of a number of men who recklessly and in some cases, even willfully transmit HIV to their sex partners. Twenty-six years ago it was Gatean Dugas, or Patient Zero, a gay male who, over three years knowingly infected an untold number (probably 50) of gays across the United States.

In 1997, there was Nushawn Williams, age 21, who in mid-1997 admitted to having unprotected sex with 50 to 75 women after he was told he was HIV positive. Most of them were teenagers ages 13 and up living in New York's Chautauqua County and in New York City. To date, 13 in Chautauqua are infected, the youngest was age 13; others were ages 15, 16, 18, and 21. After the newspaper and TV carried this story, 625 people showed up at the county health department for HIV testing. There are now 16 HIV-positive people who are linked to Williams. In April 1999, Williams was sentenced 14 years in prison. Only two women agreed to testify against him.

In February 2002, the San Francisco Superior Court Commissioner ordered a former San Francisco health commissioner to pay his ex-lover $5 million in damages for knowingly exposing him to HIV and lying about his HIV status. This civil suit judgment is one of the largest awards to date for this kind of damage. The suit also alleged that the commissioner, who was appointed by Mayor Willie Brown to the health commission in 1997, in part to represent people with HIV, was suffering from symptoms of AIDS but told his lover that he had cancer.

In May 2002, a child molester with HIV in Kansas City, Mo., was sentenced to three consecutive life terms, plus 52 years. He pleaded guilty in December to 13 counts, including statutory rape, sodomy, child molestation, and exposing others to HIV. His victims were ages 9, 11, and 14.

In January 2003, a 39-year-old Bronx, N.Y. second-grade teacher accused of sexually abusing students while HIV positive was sentenced to 10 years in prison.

In March 2004, in what may be the first verdict of its kind, a Cook County, Ill., jury awarded $2 million to a woman who sued her fiancé's parents for allegedly covering up that he was dying of AIDS. The woman, known only as "Jane Doe," was infected through unprotected sex with her fiancé in August 1996, according to the woman's attorney. The woman's lawsuit contended that her fiancé, who died of AIDS in November 1999, did not tell her he was infected with HIV. The suit alleged his parents knew of his infection and lied to her when she asked about his deteriorating health. The suit contended that the parents' misrepresentations prevented the woman from learning that she may have been infected for almost three years, during which time she could have received antiretroviral medicine to treat HIV infection.

In May 2004, a Libyan court sentenced to death by firing squad five Bulgarian nurses and a Palestinian physician for deliberately and experimentally infecting 460 children with HIV using contaminated blood products. This sentence was handed down regardless of HIV/AIDS expert testimonies from people like Luc Montagnier, the scientist who discovered HIV, who stated the infections had to have occurred before these people became associated with these children. The sentence was appealed.

Finally, after nine years of frustrating set backs and a payout of one million dollars to each of the 460 infected children's families, Libya's High Judicial Council in July 2007 commuted the death sentences to life in prison! Prosecutors in Bulgaria extradited the six people to Bulgaria, a transfer that is permitted under a 1984 agreement between the two countries, and the president of Bulgaria pardoned them.

In June 2005, a Massachusetts woman was charged with armed robbery and assault for allegedly

BOX 8.5 (*continued*)

stabbing a security guard with a syringe after he accused her of shoplifting. Witnesses say the 21-year-old then taunted customers asking, "Does anyone else want AIDS!?!" And in November, a former D.C. government worker who had known since 1996 that he was HIV positive was sentenced to a 21-year prison term for luring women and teenage girls into sexual relationships without telling them he was HIV positive. In October 2005, a New Zealand court ruled that a man who used a condom was not legally obliged to tell a woman he was HIV positive.

In January 2007, a 35-year-old male from Bournemouth, England, was sentenced to three and a half years in prison for not telling his sexual partner that he was HIV positive. She is now HIV positive. In April 2007, a Glasgow male was sentenced to nine years in prison for HIV-infecting his girlfriend. In June 2007, a Kansas City, MO., man, who spent five years in jail for exposing his sexual partners to HIV, received a life sentence in prison for knowingly exposing at least 8 women to HIV, with three of them testing HIV positive. In the summer of 2007, parents were asked to keep their HIV-infected son from using the public shower/pool at an Alabama RV resort!

In 2008, the Ontario Superior Court sentenced a 32-year-old male to 18 years in prison for 15 counts of knowingly and secretly spreading HIV to his female sexual partners. Also in 2008, in Australia, a 36-year-old male received nine years in jail for knowingly and secretly endangering three female sexual partners. In March 2008, an airport guard in Canada stopped a group, "Positive Living North," from boarding an airplane because he believed the group placed others on the plane in danger. He later resigned from his job. In May 2008, a Dallas, Texas, court sentenced a 42-year-old HIV-positive male to 35 years in prison because he spit into the mouth and eye of a police officer during his arrest. The jury determined his saliva was a deadly weapon. In July 2008, a 43-year-old HIV-positive woman from Columbus, Georgia, was sentenced to three years in jail for spitting onto another woman's face. She said, "I hope you get AIDS, bitch." Also in May 2008, a manager at an RV resort in Alabama refused to allow an HIV-positive two-year-old child to use the swimming pool, shower, or other common areas unless the parents could provide a doctor's letter stating that the child would not put other visitors in danger. (This case is under investigation.)

Between 1987 and 2009, at least 18 HIV-infected men and 3 HIV-infected women were incarcerated in 10 states because they **bit another person.** Two of the 18 bitten people became HIV positive. The charges in these cases varied from assault with a dangerous weapon, assault with a deadly weapon, attempted murder, aggravated assault with intent to murder, felony,

reckless endangerment, and assault and reckless endangerment. Prison terms varied from 18 months for reckless endangerment to 27 years for attempted murder. In nine cases within seven states, one HIV-infected woman and seven HIV-infected men went to jail for periods of one to five years for spitting on other people. In a seventh case of spitting, in Texas, at trial, a court-recognized AIDS expert testified that HIV could be transmitted through the air! The man got a life sentence and an appeals court upheld the sentence. This man died in prison.

In July 2003, in Oklahoma, a convicted HIV-infected rapist received a life sentence for spitting on a police officer. None of the people who were spat upon contracted HIV.

Sex and HIV: If you have the first without disclosing the second, you can go to prison. In some states sex crimes and sex work can be elevated to attempted murder if the perpetrator (criminal) is HIV infected. Disclosing one's HIV status to a sexual partner may exempt one from prosecution. But not telling—even if you do protect and don't infect—is still a crime in most states in America.

These cases represent just a few of the over 600 recorded cases through 2008.

DISCUSSION QUESTION: What is your response to these issues?

1. Is knowingly transmitting HIV an act of violence?
2. Should the reckless or intentional transmission of HIV be a crime? If yes, how severe the penalty?
3. Do the cases bolster arguments for more aggressive partner notification and contact tracing? Why?
4. Do HIV confidentiality protections help or hinder efforts to alter the course of the epidemic? Why?
5. Would more ready access to condoms have helped avert these tragedies? How?
6. Who is responsible when an HIV-infected person knowingly continues to have unprotected sexual relations with others? Should the infected person be warned another time, assuming that the educational message was not heard? If so, how many times should warnings go forth? Are public health officials responsible for protecting susceptible spouses or long-term lovers of those who are infected and knowingly refuse to use condoms? Should the police become involved if protective advice is not followed, or should confidentiality remain in effect while educational messages go out that untold persons in the community are infected and all should use condoms?
7. Do such incidences support calls for more sex education, or less? Or perhaps different approaches to sexuality education? What approach might work? Why?

Most AIDS researchers agree that treating STDs, which cures genital sores and reduces inflammation, can raise the body's barriers against HIV infection. According to a study by Grosskurth and coworkers (1995), researchers working in rural Tanzania saw the number of new HIV infections plummet by 42% after they improved STD health care.

Because HIV is sexually transmitted, the association between HIV and other sexually transmitted diseases can be in part attributed to the shared risk of exposure and shared modes of transmission.

Types of STDs Most Often Associated with HIV Transmission, U.S.A.

For the purpose of understanding which STDs best promote HIV transmission, the sexually transmitted diseases can be divided into **genital ulcer** and **genital nonulcerative diseases.**

Genital Ulcer Disease (GUD)—Signs of genital ulcer disease appear as open sores on the penis, vagina, other genital areas, and at times elsewhere on the body. The most widespread genital ulcer STDs are syphilis, genital herpes, and chancroid. About 60 million people in America over age 12 have chronic genital herpes. There are about 1 million new herpes infections and 70,000 syphilis cases annually (Figure 8-9).

In early 1997, researchers from the University of Washington showed for the first time that herpes sores contain high levels of HIV, which they believe makes the virus especially easy to spread during sexual contact. Additional research by Timothy Schacker and colleagues (1998) also showed that HIV can be consistently found in herpes genital lesions of HIV-infected people. Such data suggest that genital herpes infection likely increases the sexual transmission of HIV.

Nonulcerative Disease—The nonulcerative STDs include gonorrhea, about 650,000 new cases annually, chlamydia, about 3 million new cases annually, and trichomonal infections, about 5 million new cases annually (also called discharge diseases), and genital warts. There are over 30 million people in the United States infected with genital wart virus, with about 5 million new cases annually. There are about 100 types of genital wart viruses, the human papilloma virus or HPV. HPV is one of the most common sexually transmitted agents. Current estimates are that approximately 75% of the sexually active general population ages 15 to 49 years acquires at least one genital HPV type during their lifetime. Most individuals remain asymptomatic after acquiring the infection, and only about 1% will develop clinically or histologically recognizable lesions. (Figure 8-10).

In most populations, the nonulcerative STDs are much more common than genital ulcer diseases. None causes the noticeable open sores that occur in the ulcer diseases but they do cause microscopic breaks in affected tissue, and are associated with HIV transmission (Laga et al., 1993). The most common

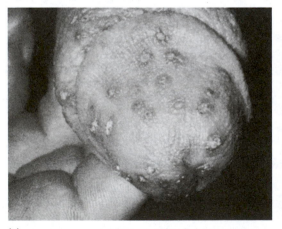

(a)

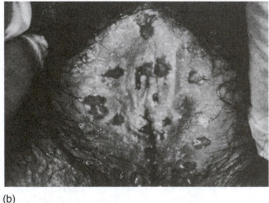

(b)

FIGURE 8-9 (a) **Genital Herpes (HSV-2) Infection of the Glans Penis.** Note these vesicles have crusted over, and thus, should no longer contain HSV-2. However, wearing a spermicide-treated condom, if involved in sexual activities at this stage, will help prevent possible transmission. (b) **HSV-2 infection of the vulva.** Note the large, superficial, ulcer-like areas on the labia. (*Photographs courtesy of the Centers for Disease Control and Prevention, Atlanta.*)

symptoms are warty growths on the genitals, discharge from the penis or vagina, and painful urination.

How Do Nonulcerative STDs Influence HIV Infection—For an example of how nonulcerative STDs may enhance HIV infection, an uninfected woman has about a 0.2% chance of being infected with HIV during vaginal intercourse with an HIV-positive partner. If her partner had gonorrhea instead, she would have a 50% to 70% chance of becoming infected.

Collectively, worldwide there are over 300 million cases a year of just seven major STDs: syphilis, herpes, and chancroid, which cause ulcers; and trichomoniasis, chlamydia, warts, and gonorrhea, do not (Figure 8-11). They occur in those ages 20–24, followed by those ages 25–29, then ages 15–19.

HIV infection and other sexually transmitted diseases share the same risk factors. The major difference between HIV/AIDS and the other STDs is the degree of cell and tissue destruction and the mortality of HIV/AIDS.

HIV is transmitted most often during sexual contact with an infected partner. There is abundant evidence that if a sexual partner has an active STD, especially one that causes an ulcer, he or she is at greater risk of becoming HIV-infected (Laga, 1991).

The types of blood cells, lymphocytes, or macrophages most likely to become infected if exposed to HIV tend to collect in the genital tract of people with STDs. This makes an STD-infected person both more likely to transmit HIV and more vulnerable to it (Laga, 1991).

Pediatric Transmission

Children can acquire HIV from their mothers in several ways. A pregnant HIV-infected woman can transmit the virus to her fetus in utero (during gestation) as the virus crosses over from the mother into the fetal bloodstream (Jovaisas et al., 1985; St. Louis et al., 1993). At least 50% of newborn infections occur during delivery by ingesting blood or other infected maternal fluids (Scott et al., 1985; Boyer et al., 1994; Kuhn, et al., 1994). If breast-fed, the newborn may also become infected from breast milk (Zigler et al., 1985; DeMartino et al., 1992; Van DePerre et al., 1993). In case reports, three women who contracted HIV by blood transfusions immediately after

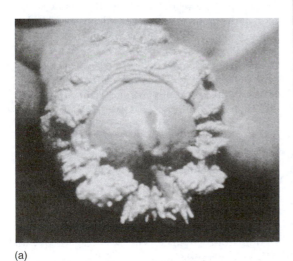

(a)

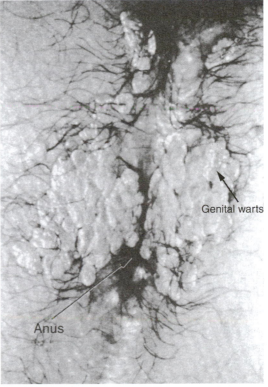

Genital warts

Anus

(b)

FIGURE 8-10 (a) **Genital Warts of the Male.** Multiple warts or condylomas that are scattered around the front edge of the foreskin and back along the penile shaft. (b) **Genital Warts of the Female.** (*Photographs courtesy of the Centers for Disease Control and Prevention, Atlanta.*)

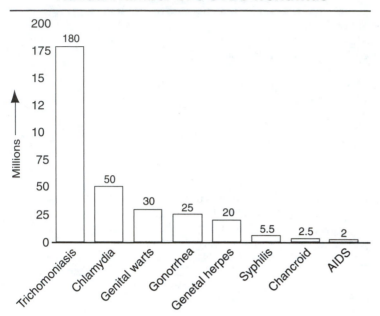

Annual Number of 8 STDs Worldwide

Millions

200
180
175
15
12
10
75
50 — 50
30
25 — 25
20
5.5
2.5
2
0

Trichomoniasis Chlamydia Genital warts Gonorrhea Genetal herpes Syphilis Chancroid AIDS

FIGURE 8-11 Global Incidence of Seven Sexually Transmitted and AIDS Disease, ages 15 to 49. According to the CDC, 50% of STDs in the United States are unreported and 50% to 90% of STDs worldwide are unreported.

birth subsequently infected their newborns via breast-feeding (Curran et al., 1988). Other studies suggest that the risk of HIV transmission through breast-feeding is increased if the mother becomes HIV-infected during lactation (Hu et al., 1992).

The relative efficiency of these three routes of infection is unknown. However, the data on mothers' milk add to the urgency of learning more about mucosal transmission. The most likely explanation for HIV transmission through breast-feeding is that the virus penetrates the mucosal lining of the mouth or gastrointestinal tract of infants. If this occurs in newborns, then what of older children, adolescents, and adults? Does the mucosal lining change with development and become HIV resistant?

HIV-Infected Babies—One major problem in perinatal transmission is how to determine which babies are truly HIV infected as opposed to just carrying the mother's HIV antibodies (which would produce a false-positive test). HIV transmission can occur during pregnancy (in utero), as well as at the time of delivery (**intrapartum**) and through breast milk. HIV transmission is more likely if virus can be cultured from the mother's blood, or if she has later-stage HIV disease, or if her T4 or CD4+ counts are low; and is more likely to occur in the firstborn than

in the secondborn of twins. A baby automatically acquires the mother's antibodies and may carry them for two or more years. Usually by 18 months of age, most of the mother's antibodies will be gone. The babies may then begin to show signs of clinical AIDS-related illness (see Chapter 13 for a discussion of nucleic acid testing of newborns).

Although the rate of perinatal and breast milk HIV transmission is unknown, evidence from 1986 into year 2009 indicates that over 90% of pediatric AIDS cases acquired the virus in utero from an HIV-infected mother after the first trimester or during the birthing process. In 1990, researchers concluded that a fetus can become infected as early as the eighth week of gestation (Lewis et al., 1990). HIV has been isolated from a 20-week-old fetus after elective abortion by an HIV-positive female and from a 28-week-old newborn delivered by cesarean section from a female who was diagnosed with AIDS (Selwyn, 1986).

Probability of an HIV-Positive Mother Infecting Her Fetus

Reports on the probability of a fetus becoming HIV infected when the **untreated** mother carries the virus vary widely. Without antiretroviral drug therapy, the most often-quoted estimate in the United States is about 30%. With drug therapy the risk to the fetus can be reduced to about 2%.

Other than viral load, there is little documented information on maternal factors that influence vertical transmission. As with other congenital infections, only one of a pair of twins may be HIV infected (Newell et al., 1990; Ometto, 1995). A mother's clinical status during pregnancy and the duration of her infection (stage of disease) may be important, but evidence remains circumstantial (see Chapter 11 for update information). Studies to determine mother-to-fetus transmission relative to stage of disease are in progress.

According to the CDC classification, children under age 13 are considered pediatric AIDS cases. They make up about 0.8% of all AIDS cases in the United States. Through 2008, about 5% of reported pediatric male AIDS cases occurred due to blood transfusions, 3% received HIV-contaminated blood factor VIII used in treating hemophiliacs, and in 2%, the cause was undetermined.

The largest numbers of pediatric AIDS cases through 2008 were in New York, Florida, California, and New Jersey, in that order. The highest incidence of all pediatric cases occurs in minority populations. By early 2009, there were over 9700 pediatric AIDS cases in the United States. Blacks and Hispanics make up 12.5% and 13% of the United States population, respectively, yet make up 55% and 20%, respectively, of all pediatric AIDS cases. Thus 75% of pediatric AIDS cases occur within two minority populations.

Vertical Infection: HIV-Infected Childbearing-Age Women

Over 100,000 women of childbearing age are estimated to be infected with HIV in the United States. The majority of these women may not know they are infected; they are identified as infected only after their children are diagnosed as having an HIV infection or AIDS. It is not uncommon for HIV-infected women to go through several pregnancies before they express HIV disease. Also, there are women who become pregnant knowing they are HIV positive. They want to have a baby regardless (see Chapter 11).

Mother-to-fetus infection or **vertical infection** could be avoided by avoiding pregnancy, but this is possible only in cases where the female is aware of her infection and takes measures to prevent pregnancy (birth control or tubal ligation). In many cases, pregnancy occurred before the mother knew she was carrying the virus. In other cases, the mother has become infected after she has become pregnant.

CESAREAN SECTION

The time-honored surgical maxim, "A chance to cut is a chance to cure," takes on new meaning in the debate now raging about **cesarean section** as a means of reducing perinatal HIV transmission. From 1998 through 2008, clinicians have shown that the use of antiretroviral drugs and cesarean section to deliver a newborn from an HIV-infected mother has reduced the risk of HIV infection to 1% or 2%. Perhaps the greatest news to come out of this pandemic to this point in time is the fact that the HIV epidemic for newborns in the United States is about over! However, each year, about 400,000 children who are under 15 become infected with HIV through mother-to-child transmission, and 90% of these are in Africa. In the worst affected countries of sub-Saharan Africa, HIV infection rates between 10% and 30% are common among pregnant women, and much higher rates have been reported in many villages. Only a relatively small number of such women currently have access to preventive measures such as antiretroviral drugs for the protection of their babies. At the United Nations Special Session on HIV/AIDS in 2001, governments from 189 countries committed themselves to halving the rate of Mother to Child Transmission (MTCT) by 2010.

Possible Antiretroviral Drugs to Prevent Maternal HIV Transmission

Current concepts on the prevention of vertical transmission now focus on the appropriate antiretroviral therapy of infected pregnant women. Despite the data from ACTG 076, zidovudine monotherapy alone can no longer be considered adequate for pregnant women because some newborns are still HIV positive. Some HIV/AIDS experts recommend the use of combination therapy that includes a protease inhibitor. In March 1999, five important studies were published regarding the use of combination antiretrovirals to reduce mother-to-infant transmission. The conclusion to be drawn from the studies is that antiretroviral prophylaxis of mother and her infant is very effective. With many women on HAART therapy during pregnancy, there were less than 100 HIV-infected infants born in the United States in 2003 through 2008. However, in developing countries, despite recent progress, there is still a great need for shorter, inexpensive, effective

BOX 8.6

HIV AND SENIOR CITIZENS

Looking at the majority of safer sex workshops and street outreach programs, one would get the impression that only the young are at risk of contracting HIV. It's true that most people with AIDS are under 49. But, according to the CDC, now about 13% of Americans who test positive for the virus are over the age of 50. It's not just with regard to prevention that over-50s are left behind. Older people with HIV are often misdiagnosed and typically learn they have the virus only later in the disease process. Medical treatment is more difficult because of both the later diagnosis and factors related to age. Few practitioners are expert both in HIV and the health problems associated with aging. When it comes to social support services aimed at their particular needs, older HIV-infected people are all but invisible. Attitudes about HIV/AIDS and aging reflect misconceptions about how people behave in the second half-century of their lives.

1. Old people are no longer interested in sex;
2. If they are interested, no one's interested in them;
3. If they do have sex, it's within a monogamous, heterosexual relationship;

4. They don't do drugs;
5. If they ever did, it's so long ago it doesn't matter.

It isn't hard to see how these misconceptions help erect barriers to effective HIV/AIDS prevention efforts, medical care, and social services for the late middle-aged and elderly. After all, if they're not doing anything risky, there's nothing to worry about, right? **WRONG,** older adults refuse to conform to the stereotypes.

GENDER AND AGE

Older women are becoming HIV infected at a higher rate than older men. No longer afraid of becoming pregnant, the postmenopausal woman who is uninformed of the danger of HIV transmission may become more sexually active, with more partners, and may give up a decades-old habit of using condoms. Even her biology increases her risk: After menopause, the vaginal walls thin and vaginal lubrication decreases. Thus, the vaginal membranes are more likely to tear during intercourse, providing easier access to HIV.

---

regimens. But the debate continues on when to begin therapy—first, second, or third trimester?

(For an excellent review of mother-to-child transmission of HIV, see the article by Peckham et al., 1995.)

CONCLUSION

Although only one new route (prechewed food) of HIV transmission has surfaced over the last 27 years of this pandemic, many people still do not believe that's all there is. People still make the arguments that: (1) Scientists do not yet know enough about this disease to be certain there are no other routes of transmission; and (2) scientists know other routes exist but are either too frightened to tell the truth, or are under political pressure not to do so for fear of creating a public panic. Many thousands of people in the United States firmly believe that in a few years they will look back and say "I told you so: You can get HIV from HIV-infected people if they breathe on you or if you touch their sweat and so on."

DISCUSSION QUESTION: How do you get everyone to believe what medical and research scientists say? Should we get everyone to believe scientific dogma?

NATIONAL AIDS RESOURCES

AIDS Action Council	1-202-547-3101
Coalition for Leadership on AIDS	1-202-628-4160
Gay Men's Health Crisis	1-212-807-6655
Mothers of AIDS Patients	1-619-234-3432
National AIDS Information Clearinghouse	1-301-762-5111
National AIDS Network	1-202-546-2424
National Association of Persons with AIDS	1-202-483-7979
Project Inform (Alternative AIDS Info)	1-800-822-7422
Public Health Service Hotline	1-800-342-2437

Centers for Disease   1-404-639-2070
    Control and Prevention
    Technical Information
American Red Cross,   1-202-639-3223
    National AIDS Education
Guide to Social Security   1-800-772-1213
    and SSI Disability
    Benefits for People
    with HIV Infection

(You can write or call for this Social Security brochure: Social Security Administration, Public Information Distribution Center, P.O. Box 17743, Baltimore, MD., 21235.)

Summary

The World Health Organization began keeping records of AIDS–like cases in 1980. Beginning 2009, there were an estimated 56 million HIV/AIDS cases in 194 reporting countries and territories. About 22 million of these have died. About 2% of AIDS cases have occurred in the United States. At the start of 2009, of the 34 million living with HIV infection worldwide, about 3% or over 1,000,000 live in the United States. It has been reported that the first cases of AIDS entered the United States via homosexual men who had vacationed in Haiti in the late 1970s. However, there is evidence of AIDS cases in the United States as early as 1952. While testing West Africans for HIV infection, a second strain of HIV was discovered: HIV-2. Both are transmitted in the same manner and both cause AIDS. However, HIV-2 appears to be less pathogenic than HIV-1.

Nearly all Americans are aware that HIV can be transmitted through unprotected intercourse, the sharing of intravenous (IV) needles, and unprotected oral sex. Less than half, however, know that having another sexually transmitted disease (STD) increases a person's risk for HIV. In addition, even after years of public education, unwarranted fears of infection through casual contact persist. For example, about one in five Americans incorrectly believes that sharing a drinking glass can transmit HIV, or are unsure about the risk of this activity. Sixteen percent believe that touching a toilet seat can transmit HIV or are unsure about the risk. Such views contribute to discrimination and stigma, which can interfere with public health efforts to encourage early testing and care.

There are two major variables involved in successful HIV transmission and infection. First is the individual's genetic resistance or susceptibility, and second is the route of transmission. Not all modes of HIV exposure are equally apt to cause infection, even in the most susceptible individual. There have been a number of studies and empirical observations that demonstrate that HIV *is not* casually acquired. HIV is difficult to acquire even by means of the recognized routes of transmission.

HIV is transmitted mainly via sexual activities involving the exchange of semen and vaginal fluids, through the exchange of blood and blood products, and from mother to child both prenatally and postnatally (breast milk). Besides a few cases of breast milk transmission, no other body fluids have as yet been implicated in HIV infection.

The current belief is that anal receptive homosexuals have a higher risk than heterosexuals of acquiring HIV because the membrane or mucosal lining of the rectum is more easily torn during anal intercourse. This allows a more direct route for larger numbers of HIVs to enter the vascular system.

Others at high risk for acquiring and transmitting HIV are injection-drug users. They infect each other when they share drug paraphernalia. Changes in sexual and injection drug use behavior can virtually stop HIV transmission among these people.

CHALLENGE YOUR ASSUMPTIONS ABOUT THE HIV INFECTED

There is an Internet game called "POS OR NOT" that aims to increase HIV/AIDS awareness. The web site, **posornot.com**, shows photographs and short biographies of men and women ages 21 to 30 and asks visitors to determine if each is HIV positive or not. The message from this exercise is that you can't judge someone's HIV status by looks, occupation, or taste in music.

PLAY THE GAME AND SEE IF YOU CAN TELL WHO IS HIV POSITIVE OR NOT

Review Questions

(Answers to the Review Questions are on pages 427–428).

1. True or False: Africa makes up the largest percentage of *reported* AIDS cases worldwide. Explain.

2. What evidence is there that HIV may have evolved in the United States and Africa at the same time?

3. Are HIV-1 and HIV-2 related? Explain.

4. True or False: HIV-1 and HIV-2 are transmitted differently and therefore are located in geographically distinct regions of the world. Explain.

5. True or False: HIV is *not* believed to be casually transmitted. Explain.

6. Name the routes of HIV transmission.

7. True or False: Deep kissing wherein saliva is exchanged is a direct route for *efficient* HIV transmission. Explain.

8. True or False: Insects that bite or suck have been claimed to be associated with HIV transmission. Explain.

9. True or False: Among heterosexuals, HIV transmission from male to female and from female to male are equally efficient. Explain.

10. True or False: If a person has unprotected intercourse with an HIV-infected partner he or she will become HIV infected. Explain.

11. What is the percentage of risk that a developing fetus with an HIV-positive mother in America will be born HIV positive, with and without zidovudine therapy? With zidovudine and C-section?

12. Despite the warnings, groups that continue to engage in high-risk sexual activity include:

    A. high school students
    B. black women
    C. injection-drug users
    D. prostitutes
    E. all of the above

13. True or False: Prior to 1985, use of blood component therapy put hemophiliacs at risk for contracting HIV.

14. True or False: Relapse to risky sexual behavior can be an important source of new HIV infection in the homosexual community.

15. True or False: The body fluids shown most likely to transmit HIV are blood, semen, vaginal secretions, and breast milk.

16. True or False: Participation in risky behaviors and not identification with particular groups puts an individual at risk of acquiring HIV infection.

17. True or False: Unprotected receptive anal intercourse is the sexual activity with the greatest risk of HIV transmission.

18. True or False: Women who are HIV infected always transmit the virus to their fetus during pregnancy or delivery.

19. True or False: A person infected with HIV can transmit the virus from the first occurrence of antigenemia throughout the rest of his/her life.

20. True or False: Women constitute the fastest-growing segment of the population with HIV infection.

21. True or False: The majority of HIV-infected women whose source of infection is known became infected through vaginal intercourse.

22. True or False: HIV infection in children is now a leading cause of death in children between the ages of 1 and 4.

23. True or False: Sexual contact is the major route of HIV transmission among black Americans.

24. True or False: Urine is one body fluid that remains an unproven route of HIV transmission.

25. Which of the following is not a recognized mode of HIV transmission?

    A. unprotected sex with an infected partner
    B. mosquito bite
    C. contact with infected blood or blood products
    D. perinatal transmission

26. True or False: Only drug users and gay men need to worry about becoming infected with HIV.

27. You can become infected with HIV by

    A. sharing utensils with or drinking from the same cup as someone with HIV.

    B. mosquito bites.

    C. hugging someone with HIV.

    D. none of the above.

28. True or False: Using protection such as a latex barrier when performing sex (vaginal, oral, or anal) lowers the risk of HIV transmission.

29. HIV is not present in

    A. semen and vaginal secretions.

    B. sweat.

    C. blood.

    D. breast milk.

30. What major role do asymptomatic people with the HIV disease play in the epidemiology of AIDS?

Preventing the Transmission of HIV

9

The best time to plant a tree is 20 years ago. The second best time is now.

African Proverb

CHAPTER CONCEPTS

- An HIV/AIDS-free generation can begin with you.
- Prevention is today's vaccine.
- HIV transmission can be prevented; the responsibility rests with the individual.
- No new routes of HIV transmission have been found after 26 years.
- Safer sex essentially means using condoms and not knowingly having intercourse with an HIV-infected person.
- Demand and supply of male/female condom, selected countries.
- Government-imposed warning labels on male condoms.
- Obstacles to condom education and distribution.
- The female condom (vaginal pouch) was FDA-approved in 1993.
- Oil-based lubricants must not be used with latex condoms.
- Plastic condoms are now available.
- Polymer gel condoms are being developed.
- Microbicides, their time come?
- Free syringe and needle exchange programs claim to help lower the incidence of HIV transmission.
- Blood bank screening to detect HIV antibodies began in 1985.
- Universal precautions and blood and body substance isolation are techniques to help healthcare workers prevent infection.
- Universal precautions require certain body fluids from all patients to be considered potentially infectious.
- Blood and Body Substance Isolation (BBSI).
- Partner notification is a means of notifying at-risk partners of HIV-infected individuals.
- Vaccines, the Holy Grail against disease.
- Vaccines are made from whole or parts of dead microorganisms, inactivated viruses, or attenuated viruses, microorganisms, and naked DNA.
- Experimental subunit vaccines are prepared using recombinant DNA techniques.
- There is no effective vaccine for prevention of HIV infection. All experimental vaccines to date have failed.
- Russian and Indian scientists believe they will have an effective HIV vaccine in the next 10 to 15 years.
- Global AIDS vaccine trial sites.

Don't walk in front of me, I may not follow. Don't walk behind me, I may not lead. Just walk beside me and be my friend.

Albert Camus

The first major HIV/AIDS benefit song was "That's What Friends Are For."

Carole Bayer Sager
Sung by Dionne Warwick,
Radio City Music Hall,
New York City, March 17, 1990

An HIV/AIDS-free generation can begin with you! LEARN: EDUCATE–DONATE–PARTICIPATE: VOLUNTEER

THE AIDS GENERATION: "I KNEW EVERYTHING ABOUT IT, AND I STILL GOT IT!"

The "magic bullet" to cure or prevent HIV infection has not been found, and too many people with or affected by HIV/AIDS are isolated by cultural, geographic, and economic barriers. HIV is a preventable disease and the first step in preventing disease is the transformation of information into knowledge and getting people to use that knowledge. For example, the slogan "Practice Safer Sex" is now as common as "Buckle Up For Safety" and "Just Say No To Drugs," but HIV infections among age groups over 12 continues at an alarming pace.

Educated people know how HIV is spread and what to do about it, but nevertheless they get carried away and ignore precautions in the heat of passion. As it is written, "Hormones will always trump neurons." A teenager who was told her drug-addicted boyfriend was HIV positive said, "I know he loves me and would never do anything to hurt me." In the face of such emotional responses, what chance do precautions or prevention have in succeeding?

Some scientists have convinced themselves that AIDS is not caused by HIV but by antiretroviral drugs. Worse yet, they have succeeded in convincing politically powerful figures, setting back HIV/AIDS control programs for years as in the case of South Africa. That country's leaders have changed their views, but the damage has been done. (See Chapter 2 for a discussion on AIDS dissidents.)

Nothing can be more important to a state than its public health; the state's paramount concern should be the health of its people.

Franklin Delano Roosevelt
32nd President of the United States

PREVENTION, NOT TREATMENT, IS THE LEAST EXPENSIVE AND MOST EFFECTIVE WAY TO STOP THE SPREAD OF HIV/AIDS

"How we define the problem determines our solution."

Jonathan Mann
(Former head of the World
Health Organization's Global
Program on AIDS, deceased).

Twenty-seven years into one of the worst health disasters in human history, the HIV/AIDS pandemic continues to grow exponentially, outstripping prevention efforts and treatment programs; every day it kills about 6,000 people and infects about 7,000 more. The global effort is inadequate to check its spread or stop the deaths. **The HIV/AIDS pandemic is almost, if not actually, incomprehensible in size and scope. And in the developing world, this pandemic may be in its early stages! Two things are now clear: the first is that treatment will not greatly effect the transmission or spread of HIV, and second, treatment/prevention is not an either/or choice—both are vital. But, what can be done now that will change the course of this pandemic? Something has to be done! What can be done and by whom? The world must engage in the largest possible dissemination of HIV prevention strategies and develop a vaccine.**

Primary Goal of HIV Prevention

The primary goal of HIV prevention is to prevent as many infections as possible. This requires allocating HIV prevention resources according to cost-effectiveness principles: Those activities that prevent more infections per dollar are favored over those that prevent fewer. This is not current practice in the United States, where prevention resources from the federal government to the states flow in proportion to reported AIDS cases. Although such allocations might be considered equitable, more infections could be prevented for the same expenditures were cost-effectiveness principles invoked. The downside of pure cost-effective allocations is that they violate common norms of equity. In 2009 the CDC wants to allocate about $900 million for HIV prevention programs in the United States.

GLOBAL PREVENTION

"I think we have to divide the world as we would like it to be from the world as it is."

Thomas R. Frieden
Health Commissioner,
New York City, 2002

When it comes to HIV/AIDS, there is no first world or third world. This is one global pandemic that requires a commitment to science-based methods of prevention and therapy to address the biologic process of infection and disease. Because we live in a global village, the public health of Africa, Asia, and elsewhere affects the public health of the United States. As there is one global economy, there is one global public health. Prevention of infectious diseases in any country is prevention for all. In each of the years from 1998 through 2008, on average, an estimated 1.5 million people died from AIDS. Worldwide by the end of 2009, about 24 million people will have died of AIDS. About 80% of these deaths will be in Africa. While waiting for an effective vaccine, how can the out-of-control spread of HIV be slowed? How can people everywhere be saved from HIV infection? In a word, **prevention** is the only hope short of a vaccine.

First: No magic bullet exists for preventing HIV/AIDS. The global HIV epidemic cannot be reversed, and gains in expanding treatment access cannot be sustained, without greater progress in reducing the rate of new HIV infections.

Second: Existing prevention strategies can be effective in reducing the risk of HIV exposure, but prevention programs, especially in countries with concentrated epidemics, fail to reach many people at high risk of exposure to HIV, including a majority of men who have sex with men and injection-drug users.

Third: Young people aged 15 to 24 account for 45% of all new HIV infections in adults, and many young people still lack accurate, complete information on how to avoid exposure to the virus. While HIV testing, condom use, and abstinence are important, it is more likely that promoting partner reduction and male circumcision will prove to be the more effective prevention choices.

Fourth: Sustaining prevention gains represents one of the great challenges in HIV prevention. To maintain a robust prevention response, countries need to nurture a "prevention movement," build the hu-man and technical capacity needed to sustain prevention efforts, and work to simulate greater demand for prevention services. (UNAIDS, August 2008)

Stop, listen, and learn all you can about HIV/AIDS. Prevention and life—it's your choice!

Investing in Prevention

Spending money on prevention is a smart investment. For example, in America, the CDC's goal is to lower the HIV infection rate from their estimated 56,000 each year to 28,000. A 2003 study by HIV economists at Emory University estimated that preventing 50% of new HIV infections yearly would save about $22 billion in medical costs by 2010. Current prevention efforts have already averted at least 250,000 HIV infections in America over the last 26 years. That would translate into about $35 billion to $70 billion already saved in medical costs. The potential for HIV prevention interventions to save lives and dollars emphasizes the need to spend money now rather than later, and to maintain consistent, if not increasing, funding to protect those at high risk. At the 2002 Fourteenth International AIDS Conference, Michael Saag reported that in the United States, health care for each patient in the advanced stages of AIDS costs an average of $34,000 a year. Antiretroviral medicines make up the largest part of the cost. The cost of treating the average patient with HIV is about $14,000. Overall, medication costs were about $11,000–$24,000. Hospital costs were second, ranging from an average of $1700 for early stage patients to $7800 for those with advanced AIDS. Taking the average of $14,000 and $34,000 or $24,000 times 1.2 million people living with HIV/AIDS in America comes to about $29 billion! Estimates are that about 700,000 people in 2008 received some measure of care for their HIV infection. Their total healthcare cost is estimated to be $13.8 billion a year (see Figure 14-9 for year 2008 federal dollars allocated to HIV/AIDS). America's prevention budget for 2009 is near $1 billion. The bottom line is, governments and their people must invest in prevention.

At the moment, globally about two plus million people are receiving antiretroviral drugs, but each year between two million and three million people become newly infected—so, for every case that goes into treatment, two or three more people join the back of the line that will require therapy. **Question; Are the prolonged care and costs of** therapy **sustainable over the next 20 to 50 years even if a vaccine is found?** The estimated cost for care programs, prevention, and therapy by 2010, just in the United States, is over $25 billion and rising annually thereafter.

ANTIRETROVIRAL DRUGS HAVING AN IMPACT ON PREVENTION, BUT WE CAN'T TREAT OUR WAY OUT OF THIS PANDEMIC

Drug Therapy Benefits Prevention

There is a variety of evidence supporting HAART's beneficial effect on HIV prevention, both in preventing HIV infection of HIV-negative persons and in the transmission of infection from HIV-positive persons to others.

Some Examples:

- **First,** the provision of antiretroviral treatment to HIV-infected women and their infants around the time of delivery has been shown to significantly reduce mother-to-child transmission.

- **Second,** follow-up of healthcare workers exposed to HIV through needle stick injuries or other accidental contact with body fluids found that persons taking antiretroviral post-exposure prophylaxis (PEP) were less likely to become infected compared to those who did not. The concept has now been extended to the general public. (See chapter 4 for discussion.)

- **Third,** this point is a bit less direct. HAART can dramatically reduce the levels of virus in the blood. The lower blood levels of HIV lowers the chance of HIV being sexually transmitted.

- **Fourth** is the value antiretroviral therapy has in promoting HIV testing. A precondition of reducing your risk is knowing your HIV status. With the availability of antiretroviral therapy and its ability to extend lives, people now have reason to be tested.

- **Fifth:** Increasing use of antiretroviral drugs, by high-risk people prior to engaging in sexual activities, is needed to prevent infection or pre-exposure prophylaxis (PrEP)—see Chapter 4 for discussion.

  One of the most important preventive measures available is for people to get tested, to learn their HIV status. This information (a) helps those infected to seek proper care and (b) helps the infected protect their sexual partners. Drug therapy, HIV testing, and risk prevention are a dynamic trio.

Drug Therapy Harming Prevention?

Increases in sexual risk behavior in recent years have led to heated discussion on the role of treatment in HIV transmission. In other words, HAART has dramatically improved the length of survival and the physical well-being of persons living with HIV/AIDS and thus has increased their opportunity to transmit HIV to others.

CONCLUSION—The trade-offs between the potential benefits of HAART in reducing the likelihood of HIV transmission and the potential harm resulting from increased risk behavior are very complex and involve moral, ethical, and economic considerations.

Prevention Is a Matter of Choice

"Being a man or a woman is a matter of birth. Being a person who makes a difference is a matter of choice."

Byron Garrett

Prevention is a hard sell. It is easier to get thousands of dollars to rescue a baby down a well than it is to get a few hundred dollars to cover old wells.

The fact that there is no cure for HIV/AIDS, no vaccine in the immediate future, and that drugs are costly and cause severe side effects, makes prevention crucial. CDC researchers reviewed 83 studies from 1978 through 1998. They found that as soon as prevention education began in the early 1980s, the rate of new HIV infections plummeted and that it has remained relatively stable, at about 56,000 new infections a year.

The means of preventing HIV infection exist. They must be used effectively to make an impact on this escalating pandemic. **HIV prevention does not have to be perfect to be effective.** The existing methods of HIV prevention are presented in this chapter.

Prevention, Is Anyone Listening?

Why do people knowingly engage in sexual behavior that can lead to a slow and painful premature death? Why do the best-intentioned HIV prevention programs often have so little impact?

WHY ARE THE EXPERTS SAYING THAT CURRENT PREVENTION METHODS ARE FAILING, THAT NEW PREVENTION MESSAGES MUST BE BROUGHT OUT WITH RENEWED VIGOR?

If the global approaches to HIV/AIDS prevention are working, then how do we account for the annual two to three million people who will become infected with HIV and the two million others who will die? This latter figure may not register very well, but it is the equivalent of about twenty 747s crashing every day into a mountain. Unless we address the underlying causes of HIV/AIDS, society can look ahead to an expansion of the pandemic over the next 20 years, especially in countries like China, India, and Russia. Some epidemiologists forecast 100 million people infected by 2025, mostly through sexual transmission and nearly all in poor countries. (And add to this scenario that many millions of HIV- negative people are and will be impacted by this disease.) To escape that fate, all countries must support measures that help women achieve an equal place in society and must seriously underwrite social and economic progress. Strong support for community-driven structural interventions is desperately needed now to turn back this pandemic, which threatens the health and stability of women in many poor countries, and by extension, the whole world.

SO WHAT'S WRONG WITH WHAT WE'VE BEEN DOING?

Globally, for decades HIV/AIDS program planners have been developing prevention interventions to modify the behaviors that put people at risk. Typically, they have been limited in scope and duration. Efforts focus on prostitutes and their clients, homosexual men and intravenous drug users, each with its own label and built-in potential for stigma and discrimination. Promotions of abstinence, being faithful, or using condoms (ABC) are now common in many programs. But the same behavior change strategies don't work for everyone, especially the millions of women who have no risk factor other than being married. Studies in communities across Africa and Asia reveal that as many as three out of four HIV-positive monogamous women are infected by their husbands. For 22 years, HIV/AIDS mainly affected men. Over the next six years, half the people in the world living with HIV were women and, in some areas, as many as 60% are women. In short, the main factors that make women, especially young women, more vulnerable to HIV/AIDS are widespread gender inequality, i.e., their low social status combined with the effects of severe poverty. These structural factors explain why HIV/AIDS prevention interventions that focus on behavior and risk alone will, in the long run, fail. Designing prevention interventions without aggressively addressing the structural factors of inequality and poverty is essentially akin to applying band-aids to a hemorrhage or believing that you can change the global tides by running your tap water down your drain.

UNITED STATES

Progress in the diagnosis and prevention of HIV in the United States has stalled. Over the past 27 years more than half a million Americans have died of HIV/AIDS. But, while mortality rates decreased by a remarkable 75% with the advent of antiretroviral therapy, there has been no improvement in stopping new HIV infections. What is the current reality? New HIV diagnoses are slightly rising. Late diagnoses are common, as is high-risk behavior. Partner notification is rare, as is counseling of HIV-positive patients to avoid transmission of the disease. Put it all together and you have over 56,000 new cases of HIV each year, wherein 20% of the infected caused about 80% of the new infections, and 40% of these will exhibit AIDS within one year of their very late diagnosis. Yet, it is estimated that one-half to two-thirds of all of these new cases are preventable. In New York City, where one in every six HIV/AIDS patients lives, only one-third of adults with three or more sexual partners in the past year had been tested for HIV in the prior 18 months. A New York study of more than 4000 HIV patients revealed that less than 20% of partners had been notified, and less than 5% of partners had been tested. Yet, studies indicate that risky behavior declines by half in those who know they are HIV positive.

A UNIVERSAL APPROACH TO HIV/AIDS PREVENTION?

A universal approach to prevention could include early partner notification, risk-education counseling, comprehensive quality care, including mental health and substance abuse treatment, CD4 level monitoring and reporting, drug resistance monitoring, and mandatory HIV testing. As has recently been suggested by the CDC, it could also include routine HIV testing for those between ages 13 and 64, to allow population surveillance and treatment. Is this feasible on a global basis? Probably not. But it could be accomplished in the developed nations, especially the United States, if HIV/AIDS were treated like any other sexually transmitted disease. (CLASS DISCUSSION, PRO/CON)

Robert Smith of HIV Edmonton, Canada, and Michael Yoder, chairman of the Canadian AIDS society reported at the Fourteenth International AIDS Conference that North American prevention programs are failing. They believe it's back to the drawing board for the AIDS community that has discovered, to its horror, that no one seems to care about safer sex anymore. (Safer sex means any sexual activity that prevents HIV or other STDs within semen, vaginal fluid, or blood from entering the bloodstream of another person.) People are not listening: **Too few are getting tested.** After 27 years of being bombarded with safer sex messages, you'd think everyone in North America would know how to protect themselves from HIV and other sexually transmitted diseases. As health professionals are becoming increasingly aware, getting the facts out is one thing—doing it in a way that changes people's behavior is another.

Among the depressing reports out of the 2002 International AIDS Conference in Spain is a study showing that most of the young, gay, HIV-positive men in major U.S. cities are unaware that they're infected. More than half the HIV-positive men who didn't know they had the virus considered themselves at low risk of HIV infection and nearly half of them reported they didn't use condoms. They concluded that in North America, young people seem to be fed up with hearing about AIDS. These data remain true through 2008.

Internationally, it seems, there is similar skepticism. At the same conference, the Joint United Nations Program on HIV/AIDS (UNAIDS) quoted grim statistics on a pandemic still in its early stages, with no stabilization of the epidemic in Africa and with exploding epidemics in Eastern Europe and Central Asia. Although the conference was full of stories about how prevention programs across the world are making a difference, the overall message focused on the staggering numbers of people living with HIV and the need for prevention and improved care. This message has been repeated at every International AIDS conference since 2002.

A Virtual Vaccine to Prevent HIV/AIDS: Education

With regard to HIV infection, there is no available vaccine against the virus, but there is a **virtual vaccine** (meaning a procedure as effective as a preventative vaccine): **education.** Thus, the leading primary preventative is education: teaching people how to adjust their behavior to reduce or eliminate HIV exposure. Because the vast majority of HIV infec-

tions are transmitted through consensual acts between adolescents or adults, the individual has a choice as to whether to risk infection or not.

Despite widely supported educational efforts at both institutional and street levels, a large number of gay males, drug abusers, and heterosexuals continue to participate in **unsafe sexual practices.** Unsafe sex is defined as having sex without using a condom. This allows the exchange of potentially infectious body fluids such as blood, semen, and vaginal secretions. Unsafe sex most often occurs among gay men and with injection-drug users, by bartering sex for drugs, and by having sex with multiple partners. The sharp increase in the use of crack cocaine and its connection to trading sex for drugs has led to a dramatic rise in almost all sexually transmitted diseases.

Safer Sex

The idea of *safer* **sexual practices** began in the early 1980s and now refers almost exclusively to the use of a latex or plastic condom with or without a spermicide. It should be remembered that for many generations of people in the United States, unsafe sex was the norm, but since HIV, people are asked to make safer sex the norm.

Among the severely drug addicted, concerns about personal safety and survival are secondary to drug procurement and use. Thus, their range of unsafe behaviors leads to random sex and sex without condoms. These behaviors are in part responsible for the increased incidence of HIV and other sexually transmitted diseases (Weinstein et al., 1990).

Comparing HIV/AIDS Prevention to Cancer

AIDS prevention is, in a sense, more essential than, say, cancer prevention. Preventing one HIV infection now will not simply prevent one death from AIDS, as preventing one incurable cancer would prevent one cancer death. Preventing an HIV infection now will help break the chain of transmission, averting the risk that the infected person will knowingly or unknowingly pass the virus on to others who in turn might infect a still wider circle of people.

ADVANCING HIV PREVENTION: NEW STRATEGIES FOR A CHANGING EPIDEMIC

In April 2003 the Centers for Disease Control and Prevention (CDC), in partnership with other U.S.

HIV/STD PREVENTION EDUCATION—UNITED STATES

THE FOUR Cs OF PREVENTION EDUCATION: THE MESSAGE MUST BE CLEAR, CONSISTENT, COMPELLING, AND COORDINATED.

Eliminating all unsafe sex is not a reasonable goal. Preventing all future HIV and STD infections is impossible, but striving for anything less is unacceptable.

Since 1988, CDC has provided fiscal and technical assistance to state and local education agencies and national health and education organizations to assist schools in implementing effective HIV and STD prevention education for youth. These agencies and organizations develop, implement, and evaluate HIV/STD prevention policies and programs and train teachers to initiate effective prevention efforts and implement curricula in classrooms. As a result of these and other efforts, school-based HIV/STD education is widely implemented in the United States. From 1987 through 2008, the number of states requiring HIV/STD prevention education in schools increased from 13 states to 40 states plus the District of Columbia. This high level of policy support is consistent with public support; 93% of U.S. residents in a 2004 survey reported that information about AIDS and STDs should be provided in school.

The findings in this survey indicate that, despite wide implementation of HIV/STD prevention education in U.S. schools, improvements in prevention programs are still needed. In particular, efforts are needed to increase the percentage of teachers who teach HIV/STD prevention in a health education setting and who receive inservice training on HIV/STD prevention.

THE 10-LETTER SOUP OF PREVENTION: ABCCDEFGH AND I

Gita Ramjee of the South African Medical Research Council said, "I would like to believe that HIV prevention is more than ABC—Abstinence, Be faithful, if not use a Condom." He wants to add one more C for circumcision (see Chapter 8); add D for diaphragm; E for pre- and post-exposure drugs (Chapter 4); F for female microbicides (Chapter 9); G for genital tract infections; H for herpes virus suppression (Chapter 8); and I for immunity by vaccines (Chapter 9).

Department of Health and Human Services agencies, other government agencies, and nongovernment agencies (NGOs) decided to change their **primary** prevention strategy, in use for the past 23 years—preventing HIV infection among the at-risk uninfected, to the **secondary** prevention strategy of preventing HIV transmission by those who are infected and their sexual partners. The secondary prevention mission involves a large federal monetary investment in initiatives that offer HIV testing and counseling to the HIV infected. This marks a substantial shift in priorities. At stake is some $90 million that the federal government provides to community groups for HIV prevention each year.

The new strategy, now in place, is aimed particularly at the estimated 300,000 people who have HIV but do not know it and may be passing it to others unwittingly. The major reasons for this shift in prevention strategy are (1) efforts to reduce the number of annual HIV infections in America have either, depending on one's point of view, stalled or failed. New infections dropped to about 40,000 cases each year in 1988 and then at least from 2002 through 2008 **increased** to about 56,000 new infections per year and (2) the advent of antiretroviral drug therapy in 1995 and its continued success at prolonging the lives of the HIV infected has made a significant increase in numbers of healthy HIV infected who, along with those who do not know they are infected, continue the transmission of HIV. The new prevention strategy began in July 2004.

Global Prevention Concerns—It is not certain that other countries, even if they have the ability, will follow the prevention strategy shift occurring in the United States. Most countries, at least through 2008, stayed with the primary prevention strategy. It is estimated that in order for the secondary strategy to be effective globally, it will require some $15 billion a year for at least the next 10 years. Where will that money come from? This money does not include the additional monies needed for medical care and living facilities, etc.

DISCUSSION QUESTION: Do you agree with the strategic shift in prevention the CDC started in July 2004? Support your decision with known data/facts that can be found within this book or from other sources (see Box 14.3, AIDS Programs: An Epidemic of Waste?), and ask yourself if the CDC is using expanded testing/counseling

to dodge the criticism it has received from conservative politicians about funding "safe sex" programs. Do you hold much hope for a successful prevention program in developing countries? Why?

PREVENTING THE TRANSMISSION OF HIV

The News Is Mostly Bad

We are now into the twenty-seventh year of a pandemic that has touched—directly or indirectly—virtually every person on the planet. We know so much about the virus, yet despite our knowledge, our only option is to *prevent* the initial infection. Prevention is foremost because there is no vaccine, no cure, and, even using the best AIDS drug cocktails available, long-term survival remains questionable, even for those who can tolerate and afford the drugs. As the world faces this realization, alarming statistics continue to emerge about the spread of HIV infection.

In San Francisco, estimates suggest that about 50% of homosexual black American men are infected with HIV. Unsafe sexual practices that could lead to HIV transmission are common among adolescents, young adults, and senior citizens. Tens of millions of persons in developing countries will become HIV infected and most likely die. Entire generations are threatened with extinction in these countries.

The Hard Questions

How can reputable HIV/AIDS scientists explain to the public that the world is being consumed by a disease that is preventable and have it make sense?

The political, social, cultural, economic, and biological factors that have led to the HIV pandemic seem overwhelming. How can a drug user be persuaded to use clean needles to prevent an infection that may kill him in 10 years, when he faces an immediate struggle in a violent environment every day? How can condom use be promoted in countries with inadequate supplies of condoms or resources to provide even basic immunizations? Why should young women on the streets of New York, San Francisco, New Delhi, or Bangkok who depend on the sex industry for daily survival care about safer sex when it might lead to rejection by their customers and an end to their livelihood?

DISCUSSION QUESTION: How would you answer the hard questions?

Gender Power

In many societies, there is a large power differential between men and women. Socially and culturally determined gender roles bestow control and authority on males. The subordinate status of women is reinforced by the fact that men are the main or only wage earners in the majority of families. This is compounded further by age differences: In most heterosexual relationships, the man is the older partner.

Wives in many cultures are expected to tolerate infidelity by their husbands, while remaining totally faithful themselves. But AIDS has raised the price of such tolerance, as it puts women at great risk of infection by their husbands. Many women feel powerless to ask their husbands to use condoms at home. Even when they can do this, their need to protect themselves may conflict with a social or personal imperative to have children.

Is There Hope?

Hopelessness threatens reason, but there is reason to believe that education may reduce the number of new HIV infections. In San Francisco, gay men organized grassroots efforts to educate themselves about HIV transmission, and the results are impressive: Less than 1% of the gay male population was infected with HIV after 1985, compared to 10% to 20% in the preceding years. People can change their behavior when educated about the risks of transmission.

Educators Given the Job of Prevention: Spread Knowledge, Not HIV

HIV has just as much potential to kill someone infected in 2009 as it did in 1981, but today's sixth graders and older are hearing much less about HIV/AIDS as did students from the late 1980s through the late 1990s. The great irony is that our fear of HIV now stands in inverse proportion to the damage it does. AIDS is killing millions of people a year—"but those people are in Africa and Asia, so they don't count." To dismiss AIDS as someone else's or some other country's problem is to deny the fundamental reality: Sex is one of the few things that can link you to anyone else on this planet. Remember the 1990s bromide, *If you have sex with someone, you're having sex with everyone they ever had sex with?* It's still true.

Importance of Prevention

The importance of prevention is especially clear as one comes to understand the limitations in HIV/AIDS therapy. Regardless of what can be medically done for patients with HIV disease, there is no cure. Thus officials from the Centers for Disease Control and Prevention (CDC), the World Health Organization (WHO), the United Nations Joint HIV/AIDS Program (UNAIDS), and the American Health Organization (AHO) have placed the responsibility of prevention in the hands of educators, which include healthcare professionals, parents, and teachers. (See Figure 9-1.)

Current Success of Education Prevention Programs

What HIV/AIDS Prevention Method Lasts A Lifetime?

Education

A growing number of countries have documented the success of their education prevention efforts through careful program evaluations and well-designed surveys. There should be no doubt in anyone's mind that education prevention programs can reverse a major epidemic, as has been seen in Uganda and Zambia; can contain an emerging epidemic as has occurred in Thailand and Brazil; and can avoid an epidemic altogether, as has been well documented in Senegal.

Complacency: The Success of Highly Active Antiretroviral Therapy—HAART

The success of HAART is good news for the people living longer, better lives because of it, but the availability of treatment may lull people into believing that preventing HIV infection is no longer important. This complacency about the need for prevention adds a new dimension of complexity for both program planners and individuals at risk. **First,** while the number of AIDS cases is declining, the number of people living with HIV infection is growing. This increased prevalence of HIV in the population means that even more prevention efforts are needed, not fewer. For individuals at risk, increased prevalence means that each risk behavior carries an increased risk for infection. This makes the danger of relaxing preventive behaviors greater than ever. **Second,** past prevention efforts have resulted in behavior change for many individuals and have helped slow the epidemic overall. However, many

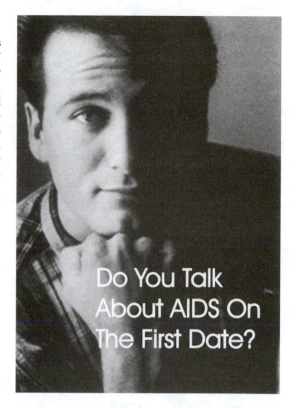

FIGURE 9-1 Do You Talk About AIDS on the First Date? (*Courtesy of the Centers for Disease Control and Prevention, Atlanta*)

studies find that high-risk behaviors, especially unprotected sex, are continuing at far too high a rate. This is true even for some people who have been counseled and tested for HIV, including those found to be infected. **Third,** the long-term effectiveness of HAART is unknown. HIV develops resistance to these drugs. If the development of drug resistance is coupled with a relaxation in preventive behaviors, resistant strains can and are being transmitted to others and spread widely. It is very important to note that society must not let the advances in ART over the past 12 years make us complacent about the global pandemic. Prevention ultimately remains the answer to eradicating this epidemic and to ending all of the associated costs, especially the devastating human costs.

Prevention Works—Pay Attention!

Sustained, comprehensive prevention efforts begun in the 1980s have had a substantial impact on slowing the

HIV/AIDS epidemic in developed countries. While it is difficult to measure prevention—or how many thousands of infections did not occur as a result of efforts to date—in the United States the epidemic was growing at a rate of over 80% each year in the mid-1980s and has now stabilized. While the occurrence of approximately 56,000 new infections annually is deeply troubling, tremendous progress has been made. Also, there is now scientific evidence on which prevention programs are most effective. There is no question that prevention works and remains the best and most cost-effective approach for bringing the HIV/AIDS pandemic under control and saving lives. (See Point of View 9.1, Figure 9-2.)

Grim Reality

Steven Findlay (1991) wrote that burying those who have died from AIDS has become almost routine. With a 27-year death toll estimated at about 595,000 beginning year 2009, most Americans are

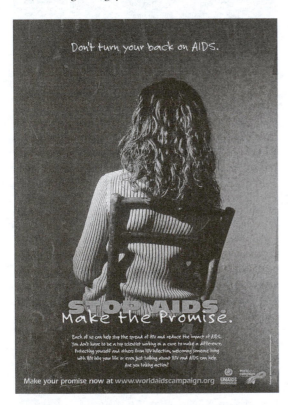

FIGURE 9-2 Prevention Can Work. The world must face the problem: The HIV/AIDS pandemic. *(Source: United Nations Program on AIDS)*

indeed becoming accustomed to HIV/AIDS-related deaths. But how many will have died, say, ending in the year 2015 or 2025 in America or worldwide? Will a cure or preventive and therapeutic vaccines be produced? Will our healthcare system become swamped and ineffective? The best guess by scientists is that neither an effective vaccine nor a cure will be found in the near future. Through the year 2009 it is projected that worldwide about 24 million people will have died of AIDS. San Francisco may lose 3% of its population; New York 2%; Central Africa 10% to 15%. To avoid the realization of these projections, people of the world must work on HIV/AIDS prevention.

What We Know

Based on over 27 years of intensive epidemiological surveys, scientific research, and empirical observations, it is reasonable to conclude that HIV is not a highly contagious disease. HIV transmission occurs mainly through an exchange of body fluids via various sexual activities, HIV-contaminated blood or blood products, prenatal events, and in some cases postnatally through breast milk. Since 1981, only one new route of HIV transmission has been discovered, giving babies pre-chewed food. (See Chapter 8 for discussion.)

HIV Is a Relatively Fragile Virus: Life Span of HIV in Different Environments

The virus is fragile and, with time, self-destructs outside the human body.

The most recent data show that HIV remains active for up to five days in dried blood, although the number of virus particles (titer) drops dramatically. But it is dangerous to assume that there are no infectious viruses remaining in the dried blood or stored body fluids from an HIV/AIDS patient. In cell-free tissue culture medium, the virus retains activity for up to 14 days at room temperature (Sattar et al., 1991). According to a recent study, HIV was found to survive between two and four days in glutaraldehyde, a lubricant used to clean surgical instruments. This finding has serious implications for instruments too delicate to be autoclaved (high-pressure steam sterilization), such as endoscopes (Lewis, 1995).

Joseph Burnett (1995) reported that HIV can survive 7 days storage at room temperature, 11 days at 37°C (98.6 degrees Fahrenheit) in tissue culture extracellular fluid, and can still be infectious in refrigerated postmortem cadaver tissue for 6 to 14 days.

Nadia Abdala and colleagues (1999 updated) reported that HIV recovered in the blood from used syringes can remain active up to at least six weeks. The bottom line is HIV is more resistant to the environment than originally believed.

SEXUAL RISK TAKING DEPENDS ON SEXUAL ACTIVITY

Perhaps the most difficult area of HIV/AIDS prevention lies in the area of sexual behavior. Sexual behavioral as change is certainly difficult to inspire and extremely hard to measure. Furthermore, the theoretical basis for sexual behavioral change has been difficult to characterize.

It appears that HIV transmission can be prevented by individual action but it will require change in social sexual behaviors. The best way to protect against all sexually transmitted diseases is **sexual abstinence.** The next best way is a mutually monogamous sexual relationship. Following these two options is the use of a barrier method during sexual activities—male and female condoms or rubber dental dams.

For the foreseeable future, prevention through sexual behavioral change is the only way to slow this epidemic.

Types of Behavior Most Difficult to Change: Sexual and Injection-Drug Use

Sexual transmission accounts for the majority of HIV infection in the developing world, but this is the most difficult type of transmission to prevent. The use of condoms, reducing numbers of partners, and abstinence remain the mainstays of preventing sexual transmission of HIV, but they will not be enthusiastically adopted just because health authorities tell people to do so.

Sexual behavior has changed in many populations: among gay men in San Francisco, among injecting-drug users in Amsterdam and New Haven, Conn., and among sex workers and their clients in Nairobi, to name a few. In most of these examples it is not clear how the behavioral change took place. Even so, success stories in HIV/AIDS prevention seem to have some elements in common, including consistent and persistent intervention measures over a period of time, a clear understanding of the realities of the target population, and involvement of members of that population in prevention efforts.

Successful interventions do far more than provide information: They teach communication and behavioral skills, change perceptions of what is **preventive behavior,** and ensure that the means of prevention, such as condoms or clean needles, are readily available.

Table 9-1 provides a number of recommendations for preventing the spread of HIV. These recommendations place the responsibility for avoiding HIV infection on both adults and adolescents. **Lifestyles must be reviewed, choices made, and risky behavior stopped.** The public health service and the CDC have established guidelines that, if followed, will prevent HIV transmission while still allowing individuals to be somewhat flexible in their personal behaviors (*MMWR, 1989*).

Quarantine

With few exceptions, proposals to quarantine all individuals with HIV infection have virtually no public support in the United States. Given the civil liberties implications of quarantine, its potential cost, and the realization that alternative, less repressive strategies can be effective in limiting the spread of HIV infection, quarantine proposals in most countries have been dismissed. Despite claims that HIV/AIDS is similar to other diseases for which quarantine has been used, public health officials have insisted on distinguishing between behaviorally transmitted infections and those that are airborne. HIV/AIDS is not airborne.

Through year 2009, HIV prevention methods in the United States and other developed nations will remain education, counseling, voluntary testing and partner notification, drug abuse treatment, and syringe exchange programs. To date, the power to quarantine, for any disease, has rarely been used in the United States. In fact, only one country, Cuba, officially used the power of quarantine in 1986 to stem the spread of HIV. Data to date indicate that the use of quarantine of HIV-infected and AIDS persons in Cuba had been very effective. Cuba had 17 sanitoriums holding some 900 persons of which about 200 had AIDS. Cuba stopped the quarantine of HIV-infected persons in mid-1993. Controversial as the sanitoriums were because of serious civil liberties violations, the measures worked. Since 1986, about 7553 Cubans have tested positive for HIV and 3108 have developed AIDS, with about 1400 deaths.

At the beginning of 2009, about 20% of Cuba's HIV/AIDS population, by choice, live in the remain-

Table 9-1 Guidelines for Prevention of HIV Infection

I. For the General Public:

1. Sexual abstinence
2. Have a mutual monogamous relationship with an HIV negative partner (the greater the number of sexual partners, the greater the risk of meeting someone who is HIV infected).
3. If the sex partner is other than a monogamous partner, use a condom.
4. Do not frequent prostitutes—too many have been found to be HIV infected and are still "working" the streets.
5. Do not have sex with people who you know are HIV infected or are from a high-risk group. If you do, prevent contact with their body fluids. (Use a condom and a spermicide from start to finish.)
6. Avoid sexual practices that may result in the tearing of body tissues (for example, penile-anal intercourse).
7. Avoid oral-penile sex unless a condom[a] is used to cover the penis.
8. If you use injection drugs, use sterile or bleach-cleaned needles and syringes and *never* share them.
9. Exercise caution regarding procedures such as acupuncture, tattooing, ear piercing, and so on in which needles or other unsterile instruments may be used repeatedly to pierce the skin and/or mucous membranes. Such procedures are safe if proper sterilization methods are employed or disposable needles are used. Ask what precautions are being taken before undergoing such procedures.
10. If you are planning to undergo artificial insemination, insist on frozen sperm obtained from a laboratory that tests all donors for infection with the AIDS virus. Donors should be tested twice before the sperm is used—once at the time of donation and again six months later.
11. If you know you will be having surgery in the near future and you are able to do so, consider donating blood for your own use. This will eliminate the small but real risk of HIV infection through a blood transfusion. It will also eliminate the more substantial risk of contracting other transfusion blood-borne diseases, such as hepatitis B.
12. Don't share toothbrushes, razors, or other implements that could become contaminated with blood with anyone who is HIV infected, demonstrates HIV disease, or has AIDS.

II. For Healthcare Workers:

1. *All* sharp instruments should be considered potentially infective and be handled with extraordinary care to prevent accidental injuries.
2. Sharp items should be placed into puncture-resistant containers located as close as practical to the area in which they are used. To prevent needle stick injuries, needles should not be recapped, purposefully bent, broken, removed from disposable syringes, or otherwise manipulated.
3. Gloves, gowns, masks, and eye coverings should be worn when performing procedures involving extensive contact with blood or potentially infective body fluids. Hands should be washed thoroughly and immediately if they accidentally become contaminated with blood. When a patient requires a vaginal or rectal examination, gloves must always be worn. If a specimen is obtained during an examination, the nurse or individual who assists and processes the specimen must always wear gloves. Blood should be drawn from all patients—regardless of HIV status—only while wearing gloves.
4. To minimize the need for emergency mouth-to-mouth resuscitation, mouthpieces, resuscitation bags, or other ventilation devices should be strategically located and available for use where the need for resuscitation is predictable.

III. For People at Risk of HIV Infection:

1. See the recommendations for the general public.
2. Consider taking the HIV antibody screening test.
3. Protect your partner from body fluids during sexual intercourse.
4. Do not donate any body tissues.
5. If female, have an HIV test before becoming pregnant.
6. If you are an injection-drug user, seek professional help in terminating the drug habit.
7. If you cannot get off drugs, do not share drug equipment.

IV. For People Who Are HIV Positive:

The prevention of transmission of HIV by an HIV-infected person is probably lifelong, and patients must avoid infecting others. HIV-seropositive persons must understand that the virus can be transmitted by intimate sexual contact, transfusion of infected blood, and sharing needles among injection-drug users. They should refrain from donating blood, plasma, sperm, body organs, or other tissues. HIV-infected people should:

1. Seek continued counseling and medical examinations.
2. Do not exchange body fluids with your sex partner.

Table 9-1 (*Continued*)

3. Notify your former and current sex partners, and encourage them to be tested.
4. If an injection-drug user, enroll in a drug treatment program and do not share drug equipment.
5. Do not share razors, toothbrushes, and other items that may contain traces of blood.
6. Do not donate any body tissues.
7. Clean any body fluids spilled with undiluted household bleach.
8. If female, avoid pregnancy.
9. Inform healthcare workers on a need-to-know basis.

V. Practice of Safer Sex:

Safer sex is body massage, hugging, mutual masturbation, and closed-mouth kissing. HIV-seropositive patients must protect their sexual partners from coming into contact with infected blood or bodily secretions. Although consistent use of latex condoms with a spermicide can decrease the chance of HIV transmission, condoms do break. (Also see 1 through 6 under "For the General Public" in this table.)

[a] Tests show that HIV can sometimes pass through a latex condom. Experts believe that natural-skin condoms are more porous than latex and therefore offer less effective protection. Never use oil-based products such as Vaseline, Crisco, or baby oil with a latex condom because they make the latex porous, causing latex deterioration and breakage, thus nullifying the protection the condom provides against the virus.

ing 14 sanitoriums. The rest live outside and receive care at a few specialty centers. A key criterion for living outside the sanitoriums is disclosure of one's sexual partners and providing evidence to health authorities that one is sexually responsible. The authorities actively pursue contact tracing and HIV testing of sexual partners, strategies borrowed from their TB program. There is also mandatory HIV testing of pregnant women, soldiers, and blood donors, but anonymous testing is available for the general public. Last year, over 1 million HIV tests were done in Cuba, out of a population of 11.4 million.

Cuba has screened all blood donors for HIV since 1986. Jorge Perez, who diagnosed the country's first AIDS patients and helped shape the policies of the Santiago sanatorium as its director for 12 years, said, "The Cuban point of view is that you have the right to be sick, but not to transmit it to anyone else." Currently, Cuba has the distinction of having one of the smallest HIV infection rates in the world in a region with one of the highest.

NEW RULES TO AN OLD GAME: PROMOTING SAFER SEX—NOBODY HAS A BODY TO DIE FOR!

The use of barrier methods is one of the few behavioral strategies that individuals can adopt to protect themselves against sexually transmitted diseases. Male, and in some countries female, condoms are currently the only barrier methods widely available. However, there are many cultural, gender, economic, and service-delivery barriers that impede the wide-scale and consistent use of barrier methods for preventing the transmission of HIV and other sexually transmitted diseases.

Barriers to HIV Infection

The two most effective barriers to HIV infection and other sexually transmitted diseases are **(1) abstinence,** which can be achieved by saying *no* emphatically and consistently; and **(2) forming a no-cheating relationship with one individual, preferably for life.** These solutions to the danger of HIV infection may not be "cool," but they do work. These two apparently safe approaches are endorsed by the surgeon general as the preferred methods. For those who do not practice abstinence, barrier methods are necessary to prevent HIV infection/transmission.

Barrier Methods

The barrier methods used to prevent HIV infection are the same methods used to prevent other sexually transmitted diseases and often contraception or pregnancy. They include latex condoms, plastic condoms (new in 1995), and latex dental dams and diaphragms used in conjunction with a spermicide. Barrier dams or dental dams are thin sheets of latex or similar material placed over the vagina, clitoris, and anus during oral sex. (Ask your dentist to show you a dental dam.) **Spermicides** are chemicals that kill sperm. These same chemicals have also been shown to kill some bacteria and inactivate certain viruses that cause STDs. Spermicides are commercially available in foams, creams, jellies, suppositories, and sponges. Use of these products may provide protection against the transmission of STDs, but the only recommended barrier protection against HIV infection is a condom. National Condom Week is February 14–21. National Condom Day is always on Valentine's Day.

Condom—A Medical Device?

Condoms are classified as medical devices. Every condom made in the United States is tested for defects and must meet quality control guidelines enforced by the federal Food and Drug Administration (FDA).

Theoretical Basis for Protection—Condoms can be expected to provide different levels of protection for various sexually transmitted diseases, depending on differences in how the diseases are transmitted. Because condoms block the discharge of semen or protect the male urethra against exposure to vaginal secretions, a greater level of protection is provided for the discharge diseases. A lesser degree of protection is provided for the genital ulcer diseases or HIV because these infections may be transmitted by exposure to areas—for example, infected skin or mucosal surfaces that are not covered or protected by the condom.

From the CDC: Sexually Transmitted Diseases, Including HIV—Latex condoms, when used consistently and correctly, are highly effective in preventing the transmission of HIV, the virus that causes AIDS. In addition, correct and consistent use of latex condoms can reduce the risk of other sexually transmitted diseases (STDs), including discharge and genital ulcer diseases. While the effect of condoms in preventing human papillomavirus (HPV) infection is unknown, condom use has been associated with a lower rate of cervical cancer, an HPV-associated disease.

Choosing the Condom: Manufacturers, Colors, and Shapes

Condoms are intended to provide a physical barrier that prevents contact between vaginal, anal, penile, and oral lesions and secretions and ejaculate.

At least 50 brands of condoms are manufactured in the United States (Figure 9-3). There are colored condoms—pink, yellow, and gold; flavored condoms; and condoms that are perfumed, ribbed, stippled, and glow in the dark. This assortment of condoms ex-

poses the user and his partner not only to rubber but also to a variety of different chemicals—some that can cause allergic skin reactions **(contact dermatitis).** One to two percent of people are sensitive to latex rubber and demonstrate contact dermatitis.

Condoms are also called rubbers, prophylactics, bags, skins, raincoats, sheaths, and French letters. They can be lubricated or not, have reservoir tips or not, and can contain spermicide.

Condom Size

Most brand name condoms are made in four different lengths and widths (sizes). There is no standard length for condoms, though those made from natural rubber will stretch if necessary to fit the length of the man's erect penis. The width of a condom can also vary. Some condoms have a slightly smaller width to give a closer fit, while others will be slightly larger. Condom makers have realized that different lengths and widths are needed and are increasingly broadening their range of sizes. An Internet retailer now advertises 95 sizes of "They Fit" condoms whose length ranges from 3 inches to 10 inches.

History of Condoms

Condom use can be traced back to 1000 B.C. when Egyptian men used linen sheaths or animal membranes as a sheath to cover their penises (Barber, 1990). Animal intestines were flushed clean with water, sewn shut at one end and cut to the length of the erect penis. In 1504, Gabrielle Fallopius designed a medicated linen sheath that was pulled on over the penis to prevent syphilis infection. A Japanese novel written in the tenth century refers to the uncomfortable use of a tortoise shell or horn to cover the penis.

It is interesting to note that condoms were used far more often throughout history as protection against STDs than as contraceptives. For example, an eighteenth-century writer recommended that men protect themselves against disease by placing a linen sheath over the penis during intercourse.

The term "condom" came into common usage in the 1700s. According to accounts in the early 1700s, condoms were sold and even exported from a London shop whose proprietress laundered and recycled them in a back room (Barber, 1990). Condoms became more widely available after 1844. The latex condom was first manufactured in the 1930s.

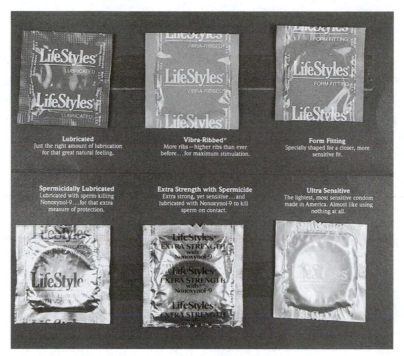

(a)

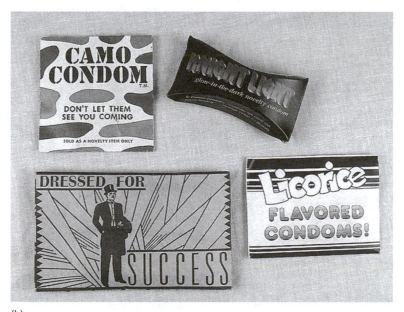

(b)

FIGURE 9-3 (a) Types of Condoms Available in the United States. (b) Types of Novelty Condoms. *(Photos by Michael Muyres)*

Condoms have been available in the United States for about 150 years, but have never been as openly accepted as they are now. Their sale for contraceptive use was outlawed by many state legislatures beginning in 1868 and by Congress in 1873. Although most of these laws were eventually repealed, condom packages and dispensers until only a few years ago continued to bear the label "Sold only for the prevention of disease," even though they were being used mainly for the prevention of pregnancy.

After the advent of nonbarrier methods of contraception during the 1960s (mainly the use of the birth control pill) there was an ensuing epidemic increase in most sexually transmitted infections. Condoms once again are being marketed for the prevention of disease (Judson, 1989) (Table 9-2).

Safer Sex, the Choice of Condom

Although a variety of preventative behaviors have been recommended (Table 9-1), the responsibility of safer sex, with a condom, is a personal choice. If one decides to use a condom, then the choice is what kind, and whether or not to use a spermicide.

THE MALE CONDOM

The American-made condom most often sold is made of latex, is about 8 inches long, and in general, one size fits all. About 500 million condoms are sold annually in the United States. Ten to 15 billion are sold annually worldwide but about 30 billion more are needed and most of them in Asia (Grimes, 1992 updated). Regardless of what appears to be a large number of condoms sold worldwide, globally, consistent male condom use remains a minority strategy because of moral objections, limited consumer acceptability, or logistic reasons. The costs of condom use—including financial, interpersonal, aesthetic, and social costs—are too high for most people. Instead, many people in different settings adapt their sexual practices in ways that do not include male condoms, often with unknown or only marginal benefit for HIV or STD prevention.

Intact latex condoms provide a continuous mechanical barrier to HIV, herpes virus (HSV), hepatitis B virus (HBV), *Chlamydia trachomatis,* and *Neisseria gonorrhoeae.* A recent laboratory study indicated that latex and **polyurethane condoms** are the most effective mechanical barriers to fluid containing HIV-sized particles (0.1 μm in diameter) available. The male polyurethane condom is thinner than the latex condom, which makes them more agreeable in feel and appearance to some users. However, they also break more easily during use.

Three prospective studies in developed countries indicated that condoms are unlikely to break or slip during proper use. Reported breakage rates in the studies with latex condoms were 2% or less for vaginal or anal intercourse (*MMWR,* 1993; Spruyt et al., 1998).

TABLE 9.2

Table 9-2 Demand and Supply of Condoms in Select Countries Annually Beginning 2006[1,2]

Population	Country	Male Condoms/Year	Introduction of Female Condoms
1.3 billion	China	305 million[3]	2005
1.1 billion	India	1.6 billion	2004
730 million	Europe	913 million	2002
300 million	United States	365 million	1993(FDA-Approved)
180 million	Brazil	1.5 billion	1997
47 million	South Africa	400 million	1996

[1]About 18 billion condoms were required in the developing world in 2006, but only three billion were available. In sub-Saharan Africa, for example, men had access to three condoms per year!

[2]For each country, the condoms were provided by their governments. India will provide 3.5 billion annually begining in 2008 through 3 million distribution outlets.

[3]Condoms are widely unacceptable by the Chinese population. The Chinese Ministry of Health has called for 100% condom use throughout China in 2007. The campaign slogan: "no condom, no sex."

study of a product which contains nonoxynol-9 (N-9). The study found that the spermicide N-9 did not protect against HIV infection and may have increased the risk of transmission. Women using N-9 gel became infected with HIV about 50% more often than women who used the placebo gel.

Buying Male Condoms—Women are taking a more active role in buying condoms. In 1985, women bought about 10% of the condoms sold. Now they purchase 40% to 50%. According to surveys, most women buying condoms are single, and their concern is about HIV infection rather than pregnancy. The fact that more women are willing to buy condoms is evidence that HIV education is working to some degree.

Many condoms are purchased from vending machines. The FDA recommends the following guidelines when purchasing condoms from a vending machine:

1. Is the condom made of latex or polyurethane?
2. Is the condom labeled for disease prevention?
3. Is the spermicide (if any) outdated?
4. Is the machine exposed to extreme temperatures or direct sunlight?

In mid-1992, the first drive-up "Condom Hut" opened in Cranston, R.I. With each purchase the customer receives a brochure on safer sex.

It is generally recommended that condoms be stored below 25° C (77° Fahrenheit; room temperature is 72° F or 22.2° C). The packaging should be impermeable to both sunlight and gas. If air, which includes ozone, enters the package, it will affect the condom very quickly—ozone is like rust to a condom. Latex is a natural product—it will go bad if you don't treat or store it properly.

Condoms in Public Schools?

Condoms are now being dispensed without charge in most college and university and public health clinics, and in at least 400 high school health offices in the United States. Some cities in Canada have been providing access to free condoms in high schools since 1984.

In December 1999, the American Medical Association (AMA) adopted a policy that advocates handing out condoms in schools and minimizes the value of abstinence-only sex education. While some doctors and groups have called the policy medically irresponsible, it is supported by the U.S. surgeon general. The policy, based on studies, concluded that safer sex programs are effective in delaying sex in

Choice—The best choice for preventing STDs and pregnancy is condoms that are made of **latex** or **polyurethane (plastic)** and contain a **spermicide.** The spermicide is added protection in case the condom ruptures or spills as it is taken off. Although some laboratory evidence shows that some spermicides can inactivate HIV, researchers have found that these products cannot prevent a person from becoming HIV infected.

During the Thirteenth International AIDS Conference held in Durban, South Africa, July 9–14, 2000, researchers from the Joint United Nations Program on AIDS (UNAIDS) presented the results of a teenagers, and that abstinence-only programs have limited value.

Are Policies or Studies Reality?

Regardless of educational programs on safer sex and condom usage, recent studies indicate that adults and teenagers still refuse to use condoms. What they know is not equal to what they do! Based on their findings, the researchers said information-oriented school- and community-based AIDS prevention programs will not succeed in getting some adults and adolescents to use condoms because there is no association between knowledge and preventive behavior.

Equally discouraging is a recent study in the United States. A 2004 online survey by the American Social Health Association of 1155 people ages 18 to 35 indicated about 84% believed they adequately protected themselves against HIV and other STDs, but nearly half engage in unprotected sex. Approximately 47% of the respondents never used protection for vaginal sex, 82% never used protection for oral sex, and 64% never used protection for anal sex. The survey showed that 93% believed their current or most recent partner did not have an STD, yet one of three people have never discussed HIV or STDs with their partner, while 68% did not think they would contract HIV or an STD.

Religion Prohibits Use of Condoms—The Catholic church teaches that the conjugal act must always leave open the possibility of conception. It is the purpose of devices such as condoms to rule out impregnation. Consequently, the church holds that the use of contraceptives in order to prevent the origination of new life is immoral. Peter Piot, executive director of UNAIDS, said, "Catholicism has had a major role in virtually all aspects of the global response to AIDS since the disease was identified. With its hospices and hospitals, orphanages and parish outreach, the Catholic church provides more direct care for people with AIDS and their families and communities, particularly in Africa and Latin America, than any other institution. Yet, while the UN, most governments and governmental agencies, and almost all of the international organizations working in AIDS agree that condoms are the most effective means of slowing the spread of HIV, the Vatican has remained steadfast in its opposition to their use." In 2006 and 2007 the new Catholic Pope, Benedict XVI, reiterated the Catholic Church's opposition to condom use as a way to prevent the spread of HIV. The church promotes a moral educa-

tion to protect its members. Given that over 1.1 billion people worldwide are Catholics and that not all

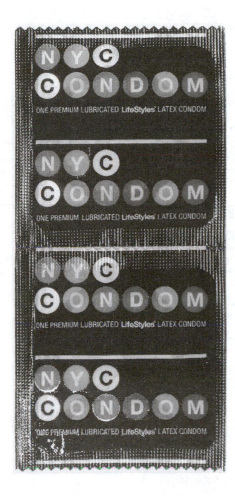
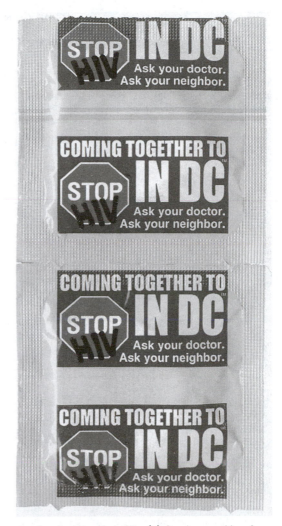

FIGURE 9-4 Free Condom Distributions. (a) Condom packaging for New York City. (b) Condom packing for Washington D.C. See Text for details.

are low-risk individuals, the sanction against condom use presents a difficult problem in slowing the transmission of HIV.

In October 2003, Cardinal Alfonso Lopez Trujillo, president of the Vatican's Pontifical Council for the Family, said on the British Broadcasting Corporation's *Panorama* program "Sex and the Holy City" that "HIV can easily pass through the net that is formed by the condom. Sperm pass through the net and HIV is 450 times smaller than sperm. Condoms do not reduce the risk of HIV infection." The cardinal also said, speaking of condoms, that "safe sex is a form of Russian roulette." Other Catholic leaders on the pro-

gram claimed that because of condom permeability, condoms can spread HIV.

DISCUSSION QUESTION: HIV/AIDS scientists worldwide disagree with Cardinal Trujillo and other Catholic leaders that the HIV easily passes through condoms. In October 2007, Mozambiquan Archbishop said, "Condoms and even antiretroviral drugs are purposely infected with HIV in order to destroy Africans." Absolute evidence supports the scientists' belief that the use of condoms can stop HIV transmission. What should, could, or ought to be done to resolve this conflict of

CLARIFYING THE ISSUES OVER CONDOM USE

Two major issues surface in the debate over advocating condom use in the prevention of HIV infection: One concerns the concept of efficacy, the condom's ability to stop the virus from passing through, and the other, the fear that making condoms available will encourage early sexual activity among adolescents and extramarital sex among adults.

EFFICACY (DO THEY WORK?)

No public health strategy can guarantee perfect protection. For instance, the influenza vaccine is only 60–80% effective in preventing influenza, but thousands of deaths could be prevented annually through the wider use of this less than perfect vaccine. The real public health question is not whether condoms are 100% effective, but rather how can we more effectively use condoms to help prevent the spread of disease?

All condoms are not 100% impermeable; they are not all of the same quality. Investigators using different testing methods have reported that latex condoms are effective physical barriers to high concentrations of *Chlamydia trachomatis, Neisseria gonorrhoeae,* the herpes and hepatitis viruses, cytomegalovirus, and HIV (Judson, 1989). But for maximum effectiveness condoms must be properly and consistently used from start to finish (Table 9-3).

Because the condom covers only the head and shaft of the penis, it does not provide protection for the pubic or thigh areas, which may come in contact with body secretions during sexual activity.

Norman Hearst and colleagues (2004) used computerized searches of peer-reviewed scientific literature, and other publications of national and international organizations, to determine the most likely probability that condoms will prevent HIV transmission. Hearst determined that if a condom was used properly, it was 90% effective in stopping the transmission of HIV.

In 2005, the American Foundation for AIDS Research (AMFAR), a well-respected AIDS organization, issued an analysis of the effectiveness of male and female condoms in preventing the transmission of HIV. The analysis revealed that when used consistently and correctly, male condoms are 80% to 95% effective in reducing the risk of HIV infection, while female condoms are 94% to 97% effective in reducing the risk. AMFAR's analysis concludes that the scientific evidence does not support recent governmental policy changes that stress a lack of condom efficacy in preventing HIV transmission. Thus, AMFAR concludes that condoms are "highly effective" in blocking HIV infection/transmission. These data are sure to fuel the ongoing debate. In spite of the argument, pro and con on the use of condoms, next to abstinence, condoms are about the only mechanical device available for safer sex. The bottom line is that condoms reduce some of the risks in preventing the transmission of HIV and other STDs, thus condoms are used for safer sex but they cannot guarantee safe sex.

MAJOR CAUSE OF CONDOM BREAKAGE

Nicholas White and colleagues (2008) reported that 90% of condom breakage is not caused by misuse. Their findings show that mostly condom breakage is caused by "blunt puncture," where the tip of the

---

Table 9-3 Proper Placement of a Condom on the Penis[a]

1. Open the packaged condom with care; avoid making small fingernail tears or breaks in the condom.

2. Place a drop of a water-based lubricant inside the condom tip before placing it on the head of the penis. Be sure none of the lubricant rolls down the penis shaft as it may cause the condom to slide off during intercourse.

3. Hold about half an inch of the condom tip between your thumb and finger—this is to allow space for semen after ejaculation. Then place the condom against the glans penis (if uncircumcised, pull the foreskin back).

4. Unroll the condom down the penis shaft to the base of the penis. Squeeze out any air as you roll the condom toward the base.

5. After ejaculation, hold the condom at the base and withdraw the penis while it is still firm.

6. Carefully take the condom off by gently rolling and pulling so as not to leak semen.

7. Discard the condom into the trash.

8. Wash your hands.

9. Never use the same condom twice.

10. Condoms should not be stored in extremely hot or cold environments.

[a]Males should practice putting on and removing a condom prior to engaging in sexual intercourse.

thrusting penis progressively stretches one part of the condom until it breaks.

Condoms used in the study were Durex and SSL (Seton Scholl and London).

DO CONDOMS ENCOURAGE SEXUAL ACTIVITY?

Many persons assert that those who promote condom use to prevent HIV infection appear to be condoning sexual intercourse outside of marriage among adolescents as well as among adults. In 2006, Natalie Smoak and colleagues presented an overall assessment of 174 studies published on whether condoms encourage sexual activities; beginning sex at an earlier age, having sex more frequently, or having more sexual partners. Bottom line, they report that condoms do not promote any of these sexual behaviors. Administrators of these studies feel that condoms no more cause sexual activity than umbrellas cause rain.

ANECDOTE: HUMOR

Presenting facts without understanding won't work. Here is a simple story to emphasize the point: "A min-ister, following his custom, paid a monthly call on two spinster sisters. While he was standing in their parlor, holding his cup of tea, engaged in their usual chit chat, he was startled by something that caught his eye. There on the piano was a condom! 'Ladies, in all the years we've known each other I have never intruded into your private lives, and never felt the need to. But now I am forced to ask what is that thing doing there?' One of the ladies replied, 'Oh, that's a wonderful thing, pastor, and they really work!' The minister was agitated: 'I'm not talking about their value or effectiveness. I just want to know what that thing is doing on your piano.'"

"'Well, my sister and I were watching television. We heard this lovely man, the surgeon general of the whole United States. He said that if you put one of those on your organ, you'll never get sick. Well, as you know we don't have an organ, but we bought one and put it on the piano, and we haven't had a day's sickness since!'"

information? Lives are in jeopardy because of HIV infection/transmission.

In mid-2006, Pope Benedict asked the Pontifical Council for Health and Pastoral Care to study condom use as a means of HIV prevention **only** among married couples in which one of the partners is HIV positive. Ending 2008 the council has not released its findings.

Food and Drug Administration (FDA) Requires a Warning Label on Condoms

In 2006, the FDA stated that all latex condom manufacturers must include the following information on their condom packages: "Condoms Greatly Reduce, But Do Not Eliminate The Risk Of Pregnancy And HIV Infection When Used Correctly During Sexual Intercourse." Manufacturers had one year to comply. They did!

Polyurethane (Plastic) Condoms—For the 1% of the general population that is sensitive to latex and for those who have a variety of other reasons not to use a latex condom, there is now a clear, thin, FDA-approved polyurethane (plastic) condom for sale in the United States. The condoms are colorless, odorless, and can be used with any lubricant. The current cost is about $1.80 each. A report by Ron Frezieres and colleagues (1999) states that although polyurethane and latex condoms provide equivalent levels of contraceptive protection, the polyurethane condom's higher frequency of breakage and slippage suggests that this condom may confer less protection from sexually transmitted infections than do the latex condoms.

Why Some Men Don't Use Condoms: Male Attitudes About Condoms and Other Contraceptives—This is the name of a study published by the Henry J. Kaiser Family Foundation (1997). The study shows that men, especially teenage males, don't use condoms mostly because of embarrassment: buying the condom, talking about the condom with their sexual partner, putting the condom on in front of their sexual partner, offending or scaring their sexual partner, losing an erection while putting the condom on, and the reduction of sexual pleasure. (This free report can be obtained at 1-800-656-4533 monograph #1319.)

EXAMPLES OF CONDOM INNOVATIONS AND ADVERTISING REPORTED IN 2007

Wellington, New Zealand—Hell Pizza company sparked a storm of protest after putting 170,000 condoms in mailboxes with leaflets promoting a new meat-lover's pizza called "lust." **Motivation?** New Zealand has the third-highest rate of teenage pregnancies in the developed world.

Capetown, South Africa—The new Pronto condom, whose promoters say can be put on in just one second thanks to special packaging, is now on sale in South Africa. The condom's designer, Willem van Rensburg, noted that low condom use is a major factor in the nation's HIV/AIDS epidemic and that many people report condoms are difficult to use. Roelf Mulder, van Rensburg's former business partner, said, "People find it's a passion-killer, so they're willing to take their chances. By the time the condom is on, the mood is halfway out the window. If you're slow, it'll take you three seconds. You can really do it in one. The Pronto condom can only be applied one way. The packaging is clearly marked and there are dents where it must be gripped to roll it down." The condom is put on without removing it from the wrapper. The wrapper is simply snapped open in the middle, and the two sides gripped to roll the condom directly over the penis, pulled off and discarded. To date, Pronto condoms are available only in South Africa.

Zaporozhye, Ukraine—Grigorly Chausovsky said his condoms come fitted with a special sensor that registers when the condom is put on. It transmits a signal to a miniature speaker in the base of the condom, which plays a melody. As the sex becomes more passionate, it registers the increased speed of the movements and plays the melody faster and louder.

THE FEMALE CONDOM OR FEMIDOM (VAGINAL POUCH)

The female condom was FDA-approved in May 1993, and has become available to the general public. Before giving the Reality condom final approval, the FDA asked that two caveats be put into the labeling. First, the agency required a statement on the package label that male condoms are still the best protection against disease, and second, that the label compare the effectiveness of female condoms with that of other barrier methods of birth control. According to the FDA, in a study of 150 women who used the female condom for six months, 26% became pregnant. The manufacturer contends that the pregnancy rate was 21%—and only because many women did not use the condom every time they had sex. With "perfect use," company officials say, the rate is 5%, in contrast to 2% for male condoms. Both conditions were met to the FDA's satisfaction.

Design of the Female Condom

The female condom is now called the **vaginal pouch.** However, the female condom is being used by gay men for anal sex. A report from gay men using this condom says that they are having problems with the condom's design and experience usage difficulties. In short, of the gay men interviewed, none believe the female condom will replace their use of the male condom for anal sex.

Description of the Female Condom

The female condom is 17 cm (about 6-3/4 inches) long and consists of a 15 cm polyurethane sheath with rings at each end (Figure 9-5). The closed end fits into the vagina like a diaphragm. The outer portion is designed to cover the base of the penis and a large portion of the female perineum (the area of tissue between the anus and the beginning of the vaginal opening) to provide a greater surface barrier against microorganisms. Studies of acceptability, contraceptive effectiveness, and STD prevention are currently underway. Potential advantages of this product are: (1) it provides women with the opportunity to protect themselves from pregnancy and STDs; (2) it provides a broader coverage of the labia and base of the penis than a male condom; (3) its polyurethane membrane is 40% stronger than latex; and (4) it is more convenient; it can be inserted hours before sexual intercourse. Disadvantages are (1) not aesthetically pleasing and (2) can be difficult to insert and remove.

Because of the polyurethane used to make it, the female condom is both strong and durable. No special storage arrangements have to be made because polyurethane is not affected by changes in temperature and dampness. The expiration date on the female condom is 60 months (5 years) from the date of manufacture.

Global Use of the Vaginal Pouch (Female Condom)—Female Health Company (FHC) of Chicago is the sole manufacturer of the female pouch. Under agreement between UNAIDS and FHC the female pouch is sold for between 50 and

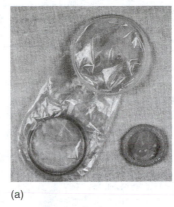

(a)

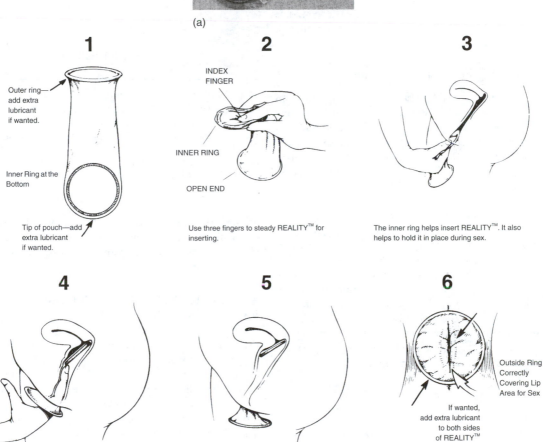

1

Outer ring—
add extra
lubricant
if wanted.

Inner Ring at the
Bottom

Tip of pouch—add
extra lubricant
if wanted.

2

INDEX
FINGER

INNER RING

OPEN END

Use three fingers to steady REALITY™ for
inserting.

3

The inner ring helps insert REALITY™. It also
helps to hold it in place during sex.

4

It is important for the inner ring to be up by
the bone. If it is not in place, you or your
partner could feel it during sex.

(b)

5

6

Outside Ring
Correctly
Covering Lip
Area for Sex

If wanted,
add extra lubricant
to both sides
of REALITY™
for more comfort.

FIGURE 9-5 (a) The Vaginal Pouch compared in size to the male condom. (b) The 7-inch female condom or vaginal pouch is made of light-weight, lubricated polyurethane and has two flexible rings **(1)**, one at each end. It is twice the thickness of the male latex condom. The inner ring **(2)** is used to help insert the device and fits behind the pubic bone. The outer ring remains outside the body. Unlike the diaphragm, the vaginal condom protects against the transmission of HIV, which can penetrate the vaginal tissues. The pouch can be inserted anytime from several hours to minutes prior to intercourse. The vaginal pouch is inserted like a diaphragm and removed after sex. FDA-approved in May 1993. *(A, photo by Michael Muyres; B, Courtesy of Female Health Co., Chicago)*

90 cents (U.S.) in the developing world to encourage its use and provide greater access to women. It is also marketed in the Americas and Europe for about $2.50 (U.S.). In March 2002, France unveiled its first female pouch (condom) machines, blue for men and pink for women. Currently about **14 million** female condoms are distributed on an annual basis to women in developing countries. By comparison, between **6 and 9 billion** male condoms per year are distributed to men! Female condoms were distributed in 88 countries in Africa, Asia, and Latin America. Distribution began in India in early 2004. They cost Third World governments 12 cents each. Male condoms cost 3 cents each! UNAIDS hopes to get the pouch into all developing nations.

Redressing the Balance of Power

The symbolic importance of the female condom should not be understated: It is the first woman-controlled barrier method officially recognized as a means for the prevention of sexually transmitted disease. The female condom allows women to be able to deal with the twin anxieties—AIDS and unwanted pregnancy—with a method that is under their own control.

Many women become HIV-infected not because of their own behavior, but because of their partner's. Because of the nature of gender relations, women may have little influence over their partner's sexual behavior. **Commentary:** Positive messages for women have been spread worldwide on the advantages of using the female condom. But convincing women, in large numbers, to use this relatively new device may not be so easily accomplished. For example, it took 17 years before women in developed countries accepted and began to routinely use the tampon.

Condom Lubricants

It has been demonstrated that petroleum or vegetable oil-based lubricants should not be used with latex condoms. Latex condoms exposed to mineral oil for 60 seconds demonstrated a 90% decrease in strength (Anderson, 1993). There are a number of water-based lubricants that do not adversely affect latex condoms; these should be the lubricants of choice (Table 9-4). **DISCUSSION QUESTION: Reaching this point in the text and having just read the section on male and female condoms, do you think the danger for life, with respect to HIV and other life-threatening STDs, is high**

Table 9-4 Water-Based[a] and Oil-Based[b] Lubricants Often Used With Latex Condoms

Lubricants Recommended	Lubricants Not Recommended
Aqualube	Petroleum jellies
Astroglide	Mineral oils
Cornhuskers Lotion	Vegetable oils
Forplay	Baby oil
H-R Jelly	Massage oil
K-Y Brand Jelly	Lard
RePair	Cold creams
Probe	Hair oils
Today Personal Lube	Hand lotions containing vegetable oils
	Shaft
	Elbow Grease
	Natural Lube

[a]Water-based lubricants can be used with latex condoms.
[b]Oil-based lubricants will chemically weaken latex, causing it to break.
These lists are not exhaustive of all available lubricants used by consumers.
(Source: The STD Education Unit of the San Francisco Department of Public Health, 1994)

enough that condoms should be as familiar to everyone as are toothpaste and toilet paper and also as available? Defend your view with credible information.

AN ALTERNATIVE TO CONDOMS: VAGINAL MICROBICIDES

Eighteen years ago, a Ugandan woman, a peer educator in her community, stood up at the 1991 AIDS Prevention Conference and asked, "If they can put a man on the moon, why can't they make something we can use to protect ourselves from HIV?" Since then, researchers and advocates have tried to answer her call. In a world where most new HIV infections occur among women and where a young African girl is now much more likely to get HIV than an African boy, finding new, effective methods of HIV prevention has never been more urgent.

One of the answers may be found in microbicides. Microbicides are substances that can prevent HIV (and possibly other sexually transmitted infections) from spreading. Some are designed for vaginal use and some for rectal use. They may take the form of gels, creams, suppositories, films, lubricants, or even a sponge or vaginal ring. (For more information on microbicides, visit www.global-campaign.org.)

The term *microbicide* is a generic term applied to anything designed to prevent infection by HIV and other sexually transmitted pathogens when applied in the vagina or rectum. Because HIV and STI (sexually transmitted infection) pathogens can attack the body in multiple ways, an effective microbicide will have to stop this attack at one or more stages in the infection process. Microbicides are designed primarily to provide protection to receptive sex partners, be they male or female, HIV positive or HIV negative. The first generation of microbicides (those are farthest along in the clinical trials and likely to come to market first) are designed for vaginal use. But researchers and developers clearly recognize that both men and women have anal intercourse and that rectal microbicides are needed. Many of the candidate microbicides now in development are likely to be bi-directional—that is, capable of disabling HIV in both semen and vaginal secretions. These would give HIV-positive women a way to reduce their male partner's risk of infection even if he chooses not to use condoms.

The Ideal Vaginal Microbicide (mi-cro-bi-cide)

An ideal vaginal microbicide would be safe and effective, and also tasteless, colorless, odorless, nontoxic, stable in most climates, and affordable. It must be pointed out that like condoms, microbicides will not protect injection-drug users.

It will take generations to change male sexual behaviors, and women, especially in the underdeveloped nations, do not have generations—they are dying now in very large numbers 24 hours a day, seven days a week, 365 days a year! The idea that women will have a way of reasserting control over their own sexuality, the idea that they will be able to defend their bodily health, the idea that women will have a course of prevention to follow which results in saving their lives, the idea that women may have a microbicide which prevents infection but allows for conception, the idea that women can use microbicides without bowing to male dictates, the idea that men will not even know the microbicide is in use—these are ideas whose time has come.

If used by only 30% of women, microbicides could save 6 million lives over five years. These data are based on a microbicide that is 60% effective. But, the first generation of vaginal microbicide is not expected to receive FDA approval until 2012.

Developing A Microbicide?

Microbicides are chemical substances that, when applied to the skin, help prevent the spread of disease. When applied in the vagina or the rectum, hopefully, they would substantially reduce the transmission of HIV or other STDs. They could be produced in many forms, including gels, creams, suppositories, films, or as a sponge or vaginal ring.

In developing a vaginal microbicide, scientists must be sure that the substance is safe, does not kill microbes naturally present in the vagina that benefit female hygiene, and does not impair a woman's ability to conceive. Any microbicide will have to be tested to determine whether it damages spermatozoa, which could result in birth defects.

The Hi-Tech Microbicides

In 2003 and 2004, at the Tenth and Eleventh Retrovirus Conferences, a number of investigations in progress toward more chemically sophisticated HIV-specific microbicides were presented. The new hi-tech microbicides incorporate already-developed or very new and experimental anti-HIV drugs. Some, even have a systemic effect, meaning that they block HIV-infection sometime after application by protecting cells against HIV rather than by acting as a simple barrier. One trial already incorporates a currently available HIV drug into a microbicide. Tenofovir is under investigation in gel form as a possible vaginal microbicide. Tenofovir gel has undergone Phase I and II human safety study among U.S. women and is about to start a Phase III African trial. Two candidate microbicides incorporate non-nucleoside HIV drugs (NNRTIs). The highest tech end of microbicide research is starting to look at what could be topical vaccines that actually incorporate anti-HIV antibodies. To date, some 60 microbicides are under investigation, 16 of which are being used in five clinical trials involving 12,000 women in South Africa. Certain of these trials will end in 2008. In the United States, Carraguard, Savvy, Buffergel, Usherall and Pro 2000 are in Phase III clinical trials. In early 2007, microbicide trails using **Ushercell** (cellulose sulfate) were stopped because there was a higher rate of HIV infections in the women using Ushercell than in those in the placebo (non–Ushercell-using) group. In early 2008, studies using the microbicide **Carraguard** were stopped because it proved ineffective. An effective microbicide could be available sometime in 2012. To date 10 microbicide trials have failed.

QUESTIONS AND ANSWERS ABOUT THE FEMALE CONDOM

1. **Does one have to be fitted for the use of a female condom?** The female condom is offered in one size and is available without prescription. Unlike using a diaphragm, the female condom covers not only the cervix but also the vagina, thereby containing the man's ejaculate.

2. **Should a lubricant be used with the female condom?** A lubricant is recommended for use with the female condom to increase comfort and ease the entry and withdrawal of the penis. The female condom is prelubricated on the inside with a silicone-based, nonspermicidal lubricant. Additional water-based lubrication is included. The lubricant can be placed either inside the female condom or on the penis.

3. **Can oil-based lubricants be used with the female condom?** The female condom is made of polyurethane, which is not reported to be damaged by oil-based lubricants.

4. **Can a spermicide be used with the female condom?** Use of a spermicide has not been reported to damage the female condom.

5. **How far in advance of sexual intercourse can the female condom be inserted?** The female condom may be inserted up to 8 hours before sexual intercourse. Most women insert it 2 to 20 minutes before engaging in vaginal intercourse.

6. **Can the female condom be reused?** Ideally, no. A new female condom must be used for each act of vaginal intercourse. After intercourse, the condom must be removed before the woman stands, to ensure that semen remains inside the pouch. Despite the fact that the World Health Organization (WHO) does not recommend reuse of the female condom (FC), it has developed a protocol. This protocol recommends that the FC not be reused more than five times, and that it be sterilized in weak bleach solution (1:20 parts water), rinsed in water, and patted dry. The reason the WHO has developed a protocol for reuse is that in a number of developing African/Asian countries, the high cost of the female condom is forcing women, particularly commercial sex workers, to reuse the device to save money, despite the risks associated with reuse. Because of cost, commercial sex workers have revealed that many of the women were reusing the condom after cleaning it with substances such as beer, urine, water, and detergent.

7. **Should a female condom and a male condom be used at the same time?** The female condom and male condom can be used at the same time but it is not recommended, because the condoms may not stay in place due to friction between the latex in the male condom and the polyurethane in the female condom.

8. **Does Medicaid cover the female condom?** Currently Medicaid covers this device in 40 states, as it does the male condom, spermicide, and other barriers. *(Information provided by the New York State Department of Health AIDS Institute Division of HIV Prevention, Info Bulletin, Jan. 1994, Number Five Updated)*

9. **What is the main problem for women in using the female condom?** Ninety percent of women who found their first experience using the condom difficult had trouble with insertion. As an aside, young girls in Lesotho, Africa strip the rings out of the condoms and use them as bangles.

10. **Gay Men and Female Condoms?** Cristina Renzi (2003) reported that of men trying the female condom for anal sex, one in five (20%) of active or passive partners promote their use. Problems reported were: spillage and slippage during removal was reported more frequently with female condoms than with male latex condoms. Receptive partners more frequently reported pain or discomfort and rectal bleeding using female condoms than with male condoms.

11. **Materials on the Web** The following materials are available from UNAIDS at http://www.unaids.org/publications/documents/care/index.html#female:

The Female Condom: A Guide for Planning and Programming Information Update on Re-use of the Female Condom

Launching and Promoting the Female Condom in Eastern and Southern Africa

Use of the Female Condom: Gender Relations and Sexual Negotiations

The Female Condom and AIDS

INJECTION-DRUG USE AND HIV TRANSMISSION: THE TWIN EPIDEMICS

About 25% of the estimated 1.7 million (at the start of 2009) U.S. AIDS cases recorded since 1981 were transmitted through injection-drug use. Now about half of all new HIV infections occur from IDU. About 75% of all people with IDU-related AIDS are either black (50%) or Latino (24%).

Syringes and needles used to inject drugs or steroids, or to tattoo the body or to pierce the ears, should *never be shared*. If an individual is going to assume the risk of HIV transmission through needle sharing, the risk can be marginally reduced by sterilizing the needle and the syringe in undiluted chlorine bleach. The needle and syringe should be flushed through twice with bleach and rinsed thoroughly with water. Although using bleach to clean syringes after use may offer some protection, it has now been shown that using bleach and water is not nearly as effective as believed through the mid-1990s. Since then several studies have questioned the value of using bleach for disinfection of syringes. Collectively, these studies report that bleach has little or no protective effect (Abdala et al., 2001).

Both injection-drug use and HIV infection are on the increase. They are twin epidemics in the United States and Europe because the virus is readily transmitted by injection-drug users and then from infected drug users to their non-infected sexual partners. Stopping injection-drug-associated HIV transmission in theory is easy—just avoid injection-drug use. But, that is a difficult proposition for most of the estimated 8 million IDUs worldwide (2.5 million in the United States). The number of countries reporting IDU in 1989 was 80, in 2008, 148. IDUs will remain a major HIV connection to the homosexual, heterosexual, and pediatric populations.

HIV PREVENTION FOR INJECTION-DRUG USERS

What can be done and what is being done to prevent HIV transmission by this population? Available drug rehabilitation programs are far too few. It is estimated that only 15% of injection-drug users in the United States are receiving treatment at any given time. Many addicts want to quit their habit but may become discouraged because of having to wait so long before getting treatment because of lack of money and treatment centers. Even if there were a sufficient number of treatment centers, there will always be the hard-core IDUs who will not enter a program (Figure 9-6).

IDUs have an economic motive to share equipment. At the beginning of 2009, studies continue to show that over 50% of IDUs share the equipment. Perhaps the most important drawback may be that IDUs have little interest in health care or changing their behaviors. In addition, there is always the problem of legality. IDU is illegal throughout the United States.

IDUs know this and fear incarceration without the possibility of a "fix." A catch-22 situation also exists for those who want to help make injection-drug use safer: Many governmental agencies and law enforcement officers interpret the intention of making drug use safer as advocating drug use. As a result, many proponents of safer drug use have avoided becoming involved in the issue. The 2000 Kaiser Family Foundation National

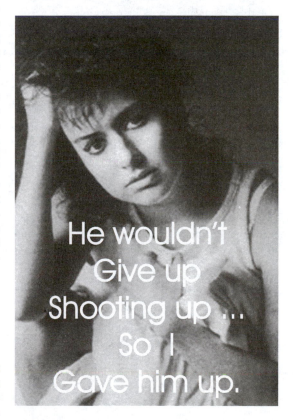

FIGURE 9-6   He wouldn't Give up Shooting up... So I Gave him up. (*Courtesy of the Centers for Disease Control and Prevention, Atlanta*)

Survey of Americans showed that 58% of those polled were in favor of syringe exchange programs. Beginning 2009, federal money could still not be used to fund needle exchange programs (NEPs).

Peter Lurie and colleagues (1998) state that each year, over 1 billion syringes would be required for IDUs to have a sterile syringe for each injection. **(Note: From this point forward, NEP stands for needle exchange programs and involves a needle and a syringe.)**

The Needle Exchange Program (NEP) Strategy

The idea of syringe-needle exchange program is based on the established public health policy of eliminating from any system potentially infectious agents or, where possible, carriers of infectious agents. The rationale of NEPs is similar, wherein active injection-drug users exchange used, potentially contaminated syringes for new, sterile syringes (Figure 9-7). In general, these exchanges are done on a one used needle and syringe for one new needle and syringe basis, though some programs will add an additional number of needles and syringes on top of those already exchanged. NEPs also provide other paraphernalia and supplies including cotton, cookers, water, and sterile alcohol prep pads. In addition, NEPs offer a variety of other services to IDUs including education, HIV testing and counseling, referrals to primary medical care, substance abuse treatment, and case management.

The world's first NEP on record began in 1984 in Amsterdam, The Netherlands. It was started by an IDU advocacy group called the Junkie Union.

Jon Parker is believed to be the first person in the United States to distribute free drug injection equipment publicly. He did so in North Haven, Conn., and in Boston in November 1986.

Evaluation of Needle/Syringe Exchange Programs

Entering year 2009, about 200 NEPs operating in American cities were exchanging about 30 million syringes annually. An IDU makes about 1000 drug injections each year (*MMWR,* 1997). The San Francisco AIDS Foundation operates the largest NEP in the United States. There are too many NEPs to list, but a few are presented here.

Tacoma, Washington—Their NEP began in August 1988. It began as a one-man program by Dave Purchase, a 20-year drug counselor.

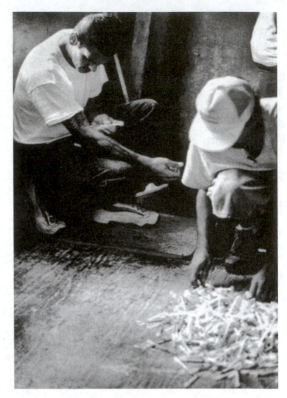

FIGURE 9-7 Getting a Fix. An injection-drug user shoots up in a shooting gallery in the La Perla neighborhood of Old San Juan, Puerto Rico. Another man sorts used syringes to be exchanged for new. (*Photo by Enrique Valentin/South Florida* Sun-Sentinel)

The NEP in Tacoma held the HIV infection rate to under 5% over a five-year study period (1988–1992). During that same five-year study period, the prevalence of HIV infection among IDUs in New York City, with few syringe exchange programs, increased from 10% to 50%! About 1.5 million syringes are exchanged annually.

New York City—In November 1988, after many delays, New York City began its NEP. The program was canceled in early 1990—the reason: because over 50% of NYC's 240,000 IDUs were HIV infected, the program offered too little too late to have an impact. IDUs make up about 38% to 40% of NYC AIDS cases. The NEP was resumed in 1992. In 1998 there were at least five NEPs operating in New York City. In May 2000, New York State passed a law making it legal to buy needles without a prescription, the forty-third state to do so. About 3 million syringes are exchanged annually.

New Haven, Conn.—Their 14-year-old program has demonstrated that NEPs dramatically slow the rate of infection without encouraging new injection-drug use. Some indicators even suggest that the program has been responsible for a decrease in both crime and the amount of drugs used illegally. These results have enabled policymakers elsewhere to call for NEPs.

After the passage of a 1992 law permitting pharmacies to sell syringes without a prescription, syringe sharing has dropped 40% in the state of Connecticut. Seventy-five percent of AIDS cases in Connecticut occur among IDUs, their sex partners, and their children.

California—Each year about 8000 Californians are infected with HIV, and injection-drug use is the second leading cause of those infections. In October 1999 a law was passed that would allow cities and counties to establish NEPs. Entering 2008 at least 14 cities and counties had funded NEPs. About 4 million syringes are exchanged annually.

Hawaii—In 1990, Hawaii became the first state to legalize a statewide NEP. The state legislature felt it was necessary to stem the rate of HIV infection in women and newborns. About 1 million syringes are exchanged annually.

Beginning 2008, all 50 states have some type of NEP system in place.

Needle Exchange Programs in Other Countries

There are an estimated 16 million IDUs worldwide. Many countries are now involved in NEPs to lower the spread of HIV.

Needle exchange program results from England, Austria, The Netherlands, Sweden, and Scotland, presented at the Fourth International AIDS Conference (1988), suggest that the European programs attracted IDUs who had no previous contact with drug treatment programs; and that IDUs were drawn from NEPs into treatment programs, thus the decrease in drug use. There was no indication in these studies of an increase in injection-drug use in cities with exchange programs. Where HIV testing had been done, the rate of HIV infection showed a marked decline after the introduction of NEPs (Raymond, 1988; Hagen, 1991).

Some of the countries with active NEPs are: Canada, England, France, Ireland, The Netherlands, Australia, New Zealand, Italy, and China.

Some countries, instead of offering NEP, offer IDU treatment centers. Switzerland is currently providing IDUs with heroin three times a day in 18 treatment centers across the country. So far Swiss health authorities say the program has reduced criminal activity among the participants by about 60%. The program also reduced their rate of homelessness from 12% to zero and their death rate by 50%. Entering 2008, following Switzerland's lead, Germany, The Netherlands, Spain, Portugal, Australia, Luxembourg, and Vancouver, British Columbia (North America's first consumption room) have implemented consumption or injection rooms for the legal use of heroin. There are about 50 legal heroin consumption rooms or clinics worldwide. Requests for heroin consumption rooms in Austria and the United States have been denied.

DISCUSSION QUESTION: The United States has zero tolerance for such activities and will not become involved in what the Swiss term "an innovative program." Do you think the United States should, based on the Swiss data, offer heroin to the addicted in a controlled environment similar to the Swiss? Present credible reasons/data to support your stand.

LIFTING THE BAN ON THE USE OF FEDERAL FUNDING TO SUPPORT NEEDLE EXCHANGE PROGRAMS

Since 1990, seven national reports have reviewed the scientific evidence and recommended that the federal ban for NEP funding be lifted. In April 1998, Health and Human Services Secretary Donna Shalala informed President Clinton that scientific research had proven that NEPs effectively prevent the transmission of HIV and hepatitis and do not lead to increased drug use. Her long-awaited action cleared the way for the president to lift the 10-year ban on federal funding for NEPs. Clinton accepted the findings, but stated that in spite of them he would continue to block the use of federal funds for NEPs. President George Bush continued that ban. As of the start of 2009, the ban remains in effect.

DISCUSSION QUESTION: Do you agree with current federal policy on money for NEPs? List any scientific facts or studies that could be used to support President Bush's action. List any that disagree with his decision.

Summary

Entering 2009, 85% of IDUs in Glasgow, 83% in Lund, 85% in Sydney, 74% in Tacoma, and 88% in Toronto reported they had changed their behavior in order to avoid HIV/AIDS. The most commonly mentioned specific behavior change: reduced sharing of injection equipment.

PREVENTION OF BLOOD AND BLOOD PRODUCT HIV TRANSMISSION

A combined fear of disease and lawsuits have led most wealthy developed nations to adopt a zero tolerance policy regarding HIV contamination of the blood supply. However, 10% of all new HIV infections in developing countries are due to transfusions of tainted blood. In the early 1980s, 1 of every 50 bags of blood collected in San Francisco contained HIV. The chance of acquiring either HIV or hepatitis C from a blood transfusion, in America, is now about 1 in 1 million.

Blood Donors

In the United States, there are at least 52 medically related restrictions for donating your blood. Thirteen of these reasons place a person on permanent restriction from donating blood—for example, being HIV positive, having multiple sclerosis, being a hemophiliac, men having sex with other men since 1977 (even once), having used injection drugs (even once), or having had a stroke.

There should be no risk in the United States or in other developed nations of contracting HIV by donating blood if blood centers use a new, sterile needle for each donation. Yet a 1998 survey revealed that 25% of those polled believed that they could become HIV infected by **donating blood.**

Blood Collection and Screening Blood for HIV

Testing blood for infectious diseases began with syphilis screening in the 1940s. Hepatitis B antibody screening was added in the 1970s, HIV antibody screening in 1985, the hepatitis B-core antigen in 1986, HTL V-1 and II-antibodies in 1988, and hepatitis C antibodies in 1990. Inclusion of the HIV antigen (p24) test in 1996 provided detection of HIV infection sooner than antibody testing. At least eight tests for infectious diseases are now routinely performed on each unit of blood collected.

No Blood Purchases for Transfusion—All blood transfused in the United States comes from volunteer donors. Blood from paid donors is used for pharmaceuticals such as Rh Ig, albumin, and intravenous immunoglobulins. Under the current standards for blood banks and transfusion services of the American Association of Blood Banks, all units must be clearly labeled volunteer, paid, or autologous (donated for self-use).

U.S. FDA Approves Blood Screening Test for HIV—Blood screening for HIV and HIV-testing procedures are presented in Chapter 13. The risk of becoming HIV infected from a blood transfusion has dropped by more than 99% from 1983 to 2003. Regardless, a male living in Durango, Tex., received contaminated blood during heart bypass surgery in August 2000. This is reported to be the first case of HIV-positive blood transfusion since restrictive blood-screening tests for HIV were put in place in April 1999. In 2002, two people became HIV infected from blood transfusions in Florida's Tampa Bay area. Tracing the infectious blood back to its donor source revealed that, in both incidents, the donors were in the **window period;** they were infected but the blood test failed to detect the virus.

Blood Transfusions Worldwide—Twenty-three years after the industrialized world began to screen all blood used in transfusions for HIV, about 1 in 10 people in developing countries are still being infected through this route.

A combination of the lack of screening with high levels of infected donors turns transfusion into a form of roulette. As 2009 began, blood transfusions accounted for 5% to 10% of HIV infections worldwide.

Blood Safety—From 1985 into 2009, over 500 million units of blood or plasma have been screened for HIV antibody in the United States. By excluding those who test HIV positive and by asking people from high-risk behavior groups not to donate blood, the incidence of HIV transmission from the current blood supply is relatively low. With faster and more accurate testing procedures now in use, the risk is becoming even lower. However, the probability or risk of receiving HIV-contaminated blood will never be zero. The reason a small risk still exists is because some people infected with HIV may donate blood during what is known as the window period. During that period, a person may be infected with the HIV, but the test cannot yet detect the infection. And, the test is not 100% accurate.

INFECTION CONTROL PROCEDURES

With no cure or vaccine for HIV/AIDS, prevention of infection is of paramount importance. With the advent of the HIV/AIDS epidemic, healthcare workers and others who are occupationally exposed to body fluids, especially blood, are understandably concerned about the risk of becoming HIV infected. However, when precautions are observed, the risk is very small, even for those treating HIV/AIDS patients.

Two sets of infection control procedures are in use in hospitals, medical centers, physicians' offices, and units that deal with people in medical emergencies. One is called **universal precautions,** the other is **blood and body substance isolation.**

Universal Precautions (UP)

Universal precautions (Table 9-5) are standard practices that workers observe on the job to protect themselves from infections and injuries. These precautions or safety practices are called **universal** because they are used in all situations even if there seems to be no risk. Universal precautions had their

---

Table 9-5 Universal Precautions: Protection from Infections

DEFINITION

Universal precautions (UP) are a set of infection control practices developed by the Centers for Disease Control and Prevention in which healthcare workers (HCWs) appropriately utilize barrier protection (gloves, gowns, masks, eyewear, etc.) for anticipated contact with blood and certain body fluids of *all* patients.

1. The hands and skin must be carefully washed when contaminated with blood or certain body fluids.

2. Particular care is taken to prevent injuries caused by sharp instruments.

3. Resuscitation devices should be available where the need is predictable.

4. HCWs with exudative lesions or weeping dermatitis should refrain from patient care until the condition resolves.

BLOOD AND BODY FLUIDS TO WHICH UP APPLY

Blood is the single most important risk source of HIV, HBV, and other blood-borne pathogens in the occupational setting. Prevention of transmission must focus on reducing the risk of exposure to blood and other body fluids or potentially infectious materials containing visible blood.

1. UP should be used when exposure to the following body fluids may be anticipated:
   a. Blood
   b. Serum plasma
   c. Semen
   d. Vaginal secretions
   e. Amniotic fluid
   f. Cerebrospinal fluid (CSF)
   g. Synovial fluid
   h. Pleural fluid
   i. Vitheous fluid
   j. Peritoneal fluid
   k. Pericardial fluid
   l. Wound exudates
   m. Any other body fluid containing visible blood (but not feces, urine, saliva, sputum, tears, nasal secretions, or sweat, unless they contain visible blood).

2. Note: Blood, semen, and vaginal secretions have been shown to transmit HIV. The others, with the exception of fluids containing visible blood, remain a theoretical risk.

RATIONALE

1. UP reduces the risk of parenteral, mucous membrane, and skin exposure to blood-borne pathogens such as, but not limited to, HIV and HBV.

2. For several reasons, focusing precautions only on diagnosed cases misses the vast majority of persons who are infected (many of whom are asymptomatic or subclinical) and who may be as infectious as the diagnosed cases. Persons who have seen a physician and have been diagnosed with acute or active disease represent only a small proportion of all persons with infection. Infectivity always precedes the diagnosis, which often is made once symptoms develop.

(Adapted from Mountain-Plains Regional AIDS Education Training Center HIV/AIDS Curriculum, Nov. 1994.)

beginnings in 1976 when barrier techniques were first recommended for the prevention of hepatitis B infection. Precautions required the use of protective eyewear, gloves, and gowns, and careful handling of needles and other sharp instruments. In 1977, hepatitis B immunoglobulin was recommended for those exposed to hepatitis B through needle sticks. In 1982, hepatitis B vaccine became commercially available and recommended for all healthcare workers exposed to human blood.

Under universal precautions, the blood and certain body fluids of all patients are considered potentially infectious for HIV, hepatitis B virus (HBV), and other blood-borne pathogens.

Universal precautions are intended to prevent parenteral (introduction of a substance into the body by injection), mucous membrane, and broken skin exposure of healthcare workers (HCWs), teachers, or any other person who may become exposed to blood-borne pathogens. In 1987, the CDC also published a report that got the immediate attention of most, if not all, informed healthcare workers. The report stated that three healthcare workers who were exposed to the blood of AIDS patients tested positive for HIV. What was so startling was that until that time, needle punctures and cuts were thought to be the only dangers in a clinical setting. These three cases appeared to involve only skin exposure to HIV-contaminated blood. One of the three cases involved a nurse whose chapped and ungloved hands were exposed to an AIDS patient's blood.

The second case involved a nurse who broke a vacuum tube during a routine phlebotomy on an outpatient. The blood splashed on her face and into her mouth. A blood splash was also involved in the third case. The worker's ungloved hands and forearms were exposed to HIV-contaminated blood (Ezzell, 1987).

An Important Wake-Up Call

These three cases of HIV infection informed healthcare workers in the most dramatic way that they were all vulnerable. Perhaps these three cases produced a fear among healthcare workers out of proportion to the actual risk of their becoming infected. Although calculations show that the risk of HIV infection after exposure to blood from an HIV/AIDS patient is about 1 in 200, if you are that one, probability is meaningless.

Who Is Affected by Universal Precaution Mandate?

The universal precautions as published by the CDC currently apply to some 5.3 million healthcare workers at 620,000 work sites across the United States and another 700,000 Americans who routinely come in contact with blood as part of their job, for example, people in law enforcement, education, fire fighting and rescue, corrections, laboratory research, and the funeral industry.

In summary, the concept of universal precautions assumes that all blood is infectious, no matter from whom and no matter whether a test is negative, positive, or not done at all. Rigorous adherence to universal precautions is the surest way of preventing accidental transmission of HIV and other blood-borne pathogens.

Blood and Body Substance Isolation (BBSI)

An alternative, and some believe superior, approach to the CDC's universal precautions in areas of high HIV prevalence is the system referred to as **body substance precautions or Blood Body Substance Isolation (BBSI)** (Gerberding, 1991).

In practice, these precautions are similar to universal precautions, in that prevention of needle stick injury and use of barrier methods of infection control are emphasized. Philosophically, however, the two are quite different. Whereas universal precautions place a clear emphasis on avoidance of blood-borne infection, body substance precautions take a more global view. Body substance isolation (BBSI) requires barrier precautions for all body substances (including feces, respiratory secretions, urine, vomit, etc.) and moist body surfaces (including mucous membranes and open wounds). BBSI is designed as a system to reduce the risk of transmission of all nosocomial (hospital-associated) pathogens, not just blood-borne pathogens. Gloves are worn for any anticipated or known contact with mucous membranes, nonintact skin, and moist body substances of all patients.

SEXUAL PARTNER NOTIFICATION: DISCLOSURE

One of the most controversial issues in HIV prevention is **contact tracing, partner notification, or disclosure** of sexual contacts mostly because HIV/AIDS is considered an incurable disease with a great deal of stigma attached to the infected. Disclosure can cause an increase in stigma and discrimination, but it is also, paradoxically, an essential step in fighting stigma and discrimination.

Partner notification is the practice of identifying and treating people exposed to certain communicable diseases. The term "partner notification" rather than disclosure is used by the CDC and some healthcare providers because it more comprehensively describes the process by which the physician, other healthcare workers such as Disease Intervention Specialists (DIS, someone who is specially trained in STD work), and the infected person may provide information to at-risk partners and sometimes to family, friends, or care providers.

How Does One Communicate in Partner Notification: Disclosure?

There are two very different approaches to informing unsuspecting third parties about their potential exposure to medical risk.

Each approach has its own history, including a unique set of practical problems in its implementation, and provokes its own ethical dilemmas. The **first** approach, involving the moral **duty to warn,** arose out of the clinical setting in which the physician knew the identity of the person deemed to be at risk. This approach provided a warrant for disclosure to endangered persons without the consent of the patient and could involve revealing the identity of the patient. The **second** approach—that of contact tracing—emerged from sexually transmitted disease control programs in which the clinician typically did not know the identity of those who might have been exposed. This approach was founded on the voluntary cooperation of the patient in providing the names of contacts. It never involved the disclosure of the identity of the patient. The entire process of notification was kept confidential (Bayer, 1992).

THE U.S. FEDERAL GOVERNMENT HAS NOW ADOPTED PARTNER NOTIFICATION AS ITS CORNERSTONE IN ITS EFFORT TO HELP CONTROL THE SPREAD OF HIV

A major reason for the federal government's push for partner notification is that it is a more efficient and focused way to test for HIV. Studies show that routine testing and counseling among the general population typically turns up new infections in less than 1% of those tested. But among the sexual partners of HIV-positive people, infection rates are around 20%. Partner notification concentrates on a group most likely to have previously undetected infections.

History of Sexual Partner Notification

The concept of partner notification was proposed in 1937 by Surgeon General Thomas Parran for the control of syphilis (Parran, 1937). By tracing and treating all known contacts of a syphilitic patient, the chain of transmission could be interrupted. According to George Rutherford (1988), contact tracing has been successfully used for a number of STDs beginning in the 1950s. It is still used in cases of syphilis, endemic gonorrhea, chlamydia, hepatitis B, STD enteric infections, and particularly in cases of antibiotic-resistant gonorrhea.

In 1985, when the HIV antibody was first used in screening the blood supply, notification of blood donors and other HIV-infected individuals and their contacts became possible. The strategy in HIV partner notification is the same as that used for the other STDs: to identify HIV-infected individuals, counsel them, and offer whatever treatment is available. In asymptomatic HIV-infected people only counseling is given.

Partner Notification Depends on Cooperation

Partner notification depends on HIV-positive people to give the names of their partners; but they may be reluctant to do so fearing that their identification may result in physical abuse and loss of jobs and housing. For a review of partner notification read the article by Kevin Fenton et al., 1997. Those who oppose the use of partner notification call the investigators "sex police."

Examples in the Use of Sexual Partner Notification/Contact Tracing

One—In April 1993 an incarcerated male asked for an HIV test. The diagnosis was positive. Contact tracing turned up a network of 124 persons; all were linked by syringe sharing and syringe sharing with sex. One hundred twenty-one were contacted and offered an HIV test; 118 accepted the test; 44 were positive. One hundred thirteen of the 124 lived in the same county. The estimated cost for partner notification in this network was $13,969 (*MMWR, 1995*).

BOX 9.2

CHELSEA GULDEN, AGE 24, MOTHER AND PREVENTION DISCLOSURE ADVOCATE

Chelsea Gulden is a 24-year-old HIV-positive mother and prevention/disclosure advocate (Figure 9-8). She was diagnosed in 2003 while she was a student in the University of North Carolina system. "My boyfriend and I tested positive in 2003. The first thing that came to mind was I couldn't have kids. But I had only two or three days to stress out. I went back to the doctor and I learned I was five weeks pregnant. I didn't know much about HIV. I kept asking myself what it meant for my quality of life and immediately became concerned about my pregnancy. I had to stop and make sure that my motives for wanting a child were the right ones. For instance, was I really ready for a baby? Was I in a place where I could take care of a child both emotionally and physically?"

CHELSEA'S BIG DECISION

After discussions with her physician and learning as quickly as possible all that she could about HIV/AIDS, Chelsea decided to keep her pregnancy. After her decision, her pregnancy, delivery, and newborn were labors of love. Her cherished son, who is HIV negative, is now three and a half years old and without a doubt the greatest joy in her life.

HER MAJOR FEARS

She worries that her health and economic budget may not last long enough for her to mother her son through college. She would like more children if she can find the right person, but again she fears that she may not be there in the long run. Another concern is how other children may treat her son when they find out his mother is HIV positive.

POST-DIAGNOSIS ADVENTURES

Since diagnosis, Chelsea has worked on spreading awareness and HIV education across the Carolinas and abroad. She is currently responsible for implementing programs for HIV-infected youth in the Charlotte area. This effort was started to assist with keeping a continuum of medical care and support as these youth learn to cope with their diagnosis. Her presentations have taken her many places. She has spoken at many HIV/AIDS gatherings and conferences. In October 2006, an appearance in *HIV Plus* and on the *Oprah Winfrey Show* boosted Chelsea's speaking career. In 2007, Chelsea made the cover of

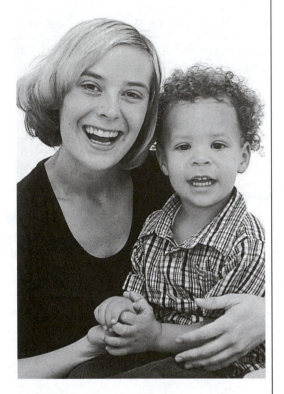

FIGURE 9-8 Chelsea Gulden. Going into her senior year of college, unexpectedly she found out that she was HIV positive. She had such faith that the HIV test would be negative, she did not return for her test results. A disease intervention specialist located Chelsea and told her she tested positive. Chelsea said, "My whole world collapsed, my heart dropped to my feet." Several days later she learned she was five weeks pregnant.
(With appreciation to Chelsea Gulden who provided the information used herein and to Emile M. Knight who granted permission and the photograph of Chelsea and her son.)

POZ magazine. Her speaking circuit has taken her across the United States as an AIDS awareness speaker for the Safe Haven Project, as well as teaching sexual health at the University of North Carolina–Charlotte. As a devoted advocate for HIV/AIDS awareness prevention and disclosure, she first makes time to be a devoted and responsible mother.

HIV-POSITIVE PEOPLE CARRY THE BURDEN OF DISCLOSURE

Actually, HIV-positive people should assess the risk they pose to others at all times with respect to how HIV can be transmitted and their involvement in those situations. However, telling someone, anyone that you're HIV positive is not an easy task.

TELLING SOMEONE YOU ARE HIV POSITIVE

In an ideal world, everyone would recognize that sexual safety and health is an obligation and responsibility of all parties involved. Asking about HIV and STD status and being prepared for safer sex would be expected of everyone. Unfortunately, because so many people are uneducated about HIV, STDs, and safer sex, the ideal world doesn't exist. HIV-positive people carry the burden of assessing the level of risk they engage in and/or subject others to.

Telling someone that you're HIV positive is rarely easy. If the person you're telling is a potential sex partner it can become even more challenging. When you disclose your HIV-positive status to a potential

sex partner, you run the risk of rejection. A lot depends upon the person that you are disclosing to and your relationship with them. Because of the stigma that comes with the HIV infection, people may reject you, gossip about you, openly or secretly discriminate against you or your family, or even threaten you. Revealing your status to someone else can be scary, isolating, and overwhelming. For those who are in denial about their HIV-positive status, it will be difficult to admit it to someone else or to disclose to or protect a sexual partner. Others who are bound by fear, shame, and distrust may even lie about their status. Some HIV-positive people believe in the "don't ask, don't tell" policy—if your partner doesn't ask, then you don't have to tell. Your only obligation is to do everything in your power to keep him or her safe. Others pick and choose those whom they feel that they can trust with this information. Still others are open about their status and disclose to family, friends, and sexual partners with little hesitation.

Two—During a five-month period (February through June 1999) seven young people were diagnosed with HIV in a small rural town in Mississippi. The CDC, working with the Mississippi Health Department through partner contact investigation, defined a social network of 122 people. Persons in the network had a median age of 21 (range: 13 to 45 years). Of the 78 people tested for HIV infection, five women (median age, 16 years) and two men (median age, 25 years) were infected, all through heterosexual sex. Results of the interviews of the infected and noninfected people indicated a serious lack of HIV/AIDS prevention knowledge (*MMWR*, 2000a).

Three—At the 2004 Eleventh Conference of Retroviruses and Opportunistic Infections investigators said they found the number of new HIV infections in men from 37 southern colleges has risen rapidly in just a few years. In 2000 there were 6; in 2001, 19; in 2002, 29; and in 2003, 30. Of that total of 84 new infections, 73 were in blacks and 11 in whites. Sixty-three percent reported having sex with men only, 33% with both men and women, and 4% with women only. They attended 33 colleges in North Carolina, two in South Carolina, one in Georgia and one in Florida. The outbreak was identified in

time for the authorities to ask North Carolina's colleges to include safer sex messages during Fall 2004 orientation sessions. Stories about the outbreak, appearing in campus newspapers, contact tracing or partner notification, and free HIV testing helped reveal and tie this minor college epidemic together.

Conclusion

In January 2003, two separate studies, one by Patricia Kissinger and colleagues and the other by Tamara Hoxworth, reveal that previously held conceptions on the negative aspects of partner notifications are wrong. Their findings reveal that partner notification rarely damages relationships or promotes violence and that, if anything, exposure to partner notification contributes to safe behaviors. Partner notification did not lead to more relationship breakups among HIV-positive individuals, in comparison to syphilis-infected persons.

DISCUSSION QUESTION: With current life-sustaining antiretroviral treatments available, is there an overwhelming excuse not to use partner notification—especially when so many HIV/AIDS experts promote the "hit early"—approach to therapy?

What is your response to the reasons for partner notification and to the opposition's point of view?

The Duty to Warn

The **duty to warn** may extend to nonpatient third parties in other contexts, based on the provider's primary duty to the patient. Thus, healthcare professionals have a duty to inform patients that they have been transfused with HIV-contaminated blood and this duty may extend to third parties. A physician in one case failed to inform a teenager or her parents that she had been transfused with HIV-contaminated blood. When the young woman's sexual partner tested positive for HIV, the court upheld his claim against the physician based on the physician's failure to inform the patient. Similarly, courts have upheld that a healthcare professional's duty to inform the patient of his or her HIV infection may extend to those the patient foreseeably puts at risk, such as a spouse or family member caregiver. On the other hand, courts have ruled that disclosure is wrongful in cases in which the third party, such as a family member, is not at actual risk of infection, or the physician has no knowledge that the patient has failed to disclose to the partner (Gostin et al., 1998).

At the end of 2008, at least 39 states in America have enacted partner notification laws that provide for penalties that range from a misdemeanor (a crime less serious than a felony, which is a serious crime) to attempted murder for anyone who does not reveal to a sexual partner that he or she is HIV positive. At least 44 states passed laws requiring or permitting workers (mostly healthcare workers or public safety employees) to be notified of potential exposure of HIV. In some cases, the laws allow testing of the source patient. To date, Arkansas and Missouri are the only states that require patients to notify healthcare providers of their HIV status before receiving care. All 50 states are now somewhere in the process of establishing the capacity for contact tracing at the request of a patient.

DISCUSSION QUESTION: If a law were passed that made persons who practiced high-risk behaviors and who contracted HIV/AIDS pay for their care and treatment or forego medical help—do you think these people would continue to engage in high-risk behaviors? Would this law be an effective means of HIV transmission prevention? Present examples to support your position. (Can you relate this scenario to those who smoke and develop cancer?)

For a detailed report on partner notification published by the WHO and UNAIDS see: http://www.who.int/asd/knowledge/rptngdiscl.html.

THE FIRST HUMAN VACCINE: THE IMPACT OF VACCINES ON INFECTIOUS DISEASES

The first human vaccine was developed in 1796 by Edward Jenner to prevent smallpox. With the exception of clean drinking water, no other human health intervention has had the impact of vaccination on reducing infectious diseases. Every year, vaccines prevent about 3 million deaths and save about a million children from disabilities caused by infectious diseases. Vaccines have been documented to be the most cost-effective means of improving human health. No human vaccine is 100% effective, but most vaccines protect between 70% and 95% of those vaccinated against the targeted disease.

HIV VACCINE DEVELOPMENT AND ITS ROLE IN PREVENTION

> Several lines of evidence indicate that development of an effective vaccine for HIV is going to be, at best, extremely. difficult. The inability to solve fundamental scientific questions is the root cause for why a successful vaccine is not currently within our grasp. A renewed, organized, focused effort is needed to overcome these scientific obstacles. The immediate prospects for hitting on a worthwhile HIV vaccine would possibly be like hitting a baseball blindfold.
>
> Roaald C. Desrosiers, 2007
> Immunologist, New England
> Primate Research Center

Despite the effectiveness of antiretroviral therapy and considerable success in reducing the price of the drugs in resource-poor settings, the relentless spread of HIV continues to overwhelm all efforts to contain it. AIDS cannot be stopped without an effective means of preventing future infections. Unfortunately, the quest for a vaccine continues to elude our best scientific efforts. The new vaccines that looked so promising a few short years ago have produced disappointing results. Some scientists argue that there is no guarantee we will ever have a vaccine, while others are more optimistic but recognize that HIV presents a uniquely difficult challenge. Yet even if a perfect vaccine were created today, it would take roughly 10 years to provide it to all those who need it. It is difficult to overstate the damage that another 10 years without a vaccine will do. To better understand what a vaccine is, how they have been made and used, and why we do not have a vaccine for HIV, the following information on vaccines is presented.

A vaccine is considered the Holy Grail in the battle against disease. The Holy Grail of HIV/AIDS prevention is a single-dose, safe, affordable oral vaccine that gives lifelong protection against all subtypes of HIV.

It is always better to prevent disease than to treat it. Vaccines protect those or disease bearing agents that come into contact with unvaccinated individuals or disease-bearing agents that carry the disease.

Historically, vaccines have provided a safe, cost-effective, and efficient means of preventing illness, disability, and death from infectious diseases through the use of vaccinations.

It is now abundantly clear that no pharmacologic agent, no educational efforts directed to safer sex (regardless of how vigorously implemented), and no nutritional modification will stop nor prevent this pandemic from continuing. Halting the spread of HIV requires an effective vaccine. Entering 2009, an estimated 56 million people will either be living with HIV or will have died from it.

Vaccine—Its Impact on Prevention

An effective HIV vaccine cannot take the place of HIV-prevention efforts, any more than prevention efforts can take the place of a vaccine. The best way to address the HIV pandemic is using multiple interventions at multiple levels. The protective power of a vaccine, if one is found, will be of enormous benefit in HIV prevention. But there have been increases in sexual risk behavior in men who have sex with men (MSM) since the advent of ART (antiretroviral treatment). There is concern that when a vaccine becomes available there could be similar increases in risk behavior among people who receive the HIV vaccine because they feel they can't become infected with HIV.

Dispelling What Vaccine Scientists Thought They Knew About Creating Vaccines for Disease Prevention

One benefit from all of the HIV-vaccine research to date is that scientists found out that they know far less than they thought they knew about producing specific prevention vaccines. Almost all previously developed vaccines were made empirically. From

POINT OF INFORMATION 9.3

THE GOAL OF DEVELOPING AN HIV VACCINE

PAST PRESIDENT CLINTON SETS A VACCINE GOAL

Speaking to the graduating class at Morgan State University on **May 18, 1997**, President Clinton invoked the legacy of John F. Kennedy's 1960s race to the moon and set a national target of developing an AIDS vaccine within the next 10 years (2007). This was the first annual Vaccine Awareness Day in America. The president said, "We dare not be complacent in meeting the challenge of HIV, the virus that causes AIDS." He then announced the creation of a research center at the National Institutes of Health in Bethesda, Md., to complete the task. However, Clinton's goal for a preventive HIV vaccine by year 2007 failed.

In June 2001, Health and Human Services Secretary Tommy Thompson told scientists at a Geneva gathering that an HIV vaccine will be available within three to five years. There was a collective audible groan from his audience as they must have recalled a similar comment by Margaret Heckler on April 23, 1984.

With the failure of a third human HIV vaccine, in which there was so much hope (see POV 9.4), there is a real fear that there may never be an acceptable HIV vaccine! However, it must be cautioned that historically, it has taken decades and more setbacks than advances from the discovery of a virus or bacterium until an effective vaccine is licensed. Typhoid was discovered in 1884 but there was no vaccine until 1989, over 100 years later. The measles vaccine took 42 years to develop. Malaria was discovered in 1893 but still has no vaccine. In the 1930s, two experimental polio vaccines failed because they were determined to be unsafe, and polio vaccines were almost abandoned. At the time, we understood how to prevent infection by sanitation and avoiding public swimming areas, just as we know how to stop HIV infection today. We needed new tools then, and we need them now.

May 18, 2008—The Eleventh anniversary—has passed.

Predictions Continue for an AIDS Vaccine (HIV)

Now the date for a vaccine has been pushed to 2020 at the earliest, some 40 years following the announcement by the CDC of a new and baffling disease affecting gay men in the United States. It is important to understand that even if an AIDS vaccine is found now, the vaccine will have no impact on the approximately 24 million new infections estimated to occur by 2020. Because there are no current prospects for a medical cure for AIDS, the only remaining strategy for slowing the next 24 million infections is through prevention efforts.

smallpox to measles, most FDA-approved vaccines have been developed through trial and error: substitute, kill, attenuate, fragment, mix, and test for the one that works. For example, scientists believed that vaccines work simply by producing antibodies, right? Well, probably not. This misconception coupled with basic ignorance of how they do work is stalling the urgent quest for an HIV/AIDS vaccine. No one yet has found out how highly successful vaccines like polio, measles, and hepatitis B actually protect people from disease. Phillippe Kourilsky, director of the Pasteur Institute, said, "We've had many successful vaccines over the past decades but we've missed a chance to see how these vaccines work. Each time a vaccine works the scientific community wanders off and leaves it to the public health workers to use it—and fails to invest in the research. If we had done that we would have been in a much better position to tackle the AIDS vaccine problem." Scientists are, for the first time, learning about the mechanisms of viral-host pathologies necessary to produce preventive vaccines.

What Is a Vaccine?

A vaccine is a suspension of whole microorganisms, or viruses, or a suspension of some structural component or product of them that will elicit an immune response after entering a host. In brief, vaccines mimic the organisms, virus, or other agents that cause disease, alerting the immune system to be aware of certain viruses or bacteria. Because of this advance warning system, when the real organism or virus invades the body, the immune system marshals a response before the disease has time to develop. That is, the immune system, by previous exposure, has learned or been trained to defend itself against a disease-causing agent.

Ideally, the body will make **neutralizing antibodies** (antibodies that prevent infection by neutralizing—cancelling out—HIV's ability to cause infection; an effective neutralizing antibody is the "Holy Grail" of preventing HIV infection) that bind to and disable the foreign invader **(humoral immunity)** and trigger white blood cells called T cells to organize **attack cells** in the body to destroy those cells that have been infected by viruses **(cellular immunity).** Once the immune system's T cells and B cells are activated, some of them turn into **memory cells.** The more memory cells the body forms, the faster its response to make antibody. (See Chapter 5 for a discussion of the human immune system.) To date all successful vaccines prevent disease through the production of neutralizing antibodies.

The Use of Weakened or Inactivated Agents to Trigger Humoral and Cellular Immunity

Some vaccines, such as those against smallpox, polio (Sabins), measles, mumps, and tuberculosis, contain genetically altered or weakened organisms or viruses that are reproduced in the body after being administered but do not generally produce disease. Yet since the virus or bacterium is still alive, there is a small risk of developing the disease.

Whooping cough, cholera, and influenza vaccines are made of inactivated whole organisms and viruses or pieces of them. Because killed organisms and inactivated virus do not replicate inside the recipient, the vaccines confer only humoral immunity (the production of antibody), which, in some cases, are short-lived.

What Then Is the Goal of an HIV Vaccine?

The goal of an HIV vaccine is to teach the immune system new and hopefully better ways to win the battle against the virus. HIV vaccines exploit the side of the immune system that is learned (acquired) by providing information to cells in new ways in hopes of enhancing their learning and making them more effective fighters. Why the human immune system cannot learn to make neutralizing antibodies from the current group of vaccines in clinical trials is the "billion dollar question." At the beginning of 2009 there were over 30 clinical trials ongoing, using about 40 different vaccines, in four continents involving 24 countries (Figure 9-9). The most advanced vaccine trial that got under way in 2005, the adenovirus-5 vector, vaccine failed. (See Point of View 9.3)

Types of HIV Vaccines

Scientists are attempting to design three types of HIV vaccines: (1) a **preventive** or **prophylactic vaccine** to protect people from becoming HIV infected (chance of success—doubtful). Historically, primary prevention is most often referred to as sterilizing or 100% immunity, in which a vaccine is given to those who have not yet been exposed to the infectious agent. This was the focus of many earlier vaccine searches and remains a target even though researchers will now accept far less than a 100% effective HIV vaccine and still feel successful. (One hundred percent immunity is an ideal. In reality, most vaccines licensed in the United States are between 70% and 95% effective.) (2) A **therapeutic**

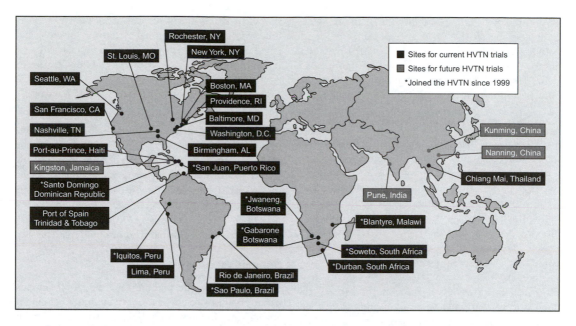

FIGURE 9-9   Sites of HIV Vaccine Trials—2009. Ongoing AIDS Vaccine Trials Organized by the HIV Vaccine Trials Network (HVTN). Worldwide, this is the largest clinical trials program devoted to the development and testing of preventive HIV vaccines. The HVTN is committed to coordination, information sharing, and global collaboration to find an effective HIV vaccine—exemplified by the participation of senior HVTN investigators in the Genesis of the Global HIV Vaccine Enterprise.

vaccine (this is not a true vaccination, but a postinfection therapy to stimulate the immune system; the term "vaccination" is reserved for preventive strategies) for those who are already infected with HIV to prevent them from progressing to AIDS (chance of success in the next 10 years—good); and (3) a **perinatal vaccine** for administration to pregnant HIV-infected women to prevent transmission of the virus to the fetus (chance of success in the next 10 years—good).

What Is an Effective Viral Preventive Vaccine?

An effective preventive viral vaccine usually blocks viral entry into a cell, but vaccines are generally *not* 100% effective. For example, measles vaccine is 95% effective, tetanus 90%, hepatitis B 85%, and influenza 50% to 70%. Vaccine researchers attending the Seventh Conference on Retroviruses and Opportunistic Infections in February 2000 said that they may have to lower their sights regarding an HIV vaccine and settle for one that does not completely prevent HIV infection. Based on recent calculations, it has been estimated that a vaccine that is

30% effective against HIV can begin to eradicate the virus if it is widely administered and accompanied by prevention education.

Why Is There No Preventive HIV Vaccine?

Because HIV, once inside the cell, is capable of integrating itself into the genetic material of infected cells, a vaccine would have to produce a constant state of immune protection, which not only would have to block viral entry to most cells, but also would continue to block newly produced viruses over the lifetime of the infected person. Such complete and constant protection has never before been accomplished in humans, but it has been accomplished in cats that are vaccinated against the feline leukemia virus, also a retrovirus. Perhaps more pertinent explanations for why there is still no HIV vaccine nor is one likely to be available soon are the facts that scientists lack sufficient understanding of HIV infection and the biology of HIV disease/AIDS is very complex.

Scientists know that the body defends itself against HIV in the early years of infection. But the great mystery has always been why it cannot neutralize

HIV completely. One possibility is that the body has trouble seeing all the variant viruses. Like a Stealth fighter plane, some HIV may have hidden parts that do not show up on the immune system scanner. As a result, the immune system may not produce the right kind of antibody to neutralize all the variant HIVs.

Requirements for an HIV-Specific Vaccine

Scientists agree that blocking an infection requires the production of neutralizing antibodies. This is how standard vaccines work: They show the immune system a protein that is unique to the virus or bacterium. If they ever get into the body, the defenses will quickly make antibodies that latch onto that protein, blocking and destroying it. HIV, however, presents a changing target. It mutates so fast that it constantly changes the proteins on its surface. So a vaccine that triggers an attack against one strain of HIV may be powerless against another, (recall the discussion of "Original Sin" in Chapter 8). Furthermore, the virus covers its surface with sugar, which hides its proteins from antibodies.

Is an HIV/AIDS Vaccine Really Possible?

However long it takes, only an effective preventive vaccine has any reasonable prospect of eliminating HIV as a global public health problem.

TYPES OF EXPERIMENTAL HIV VACCINES

To make vaccines, scientists use either **dead microorganisms** and **inactivated** or "killed" **viruses** (examples are influenza and rabies) or **attenuated viruses** (examples are measles, mumps, and rubella) and **microorganisms.** Attenuated (at-ten-u-ate-ed) means that viruses and other microorganisms are modified; they are capable of reproducing and invoking the immune response but lack the ability to cause a disease.

Use of Attenuated HIV Vaccine—In 1997 data from several labs revealed that a vaccine made from weakened or attenuated SIV-HIV's simian analog can cause AIDS-like symptoms in adult monkeys. These findings have worried some investigators about attempting to use an attenuated HIV vaccine in humans. Robert Gallo, director of the Institute for Human Virology, believes that a live HIV vaccine is too dangerous. He said that "live, low-replicating

retroviruses almost always cause disease; that's been our experience in all animal systems. If those vaccinated do not get the disease in three years, it will not tell you what will happen in 10 years or 30 years."

Use of Whole Inactivated or "Killed" Viruses

To inactivate viruses for use in vaccines, the viruses are treated with formalin (for-mah-lin, a strong disinfectant) or another chemical. There is a danger in using inactivated viruses—**they may not all be inactivated.** Inactivated virus vaccines have been made against hepatitis B, rabies, influenza, and polio (Salk vaccine). Salk's first vaccine killed a number of recipients in the late 1950s because not all the polio viruses were destroyed; that is, some could still replicate.

Subunit Vaccines

Subunit vaccines are made from antigenic fragments of an organism or virus most suitable for evoking a strong immune response. Specific subunits can be mass produced and used in pure form to make a specific vaccine. Vaccine against hepatitis B is made from a subunit of the hepatitis B virus and produced in quantity in yeast.

In the United States, researchers are currently basing their vaccine strategies on the use of subunit proteins, gag/pol and nef gene products of HIV. (See Chapter 3 for HIV protein discussion.)

DNA VACCINE

What Is a DNA Vaccine?

To make a DNA vaccine, a gene (or length of DNA) that is responsible for making a protein in the infectious virus or organism is inserted into a bacterial plasmid (a circular length of DNA that can replicate by itself inside a bacterial cell). Plasmids carrying the gene of choice are replicated in trillions of bacteria; the bacteria are then broken open and the trillions of plasmids, each carrying a copy of the gene, are purified. The purified genes/DNA are then given to a patient. Cells of the person take up the DNA and begin to make the exact protein the gene made while it was in the virus or microorganism from which it was taken. Such a protein is considered an antigen by the body and the immune system mounts a defense against it. Entering 2009, there are at least nine DNA vaccines in human trials.

At the 2008 annual American Association for the Advancement of Science (AAAS) meetings, AAAS President David Baltimore (Figure 7-9) said, "Scientists are no closer to developing an HIV vaccine now than they were when vaccine research began." But, he said, "I want to take an optimistic stance and say this is too important to give up on." Baltimore told his audience that the HIV-vaccine development community is depressed after recent failed attempts to develop a vaccine but said that will not halt HIV vaccine research. The HIV-vaccine community needs to begin thinking about vaccine development in a very different way, he said, adding that "scientists are beginning trendy and difficult research involving gene therapy, immunotherapy, and stem cell therapy." He also said that researchers are trying to design vectors than can carry genes that will be of therapeutic advantage.

No Way Out—antiretroviral therapy (ART) for those infected with HIV or who have developed AIDS is critical, but no one should forget that there is no way out of the AIDS epidemic without a vaccine. There is no way to stop unprotected or unsafe sex, sharing needles by injection-drug users, or childbearing and breast feeding by HIV-infected women.

FAILURE OF HIV VACCINES AND RESULTING IMPACT

Between 2001 and 2008, three candidate HIV vaccines failed to benefit those participating in the vaccine trials: the 2001 ALVAC canarypox vector vaccine, the 2003 VaxGen or AIDSVAX (a modified version of an earlier Genentech rgp 160 vaccine), and the 2004 Merck adenovirus-based vaccine (MRKad-5 HIV-1 gag/pol/nef trivalent vaccine). (The ad-5 trial, called the **STEP** trial, was stopped in September 2007 because it was not effective in preventing HIV infection or stopping viral load increase in human test subjects.) The adenovirus is a common cold virus. The shell of the adenovirus was used as a vector (means) to deliver three pieces of HIV-DNA taken from HIV's Gag, Pol, and Nef genes (discussed in Chapter 3). The resulting product is unable to replicate, so that while it initially infects a CD4 cell, it can't produce new HIV. However, it was hoped it would stimulate a cellular immune response that would destroy HIV after infection. This was a major setback!

Several candidate vaccines that are modeled on the ad-5 system have now been postponed or canceled. For some scientists this has been the failure of a specific product but not of the concept. For other scientists this failure spells doom for vaccine research as it is currently practiced. Currently, about $1 billion is spent each year on HIV vaccine research, but there is not likely to be a useful product any time soon. The estimated cost for the ALVAC vaccine and trials was $130 million; for the AIDVAX, it was $185 million and for the Merck ad-5, $200 million.

Is Time and Money Being Wasted on Vaccine Research?

You have read what David Baltimore thinks current vaccine research has to offer—very little. "We need to go back to square one and begin thinking in a different way."

Ronald Desrosiers (2008) of the New England Primate Research Centre at Harvard University and Neal Nathanson of the University of Pennsylvania have eloquently condemned of the current approach to HIV vaccine research. Both argue that researchers must return to basic science instead of generating similar pipeline products to be tested in wasteful and expensive human trials. Desrosiers said that the enormous genetic diversity of HIV, its ability to replicate unrelentingly despite everything the immune system can throw at it, the fact that the immune system cannot protect against superinfection, and the fact that we do not currently know what constitutes an immune response to HIV all persuaded him that at the current time an effective HIV vaccine "is not feasible." Agreeing with Baltimore's views, Desrosiers urged a return to basic discovery research and to work being done with artificial viral vectors that generate broadly neutralizing antibodies against HIV (beginning to be recognized as essential in a vaccine) themselves, instead of trying to stimulate the body to make them.

Neal Nathanson (2008) basically agrees. He said that he and other researchers had long ago defined HIV as a virus that defies vaccination. He, too, urged a return to basic science, such as the devising of genetic assays to search for broadly neutralizing antibodies, and said that the marginal effects seen so far in lowering HIV viral load in human volunteers did not justify further large human studies as currently proposed. For example, the $130 million **PAVE** (a consortium of government-funded agencies involved in HIV vaccine research) 100 trials (similar to ad-5 trials) were to begin in January 2008. They have been postponed. A smaller trial will begin some time in early 2009.

In June 2008, the National Institute of Allergy and Infectious Diseases (NIAID) created an HIV Discovery Branch to promote synergy between basic HIV researchers and vaccine designers. This new branch will build bridges between the two groups and monitor HIV developments in multiple fields related to HIV vaccine discovery. In mid-2008, Russian and Indian scientists announced that they should have an effective HIV vaccine in the next 10 to 15 years.

The Early Years and Producing an HIV Vaccine

On April 24, 1984, Margaret M. Heckler, who was then secretary of the Department of Health and Human Services, announced the discovery of the AIDS virus. She predicted an AIDS vaccine within two years. Even though the prediction proved wrong, very wrong, research was guided by the idea that finding the virus was the hard part, and vaccines could be made by simply injecting people with crucial viral proteins. Her optimism was most likely based on the success of the polio, measles, and flu vaccines. The approach to combating these diseases was: Isolate the virus, develop a vaccine, and prevent the disease! Since then, in the rush to develop new vaccines, scientists have only belatedly understood that their technical ability to mass-produce vaccines has failed to match their knowledge about the cellular and molecular processes used by the body to protect itself from invading pathogens.

PROBLEMS IN THE SEARCH FOR HIV VACCINE

In retrospect, in the movie *Rocky,* Rocky Balboa had it easy. Downing raw eggs at 5 A.M., sprinting through the streets of Philadelphia, pummeling sides of raw beef and pumping out one-armed pushups prepared him to go the distance against world heavyweight champion Apollo Creed. Brute force was what it took. He eventually won! With regard to developing an HIV/AIDS vaccine, brute force is just one of the ingredients essential to winning.

HIV poses some unique problems for making a human vaccine. **First,** Scientists have not established what immune responses are crucial for protecting the body against HIV infection. Studies over the last couple of years have shown that the cell-mediated arm of the immune system may be more important than the HIV antibody response. If this turns out to be true, investigators will have to regroup with respect to producing an HIV vaccine—most vaccines in field trials now are geared toward producing sustained HIV antibody responses.

Second, predictably, money—or rather, lack of it—is an important obstacle. Even though vaccines are among the most cost-effective medical interventions ever devised, they are not big money-makers. **Drug companies are traditionally reluctant to invest in any form of vaccine development that carries high costs, low profits, and big risks of costly legal suits should accidents occur.** Their

current analysis of the state of HIV/AIDS vaccine research is particularly bleak. Of the estimated **$30 billion to $40 billion spent globally each year** on HIV/AIDS research, care, and prevention, about **$1 billion** goes into vaccine research.

In mid-2006 the Bill and Melinda Gates Foundation gave $287 million for funding HIV vaccine research. The money was allocated in 16 grants to 16 scientific teams in 19 countries. The goal is to foster international collaboration in finding the vaccine.

Third, the science is very tough. Animal models used to test HIV vaccines have severe limitations; no researcher has successfully demonstrated which immune responses correlate with protection from HIV.

Fourth is time. All of the preceding items require enormous amounts of time to accomplish; the process of scientific discovery, raising money, or creating an animal model. Linking together all of the people necessary to achieve success in vaccine research is much like linking together all of the people necessary to build the old cathedrals. Linking the builders of these cathedrals took generations of time. It was considered an honor to contribute your work on that cathedral, a piece at a time, even though one knew it would not be finished in their lifetime or perhaps their children's lifetime. The Washington Cathedral in Washington, D.C. was started in 1907. It was completed in 1990—83 years of progress to success. Similarly, vaccine researchers are progressing, one piece of information at a time, toward a successful vaccine.

HIV Vaccine: The Costs

Perhaps the most difficult moral question is the cost of the vaccine. A successful vaccine that sells for a high price will be of little use to poor and uninsured Americans and most people of developing nations, who have no more than a few dollars a year to spend on health care. Eighteen years have passed since the discovery of a vaccine for hepatitis B, a viral disease that is also spread by sexual contact and the sharing of hypodermic needles. But the product has yet to reach many poor people in the United States and Third World countries largely because it costs about $120 for a series of three injections.

Current Costs For Vaccine Development

In 2005 through 2008, the U.S. federal government and private corporations spent about $800 million annually. AIDS vaccine investigators estimate that this is about 1% of monies spent on all other aspects of the AIDS pandemic. The pharmaceutical sector estimates a cost of $50 million to $100 million, just to get to the point of identifying an effective vaccine. To build a production plant could cost between $100 and $200 million. How much it then costs to make the vaccine and deliver it is probably going to vary, depending on the size of the manufacturing plant and the type of vaccine that's made. Before a successful vaccine is found, produced in mass quantity, and made available to the market, the price will be several billion dollars.

Infrastructure—While making, purchasing, and bringing vaccines to developing countries is a daunting task, many experts say that the real challenges start at the airport, after the vials have been unloaded for distribution throughout the country. It's here that the issue of uptake—demand with a reality check—comes into play. Are there sufficient refrigerators, trucks, syringes, and syringe disposal facilities for the vaccine dispensaries? Are there trained personnel at these dispensaries? Is there capacity for community outreach and for follow-up to individuals who do not complete their immunization course? In short, is the necessary infrastructure in place? If the answer is no, then it will not matter whether a country has an explosive epidemic or an early one that could be stopped with a relatively small-scale immunization campaign. Without infrastructure, there is an unbridgeable gap between need and demand. The scientific consensus is that an effective HIV vaccine can be developed, but infrastructure is a challenge that must be confronted.

The Future for a Preventive Vaccine

Vaccine programs in the United States and in other nations are led by some of the most talented and dedicated scientists in the world. One must admire them and the dedicated public and private teams developing each vaccine candidate. Together they recognize that a preventative vaccine is our best long-term hope to control the pandemic, although it will not be a magic bullet replacing other preventive interventions.

In 1995 the International AIDS Vaccine Initiative (IAVI) was constituted in the United States as a nongovernmental organization sponsored by various U.S. foundations and donors. A group of the best minds in immunology joined the IAVI because global efforts to create a preventive HIV vaccine were in trouble. This group, led by Seth Berkley, is in large part responsible for the many ongoing clinical HIV vaccine trials. In 2005 a second team of AIDS researchers from four universities, led by Barton Haynes, received $300 million from the National Institute of Allergy and Infectious Diseases (NIAID) to explore the immunologic mysteries confronting the field of HIV vaccine studies. They work at the newly formed Center for HIV/AIDS Vaccine Immunology (CHAVI) at Duke University Medical Center.

Disclaimer: The author of this book cannot be held responsible for any inaccuracies found in the inclusion of information by any organization, treatment, therapy, or clinical trial. The use of their information is not an endorsement of their facts or data. Any information found within this textbook should always be used in conjunction with professional medical advice.

For additional information about the search for an HIV/AIDS vaccine, the following literature is recommended.

AIDS Vaccine Research
Flossie Wong-Staal and Robert C. Gallo, Eds.
Marcel Dekker, 2002

Shots in the Dark: The Wayward Search for an AIDS Vaccine
by Jon Cohen
W.W. Norton, 2001

HIV and Molecular Immunity: Prospects for the AIDS Vaccine
by Omar Bagasra
Eaton Publishing, 1999

The Search for an AIDS Vaccine: Ethical Issues in the Development and Testing of a Preventive HIV Vaccine (Medical Ethics Series)
by Christine Grady
Indiana University Press, 1995

AIDS Vaccine Resources on the Internet

www.avac.org
www.niaid.nih.gov/daids/vaccine/default.htm
www.fhi.org/en/aids/hivnet/hivnet.html
www.vaccinealliance.org
www.vaccineadvocates.org/avacsite/inde.htm

These addresses will list most of the important vaccine Internet addresses and serve as linkage to others.

Summary

We should be winning HIV prevention. There are effective means to prevent every mode of transmission; political commitment on HIV has never been stronger, and financing for HIV programs in low- and middle-income countries increased eightfold between 2001 and 2009. However, while attention to the pandemic, particularly for treatment access, has increased in recent years, the effort to reduce HIV incidence is faltering. For every patient who initiated antiretroviral therapy in 2008, three other individuals became infected.

The numbers become so large that the individuals suffering and the personal, societal, and economic losses become impossible to measure or to even attempt to estimate. While there have been successes in slowing the epidemic in some communities and dramatic advances in survival in developed countries due to combination antiretroviral therapy, it is very important that people do not become complacent and focus on false beliefs that the pandemic is declining, that individuals are becoming less infectious, or that HIV control will be much better in the twenty-first century. If anything, the limited success in prevention should encourage a continued effort to work harder at educating more people about how best to prevent further transmission through safer sex practices, antiretroviral therapy during pregnancy, treatment of STDs, provision of condoms, screening of the blood supply, the use of sterile needles, or many of the other avenues that can help to slow the pandemic until a vaccine can be developed.

Historically, most prevention programs were designed to address the needs of persons who were at risk for contracting HIV. During the first decade of the epidemic, fewer prevention programs focused on persons living with HIV. Then in 2001, CDC introduced the Serostatus Approach to Fighting the HIV Epidemic (SAFE), which defined a framework for improving the health of persons living with HIV and preventing transmission to others. In 2003, CDC implemented the Advancing HIV Prevention (AHP) initiative, which formally adopted prevention measures for persons living with HIV as a core element of a comprehensive approach to HIV preventions. Despite considerable success, many prevention challenges remain. Racial/ethnic disparities have increased during the past 27 years, especially among black men and black women. HIV prevalence remains high among MSM overall.

The key to stopping HIV transmission lies with the behavior of the individual. That behavior, if the experience of the past 27 years can be used as an indicator, has proven to be very difficult to change. Behavioral prevention can only achieve so much. Safer behaviors are *not* sustainable 100 percent of the time.

Changing sexual behavior and using a condom is referred to as **safer sex.** The latex condom is the only condom believed to stop the passage of HIV, and a spermicide should be used with the condom. Oil-based lubricants must not be used because they weaken the condom, allowing it to leak or break under stress. Water-based lubricants are available and should be used. There is at least one female condom, called a vaginal pouch, approved by the FDA and sold worldwide. It is inserted like a diaphragm. It offers protection to both sexual partners.

A test developed in 1985 to screen all donated blood in the United States has reduced the risk of HIV transfusion infection. But blood bank screening has reduced the size of the blood donor pool. Many hospitals are encouraging people who know they might need an operation to donate their own blood for later use—autologous transfusion.

Entering 2009, the only FDA-approved HIV vaccine trials have failed. Many top HIV/AIDS scientists have ruled out the use of an attenuated HIV vaccine. Inactivated whole virus vaccines are also being held back because there is no 100% guarantee that all HIV used in the vaccine will be inactivated.

Even if a vaccine does well in Phase III trials, will it be effective against all the HIV mutants in the HIV gene pool? Can the threat of vaccine-induced enhancement of HIV infection be overcome? How are vaccine testing agencies going to handle the ethical question of vaccine seroconverting normal subjects to positive antibody status? The social repercussions may be devastating for those who, when tested, test HIV positive even though they are HIV-free.

There are some 5.3 million healthcare workers in the United States. It is crucial that they adhere to the Universal Protection Guidelines set down by the CDC, as a significant number of them are exposed to HIV annually. The risk of HIV infection after exposure to HIV-contaminated blood is about 1 in 200.

Some states have implemented HIV partner notification; other states are beginning to experiment with HIV partner notification or contact tracing programs. It is too early to tell how successful locating and testing high behavioral risk partners will be, or the cost-to-benefit ratio. If these programs are to be successful, they will have to ensure confidentiality to those who are traced. Partner notification or contact tracing continues to work well for other sexually transmitted diseases.

In short, considerable success in the prevention of HIV infection in the United States has been achieved. HIV testing and donor deferral have markedly increased the safety of the nation's blood supply. Perinatal transmission of HIV has been greatly reduced. Reductions in needle sharing have resulted in a substantial decrease in HIV transmissions associated with injection-drug use. These and other prevention successes have reduced the incidence of HIV infection from more than 150,000 cases per year in the mid-1980s to over 56,000 cases per year since at least 2002.

Review Questions

(Answers to the Review Questions are on page 428.)

1. Which is the better condom for protection from STDs, one made from lamb intestine or one made from latex rubber? Explain.

2. Which lubricant is best suited for condom use? Explain.

3. Briefly explain safer sex.

4. True or False: If a person has unprotected intercourse with an HIV-infected partner, he or she will become HIV infected. Explain.

5. Yes or No: If injection-drug users (IDUs) were given free equipment—no questions asked—would this stop the transmission of HIV among them. Explain.

6. What is the current risk of being transfused with HIV-contaminated blood in the United States?

7. What do you think should happen in cases where a person who knows he or she is HIV positive lies at a donor interview, and donates blood?

8. Why do most scientists wish to avoid using an attenuated HIV vaccine or an inactivated HIV vaccine?

9. What is the advantage of using recombinant HIV subunits in making a vaccine?

10. What are universal precautions? Who formulated them?

11. True or False: Latex condoms eliminate the risk of HIV transmission.

12. True or False: Partner notification is usually performed by the infected individual or a trained and authorized health department official.

13. True or False: The Centers for Disease Control and Prevention estimates that as many as 1 in 100,000 units of blood in the blood supply may be contaminated with HIV.

14. True or False: The three types of vaccines that scientists are interested in developing are preventive, therapeutic, and perinatal vaccines.

15. True or False: Used disposable needles should be recapped by hand before disposal.

16. True or False: Prompt washing of a needle stick injury with soap and water is sufficient to prevent HIV infection.

17. True or False: The FDA approved the first vaccine for broad-scale testing in the United States in 1997.

18. HIV/AIDS is not curable, but it is preventable. Write a short essay on the best methods of prevention.

Prevalence of HIV Infections, AIDS Cases, and Deaths Among Select Groups in the United States and in Other Countries

CHAPTER CONCEPTS

- HIV/AIDS is a new plague.
- UNAIDS defines a generalized epidemic.
- Worldwide, ending 2009, heterosexuals will make up about 95% of people living with HIV/AIDS.
- Worldwide, 50% of new HIV infections are in people under age 25.
- Worldwide, about 7,000 new HIV infections occur daily.
- Worldwide, women represent about 45% of all HIV-infected adults and about 50% of AIDS deaths.
- In sub-Saharan Africa, 59% of the HIV infected are women.
- AIDS is the world's leading cause of death by an infectious disease.
- AIDS is ranked fourth in causes of death worldwide.
- In the United States, men make up an estimated 76.5% of all AIDS cases; 23.5% are women.
- The majority of people with HIV/AIDS can be associated with certain lifestyle behaviors.
- HIV/AIDS can be associated with single or multiple exposure behaviors.
- HIV/AIDS cases can be separated by sex, age group, race, ethnicity, and sexual preference.
- Risk is strongly tied to social behavior.
- At-risk groups include homosexual and bisexual men, injection-drug users (IDUs), hemophiliacs, transfusion patients, and the sex partners of these people.
- HIV infection is strongly associated with injection-drug use and men having sex with men.
- About 54% of new HIV infections occurred in the black population.
- All military personnel are tested for HIV.
- Two per 1000 college students are HIV infected.
- Ending 2008, all states reported the HIV infected by name.
- High rates of HIV infection have been found among prisoners.
- Difference between prisons and jails explained.
- The greatest HIV threat to healthcare workers is needle stick (syringe) injuries.
- All 50 states and U.S. territories must report all HIV and AIDS cases.
- The CDC updates United States HIV surveillance estimates, August 2008.
- Ending 2009: *reported* AIDS cases in the United States will reach 1.3 million, of which over 600,000 will have died.
- People do not always tell the truth when completing questionnaires, especially with regard to sexual behavior.

- By the end of 2009, an estimated 59 million people worldwide will have been HIV infected and about 24 million of them will have died of AIDS.
- Some HIV/AIDS statistics on Canada are provided.

I WISH YOU ENOUGH®

I wish you enough sun to keep your attitude bright.
I wish you enough rain to appreciate the sun more.
I wish you enough happiness to keep your spirit alive.
I wish you enough pain so that the smallest joys in life appear much bigger.
I wish you enough gain to satisfy your wanting.
I wish you enough loss to appreciate all that you possess.
I wish you enough "Hellos" to get you through the final "Goodbye."

®2001 Bob Perks

The World Trade Center (WTC) and the Pentagon were attacked on September 11, 2001. No one expected to see commercial airliners hijacked and flown into crowded skyscrapers and government buildings. Likewise, in the early 1980s, no one expected the sudden appearance of a deadly new disease spreading across the cities of America. Only a few years earlier some prominent scientists had declared that the fight against infectious disease was over. The horrible damage caused by fuel-laden airliners crashing into buildings and exploding into a fiery inferno was all but beyond our imagination. Equally beyond our imagination was this new disease that appeared 27 years ago. It was a disease that appeared without warning and seemed to lead to a painful, agonizing death in just a few weeks for some, a few months for others. The depth and scope of human destruction was so unprecedented that only a few people were quick to recognize the horror that was to come. On September 11, while the image of the jetliners with their passengers exploding into the World Trade Center was still painfully fresh, we were further stunned to see these seemingly invincible structures collapse, crushing almost 3000 men, women, and children in a vast cloud of toxic dust, rubble, and fire. A week earlier, no one would have believed that such pillars of concrete and steel could possibly collapse, let alone from the top down. In the tragedy that began to unfold in the beginning of the 1980s, scientists were puzzled and bewildered as they watched a disease that led to the collapse of the human immune system. Working from the inside out, here was a diabolically clever virus that destroyed the very system that was otherwise designed to defeat it. The beginning of AIDS in America in 1981 is the greatest plague in history to cross the globe, and the 2001 attack on the WTC and the Pentagon, the largest attack on the United States, caused the greatest loss of life since the Japanese attack on Pearl Harbor. The two have much in common. Both tragedies have appeared over and over again on television. Both require the best in people to set them right—to save lives. The United States and the world must not let terrorists or HIV determine our way of life. Both require acts of heroism and research. Both require sacrifice, resolve, and the determination to overcome. Both have placed America and the world in a race against time.

The News Media: The Result of Omission

When AIDS isn't visible in the media, it doesn't exist for many communities that rely on media to tell them what matters most. This is true not only in the West, but in Africa and in other developing nations, where stigma and discrimination against AIDS sufferers is deeply entrenched, and where silence and denial still drive many governments to cover up their frightening levels of HIV infection. Often the young people who most need to know how to protect themselves have few programs directed their way. At the same time, there are many stirring and effective responses led by unsung young heroes whose stories could inspire a greater mobilization. But who is going to tell these stories if the media doesn't? AIDS will surpass the bubonic plague or "Black Death" of Asia and Europe in the fourteenth century unless a vaccine is found. That plague killed about 40 million people. By the end of 2009, about 24 million will have died from AIDS. Each day AIDS kills over twice the number of people who died September 11, 2001, in New York City and at the Pentagon. No terrorist attack, no war or natural force of nature in our lifetime has ever killed 24 million people and threatened 35 million more with premature deaths in a quarter of a century! HIV is a virus of mass destruction.

A WORD ABOUT HIV/AIDS DATA

As most college students might say, nothing could be more boring than statistics and numbers. Regardless, if you're reading or hearing them with regard to the HIV/AIDS pandemic, the use of statistics is one of the better ways to understand the dimensions of this

— BOX 10.1 —

XVII INTERNATIONAL AIDS CONFERENCE, MEXICO CITY, MEXICO AUGUST 3–8, 2008

Jorge Saavedra's moment of truth came in the middle of a speech to 5,000 people about the paltry amount of money being spent to stop the spread of AIDS among gay men. The Mexican federal official paused, then said publicly for the first time that he was gay. As he help up a photo of himself with his partner, the crowd applauded wildly. Afterward, men from Africa and India congratulated him with tears in their eyes. Saavedra, age 48, said, "They told me that I was a hero, and that they wished they could do the same in their countries." He is infected with HIV and also heads the AIDS prevention program in a country where many gay men live in denial. His coming out at the International AIDS Conference sent a powerful message to the world: homophobia must be stamped out if AIDS is to be controlled. Fewer people are dying from AIDS, but new HIV infections among gay and bisexual men in many countries are rising at alarming rates. UNAIDS says these men receive the lowest coverage of HIV prevention services of any at-risk population. And experts say discrimination has driven gay and bisexual men in developing nations underground —turning them into one of the epidemic's hardest groups to reach. In 86 nations, homosexual sex is considered a crime, and in seven countries it is punishable by death.

Brief History of the International AIDS Conferences

The International AIDS Conferences began in 1985. The conferences were held yearly through 1994. Because the conferences became so large in attendance it was decided to hold them every other year beginning in 1996 (See Table 1.2 for a list of conferences). The conferences have provided a unique global venue of the struggle against AIDS. The next meeting will take place in Vienna, Austria in July 2010.

Conference Vision

The Conference has evolved from a relatively small scientific meeting focused on understanding an emerging epidemic to the largest and most diverse international gathering dedicated to a global health issue. Today, the Conference is as much about state of the art practice and effective utilization of available tools as it is about new scientific knowledge. As a gathering that brings together so many people and focuses on such a politically charged life and death issue, the Conference will always generate controversy. It should also be a place that concentrates attention on evidence and outcomes over rhetoric and individual or organizational agendas. It should engage people on an ongoing basis, rather than focus exclusively on the five days of the actual Conference meetings.

Conference Goals: To Reflect on How Far We Have Come and How Far We Have To Go

The goal of every International AIDS Conference is to present a forum for everybody engaged in the response to the HIV/AIDS pandemic and a platform to reach the global public. For this conference, the first conference to be held in Latin America, there was a unique opportunity to focus attention on a region that has been neglected in the global response to HIV/AIDS. Yet, almost two million people are HIV infected in Latin America and the Caribbean—more than in the U.S., Canada, Western Europe, Australia, and Japan combined. During the conference people from Latin America and the Caribbean had a chance to show the world their reality, the different kinds of epidemics and obstacles that the region is confronting. Pedro Cahn, outgoing President of the International AIDS Society, said, "AIDS 2008 is taking place at a unique moment in the epidemic when there is widespread consensus on the urgency of ensuring universal access to HIV prevention, treatment, care, and support by 2010. What we now need is action on the part of all stakeholders. As we gather in Mexico, each of us must ask ourselves: what can I do to end AIDS? In 2008, there are no longer bystanders in this global struggle."

Universal Action Now

The theme for this conference was "Universal Action Now." Universal Action Now was not just a slogan for the conference, but also a call for action by everyone to ensure that universal access to prevention, treatment, care, and support becomes a reality by 2010. This includes ensuring that governments stop criminalizing the most marginalized, vulnerable, and at risk populations, such as sex workers, men who have sex with men, people who use drugs, and people living with HIV. Without protecting their human rights, these populations will continue to be unable to access the critical services they need to protect themselves from HIV and/or maintain good health. Tangible progress from "Universal Action Now" can and will be assessed in Vienna, Austria, the site of the 2010 XVIII International AIDS Conference.

BOX 10.1 (*continued*)

Conference Goals 2008

There are three main goals to any AIDS conference. First is to call the world's attention to truly focus in on this pandemic and appreciate the many challenges this disease presents. Second is to share essential information globally and to learn from each other. Third, is to inspire and to invigorate each other, to renew a global commitment to defeating this disease.

Attendance and Presentations

There were about 22,000 participants from nearly every country in the world who delivered over 5,000 reports, 300 oral presentations, 1,000 poster sessions, 2,000 poster exhibitions, and 90 skills-building workshops. And yes, there were AIDS activist demonstrations. This was the second largest of the International AIDS meetings in its 23-year history.

Cost of the Conference

The Mexico City International AIDS Conference cost at least $20 million, about the cost for each of the six previous meetings. There has always been argument and speculation as to whether these monies could have been better spent on care and support of those with HIV/AIDS.

A Marriage Made In Mexico City, 2008: Prevention and Treatment

At this Conference it became clear that researchers, physicians, and others have moved on from the fruitless debate between prevention and treatment that plagued the past. Finally, a happy marriage between these opposing forces. Discussions about preventive benefits of treatment become more sophisticated. A key word that came about as a result of this marriage of ideas and positions is the word "combination:" combination prevention strategies tailored to decrease HIV transmission, combination antiretroviral therapy to dramatically reduce morbidity and mortality among those affected worldwide, combination antiretroviral therapy to also reduce community viral load as an aid to prevention, combination strategies to enhance HIV testing, and combination strategies to reduce poverty, homelessness, and discrimination. It became clear that although both treatment and prevention are essential, prevention is being short-changed. It is this very point, the need to drastically scale up prevention efforts, that came to dominate this conference. Every day, about 6,800 people become infected with HIV and about 5,700 die, mostly because they have no access to HIV prevention, treatment, and care services. Despite progress made in scaling up the response over the last decade, the HIV pandemic remains the most serious infectious disease challenge to global public health. From the very beginning of the global response to the AIDS pandemic, prevention has been marginalized. Treatment has dominated. This systematic imbalance in clinical and public health programs is largely responsible for the fact that about 2.5 million people become newly infected with HIV each year. The publication of a series by the Lancet on the state of the science of HIV prevention (The Lancet DOI: 10-1016/50140-6736(08)60885-5), together with a call for action by leading academics, UNAIDS, and the World Bank, signifies a new commitment to stop the virus and its consequences through the use of new and improved prevention methods.

HIV PREVENTION MUST BE THE WAY FORWARD

At past International AIDS Conferences, a session on prevention wouldn't have drawn enough attention to fill a large meeting room. In previous years, treatment dominated the conversation. But this year the theme of prevention surfaced among the tangle of panels and workshops, debates, and discussion groups. For example, a morning plenary on the topic was filled to capacity. Later, at the Lancet Series on HIV Prevention session, hundreds of people packed into the session room and many others stood outside, unable to get in. Clearly, this was not just prevention as usual. Throughout the conference, scientists and activists have called for new ways to staunch the spread of HIV throughout the world. Richard Horton, editor of The Lancet said, "Prevention has not only been marginalized, but in some places it's been suppressed for political, religious, or social purposes. We have to redefine prevention to create a new dialogue of what we mean by prevention." Given that neither a preventive or therapeutic vaccine is in the foreseeable future coupled with the fact that for every person being placed on drug therapy, four others become infected, prevention is an absolute.

BOX 10.1 (*continued*)

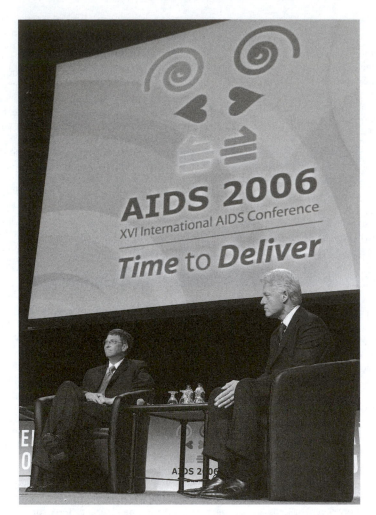

FIGURE 10–1 The Two Bills at the XVI International AIDS Conference. Former President Bill Clinton (on the right) and Bill Gates sat down before a packed house, took questions and discussed priorities in the global AIDS pandemic. Both men, who are well recognized public faces in the international fight against HIV/AIDS, set out what they saw as their priorities to end the AIDS pandemic: prevention that goes beyond abstinence, wider treatment access, fighting stigma to increase testing and the wider issues of poverty and hunger. (*Photograph © Frank Gunn AP/Wide World Photos*)

Shock And Awe For Prevention From the United States

Although the evidence of the need for all nations to make prevention methods available is overwhelming, the U.S. Center for Disease Control and Prevention (CDC) announced a 40% annual increase in the number of new infections since 2002. Instead of the CDC's annual 40,000 cases, suddenly it is over 56,000 HIV infections per year! Bill Clinton, addressing several thousand delegates, said, "This should be a wake-up call for Americans." **Question:** If the U.S., a global leader in HIV/AIDS case testing and reporting, what does this imply about HIV/AIDS surveillance and reporting from any nation, especially from the developing nations? Can there be a more shocking revelation in the pursuit of prevention?

Other Challenges For HIV Prevention Presented At The Meetings

Men Having Sex With Men (MSM)

Kevin Frost of the American Foundation for AIDS Research (AmfAR) said, "The same kinds of stigma and discrimination and institutionalized homophobia that failed gay men in America is now failing MSM in the rest of the world." An AmfAR report released at the Conference found MSM is at an increased risk of HIV. According to the report, despite a unanimous commitment that all UN member countries made in 2001 to monitor HIV among high-risk groups, 71% of countries said they did not have any information on the percentage of MSM contacted by HIV prevention groups. Of

BOX 10.1 (*continued*)

128 countries, 44% failed to provide HIV data on MSM. According to the report, Benin, Ghana, Jamaica, Kenya, and Thailand are the countries with the highest reported HIV prevalence among MSM. Although data were scarce, the study found MSM were 33 times more likely to be living with HIV than the general population in Latin America, 18 times more likely in Asia, and at least four times more likely in Africa. Sexual activity between men is criminalized in 85 countries and is punishable by death in seven countries and by imprisonment in 76 countries. It is difficult to provide services to men who have sex with men in countries where they don't acknowledge they exist.

HIV/AIDS Therapy

Antiretroviral drugs have become so effective that a 20-year-old HIV positive person in a wealthy country can now expect to live another 49 years on average. The near-miraculous effects of the drugs highlight the need to treat as many people as possible worldwide. Currently, about three million people in the developing world have access to antiretrovirals, an estimated 30% of those in need. About three million people with HIV/AIDS are taking the drugs in wealthy nations. The United Nations' goal of providing universal access to HIV drug therapy to all by 2010 will not happen.

Cost of Universal Access Therapy

According to estimates, universal access will cost $54 billion annually by 2015, a figure that could increase as people living with HIV/AIDS continue taking antiretrovirals for the rest of their lives. Seth Berkly, head of the International AIDS Vaccine Initiative, said, "If you add in the $35 billion currently being spent in the developing world, you're talking about an annual need of $90 billion."

New HIV/AIDS Treatment Guidelines

The report "Antiretroviral Treatment of Adult HIV Infection: 2008 Recommendations of the International AIDS Society—USA Panel," was published in the Journal of the American Medical Association (2008; 300(5):555-570). It calls for raising the previous threshold of 250 CD4 cells, prior to initiating therapy, to 350 CD4 cells per microliter of blood.

Adios, Hasta Luego to the XVIII International AIDS Conference 2008

This conference will be remembered for many positive events. But the more important, lasting, and meaningful events were the conference promoting push for **universal access** to:

- Prevention, education, and methodology
- Antiretroviral Therapy
- Anti-discrimination programs
- Human rights
- Partnerships among politicians, scientists, activists, social scientists, medical personnel, pharmacologists, and governments.

Looking Forward

After much was said, it was acknowledged that regardless of hope, help, and progress, perhaps the largest issue that has to be dealt with, after raising money, is that of providing heathcare workers worldwide to fight HIV/AIDS. Looking into the immediate future, four million additional health care workers will be needed in 60 countries just to fight HIV/AIDS. There is a plan: It is called "Treat, Train and Retain." The plan will cost $7.2 billion over the next five years. **Question:** Where will this money come from? One thing is very clear: The shortage of health workers is devastating public health systems, particularly in the developing world, and it is one of the most significant challenges we face in preventing and treating HIV.

Summary

The issues pertaining to this pandemic are confusing. Should we be enraged that many millions of people across the globe still know very little about HIV/AIDS. Or that in many developed countries like the U.S., the HIV infection rate has stabilized at unacceptably high numbers, yet this is a preventable disease. Or should we rejoice and celebrate the progress that has been made in such a relatively short time: 27 years? We now have life-extending drugs and decent prevention techniques for those that will practice them, and children in developed nations can be born free of HIV. In the past conferences there was always the charge of accountability. The researchers, the drug companies, the healthcare workers, or the government never did enough of what was perceived to be right. Here we are, more than 27 years later, and accountability is still perceived as a major issue at these conferences. How do we change this? With what we have learned and the lives we have saved, this conference should have and actually did unfold in a mood of relative optimism, but the question of accountability on every level continues to nag everyone dedicated to the demise of this disease.

pandemic. It's important to get a grasp of the numbers of people with HIV and AIDS so that an informed policy on economic and political issues can be made that will eventually change the scope of this pandemic.

The term *HIV/AIDS* refers to three categories of diagnoses collectively: (1) a diagnosis of HIV infection, not AIDS; (2) a diagnosis of HIV infection with a later diagnosis of AIDS; and (3) a concurrent diagnosis of HIV infection and AIDS.

The UNAIDS defines a generalized epidemic as "high-level—where adult HIV prevalence among the general adult population is at least 1% and transmission is mostly heterosexual." A concentrated epidemic is defined as "low-level—where HIV is concentrated in groups with behaviors that expose them to a high risk of HIV infection."

All HIV/AIDS data, including data from the Centers for Disease Control and Prevention (CDC), Joint United Nations Program on HIV/AIDS (UNAIDS), World Health Organization (WHO), and other organizations should be treated as broadly indicative of trends rather than accurate measures of HIV/AIDS incidence or prevalence. A large number of HIV/AIDS cases in developing countries, in particular, are underreported due to a lack of adequate medical and administrative personnel, the stigma associated with the disease, or the reluctance of countries to incur the loss of trade, tourism, and other losses that such revelations might produce.

Because morbidity and mortality of HIV/AIDS cases are multicausal, diagnosis and reporting can vary significantly, thereby distorting comparisons. The WHO and other international entities are dependent on such data despite its weaknesses and are often forced to extrapolate or build models based on relatively small samples, as in the case of HIV/AIDS. Changes in methodologies, moreover, can produce differing results; for example, the ranking of AIDS mortality ahead of TB mortality. This is partly due to the fact that HIV-positive individuals dying of TB were included in the AIDS mortality category in the most recent WHO survey. Another example is the global data on those living with HIV/AIDS. The WHO/UNAIDS global data say there are about 33.2 million such people at the end of 2007, but this estimate results from a low estimate of 30.6 million and a high estimate of 36.1 million—recognizably a large margin for error. Such data come from using a relatively simple equation that calculated low- and high-risk populations with the crude adult death rate and the HIV-infected sur-

vival rate, along with variables including the start date of HIV for that country and the demand for risky sex. The bottom line is that estimates are just that—estimates. However, estimates prove to be very useful in predicting what is occurring now and what lies ahead.

In early 2007, epidemiologists, analysts, and heads of AIDS programs from 124 countries began to refine and improve country HIV/AIDS estimates. These data for 2007 became available in early 2008, and have been updated through 2008.

THE MILLENNIUM: YEAR 2009

As we begin this ninth year of the new millennium and enter into the early years of the third decade of AIDS, it is evident that the small epidemic recognized among a handful of homosexual men in 1981 is quite different from the global pandemic of today. For developed countries, current antiretroviral regimens are allowing HIV-infected individuals to live longer, healthier lives. However, the use of these regimens may be associated with complacency and a relapse to unsafe sexual practices resulting in sustaining the HIV epidemic, as will be discussed. For developing countries the problem is far more complex. The infrastructure to support the use of antiretroviral drugs is not in place, the cost of the drugs is too high, and the vast majority of HIV-infected people do not even know they are infected. Education and condom distribution campaigns have had limited success, but they remain the primary avenues of prevention.

Developed Countries: The AIDS Crisis Is Over?

In the developed nations, too many people think the AIDS crisis is over. Think again. It is estimated that by the end of 2009, about 59 million people will have been HIV infected, with about 35 million of them alive. About ninety percent of infections are in developing nations that hold 10% of the world's wealth. There is still neither a cure nor an effective vaccine.

Entering year 2009 there does not appear to be an immediate end to either the spread of HIV infection or the devastation caused by AIDS. Who would have imagined in the mid-1980s that HIV would eventually spread to every country of the world, infecting 59 million people and resulting in about 24 million deaths by the end of 2009? And the global HIV/AIDS pandemic is not expected to peak for another 20 to 30 years (2028 to 2038).

Reporting and Underreporting AIDS Diagnosis and AIDS Deaths

Many countries have a long history of reporting AIDS cases and in some—including the U.S.A., Canada, and much of Africa—reporting of all AIDS cases is compulsory. A problem with AIDS case reporting is that different countries have different definitions of what actually constitutes AIDS. While a definition of AIDS is becoming standardized, there is still the problem that some resource-poor areas lack HIV testing facilities, and therefore they have to diagnose AIDS (and thus HIV) on the presence of several marker conditions such as the presence of tuberculosis (TB). Another problem is that people in many countries without the proper AIDS diagnosis resources die of AIDS, but are not counted as AIDS deaths.

Antiretroviral treatment has made it difficult to interpret trends in AIDS diagnoses and AIDS deaths in countries where most people have access to the drugs. Also, in countries where AIDS is highly stigmatized, doctors may be inclined to spare shame to a family by misrecording the cause of an AIDS death. Such underreporting occurs worldwide!

The Statistical Politics of This Pandemic

For over a decade the director of UNAIDS, Peter Piot, sounded the alarm of the quickly moving and horribly devastating modern day plague, the HIV/AIDS pandemic. In 2007 he said, "the pandemic and its toll are outstripping the worst predictions. It is now one of the make or break forces of this century." The developed nations responded with AIDS funding at $10 billion a year. Regardless, this was considered insufficient funding. Organizers at the WHO, UNAIDS, and other HIV/AIDS organizations insisted that many billions of dollars more will be required each year just to catch up to the growing need of funding. And then, something happened on the way to securing greater amounts of money.

What Happened?

In November of 2007, the WHO along with UNAIDS published their "AIDS Epidemic Update '07." Indeed this report presented some surprising information about this global pandemic. At first glance it appeared that the pandemic was fast fading with the devastating number of estimated HIV/AIDS cases of 2006 in free-fall. In 2006, 39.5 million people were living with HIV/AIDS. The number dropped to 33.2 million in 2007. And new HIV infections fell from 4.3 million in 2006 to 2.5 million in 2007—a drop of 42% in one year! What happened? Were the new prevention methods, new drugs preventing infections, abstention, and education finally showing huge results?

Not Exactly

What happened is that WHO and UNAIDS personally admitted that their numbers had been greatly overstated. Stephen Lewis, former special UN envoy for HIV/AIDS in Africa, stated that these organizations "had clearly been using inflated numbers for years." He accused the WHO and UNAIDS of irresponsibility. Much more on this subject can be found at the beginning of this book. Because of the 2007 AIDS Epidemic Update Report, all global HIV/AIDS numbers have been reduced accordingly.

Estimates by UNAIDS

Currently, UNAIDS reports that each day about 7,000 people become newly infected with HIV, or 5 men, women, and children per minute. Eleven percent of the newly infected people are under age 15. Over 50% of new infections are now occurring in people between ages 15 and 24, primarily due to sexual transmission. Worldwide, women now represent 50% of all people over age 15 living with HIV infection. At the end of 1998, UNAIDS reported that AIDS had become the world's most deadly infectious disease. It reached this level of human devastation in just 18 years. Of all causes of death worldwide, AIDS has moved up to fourth place. These data are a bit ironic because as Peter Piot, executive director of UNAIDS, said, "The pandemic is out of control at the very time when we know what to do to prevent its spread."

As shocking as these numbers are, they do not begin to adequately reflect the physical and emotional devastation to individuals, families, and communities coping with HIV/AIDS, nor do they capture the huge deleterious impact of HIV/AIDS on economies, on the security of nations, and on entire regions.

What About Reported HIV Infections?

Each positive HIV test means one person is infected. This method of looking at an epidemic can give a very clear picture in terms of people who have been infected. But most countries only report their AIDS cases. However, as the numbers of AIDS cases began to soar, many of the worst affected countries stopped monitoring AIDS cases because those reports grossly underestimated the number of HIV-infected people.

In general, national totals of reported HIV diagnoses are only reliable when they come from countries with well-developed voluntary testing schemes. However, even in these countries, one in every three or four people living with HIV has never been tested. And for those tested, not all test results are reported.

Another point to remember is that looking at the years in which people tested HIV positive does not say when they were infected—the HIV test itself may come many years after infection occurred. When looking at HIV statistics, it's important to keep in mind that there might be more than one reason for trends in the data. An increase in diagnoses might not mean that more people are becoming HIV infected than in previous years. It might mean that HIV testing has become more easily available than in recent years, or that stigmatization of people with HIV has declined, so more people are willing to be tested.

Overwhelming Numbers of HIV/AIDS Cases in the United States

It is easy to be overwhelmed by statistics in reporting on HIV infections and AIDS cases and to lose track of the human faces of the pandemic. But certain numbers, like the first half-million documented AIDS cases reported in October 1995 and over 600,000 dead ending 2009 take on a compelling quality of their own. Therefore, within this chapter there are many statistics presented on all facets of the HIV/AIDS pandemic. **After reading this chapter one will have gained a deeper insight into the spread of HIV and those who are affected by HIV: those who have it, and those who don't—those who will suffer and those who won't. In reality we are all impacted by this disease in one way or another.**

Prevalence/Incidence/Rate
How Many People Are HIV Positive?

The **prevalence** of a disease refers to the percentage of a population that is affected by it at a given time. **Prevalence = total number of AIDS cases at a given time divided by total population at the same time.** For example, if 1000 specific high-risk males are tested for HIV and 30 of them are found to be HIV positive, the results mean that within this population HIV prevalence is at 3%. The **incidence** means the number of times an event occurs in a given time frame, for example, the number of new AIDS

cases each month or new HIV infections each week (events that occur within a specified period of time). The two terms are similar. However, changes in HIV incidence statistics can give a better idea of whether prevention strategies are succeeding in reducing the number of new infections. A society that shows regularly declining incidence figures is one that is experiencing fewer new HIV infections.

The **rate** is the number of HIV or AIDS cases divided by the population in each group, multiplied by 100. The higher the rate, the greater the burden or impact of HIV/AIDS on each community. This burden can be directly compared across countries and racial/ethnic groups of different population sizes, since the rate assumes that each group has exactly the same population (For example, the number of AIDS cases per 100,000 people).

Although cases of AIDS appear retrospectively to have occurred in the United States as early as 1952, the **AIDS pandemic** in the United States is considered to have begun with the initial report in June 1981. Since then, the HIV/AIDS pandemic has become the most serious pandemic to occur worldwide since the Spanish flu of 1918, which killed between 30 million and 50 million people but lasted less than a year.

FORMULA FOR ESTIMATING HIV INFECTIONS

A formula proposed by the CDC for use in determining the number of HIV-infected persons in a given city is as follows:

National Number of Persons Living With AIDS (1997) Number of PLWA in Your City (1997)

$$\frac{258,000}{900,000} \times \frac{(e.g.,)\ 1000}{x} = 258,000$$

(Estimated national number of HIV-infected persons)

$$x = 900,000,000$$

$$x = \frac{900,000,000}{258,000}$$

$$= 3488$$

(About 3488 persons in this sample city are estimated to be HIV infected.)

Single or Multiple Exposure Categories

In Table 10-1, the number of AIDS cases estimated ending 2009 is presented with respect to adult/

Table 10-1 Total Adult/Adolescent AIDS Cases by Single and Multiple Exposure Categories, Estimated Ending 2008, United States

	AIDS Cases	
Exposure Category	No.	(%)
Single Mode of Exposure		
1. Men who have sex with men	542,960	(44)
2. Injection-drug use	283,820	(23)
3. Hemophilia/coagulation disorder	12,340	(1)
4. Heterosexual contact	135,740	(11)
5. Receipt of blood transfusion	12,340	(1)
6. Receipt of transplant of tissues/organs	35	(0)
7. Other/undetermined	150	(0)
Single Mode of Exposure Subtotal	**987,200**	**(80)**
Multiple Modes of Exposure		
1. Men who have sex with men; Injection-drug use	86,380	(7)
2. Men who have sex with men; hemophilia	176	(0)
3. Men who have sex with men; heterosexual contact	24,680	(2)
4. Men who have sex with men; receipt of transfusion/transplant	3,715	(0)
5. Injection-drug use; hemophilia	185	(0)
6. Injection-drug use; heterosexual contact	61,700	(5)
7. Injection-drug use; receipt of transfusion	1,610	(0)
8. Hemophilia; heterosexual contact	110	(0)
9. Hemophilia; receipt of transfusion/transplant	820	(0)
10. Heterosexual contact; receipt of transfusion/transplant	1,610	(0)
11. Men who have sex with men; Injection-drug use; hemophilia	60	(0)
12. Men who have sex with men; Injection-drug use; heterosexual contact	12,340	(1)
13. Men who have sex with men; Injection-drug use; receipt of transfusion/transplant	610	(0)
14. Men who have sex with men; hemophilia; heterosexual contact	26	(0)
15. Men who have sex with men; hemophilia; receipt of transfusion/transplant	43	(0)
16. Men who have sex with men; heterosexual contact; receipt of transfusion/transplant	261	(0)
17. Injection-drug use; hemophilia; heterosexual contact	90	(0)
18. Injection-drug use; hemophilia; receipt of transfusion/transplant	45	(0)
19. Injection-drug use; heterosexual contact; receipt of transfusion/transplant	1,120	(0)
20. Hemophilia; heterosexual contact; receipt of transfusion/transplant	45	(0)
21. Men who have sex with men; Injection-drug use; hemophilia; heterosexual contact	15	(0)
22. Men who have sex with men; Injection-drug use; hemophilia; receipt of transfusion/transplant	16	(0)
23. Men who have sex with men; Injection-drug use; heterosexual contact; receipt of transfusion/transplant	170	(0)
24. Men who have sex with men; hemophilia; heterosexual contact; receipt of transfusion/transplant	10	(0)
25. Injection-drug use; hemophilia; heterosexual contact; receipt of transfusion/transfusion	28	(0)
26. Men who have sex with men; Injection-drug use; hemophilia; heterosexual contact; receipt of transfusion/transplant	9	(0)
Multiple Modes of Exposure Subtotal	**185,100**	**(15)**
Risk Not Reported or Identified	**61,700**	**(5)**
Total AIDS Cases	**1,234,000**	**(100)**

(*Source: For exposure categories.* CDC HIV/AIDS Surveillance Report, *through 2005, 11:1–45, updated*) Pediatric AIDS cases = 9970 (*Total adult AIDS cases about 1,800,000–9970 (pediatric) = 1,190,030*)

adolescent single or multiple exposure categories. For example, under *Single Mode of Exposure,* heterosexual contact accounts for 10% of all AIDS cases. Under *Multiple Modes of Exposure,* 5% of AIDS cases occurred among injection-drug users who also had heterosexual contact. Table 10-1 lists the numbers and percentages of all reported AIDS cases broken down into seven categories of people who contracted HIV/AIDS from a single risk mode of exposure and 26 categories of people who contracted HIV/AIDS from multiple risk modes of exposure. Note that of the total number of adult/adolescent AIDS cases, 77% occurred from single risk modes of exposure. Of this 80%, 44% occurred among men who had sex with men and about 23% among injection-drug users.

A composite representation of all AIDS cases by exposure category estimated beginning 2009 is shown in Chapter 8, Figure 8-1.

BEHAVIORAL RISK GROUPS AND STATISTICAL EVALUATION

Behavioral Risk Groups and AIDS Cases

As the pool of AIDS patients grew in number during 1981–1983, individual case histories were separated into **behavioral risk groups.** The early case histories of AIDS patients clearly separated people according to their social behavior and medical needs. AIDS patients were placed into the following six risk behavior categories: (1) homosexual and bisexual men; (2) injection-drug users; (3) hemophiliacs; (4) blood transfusion recipients; (5) heterosexuals; and (6) children whose parents are at risk. Each of these groups is considered to be at risk of HIV infection based on some common behavioral denominator. That is, those within these groups represented a higher rate of AIDS cases than people whose needs or behaviors excluded them from these groups. However, because there is some mixing between individuals in behavioral risk groups, HIV infection has gradually spread to lower-risk behavioral groups. Over time the behavioral risk groups have been aligned and defined according to age, exposure category, and sex (see Table 10-1).

A review of AIDS cases by sex/age at diagnosis, and race/ethnicity in the United States, shows that white, black, and Hispanic males between the ages of 20 and 44 make up 79% of all male AIDS cases. Between ages 20 and 59, they make up 97% of all male AIDS cases. People between the ages of 25 and 44 make up over half the nation's 82 million workers.

Statistical Evaluation of Selected Risk Behavioral Group AIDS Cases

Adult/Adolescent AIDS Cases—On October 31, 1995, the United States reached a half-million (501,310) reported AIDS cases. Ending 2009, an estimated 1.3 million AIDS cases and about 610,000 AIDS-related deaths will be reported to the CDC. Cumulative through 2008 about 14% of AIDS cases have occurred among the heterosexual population, 24% occurred among injection-drug users, and 58% occurred in the male homosexual/bisexual IDU population. In 2004, for the first time since the United States AIDS pandemic began, more blacks were diagnosed with AIDS (40.2%) than whites (39.8%). Table 10-2 presents the total estimated number of AIDS cases for 2008 and their distribution based on race, sex, and exposure group.

Figure 10-2 shows that the percentage of AIDS cases for ethnic-related adult/adolescent groups is in striking contrast to the population percentages of each group. Estimating through year 2009 whites made up 67.5% of the population and represented 41% of adult/adolescent AIDS cases. Blacks made up 13.4% of the population but represented 39% of the adult/adolescent AIDS cases. Hispanics made up about 15.1% of the population but represented 19% of the adult/adolescent AIDS cases.

The CDC reported that in 2002, after seven straight years of declining AIDS cases, new AIDS cases began to increase nationally.

According to 1993 data analyzed by Philip Rosenberg (1995 updated) of the National Cancer Institute, 1 in every 92 white American men between ages 27 and 39 may be HIV infected. The findings were especially dismal for black American men, with 1 in 50 estimated to be HIV infected. The estimate was 1 in 60 for Hispanic men. The statistics were equally high for women of color. One in 130 black American women and 1 in 200 Hispanic women are estimated to be infected with HIV. By comparison, the number of white women infected with HIV was 1 in 3000. If the trends continue, Rosenberg noted, HIV/AIDS in young people and minorities must be considered "endemic in the United States."

According to estimates, ending 2008, black Americans made up about 54% of all new AIDS cases and Latinos 20%. Together blacks and Latinos will represent about 74% of all new AIDS cases, but make up 28% of the population. The two populations also represent 85% of all pediatric AIDS cases. In 2008, black women made up about 65% of new AIDS cases reported among females. White women made up 15% and Latino women 20% of new AIDS cases.

Table 10-2 Adult/Adolescent Behavioral Risk Groups, Race and Sex: Percent of Total AIDS Cases—United States, 2008

HIV/AIDS	No. of Cases[a]	% of Cases
Exposure Group		
Men who have sex with men	15,200	38
Injection-drug user (IDU)	5,600	14
Homosexual/IDU	2,400	6
Hemophiliac	82	0
Heterosexual contact	8,000	20
Transfusion related	240	0.6
None of the above	8,560	21.4
Total		100
Race/Ethnicity (all cases)[b]		
White (non-Hispanic)	12,400	31
Black (non-Hispanic)	18,800	47
Hispanic	8,000	20
Other	800	2
Sex (adults only)		
Male	30,800	77
Female	9,200	23
Age Group (yrs)		
13–19	200	0.5
20–24	1,440	3.6
25–29	5,680	14.2
30–39	18,320	45.8
40–49	10,400	26
50–59	2,920	7.3
60 and above	1,040	2.6

[a]Cumulative estimated total = 40,000 adult/adolescent plus 70 pediatric = 40,073 = 100% of cases for 2008.

[b]About one-third of the U.S. population (estimated 306 million ending 2008) or about 102 million are minorities. Blacks make up about 13.4% and Hispanics about 15.1%.

(Adapted from AIDS Surveillance Report, December 2006, updated)

In June 2004, the CDC released a study of men who have sex with other men, conducted in Baltimore, Dallas, Los Angeles, Miami, New York City, and San Francisco. The study showed that of black men tested, 46% were positive for HIV and two-thirds of them were unaware of their infection. There are myriad factors contributing to the spread of HIV among blacks. Information about the threat of AIDS has not been disseminated widely or effectively enough, particularly among those under 21 who feel they are invulnerable. An official with the New York AIDS

Coalition tells a story about a 15-year-old girl who said: "Don't tell me nothin about no AIDS cause that won't impact me. And if I was to get it, all I'd have to do is take a pill in the morning and I'll be O.K." In 2004, Cynthia Davis, a leading AIDS activist in Los Angeles, wrote to leaders of 300 black churches inviting them to a summit on the worsening problem of HIV/AIDS in the black community. She received a response from five!

Figure 10-3 is a U.S. map of estimated AIDS cases through 2009. Note that the highest incidence of AIDS cases occurs along the coastal regions.

Behavioral Risk Groups and Percentages of HIV-Infected People

Entering 2009, investigators found that HIV infection remains largely confined to the populations at recognized behavioral risks: homosexual men, injection-drug users, heterosexual partners of injection-drug users, hemophiliacs, and children of HIV-infected mothers. In the general population, rates for HIV infection include 0.04% for first-time blood donors, 0.14% for military applicants, 0.33% for Job Corps entrants, 0.19% to 0.87% for childbearing women, and 0.30% for hospital patients. Data reported by the CDC in the 1990s indicated that while the number of new AIDS cases increased by 5% in cities, it had increased by 37% in rural areas. This trend continues.

Comments on a Variety of Individual Behavioral Risk Groups

Keep in mind that because a group of people is at risk for HIV does not mean that these people are predes-

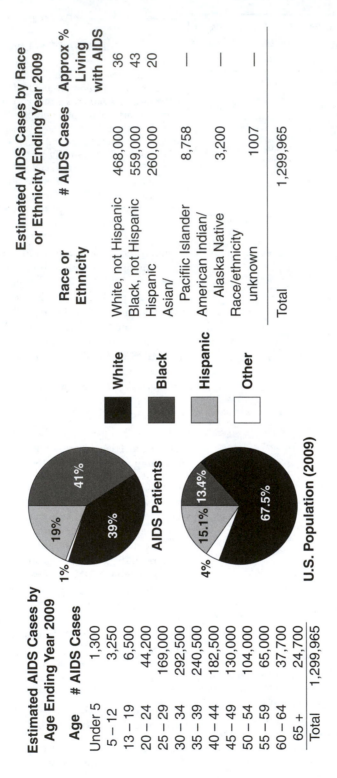

Estimated AIDS Cases by Age Ending Year 2009

Age	# AIDS Cases
Under 5	1,300
5 – 12	3,250
13 – 19	6,500
20 – 24	44,200
25 – 29	169,000
30 – 34	292,500
35 – 39	240,500
40 – 44	182,500
45 – 49	130,000
50 – 54	104,000
55 – 59	65,000
60 – 64	37,700
65 +	24,700
Total	1,299,965

Estimated AIDS Cases by Race or Ethnicity Ending Year 2009

Race or Ethnicity	# AIDS Cases	Approx % Living with AIDS
White, not Hispanic	468,000	36
Black, not Hispanic	559,000	43
Hispanic	260,000	20
Asian/ Pacifiic Islander	8,758	—
American Indian/ Alaska Native	3,200	—
Race/ethnicity unknown	1007	—
Total	1,299,965	

White · Black · Hispanic · Other

AIDS Patients — 1%, 19%, 41%, 39%

U.S. Population (2009) — 4%, 15.1%, 13.4%, 67.5%

FIGURE 10–2 Estimated AIDS Cases by Age and Racial and Ethnic Classification. Adults AIDS cases show a disportionate percentage among blacks and Hispanics. Fifty-eight percent of reported AIDS cases occur among racial and ethnic minorities. The figures reflect higher rates of AIDS in black and Hispanic injection-drug users and their sex partners. Percentages of the population are based on the numbers of AIDS cases in the United States estimated ending year 2009. U.S. population is over 300 million.

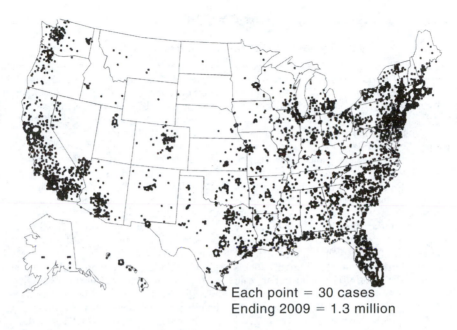

Each point = 30 cases
Ending 2009 = 1.3 million

FIGURE 10–3 United States: Estimated Cumulative AIDS Cases and Approximate Location Ending 2009. *(CDC. Atlanta Surveillance Branch)*

tined to become infected. People are placed within these groups because of their social behavior, a behavior that has been associated with a high, medium, or low risk of becoming HIV infected. Essentially, there is no zero-risk group because a scenario can always be formulated to show that under certain circumstances one or more members of that group could become HIV infected.

The point of placing people in behavioral risk groups is not to offend them but to provide a warning that certain behavior might make them more vulnerable to HIV infection. It is not race or ethnic group that places people at high or low risk for infection, it is their behavior.

The fact that AIDS was first identified in 1981 in seemingly well-defined behavioral groups (homosexual men, injection-drug users, hemophiliacs, Haitian immigrants) probably contributed to a false sense of security among people who did not belong to any of these groups. However, as information about HIV and AIDS accumulated, it became clear that HIV was transmitted in body fluids. This had grave implications for all social groups. On reflection, the people in the original high-risk groups simply had the bad luck of being in the way of a newly emerging infectious agent as it first began to spread. It is highly probable

that in the different behavioral risk groups there are lifestyle or medical history factors that increase the efficiency with which the virus is transmitted.

Men Who Have Sex With Men (MSM)—The term *men who have sex with men* (MSM) was first used in 1994 to reduce stigma. It refers to all men who have sex with other men regardless of how they identify themselves (gay, bisexual, or heterosexual). In the United States, HIV and AIDS have had a tremendous impact on MSM. In 1981, almost 100% of all AIDS cases reported to the CDC occurred in homosexual males. In the 1980s, the infection rate among gay men in San Francisco was over 60%. For the 2000s it dropped to about 30% to 40% per year.

Recent studies show that a significant percentage of gay men who had originally adopted safer sex behaviors are relapsing to unsafe sex (Lemp et al., 1994). For example, in 2004 the CDC reported an 8% increase in new HIV cases among gay men. And in a study of gay men ages 15 to 29 by Duncan MacKellar of the CDC (2005), 10% of 5600 men tested HIV positive but 77% of them were unaware they were infected. **Before being tested** the majority of these men thought they were at low risk of

ACROSS THE UNITED STATES: WASHINGTON, D.C.

In February 2006, National Public Radio (NPR) examined the state of HIV/AIDS in the nation's capital. According to NPR, the rate of new AIDS cases reported each year in the district is 10 times the national average. Of the district's more than 500,000 residents, an estimated one in 50 is living with AIDS and one in 20 is HIV positive. Cornelius Baker, former executive director of the Whitman-Walker Clinic in the district, said several factors contribute to the high HIV prevalence rate in the city. The city has a small population, with a large gay community and a majority black population that is being ravaged by HIV. In addition, there is a poor healthcare infrastructure, inadequate primary care, and high rate of drug addiction. The city's high rate of incarceration also contributes to the number of HIV/AIDS cases. Marsha Martin, the senior deputy director of the district's HIV/AIDS Administration, said HIV/AIDS has fallen "off the radar screen" in the city.

From 1997 through 2006, 66% of AIDS patients received an HIV diagnosis within one year of their AIDS diagnosis and of those, 53% were tested one month before their AIDS diagnosis! In mid-2006 Martin made condoms available in all public places that serve alcohol and has expanded the city's needle exchange program, targeted prevention messages at sexually active teenagers and college students, offered HIV testing in more physicians' offices and emergency departments, and required mandatory HIV testing of inmates during the prison intake and discharge process. Also, in June 2006, Martin launched an unprecedented city-wide campaign for routine HIV testing of every person between ages 14 and 84. The campaign targeted 400,000 people to be tested. As of mid-2007, over 20,000 had been tested with 1200 being HIV positive. A prevalence of about 6%! The slogan to begin the HIV testing campaign was "Come Together D.C., Get Screened for HIV." Washington, D.C. has the highest rate of new AIDS cases in the United States at 179 per 100,000 people. Martin wants every D.C. citizen to know their HIV status by year 2010. If this routine testing program is successful, most likely many states will choose to follow Martin's program.

UPDATE 2008—In November 2007, a new 120-page national report appeared, entitled "We're the Ones We've Been Waiting For: The State of AIDS in Black America and What We Are Doing About It!" The data is about blacks living in Washington, D.C. The data offers a look at the problem of HIV/AIDS in the black community in D.C. from 2001 through 2006. During this time frame, 80% of new infections occurred in black men, women, and children. Among women in D.C. who tested HIV positive, 9 out of 10 were black. The study shows that the disease, once considered a gay disease, has moved into the general population. Over 37% of infections were spread heterosexually in contrast to 25% of cases attributable to gay men. In 2006, 12,500 people in D.C. had HIV/AIDS. In 2008 the number had risen to 17,600. The study states that the HIV/AIDS rate in D.C. is the worst of any city in the United States, nearly twice that of New York City and four times that of Detroit, Michigan.

On any given day, a team of doctors, social workers, and outreach advocates with the Anacostia-based Family & Medical Counseling Service, Inc. (FMCSI) travels D.C. with the goal of preventing HIV/AIDS. With a staff of 75 and a mobile clinic in a Winnebago, FMCSI visits jails, churches, and festivals—anywhere the team can reach people. (Owens, 2008)

Also in July 2008, the Black AIDS Institute published a report, "Left Behind: Black America: A Neglected Priority in the Global AIDS Epidemic," about HIV/AIDS among black Americans, saying that the HIV/AIDS epidemic among blacks resembles the epidemics seen in many African countries.

The report says that HIV/AIDS should be seen as a threat to the entire black community in the United States and not just specific high-risk groups. HIV is increasingly transmitted among blacks through heterosexual activity through networks in which men have many sexual partners at the same time. The report says that almost 600,000 blacks in the United States are living with HIV and that up to 30,000 are contracting the virus annually. When adjusted for age, the death rate from AIDS-related causes among blacks with HIV is $2\frac{1}{2}$ times greater than that among HIV-positive whites. Two percent of blacks in the United States are HIV-positive, according to government estimates, and the report says that only four countries outside Africa have a higher HIV prevalence. If the U.S. black population were a separate country, it would rank 16th worldwide in the number of people living with HIV. (kaisernetwork.org, 2008)

Black AIDS Institute Executive Director Phill Wilson said that "[the U.S.] response to the epidemic in black America stands in sharp contrast to our response to the epidemic overseas." The report found that more blacks in the United States are living with HIV than in Botswana, Ethiopia, Guyana, Haiti, Namibia, Rwanda, and Vietnam—7 of the 15 countries targeted in the [President's Emergency Plan for AIDS relief]. PEPFAR is guided by a strategic plan, clear standards, and annual progress reports to Congress, but "America itself has no strategic plan to combat its own epidemic." According to Wilson, the purpose of making the comparison between PEPFAR and U.S. domestic efforts is not to criticize the global program but to call for more money and attention to domestic issues. Wilson said, "When we give aid to foreign countries, we demand that they have a national AIDS plan, but we don't have a plan in the United States."

being HIV positive, and half of them had unprotected sex during the previous six months. A 2007 CDC report states that about 46% of black gay men in the U.S. may be HIV positive.

Demographic Changes of HIV-Infected Men in the Gay Community

Data compiled by the CDC and reported in June 2001 reveals a striking change in the disease's demographics in America (HIV/AIDS Surveillance Report, 2001). Year-end data shows that 74% of HIV/ AIDS cases in white Americans, 37% in black Americans, and 42% in Latino Americans resulted from homosexual contacts. Ending 2008, of the estimated 275,000 MSM living with HIV/AIDS in America, 34% were white, 46% were black, and 20% were Hispanic.

The national level of HIV infection among gay men is over 1%. About a third of the gay men surveyed knew they were HIV infected. Ending year 2008, MSM accounted for about 52% of 1.2 million adult/adolescent AIDS cases in America and about 52% of them have died. An estimated 267,000 gay men are living with AIDS and about 330,000 are progressing to AIDS (Wolitski et al., 2001; Catania et al., 2001 updated).

Overall, of the 24 million AIDS deaths worldwide ending year 2009, about 2 million will be gay men. These data overwhelmingly make this global pandemic a heterosexual pandemic.

Injection-Drug Users—According to the CDC, as many as 33% of the nation's 1.2 million injection-drug users may be HIV infected. This behavioral risk group contains the nation's second largest group of HIV infected and AIDS patients. An association between injection-drug use and AIDS was recognized in 1981, about two years before the virus was identified. AIDS in IDUs and hemophiliacs offered the first evidence that whatever caused AIDS was being carried in and transmitted by human blood. From the reported IDU AIDS cases in 1981 through 2006, 25% of all adult/adolescent AIDS cases were associated with IDUs. Of IDUs, 74% listed IDU as their only risk factor for HIV infection; 26% were also homosexual/bisexual. It is estimated that through 2006 40% of infected women and 22% of infected men were infected through IDUs.

IDU AIDS cases have been reported in all 50 states and the District of Columbia. Among the adult/adolescent heterosexual AIDS cases, over half had sexual partners who are/were IDUs.

About 55% of all IDU-associated cases were reported in the Northeast, which represents about 20% of the population of the United States and its territories. The South reported 20% of IDU-associated AIDS cases, 5% from the Midwest, and the West reported the remaining 20%.

The rate of IDU-associated AIDS continues to be higher for blacks and Hispanics than for whites. Except for the West, where rates for whites and Hispanics were similar, this difference by race/ethnicity was observed in all regions of the country and was greatest in the Northeast.

Heterosexuals—The spread of HIV in the general population is relatively slow, yet potentially it is the source of the greatest numbers of HIV/AIDS cases. The CDC estimates there are about 150 million Americans without an identified at-risk behavior, the general population.

Data from the CDC for years 2004 through 2008 indicate that about 15% of all the AIDS cases and 35% of all new HIV infections in the United States occurred through heterosexual contact. Most of the heterosexual AIDS cases occurred in persons or the sexual partners of individuals with an identified behavioral risk. Relative to the general adult population, the number of heterosexual AIDS cases is only a fraction of 1%.

Global HIV/AIDS Cases and Heterosexuality

Worldwide ending year 2009, there will be an estimated 9 million people living with AIDS and about 24 million will have died of AIDS. According to the Worldwatch Institute, South Africa's HIV pandemic is perhaps the worst on the globe. It has engulfed the country, and "barring a medical miracle, one of every five adults will die of AIDS over the next 10 years." This unprecedented social tragedy is also translating into an economic disaster. The working-age population is being lost to AIDS. In Zimbabwe, state morgues have extended their hours to cope with the soaring death rate, mostly as a result of AIDS. An estimated 2000 people now die every week in that southern African country, nearly 70% of them from AIDS-related illnesses. The main hospital in Harare has opened its morgue around the clock and other hospital and mortuary facilities have extended closing time by four hours. At the University of Durban Westville in KwaZulu-Natal, 14% of students tested HIV positive in 1997; in 2001 it was about 40%.

Worldwide, beginning 2009, **heterosexuals** made up about 80% of the estimated 34 million living

THE LATINO COMMUNITY

The seventh annual National Latino AIDS Awareness Day, an observance sponsored by the Latino Commission on AIDS, will be held on October 15, 2009, the last day of Hispanic Heritage Month, in cities throughout the United States. Latino leaders sponsor activities that respond to the state of AIDS among Latinos in their communities. In recognition of the surging number of new infections among Latinos and young Latinos, organizers will use the day to promote and sponsor prevention activities, alert religious leaders and public officials to the need to reduce new infections, and care for Latinos infected with the virus.

"In 1983, my brother died of AIDS. It infected his wife, and a year later she died. And now we had the first set of orphans in our family. Despite everything, I saw the love and unity of my family—how we pulled together and took care of my brother and loved him. My sister left another set of orphans. My uncle, who is my godfather, lost children to HIV. His son died in a prison hospital of AIDS. His daughter died at the age of 33 and left another orphan child. My uncle wasn't around to see his daughter die because he died of suffering from watching. Last year we found out my 70-year-old uncle is infected with HIV. And that's just my family. I watch the news. I watch people talk about wars in other countries and I identify with the feelings of those people. I know they have bombs thrown at them. I know they have weapons pointed at them. But we have a weapon that is killing my community. We have to silence this weapon of AIDS, which is killing us."

The rate of infection among Latinos in the United States reflects an increasingly dire situation. Latinos represent about 15.1% of the total population. Beginning 2009 Latinos represented an estimated 19% of new AIDS cases in America. About 83,000 Latinos are currently living with AIDS and about 130,000 are HIV infected. The rate of HIV infection among Latino men is three times greater than the infection rate found among white, non-Hispanic men. Similarly, women and children in the Latino community have rates of infection that are seven times greater than the rates found among white women and children. If these trends continue, the Harvard AIDS Institute projects that by 2009 the percentage of total annual AIDS attributable to the Latino population will eclipse the percentage of such cases attributable to the white, non-Hispanic population.

AIDS is the fourth leading cause of death for Latinos ages 25 to 34, and third among those ages 35 to 44. There are over 46 million Latino/Hispanic people in America. The rate of new AIDS cases among Latinos is about four times the rate among white Americans but about three times lower than the rate for black Americans. According to the AIDS Healthcare Foundation, 45% of Latinos have never tested for HIV and 40% have never talked with a doctor about HIV/AIDS.

The HIV/AIDS Epidemic in Mexico: Mexico City was home to the XVII International AIDS Conference (see Box 10.1)

Mexico is home to 200,000 people living with HIV/AIDS, the second-highest number of people living with HIV/AIDS in Latin America. The country's HIV/AIDS prevalence rate is among the lowest in the region and has stabilized over the last decade. At the same time, HIV prevalence rates among certain populations in the country are significantly higher. The epidemic in Mexico is influenced by cultural, social, and economic factors and, similar to other countries in Latin America, homophobia, stigma, discrimination, gender inequalities, interregional migration, and poverty contribute to or exacerbate the epidemic. Among the issues unique to HIV/AIDS in Mexico is the role played by population mobility and migration along the Mexico-United States border.

Overview

- The first case of HIV/AIDS in Mexico was reported in 1983.
- Mexico had an estimated 200,000 people living with HIV/AIDS in 2007. This is the second-highest in all of Latin America—Brazil tops the list with 730,000.
- The HIV/AIDS prevalence rate in Mexico is 0.3%, which is among the lowest in the region and lower than the rate in Latin America (0.5%) and globally (0.8%).
- An estimated 11,000 Mexicans died of HIV/AIDS in 2007.
- HIV is spread primarily through sex in Mexico, accounting for about 90% of all cumulative cases of AIDS. Sex between men accounts for the largest share of HIV diagnoses recorded to date (57%). There is also an increasing trend toward heterosexual transmission in recent years.

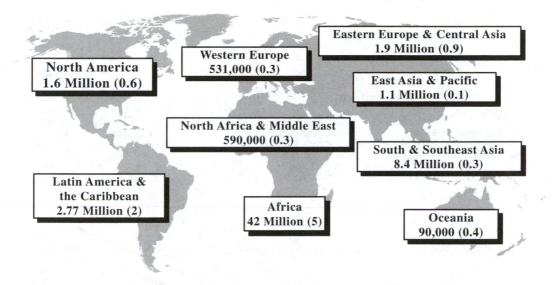

Estimated: Global Total 59 Million HIV Infections Ending 2009 and HIV/AIDS Prevalence Rates (%). Global Rate (0.8%)

FIGURE 10–4   Estimated Number of Global HIV Infections Projected using data from United Nations AIDS Program and World Health Organization. Of the estimated 59 million HIV-infected persons, about 35 million **are living** in some state of HIV/AIDS illness. About 3.8 million of these are children. Of 209 countries reporting to the WHO and UNAIDS,194 have reported AIDS cases. World population reached 6.65 billion in March 2008. *(UNAIDS Report on the Global HIV/AIDS Epidemic, December 2006 updated)* All numbers have been rounded off and may not add up to 59 million.

HIV-infected people. About 65% of these infected people live in sub-Saharan Africa. North America, Latin America, South and Southeast Asia, and Africa account for about 93% of global HIV infections (Figure 10-4). Of the 34 million living HIV-infected people worldwide, about 95% live in nonindustrial nations.

UNAIDS updated estimates are that, on average, 2.5 million new HIV infections occurred annually from 1997 through 2008. The AIDS death toll for these eleven years is estimated at 22 million of which 8.5 million were women and 5 million were under age 15 (Table 10-3). The United States will have over 1.3 million AIDS cases ending 2009—

Table 10–3 Leading Cause of Death Worldwide from 1998 estimated through 2009

Infectious Diseases	All Diseases
1. **HIV/AIDS**	1. Heart diseases
2. Diarrheal disease	2. Cerebrovascular diseases
3. Childhood diseases	3. Lower respiratory diseases
4. Tuberculosis	4. **HIV/AIDS**
5. Malaria	5. Obstructive pulmonary diseases
6. STDs excluding HIV/AIDS	6. Diarrheal diseases
7. Meningitis	7. Perinatal conditions
8. Tropical diseases	8. Tuberculosis

(Data Courtesy of the World Health Organization, 1998 updated.)

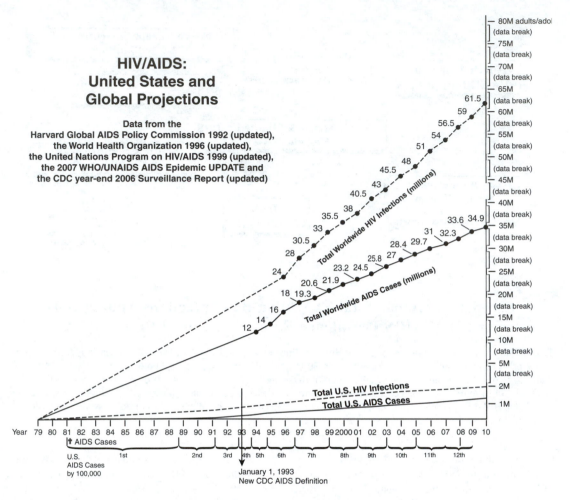

FIGURE 10–5 Estimated U.S. and Global Projections for Total Number of HIV and AIDS Cases. Ending year 2009, about 1.3 million U.S. AIDS cases will be reported to the CDC. Estimated total U.S. HIV infections through 2009 is 1.8 million. Worldwide the total number of AIDS cases is expected to reach about 33.6 million ending 2009 (24 million dead and 9.4 million living with AIDS). Through the year 2009 , about 2% of all HIV infections and 2.8% of total AIDS cases will have occurred in the United States. William Hazeltine, AIDS researcher formerly at the Dana Farber Institute, and now with Human Genome Sciences, Inc. said that if prevention does not work or a cure is not found, some *1 billion* pepole could be HIV positive by the year 2025. *(Source: Harvard Global AIDS Policy Commission 1992 and World Health Organization 1993, 1994, National Census Bureau 1998, and projected data)*

NOTE: *The true data would not give rise to the linear increments as shown, but the true data per year for HIV infections or AIDS cases globally are guesstimates or at least best estimates because of underreporting, wrongful reporting, case overlap, errors and, through 2008, the lack of complete mandatory reporting of HIV infections.*

worldwide there will be about 27 times that number (Figure 10-5).

Worldwide, it is estimated that 6 in every 100 sexually active people aged 15 to 49 is HIV infected. Ending 2009, there will be an estimated 35 million people living with HIV infection. There are over a dozen countries whose population is not equal to 35 million people!

Hemophiliacs—There are about 16,000 to 20,000 hemophiliacs in the United States. At least half are HIV positive and through 2008, about 3700 of them have died. Of those infected, over 98% received HIV in blood products that were essential to their survival. By mid-1985, an HIV blood screening test was put into effect nationally. From that point, the risk of HIV infection from the blood supply has been significantly lowered, but a small risk still exists. **Scandals** of knowingly selling HIV-positive blood for transfusions and in production of the blood factor essential for hemophiliacs, surfaced in France, Germany, the United States, Canada, and Japan in the 1990s. (For discussion, see Point of Information 8.1, Chapter 8.)

American Military—The incidence of HIV infection can be measured best in groups that undergo routine serial testing. Because active duty military personnel and civilian applicants for the service are routinely tested for HIV antibody, there is a unique opportunity to measure the incidence of HIV infection in a large, demographically varied subset of the general population.

Beginning 2004 the military began HIV testing of all personnel every two years. The current infection rate among all military personnel is about 0.02% or two per 10,000, much lower than for the general population.

College Students A study was conducted by the CDC with the American College Health Association (Gayle et al., 1988). At five campuses the rate of HIV-positive blood ranged from 4 to 9 samples per 1000. In contrast, the rate of HIV in the general heterosexual population is about 0.02% and the rate for military personnel in about the same age group tested over a similar time period was 0.14%.

The question is why college students have a rate of HIV infection about 10 times higher than the general heterosexual population. Are college students less informed than the general heterosexual population?

Surveys indicate that college students are well educated about HIV/AIDS. Why, then, the higher rate of infection? Perhaps it's the age-old dilemma of information versus behavior. **They know what to do but they don't do it.** College students have always had information on drug use, alcoholism, pregnancies out of wedlock, and sexually transmitted diseases; but this knowledge has not appreciably reduced at-risk behaviors. STDs are at an all-time high in teenage and college students.

Prisoners Anne Spaulding and colleagues (2002) estimated that about 25% of all people living with HIV infection have passed through a correctional facility in the United States. Beginning 2009, the nation's prison population is at an all-time high, over 2 million adults contained in 1300 state and 71 federal prisons. Ninety percent are men.

According to the U.S. Bureau of Justice Statistics, 2.1% of these people or 42,000 are HIV positive and of these, 17% have AIDS (Rubel et al., 1997 updated). The total number of **prisoners, parolees,** and **probationers** in 2008 was about 6.5 million with an HIV-positive rate of about 0.8% or about 50,000 being HIV positive (DeGroot et al., 1996 updated). Entering 2009, over 6000 adult inmates in U.S. state and federal prisons and jails had died of AIDS.

The Aging HIV/AIDS Population in America—The face of AIDS has changed dramatically from the 1980s into the new millennium. AIDS cases among men, in particular gay men, and IDUs predominated in the 1980s. But from the 1990s onward the numbers of AIDS cases among the elderly, women, their children, and people of color increased significantly. **The senior citizens of today did not grow up in the age of AIDS—they did not have sex and HIV in the same thought.**

Research on Older Adults with HIV (ROAH)—In 2006, key findings of ROAH (Research on Older Adults with HIV), the nation's first comprehensive study addressing the aging HIV/AIDS population, conducted by the AIDS Community Research Initiative of America (ACRIA), was released. The study examined a New York City cohort of 1000 people living with HIV. They represent the underserved, unacknowledged, yet substantial HIV-positive population of men and women of all sexual orientations and race in New York City who are growing old with this disease. ROAH looked both at their unique health needs—that is, complications that arise from or that are made worse by their age—and the complex psychological and social issues that affect these older adults. Prior to this study, many saw the face of AIDS in New York City as that of a white, homosexual male—the media archetype of the 1980s. Yet in New York City and other urban centers, the face of HIV/AIDS is that of a heterosexual-identified person over the age of 50 who is a person of color and increasingly likely to be female. The study showed that one decade after the introduction of highly active antiretroviral therapy (HAART), a dramatic decrease occurred in mortality rates, and life expectancy increased among people living with HIV/AIDS. With new HIV infection rates remaining stable, the net result is an HIV-positive population that is both aging and growing. The CDC states that about 29% of all people living with HIV/AIDS in the United States are over age 50. That is about 327,000 people! A large percentage of these people were infected prior to age 50 but are surviving because of ART. They make up about 19% of all AIDS cases, and they make up about 35% of all deaths due to AIDS. The CDC says that people over age 50 will make up the majority of living HIV/AIDS cases by the year 2015! In New York City, the HIV/AIDS epicenter of the United States, 30% of the almost 100,000 people living with HIV/AIDS are over age 50 and 70% are over age 40. Within the next decade it is probable that the majority of people with HIV/AIDS in New York City will be over age 50.

A Reality Check for New York City—Because of the ROAH study, a signal event in the history of the HIV/AIDS pandemic occurred in June 2007. The New York City Council passed a $1 million initiative to provide HIV education and prevention information to older adults. This response by the council demonstrates an awareness that conditions for the HIV infected are changing. More people are growing old with this virus. Because nearly one-third of HIV-infected New Yorkers are age 50 and older, the numbers are too large to be ignored.

Across the United States, the rate of HIV/AIDS among persons age 50 and older is 12 times as high among blacks and 5 times as high among Hispanics as it is among whites.

Florida—In Florida, a state with a large retired population, the number of recorded AIDS cases among those over age 50 rose from 6 in 1984 to about 17,000 by 2009, or about 15% of the state's cases. In Dade County, Fl., a popular destination among retirees, about 20% of people with HIV/AIDS are seniors. Forty-four percent of women over 50 in Florida with AIDS, and 18% of Florida men over 50 with AIDS are known to have become infected through heterosexual sex. These numbers are predicted to grow as the more sexually liberal baby boom generation ages.

Many seniors feel that HIV infection is just a problem for young people, homosexuals, and injection-drug addicts. Now, the use of Viagra compounds the problem. With the use of Viagra, seniors are much more sexually active and few practice safer sex. The manufacturer of Viagra is trying to incorporate safer sex messages into its advertisements.

Healthcare Workers—Healthcare workers are defined by CDC as people, including students and trainees, whose activities involve contact with patients or with blood or other body fluids from patients in a heathcare setting. They represent 7.7% of the U.S. labor force. **The risk of HIV transmission from healthcare worker to patient during an exposure-prone invasive procedure is remote. There is a greater and well-documented risk of transmission from an infected patient to a healthcare worker.**

Needle Stick Injuries—Healthcare workers are in a quandary about the possibility of becoming HIV-infected via needle sticks. Articles such as "Needle-stick Risks Higher Than Reports Indicate" or "The Risk of HIV Transmission via Needlesticks Is Low" convey conflicting impressions.

Needle sticks and penetration of sharp objects account for about 80% of all healthcare workers' exposures to blood and blood products. There are about 800,000 needle stick injuries from contaminated devices in healthcare settings each year. Of these, about 16,000 devices are contaminated with HIV (Miller et al., 1997).

Ruthanne Marcus and colleagues (1988) reported that, across the board, healthcare workers exposed to HIV-contaminated blood have about a 1 in 300 chance of becoming infected. Other more recent reports place the risk of HIV infection at 1 in 250. However, with the introduction of **P**ost **E**xposure **P**rophylaxis (PEP—see Chapter 4), the number of persons who are exposed to HIV and progress to AIDS should be significantly reduced.

ESTIMATES OF AIDS CASES AND HIV INFECTION

In 1987, Otis Bowen, then secretary of health and human services, said "AIDS would make Black Death pale by comparison."

As long as the number of newly infected people each year exceeds the number who die, the pandemic will continue to build.

Who Reports AIDS Cases and to Whom? United States

AIDS cases are reported to the CDC through the SOUNDEX system, which involves translating names into specific sets of numbers and letters. While the resulting codes are not unique, when they are combined with other information, such as birthdates, individual cases can be followed without revealing names.

AIDS Reporting Systems

Reporting AIDS cases reveals past HIV infections. When an AIDS case is reported, it is like looking at a 10- to 12-year-old photograph of the infection date (average time, without drug therapy, from infection to AIDS diagnosis is 10 to 12 years). AIDS became reportable in all 50 states, the District of Columbia, and U.S. territories to the CDC in Atlanta in 1986.

By the end of 1993, all 50 states, the District of Columbia, and four territories (Guam, Pacific Islands, Puerto Rico, and the Virgin Islands) reported adult/adolescent cases. The CDC also reported the numbers of adult/adolescent/pediatric AIDS cases per 100,000 population by state. For the 10 leading metropolitan areas of at least 500,000 population for AIDS beginning year 2009, see Table 10-4. Beginning year 2009, the 10 states reporting the highest incidence of AIDS cases for adult/adolescents can be seen in Table 10-5.

U.S. Cities with Highest AIDS Cases

The seven U.S. cities with the highest incidence of new AIDS cases beginning year 2009 were, highest to lowest: New York, Ft. Lauderdale, San Francisco, West Palm Beach, Jersey City, Newark, and Columbia, S.C. The American HIV/AIDS epidemic is now disproportionately affecting the South. Only 36% of the U.S. population lives in the South but the region is home to 41% of all people living with AIDS and 46% of newly identified cases. Of other people living with AIDS, 29% live in the Northeast, 20% in the West and 11% in the Midwest. And, while the incidence of AIDS has been increasing in the South in recent years, in other regions of the country it has either remained constant or decreased.

With the widespread use of antiretroviral drugs beginning in 1995/96 there was a decline in AIDS

Table 10-4 Ten Metropolitan Areas Reporting Highest Number of AIDS Cases Through Year 2008

Metropolitan Area	Number of AIDS Cases
New York City	183,696
Los Angeles	67,080
San Francisco	51,600
Miami	36,120
Washington, D.C.	35,088
Chicago	32,508
Philadelphia	29,928
Houston	28,844
Newark, NJ	25,800
Atlanta	25,284
	516,000 or 43% of all AIDS cases in America.

Table 10-5 Ten States Reporting Highest Number of AIDS Cases Through Year 2008

States	Number of AIDS Cases	Approximate # Living with AIDS
New York	219,648	95,040
California	189,995	76,032
Florida	122,496	60,445
Texas	82,790	39,916
New Jersey	65,894	22,429
Illinois	36,664	20,189
Pennsylvania	36,323	20,110
Georgia	34,806	18,589
Maryland	32,102	16,308
Massachusetts	23,654	10,986
	844,800 or 70.4% of all AIDS cases in America	380,160 or about 45%

cases but not in new HIV infections. Thus, it became clear that the total numbers of AIDS cases no longer accurately represent the pandemic. To track this pandemic now, it will be essential to have some form of reporting new HIV infections (Figure 10-6).

Names-Based HIV Reporting

In mid-2005, the CDC urged all state health departments toward names-based reporting. The CDC wanted a single accurate system that will provide national data to monitor the scope of HIV infections nationally (all other illnesses are reported by name). For those states who do not comply, they may lose millions of Ryan White AIDS Care dollars. All states

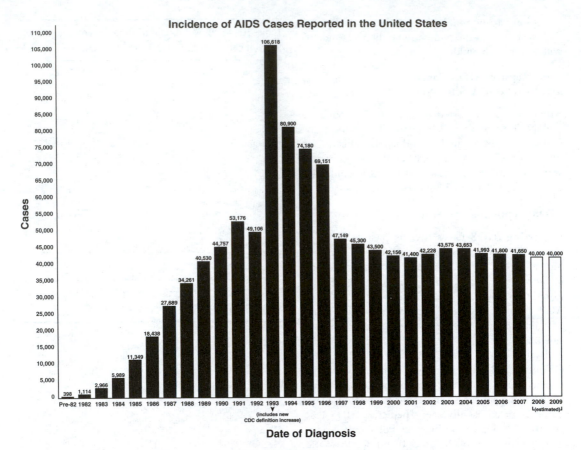

Incidence of AIDS Cases Reported in the United States

FIGURE 10-6   Incidence and Estimates of AIDS in Persons 13 and Older by Year of Diagnosis—United States, pre-1982 through 2008. The total for 1995 reflects a 9% reduction in AIDS cases from 1994 due to a drop in the backlog of persons to be identified as AIDS cases according to the 1993 definition of AIDS. AIDS cases reported in 2002 increased for the first time in 10 years, about a 2.2% rise over 2001. Data for years 2002 through 2005 reflect an increase in AIDS cases resulting from therapy failure and increases in gay males. Throughout the American pandemic, about 85% of persons wih AIDS were/are ages 20–49.

used names-based reporting ending 2008. It took almost 10 years to get all states to use name-based HIV reporting.

It is expected that HIV reporting will provide a more accurate view of recent transmission trends. The information will also help direct money to the most effective programs and could affect allocations for HIV patient care. The decision of states to report HIV cases was most influenced by the development of successful treatment, which allows many people with HIV to live healthier longer. But that progress has made it hard for statisticians to calculate backward to estimate time of infection. AIDS case reporting now has become much more of an indicator of who is get-

ting treated, who is not getting tested early, and how effective is their therapy.

NEWLY INFECTED

For the 50,000 to 56,000 plus new HIV infections occurring in 1999 through 2008 annually, the CDC estimated, on average, that 67% of the infected were men. Of these men, 42% were infected via homosexual sex, 25% through IDU and 33% through heterosexual sex. Of these men, 54% are black, 26% are white, and 20% are Hispanics. Black American men make up 75% of new HIV infections among heterosexual cases. A small

WHY THE CDC RAISED THE NUMBER OF NEW HIV INFECTIONS BY OVER 16000 CASES PER YEAR

Beginning in 2003, the CDC began reporting on new HIV infections from 33 states and 5 dependent areas that used a confidential name-based reporting system. The other 17 states did not report their new HIV infections by name. This means that 17 states did not have their new cases of HIV infections included in the annual CDC reports on the number of new HIV infections. However, AIDS cases from all 50 states and 5 dependent areas continued to be reported as usual. In fact, AIDS cases actually increased between 2002 and 2006, the period reported on in the 2006 HIV/AIDS Surveillance Report. Thus, HIV data from these 33 states and 5 dependent areas represented just 63% of the estimated total of new infections that were believed to be occurring in all 50 states and 5 dependent areas. In 2003, the CDC recommended that all 50 states use confidential name-based reporting of new HIV infections, and by 2006, 45 states and the 5 dependent areas were reporting new HIV cases via that system. Therefore, data on new HIV cases for 2006 contained new HIV infections from an additional 12 states whose HIV cases were previously unreported. Data from the 45 states and 5 dependent areas revealed that there were an estimated 52,878 new HIV infections. Still 10% of the states, or about 5% of the new HIV infections, were left out of the count. So the 2006 estimate of HIV infections is really more like 56,000 plus!

Clearly the increase in the estimate of new HIV infections for 2006 did not just happen as a singular event; the number of new HIV infections had to be greater than the 40,000 a year estimated by the CDC from 1989 through 2005, they were just not being counted! It was the history of confidential name-based reporting beginning in 2003 from 33 states and 5 dependent areas in 2005 that set the stage for the data from 45 states and the 5 areas in 2006 and the use of STARHS data (Serologic Testing Algorithm for Recent HIV Seroconversions—see Chapter 13 for an explanation for the use of STARHS) in 2006 from 22 states with name-based reporting, extrapolated to estimate the number of new HIV infections in all 50 states and the District of Columbia, provided the 56,300 HIV cases for 2006.

The updated estimates confirm that the largest proportion of new infections—53%—is occurring among gay and bisexual men. HIV incidence has steadily increased among this group since the early 1990s, while the rate of new infections among heterosexuals and injection drug users has fallen. Women accounted for 25% of all new infections.

By race/ethnicity, African-Americans account for 45% of new infections, compared with 35% among whites and 17% among Latinos. According to the revised estimates, blacks have an infection rate nearly three times higher than that of Latinos and seven times higher than that of whites (Hall et al. 2008).

A STATEMENT FROM THE CDC AUGUST 2008

The estimates from our nation's new HIV incidence surveillance system reveal that the U.S. epidemic is—and has been—worse than previously estimated and serve as a wake-up call for all Americans. Using the new technology called Serological Testing Algorithm for Recent HIV Seroconversion (STARHS) that distinguishes recent from longstanding HIV infections, CDC estimates that 56,300 new HIV infections occurred in the United States in 2006. Prior to the availability of STARHS, CDC previously estimated that approximately 40,000 new HIV infections occurred annually since the 1990s. It is important to note that the 2006 estimate does not represent an actual increase in the annual number of new infections; rather, a separate CDC historical trend analysis published alongside the incidence estimate suggests that the number of new HIV infections was never as low as 40,000 and has been roughly stable since the early 2000s. Even though the analysis shows overall stability in new HIV infections in recent years, the HIV/AIDS epidemic remains at an unacceptably high level.

The 2006 HIV incidence estimates show:

- Gay and bisexual men of all races remain the group most heavily affected by HIV, accounting for 53% of all new infections.
- The impact of HIV is greater among blacks than any other racial or ethnic group, with an HIV incidence rate that is 7 times higher than that of whites (83.7/100,000 for blacks compared to 11.5/100,000 for whites) and almost 3 times higher than that of Latinos (29.3/100,000).

Overall, levels of HIV infection in the United States are too high and have been increasing among men who have sex with men (MSM) since the early 1990s. The HIV epidemic must not continue on its current course. With more people living with HIV than ever before, there are more opportunities for transmission; however, the number of new infections has remained relatively stable.

percentage are members of other racial/ethnic groups. Of the estimated 12,354-plus new infections among women in the United States annually for 2002 through 2008, the CDC estimated that approximately 75% of women are infected through heterosexual sex and 25% through injection-drug use. Of newly infected women, approximately 64% are black, 17% are white, 17% are Hispanics, and a small percentage are members of other racial/ethnic groups. The CDC estimates that over the next four years, about 120,000 people under the age of 29 will become HIV-infected if current trends continue. The current increase in HIV infections is a reversal of prevention program successes. The overtly sick, the emaciated, and those with visible Kaposi's sarcoma are rarely seen on the streets; antiretroviral drugs have the dying going back to work. The fear of infection and death has subsided. Accordingly, new AIDS cases have increased about 8% nationwide from 2002 through 2008.

Will There Be a Heterosexual AIDS Epidemic in the United States?

A heterosexual epidemic on a scale similar to any developing nation is very unlikely now or in the future. Heterosexual AIDS epidemics in the developing nations result largely from conditions that do not exist in America or in other industrialized countries. These include large-scale population shifts, little information about HIV/AIDS prevention, many migrant workers, widespread prostitution, deep reluctance to use condoms, and frequent, untreated sexually transmitted diseases. Still, according to the CDC, heterosexual transmission will slowly increase in the United States largely due to low-income black and Hispanic women. Among the things that put them at increased risk: exchanging sex for crack cocaine and having sex with injection-drug users and bisexual men.

SHAPE OF THE HIV PANDEMIC: UNITED STATES

There is a common misconception that the AIDS pandemic is under control in the developed world. While the mortality rate associated with HIV has been sharply reduced, because of behavioral changes and antiretroviral drugs, they are imperfect solutions. Drug therapies are expensive, often toxic, and not a cure. AIDS education programs have impeded but have not stopped the epidemic. The United States has the highest rate of HIV infection among the world's most highly industrialized countries, in spite of the fact that it serves as a leader in AIDS education and prevention. About 1 in 165 people in the United States has been HIV infected. The ratio in some sub-Saharan countries is 1 in 5 and in some African villages the ratio is 1 in 2 in women of childbearing age.

It is estimated that there were about 19,000 people HIV infected in 1977, and ending 1982, 190,000. Prior to 1981, 32 were believed to have died of AIDS (Table 10-6).

HIV infections reached their peak ending 1982 and then rapidly declined. Ending 1982 there were an estimated 529,000 people infected in the U.S. No one can say exactly which factors have been responsible for bringing the HIV infection rate down from some 190,000 people in 1982 and stabilized at about 50,000 a year each year from 1988 to 2001. From 2002 through 2008 there were over 53,000 new infections per year. For a breakdown of new HIV infections, see Figure 10-7. These figures are estimates with new cases of HIV infection now reportable by federal law, and will change over the coming years.

The populations that are encompassed in the numbers of new infections are different from the past: HIV is now reaching younger people, it's reaching more women, it's reaching more communities of color. Infections in heterosexual women are increasing more rapidly than in any other group. Unless a preventive vaccine is found, the rate of new HIV infections in the United States is expected to remain between 53,000 and 56,000 annually. This may mean the new prevention campaigns, without a vaccine, will not significantly reduce new infections. Society has, in a sense, reduced new HIV infections to its lower limit.

DISCUSSION QUESTION: Is the last statement plausible—have we reached a point at which further expenditures will not significantly reduce the rate of infection—that all society can do now is wait on a preventive vaccine? What would be your solution given that we have actually reached this point and no vaccine is forthcoming?

SHAPE OF AIDS PANDEMIC: UNITED STATES

There has been a decline in new AIDS cases in every region of the United States. The decline began in 1996 and ended in 2001.

HIV Infections Ending 2009

There are an estimated 1.3 million people living with HIV in the United States, with on average, about 56,000 new infections occurring in the United States annually since about 2003.

By gender, about 75% of new HIV infections each year occur among men.

By risk, men who have sex with men (MSM) represent the largest proportion of new infections, followed by men and women infected through heterosexual sex and injection-drug use.

By race, more than half of the new HIV infections occur among blacks, though they represent about 13.4% of the U.S. population. Hispanics, who make up about 15.1% of the U.S. population, are also disproportionately affected.

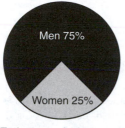

Estimates of 2009 new infections by gender (N ≅ 56,000)

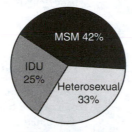

Estimates of 2009 new infections by risk (N ≅ 56,000)

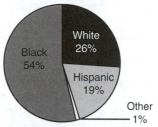

Estimates of 2009 new infections by race (N ≅ 56,000)

To better understand how the HIV/AIDS epidemic is affecting men and women, it is critical to look at race and risk by gender.

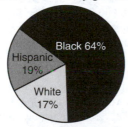

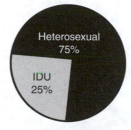

Estimates of annual new infections in women, U.S., by race and risk

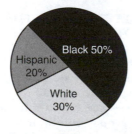

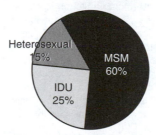

Estimates of new infections in men, U.S., by race and risk, 2009

FIGURE 10-7   A Glance at the HIV Epidemic in America. *(Source: Centers for Disease Control and Prevention updated)*

NOTE: At the time of Magic Johnson's announcement that he was HIV positive (1991), the CDC reported that one-third of AIDS cases in America were black. Black Americans now account for 54% of all new HIV diagnoses. And, for the last eight years, HIV/AIDS has been the leading cause of death for black people ages 24 to 44.

NEW YORK CITY

Beginning 2009, over 100,000 New Yorkers had been diagnosed and known to be living with HIV/AIDS. It is estimated that an additional 200,000-plus New Yorkers are HIV infected but remain unaware of their infection. About 28% of New Yorkers learned of their HIV status when they were diagnosed with AIDS. About 92% of the city's at-risk popula-ton believe they are not at risk.

THE HIV/AIDS EPICENTER

New York City remains the epicenter of the HIV/AIDS epidemic in the United States. It has the highest AIDS case rate in the United States; while it is home to less than 3% of the U.S. population, the city accounts for one in six of national AIDS cases. The AIDS case rate in New York City is four times the U.S. average, and higher than any other city in the United States. About 1.4% of the city's adults are HIV-positive.

ECONOMIC DISPARITIES AND HIV/AIDS

There are glaring epidemiologic disparities. Over 80% of new AIDS diagnoses and deaths in New York City are among African Americans and Latinos. And, as has been documented nationally, an increasing proportion of new AIDS cases are diagnosed in women, most notably women of color. Black male residents of New York City, who are nearly three times more likely to be living with HIV/AIDS than other New Yorkers, have been hit especially hard by the epidemic. Approximately one in 14 black men between the ages of 40 and 54 is living with HIV/AIDS—seven times the rate of other New York-ers. The only groups with higher infection rates are men who self-identify as gay or bisexual (one in ten are estimated to be living with HIV/AIDS) and injec-tion drug users (one in seven are estimated to be living with HIV/AIDS). The results of a 2007 survey among New York City's MSM revealed that 40% of MSM do not disclose their sexual orientation to their physicians. MSM who disclosed were twice as likely to have been HIV tested as those who did not dis-close.

Although the noticeable drop in new AIDS cases was a renewed cause for hope, the downside is that slowing the progression to AIDS and to AIDS deaths (discussed next) means more HIV-infected people with better health are available to spread HIV.

According to the CDC, beginning 2009 there were about 501,000 adult/adolescent people and 4400 children reported to be living with AIDS in the United States. The estimated number of people cur-rently living with HIV infection is about 1.2 million. The slowing of AIDS diagnosis, due to the use of antiretroviral therapy, makes tracking the epidemic difficult. However, the ability to monitor the epi-demic based on HIV infections does not, at the mo-ment, compare with the CDC's ability to track the pandemic through the reporting of AIDS cases, but it will in the next year or so.

Changing U.S. HIV/AIDS Demographics Leads to Southern Discomfort

Federal funding pays about $5625 per HIV patient everywhere but in the South, where it pays $5184. This difference in funding caused the HIV/AIDS di-rectors from 13 southern states and the District of Columbia, the Southern AIDS Coalition, to produce a "Southern States Manifesto." The major complaint within the manifesto is that the South now leads the country in new HIV infections and overall AIDS cases but receives about $400 federal dollars when compared to other HIV/AIDS regions. For example, over 200,000 people in the South have AIDS, com-pared to about 150,000 in the Northeast, 46,000 in the Midwest, and some 72,000 in the West. Still, the region is behind other areas of the nation in federal funding for HIV/AIDS programs. Blacks make up 19% of the population of the South but 53% of the region's AIDS cases. The South is home to 45% of all new AIDS cases. The manifesto was sent to Congress in 2003 for redress. To date nothing has happened.

ESTIMATES OF DEATHS AND YEARS OF POTENTIAL LIFE LOST DUE TO AIDS IN THE UNITED STATES

"All my friends are dead." This expression is unique in a lifetime and is symbolic of reaching old age—except in a time of war. Too many young people worldwide have said it over the past 27 years because of AIDS.

Deaths Due to AIDS: United States and Global

Each year in the United States there are about 2,300,000 deaths. AIDS, from 1991 through 1995,

Table 10-6 AIDS Deaths in the United States

Year	AIDS Deaths	Accumulative Deaths: 5-Year Intervals[2]
1977	—	—
1978	—	—
1979	—	—
1980	32 (before 1981)	30
1981	128	
1982	463	
1983	1508	
1984	3505	
1985	6972	12,576
1986	12,110	
1987	16,412	
1988	21,119	
1989	27,791	
1990	31,538	121,546
1991	35,616	
1992	41,094	
1993	45,850	
1994	50,842	
1995	54,670	349,648
1996	38,296	
1997	22,245	
1998	18,823	
1999	18,249	
2000	17,672	463,906
2001	17,726	
2002	16,890	
2003	16,635	
2004	16,338	
2005	16,227	547,722
2006	15,000	
Estimated Data Through 2010		
2007	14,500	
2008	14,000	
2009	13,600	604,822
2010	13,100	617,922

[1]Estimated deaths through 2010 for white people, 274,898; black, 245,321; Hispanic, 110,461.

Cumulative Deaths from AIDS in the United States from 1977 through 2006. Data for years 2007 through 2010 are estimated. AIDS deaths dropped by 75% from 1995 through year 2000. A similar or greater drop in AIDS deaths occurred in Europe over the same time period. It took from 1981 to about 1988, about 7 years, to reach the first 100,000 AIDS deaths in the U.S. Over the next 18 years (2006) there were an additional 500,000-plus AIDS deaths. The sharp decline in AIDS deaths from 1996 onward is not due to a reduction in HIV infections, but due to the introduction of combination antiretroviral drugs. Deaths from AIDS are not in the top 15 causes of death in the U.S.

caused at least 40,000 of these deaths each year and accounted for about 1.8% of all deaths for each of those years. That is, 2 people of each 100 who died, died of AIDS.

The good news is that between the end of 1995 and the end of 1996, AIDS deaths dropped in the United States for the first time since the pandemic **began—25% nationwide (about 12,600 fewer deaths).** Between 1996 and 1998 deaths had dropped by about 75% (Table 10-6). Similar data were reported from Europe. The sudden drop in expected deaths due to AIDS is believed to be associated with the use of combination drug therapy.

Beginning 2009, about 590,000 people in the United States had died of AIDS. **About 75% of these people did not live to age 45!**

And yet, the United States, after spending billions of dollars on the disease, still does not have a comprehensive national plan to guide the strategic use of AIDS-related dollars or to hold government agencies accountable for steadily improved outcomes for people living with HIV/AIDS or at risk of infection.

AIDS as a Cause of Death in the United States and Worldwide at the Beginning of 2009

United States

- AIDS is the fifth-leading cause of death among people ages 25 to 44.

- AIDS is the leading cause of death of black American men ages 25 to 44.

- AIDS is currently the fourth-leading cause of death among all U.S. women ages 25 to 44, and the second cause of death among black women ages 25 to 44.

- In the United States between five and six people per hour become HIV infected 365 days a year (53,000) and every hour about two people die (16,000). Before 1996 one person died every 13 minutes.

- Annually, from 2002 through 2008, there have been about 13,300 AIDS deaths and over 53,000 new HIV infections. Thus, the number of HIV-positive people has increased each year by about 40,000.

- Of those living with HIV infections, over 1.2 million at the start of 2009, 41% are white, 39% are black, and 20% are Hispanic. Men make up about 74% and women about 26%.

- Through year 2009, an estimated 605,000 people will have died of AIDS.

- About 618,000 adults ages 18 to 49 are living with HIV/AIDS.

- The United States has about 3.6% of the global population of adult/adolescent/children living with HIV/AIDS and about 0.76% of all AIDS deaths.

- The prevalence of HIV/AIDS cases globally is about 0.8%. In the United States it's 0.6%.

CANADA ESTIMATED HIV/AIDS CASES THROUGH 2008: POPULATION 33,310,000

- Number of HIV infections—67,591 (Females at 15.5% or about 10,476)

- Number of children HIV-positive—600

- Number of AIDS cases—21,069 total AIDS deaths at 63% or 13, 347

- Male AIDS cases, 16,012 (76%);
  (a) MSM, 73%
  (b) Heterosexual, 12%

- Female AIDS cases–(24%) 5057
  (a) IDU, 25%
  (b) Heterosexual, 57%
- Perinatal AIDS cases, 255 (82% of pediatric AIDS cases)

Estimated Worldwide beginning 2009 (See Figures 10-8, 10-9, and 10-10).

- Worldwide, about 285 people become HIV infected every hour, 365 days a year (2.5 million) and every hour about 240 people die (2.1 million).

- About 10% of new infections are due to injection drug use. Excluding Africa that figure becomes 30%.

- About 4.5 million men having sex with men (MSM) have been infected with HIV (between 5% and 10% of global HIV infections—UNAIDS, 2007). An estimated 52% have died of HIV/AIDS, or about 2,340,000.

- About 40% of all new HIV infections globally are occurring among 15- to 24-year-old people.

- About 95% of people living with HIV/AIDS reside in low- and middle-income countries.

- Ending year 2009, about 59 million people will have been HIV infected, about 95% in developing countries.

- Nine out of ten HIV-positive people are unaware they are infected.

- Women now make up about 60% of 15- to 24-year-olds living with HIV/AIDS.

- Ending 2009 about 17.5 million men and 17.5 million women will be living with HIV infection.

- Ending year 2009, about 24 million people will have died of AIDS.

- 80% of those dying from AIDS are between ages 20 and 50. These are the people who enforce laws, harvest food, work the factories, heal the sick, and raise children.

- By the end of 2010 about 26 million people will have died of AIDS. Ending 2020 between 46 and 52 million people will have died of AIDS.

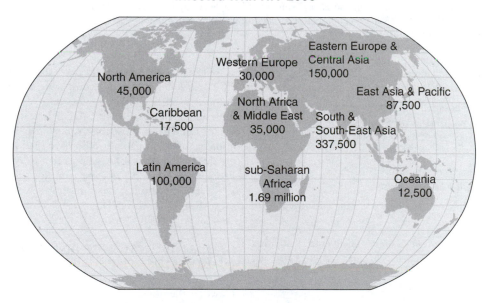

Global Estimates of Adults and Children Newly Infected With HIV 2008

North America 45,000

Western Europe 30,000

Eastern Europe & Central Asia 150,000

East Asia & Pacific 87,500

Caribbean 17,500

North Africa & Middle East 35,000

South & South-East Asia 337,500

Latin America 100,000

sub-Saharan Africa 1.69 million

Oceania 12,500

Estimates are for the entire globe.
Total: 2.5 million

FIGURE 10-8 Year 2008. Estimate for New HIV Infections. *(UNAIDS/WHO, 2007 updated)*

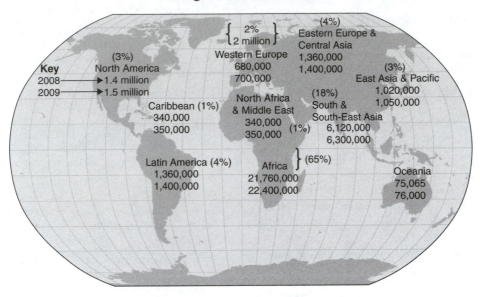

Year End Estimates: Adult/Children Living With HIV Infection

Key
2008 → 1.4 million
2009 → 1.5 million

(3%)
North America
1.4 million
1.5 million

{ 2%
2 million }
Western Europe
680,000
700,000

(4%)
Eastern Europe &
Central Asia
1,360,000
1,400,000

(3%)
East Asia & Pacific
1,020,000
1,050,000

Caribbean (1%)
340,000
350,000

North Africa
& Middle East
340,000
350,000

(18%)
South &
South-East Asia
6,120,000
6,300,000

(1%)

Latin America (4%)
1,360,000
1,400,000

Africa
21,760,000
22,400,000

} (65%)

Oceania
75,065
76,000

*Totals are estimates for the entire globe, percents for year 2008.

Total: 2008—34 million
2009—35 million

FIGURE 10-9   End-of-Year 2008 and 2009. Estimates of People Living with HIV Infection. Of the 34 million alive ending 2008, about 96% are adult/adolescent, about 50% are men and about 50% women, with 3.6% under age 15 *(UNAIDS/WHO, 2007 updated)*

- If nothing changes, there will be an estimated 20 million to 30 million new HIV infections by 2020.

- Of 196 countries reporting on adults and children living with HIV/AIDS in 2007, 34 countries had over 100,000, 2 had over 300,000, and 1 had over 500,000 HIV/AIDS cases.

- Ending 2009, about 0.9% of the world's population will be HIV infected.

- It is estimated that new HIV infections will peak in 2025.

Former Surgeon General C. Everett Koop has said on a number of occasions that "AIDS is virtually 100% fatal." Looking back over the number of AIDS cases diagnosed and comparing them to the number of AIDS patients who have died would indicate that a diagnosis of AIDS is a death sentence. Table 10-6 presents a sobering look at the numbers of AIDS patients who have died in America since those first CDC-reported cases in 1981. People with HIV/ AIDS were, through 1995, dying at the rate of about 3000 a month. Over 95% of those diagnosed with AIDS in 1981 have now died.

GLOBAL PREVALENCE AND IMPACT OF HIV/AIDS

However the impact of the disease is measured—by deaths, HIV infections, AIDS cases, or monetary losses—it is just beginning. The worldwide impact during the 1990s was 5 to 10 times that of the 1980s, and an increase in global impact will be felt,

---

LOOKING BACK 10.1

In 1987, TV talk show host Oprah Winfrey said that 50 million heterosexual Americans will have died from AIDS by 1990.

Population and HIV Infection Rates in Selected African Countries

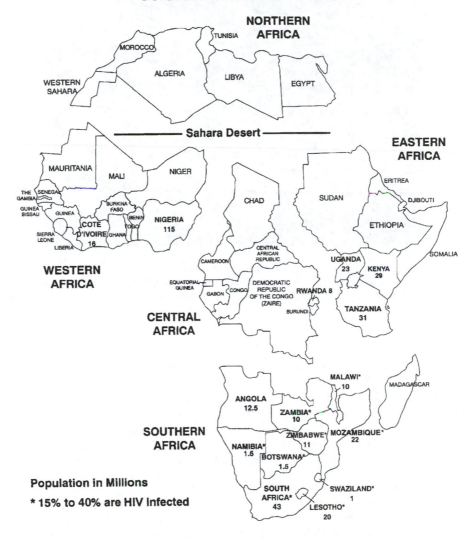

Population in Millions

***** 15% to 40% are HIV Infected**

FIGURE 10-10 Map of Africa. Population of Africa = approximately 800 million. Population of sub-Saharan Africa = about 657 million. Prevalence of HIV infection and AIDS cases is highest in South Africa. South Africa with about 47 million people ending 2009 will have an estimated 5.5 million HIV-infected people, the highest incidence of HIV infection in the world. In seven African countries over 20% of the 15- to 19-year-old population is HIV infected, from 20% in South Africa to about 40% among adults in Botswana. The lifetime risk of dying from AIDS for a boy who is currently 15 is 65% in South Africa and near 90% in Botswana. Karen Stanecki of the U.S. Census Bureau reported that in KwaZulu-Natal, a province of South Africa, HIV infection has reached 46%. In Francistown, Botswana, HIV infection among adults is at 42%. Stanecki projected that AIDS deaths will peak in sub-Saharan Africa in 2020 at 6.5 million deaths/year; South Africa in 2010 at 940,000/year; Haiti in 2017 at 39,000/year; Thailand in 2000 at 66,000/year; Myanmar (Burma) in 2015 at 97,000/year; Brazil in 2020 at 623,000/year. *(Map courtesy of Centers for Disease Control and Prevention)*

Notation: Based on the WHO/UNAIDS 07 AIDS Epidemic Update Report; Stanecki's numbers should be lowered by at least 20%.

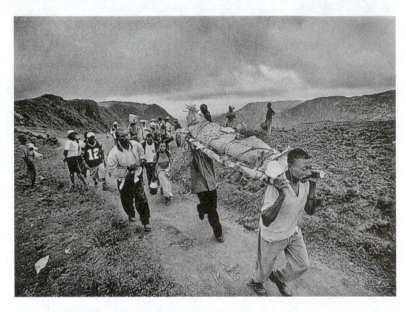

FIGURE 10-11 The Long Journey Home. Friends chant while carrying the body of their friend to his mother's home in Haiti. It is many miles up through the mountains to a small rural village where he grew up. He left home at the age of 15 to find work. He is now returned home for burial at age 28 *(Photo by Mike Stocker/South Florida Sun-Sentinel)*

even with an available vaccine, through the next 30 to 50 years. As the pandemic continues, the United States will find itself progressively more involved with prevention/treatment programs and with the political changes that HIV/AIDS will bring about in countries with a high incidence of HIV/AIDS. (See PEPFAR discussion in Chapter 14.) Although it's true that the global HIV/AIDS pandemic has apparently peaked worldwide, population growth and the life-prolonging effects of antiretroviral therapy mean that the number of HIV-infected will remain about the same over the next two decades except in sub-Saharan Africa. There the number of HIV/AIDS cases will continue to increase.

CONNECTED BUT SEPARATE

Although all nations on earth are connected in so many ways, there remains a separation of the haves and have-nots—the developed and developing nations. Two worlds: one with hope and one with over 90% of all AIDS cases and orphans. (AIDS-associated orphans are presented in Chapter 11.)

Africa, the HIV/AIDS Time Bomb: Ticking Out of Control

The first case of AIDS was identified in Africa in 1982. HIV/AIDS is almost too large a problem in Africa to fully grasp. Like the bubonic plague in Europe in the fourteenth century and the flu epidemic of 1918, the scale of the loss is staggering. HIV/AIDS is the worst human disease disaster the world has ever seen.

Africa, with about 10% of the world's population, now accounts for about 68% of all global HIV infections and for about 90% of all new HIV infections. As of 2009, about 72% of all AIDS deaths have occurred in Africa. The United Nations in 2002 reported that in Africa's 25 worst affected countries, 7 million agricultural workers have died from AIDS since 1985 and 10 million more could die by 2020. Also, unless there is some immediate relief, by 2010, most Africans will not live to see their forty-eighth birthday. Stefano Vella, president of the International AIDS Society, said in 2002, "This pandemic is not stabilizing, it is just beginning, it's just a baby beginning to grow." As a comparison, Vella said that if the United States had in proportion the same HIV infection rate as Botswana, between 35% and 40%, there would be 40 million HIV infected in America. The world and especially Africa has been living with a biological terrorist for the past 27 years with no end in sight. (1982 through 2008). AIDS will be in Africa for generations to come.

Deepening the Misery

To add to the HIV/AIDS problem in Africa, reports out of Southern Africa, where as many as 20 million people are afflicted by hunger or malnutrition, reveal that this region is experiencing the worst food shortage in nearly 60 years, and HIV/AIDS is deepening the misery. Hunger is accelerating the onset of AIDS-related illnesses and death among household breadwinners. As a result, the AIDS pandemic is compounding the food problems by leaving the elderly and children to care for the sick, plant and harvest the crops, and take odd jobs for extra income. Eight countries facing the devastating drought have HIV prevalence rates over 15%: Botswana, Lesotho, Namibia, South Africa, Swaziland, Zambia, Zimbabwe, and Mozambique.

AIDS—The Modern Plague

By any and every measure, AIDS is a plague of biblical proportion. It is claiming more lives in Africa than in all the wars waging on the continent combined. AIDS is now the leading cause of death among all people of all ages in Africa and the progression of this pandemic has outpaced all projections (Figure 10-10). Nearly all those currently HIV infected in Africa without drug therapy will die between year 2010 and 2015. In Botswana and Swaziland it is estimated that 60% of the population will die of AIDS over the next 20 years. With such overwhelming numbers, it is important to remember that the data are about people, not numbers, and not facts and figures, but faces and families (see Figure 10-11).

The HIV/AIDS pandemic in Africa is like an explosion in slow motion, a slowly moving chain reaction—no sound, no blinding flash, no intense heat, no mushroom cloud, no buildings destroyed—just one silent death after another with no end in sight. Whole generations of people are in jeopardy with so little hope to go around in the developing nations.

UNAIDS 2000 Report

"HIV will kill at least a third of the young men and women of countries where it has its firmest hold, and in some places up to two-thirds. Despite millennia of epidemics, war and famine, never before in history have death rates of this magnitude been seen among young adults of both sexes and from all walks of life." If death rates continue HIV/AIDS will kill more humans on the African continent than the 50 million who died on every front and in death camps in World War II. It is estimated that between 50 million and 70 million Africans may die from AIDS by 2025.

Life Expectancy

AIDS has sharply reduced life expectancy in 25 southern African countries, 8 Caribbean nations, and 7 members of the 12 ex-Soviet republics. For instance, in Botswana, where more than one-third of adults are infected with HIV, life expectancy is now 39 instead of 74, as it would have been without the disease. It is projected that ending 2010, life expectancy will be 27 in Botswana, 30 in Swaziland, 33 in Namibia and Zimbabwe, and 36 in South Africa, Malawi, and Rwanda. Without AIDS, it would have been around 70 in many of those countries. In the Central African Republic, Lesotho, Mozambique, Swaziland, Malawi, Zambia, and Zimbabwe, a child born in 2004 would not be expected to see his or her 40th birthday. More people died of AIDS each year from 1999 through 2008 in Africa than in all the wars on the continent during those years. About 1 in 30 people is HIV infected.

Sub-Saharan Africa: About 11% of the World's Population

The sheer number of Africans infected by HIV, about 4650 a day, is overwhelming. By the end of 2009, there will be about 22.5 million HIV-infected people living in sub-Saharan Africa, 61% of them are women. About 68 percent of all people living with HIV live here, as well as 90% of all cases of mother-to-child HIV transmission cases. About 76% of all HIV/AIDS deaths occur here. In Rwanda, it is estimated that 80% of women are HIV positive resulting from rape by Rwandan soldiers during the genocide of a million Tutsi and Hutu. Overall, 59% of HIV infections in sub-Saharan Africa occur in women. In Botswana, Namibia, Swaziland, Zimbabwe, and Mozambique, current estimates show that between 15% and 40% of people aged 15 to 49 are living with HIV. In Zimbabwe, 30% to 50% of all pregnant women are now found to be infected, and at least one-third of these women will pass the infection on to their babies. South Africa, which escaped much of the epidemic in the 1980s, is now being hit particularly hard (Figure 10-10).

South Africa

Ending 2009 about 4.6 million South Africans, roughly one in ten people (one in four adults), will be living with HIV/AIDS—and dying from it. Some 700 people die each day, and about 1200 become HIV infected. It is estimated that there were 430,000 new HIV infections in 2006 and again in 2007. Estimates are that one in five or 20% of women ages 15 to 49 are HIV positive compared to 15.4% of men in the same age group. Seventeen percent of women ages 15 to 24 are HIV positive. Some two hundred thousand children under age four are also HIV positive! South Africa's new five-year plan, 2007 through 2011, is to halve HIV infections and provide antiretroviral therapy to 80% of all people with HIV. The cost of this plan may exceed South Africa's entire health budget by 20%; the largest cost is for antiretroviral drugs (40%). However, a recent study by Rochelle Walensky and colleagues (2007) revealed that even with the fastest rate of drug treatment in South Africa, about one million AIDS deaths will occur between mid-2007 and the end of 2010. **This is a best-case scenario!** Estimates are that by the end of 2010, about 4.8 million South Africans will have died from AIDS.

Military

In South Africa, according to *Johannesburg Mail and Guardian* newspaper, between 30% and 70% of the South African National Defense Force may be infected with HIV. In one unit in KwaZulu-Natal, 90% of troops are infected. Some military units near Pietermaritzburg and on the South African/Mozambique border had HIV infection rates higher than 70%. South Africa's military infection rate is similar to neighboring countries. In Malawi, 75% of the military is HIV positive, and in Mozambique, 80% have tested positive. Forces in the Democratic Republic of the Congo and Angola also have high rates of HIV infection. Militaries in sub-Saharan Africa, in general have between 20% and 40% HIV positive rates.

WORKFORCE—SOUTH AFRICA: SOME EXAMPLES

In April 2002, NMG-Levy, Agence France-Presse reported that by 2008 over 30% of South Africa's labor force will be HIV positive. The pandemic is taking a dramatic toll on the most productive members of the population, those in their 20s, 30s, and 40s. It has been estimated that 25% of "economically active people" in South Africa will die of AIDS between 2010 and 2015!

Mining

AngloGold, a gold mining company in South Africa, reported that about 30% of its 44,000 employees are already HIV positive.

Agriculture

About 30% to 45% of agriculture workers in South Africa are HIV positive, which could have a major effect on farm production in the coming years.

Nurses

An estimated 20% or 35,000 South African nurses are HIV positive. A Netcare group nursing manager recently told delegates that half of first-year students at one of the province's four nursing colleges are HIV positive. At another of the colleges, 70% of students are attending a local HIV clinic. At another, 21% of the students have volunteered information that they are HIV positive. In addition, 200 nurses a month are going abroad. The nursing manager said, "In our organization we are losing registered nurses. We are sitting with nurses who are dying now, and the students are even worse off."

EDUCATION: TEACHERS AND STUDENTS—SOUTH AFRICA AND SOME COUNTRIES IN SOUTHERN AFRICA

Senteza Kajubi, an education official in Africa, said that about 30 million girls in sub-Saharan Africa are out of school. And that out of 100 million children in the world who do not attend school, 44 million are from Africa, the majority being girls from the sub-Saharan region.

The Impact of HIV/AIDS on Teachers, Students, and School Systems

As many teachers die every year of HIV/AIDS as qualify to teach. School districts are exhausting their annual budgets within two months by transporting deceased teachers to their homes. There is widespread closure of schools because HIV/AIDS has stripped them of their teachers. These nightmare scenarios afflict Kenya, Zambia, Botswana, Mozambique, Uganda, the Central African Republic, and South Africa. The devastating impact of HIV/AIDS on teachers and learners was a repeated concern at a national policy conference on teacher training and development convened by the Department of Education in Midrand, Gauteng, South Africa. The conference also heard that there has been an incredible 85% decrease in the number of students in pre-service teacher education programs between 1994 and 2002. These alarming trends are being identified at a time when the need for effective and widespread teacher training has never been greater.

Nelson Mandela, former president of South Africa, said in September 2000 that in South Africa, 10 teachers die every month from AIDS and 1 student dies of AIDS each week in each of the country's 74 colleges and universities—roughly 120 teachers and 3600 students a year. About one in eight teachers is HIV positive. In Durban Westville University in South Africa, about 25% of students are HIV positive. The situation since then has become much worse. In 2004 and 2005 a total of about 8500 teachers died of AIDS with another 45,000 teachers HIV infected. About one-third are between ages 25 and 34. About 25% need antiretroviral drugs. In Kenya about 15,000 teachers are dying each year from AIDS. Also, one in five secondary students and one in five college students is HIV positive in Kenya. The prevalence of HIV infection in Kenya is about 5%.

Zambia, Swaziland, and Mozambique are losing about 130 teachers/month. Two teachers die for one graduate. So the teachers are not being replaced. The pool of uneducated becomes larger as does the number of students in the classrooms that continue. In Tanzania, it is estimated that by 2010, between 15,000 and 30,000 teachers will die of AIDS. To date, in sub-Saharan Africa, about 3 million students lost their teachers to AIDS over the past several years. Many schools have closed because of a teacher shortage. In KwaZulu-Natal province about 25% of teachers are HIV positive.

In part of Malawi, Uganda, Botswana, and Zambia, over 30% of teachers are HIV positive. In the Central African Republic, 85% of teachers who died between 1996 and 1998 were HIV positive and died approximately 10 years before they were due to retire. In Mozambique 17% of teachers are HIV positive. And in Zimbabwe, about 30% of 80,000 teachers are HIV

positive. These data mirror the 27% of HIV positives for Zimbabweans ages 18 to 49.

Burying the Dead

AIDS is the leading cause of death in South Africa. In 2002 through 2008, about 40% of all adult deaths were due to AIDS.

In Soweto, South Africa, as in many South African cities and towns, burying those dying from AIDS has become a daily chore. They used to bury the dead on Saturdays. Too many are dying. "There are so many funerals, it is chaos. We don't know which funeral to attend. On some days we attend three funerals. Which neighbor or which family members' funeral should we attend? We must choose."

In Kenya, the AIDS epidemic has entered a death phase in which more people are dying of AIDS each day than are becoming HIV infected. About 120,000 die annually while about 70,000 become infected. The country is sacrificing its forest for wood to build coffins. The disappearance of the forest is becoming an environmental disaster. The solution, said the environmental minister, is to use biodegradable plastic or synthetic coffins. For now, relatives are cementing wooden coffins into the ground to prevent thieves from stealing them and reselling them; the use of less valuable plastic coffins would discourage such theft.

As AIDS continues to claim the country's young, it has transformed black neighborhoods into open-air funeral parlors and neighbors into widows, orphans, and grieving relatives. (Read Sidebar 10.2)

OTHER HIV/AIDS TIME BOMBS IN ASIA: INDIA, CHINA, AND RUSSIA

Over the past three years, 2005 through 2008, the number of people living with HIV increased in every region in the world. The most striking increases have occurred in East Asia, Eastern Europe, and Central Asia. Asia, made up of at least 37 nations, with 60% of the world's population, is now home to an estimated 5 million people living with HIV/AIDS. About 300,000 people died of AIDS in the region in 2008 and about 500,000 became newly infected. Globally, one in five new HIV infections occurs in Asia. Another 8 million could be infected by 2020. HIV/AIDS in Asia is driven by three high-risk behaviors: unsafe commercial sex, injection-drug users, and unsafe sex among gay men. In many Asian countries, adult men who pay for sex and their female partners make up the largest group of people living with HIV/AIDS. It is estimated that 10 million women in Asia sell sex to about 75 million men. Men having sex with men and injection-drug use places another 10 million men at high risk for HIV infection. The most worrying aspect of the pandemic in Asia is the sharp increase in HIV infections in China, Indonesia, and Vietnam, which together have nearly 50% of Asia's population. China and India, with 2.3 billion people between them, still have low national HIV prevalence rates—0.1% in China and 0.4% to 1.3% in India—but they have extremely serious epidemics in a number of provinces, territories, and states. Asia is a large part of the global economy. The greater the impact of HIV/AIDS in Asia, the greater the impact globally.

India: 35 States and Territories

If by 2020 just 2% of India's one billion plus population is HIV infected, that would be 20 million people (over twice the population of New York City). UNAIDS reports that about 2.5 million Indians are already infected and the virus is spreading rapidly in that country, primarily through heterosexual activities and injection-drug use.

The first case of AIDS was described in India in 1986. India is a vast, heterogeneous country. Eighty percent of the people live in the countryside where many have never heard of HIV or AIDS. Yet, about 60% of the HIV infected live in the countryside or rural areas. Some local authorities even challenge the existence of HIV or AIDS. Although it is believed that 86% of HIV infections occur through heterosexual intercourse with an infected partner, it is estimated that there will be between 1 million and 2 million HIV infections among female sex workers, their clients, and their families ending year 2009.

China

In China, HIV is present in all 31 provinces, autonomous regions, and municipalities but epidemic patterns are different in different parts of the country.

In August 2001, the deputy health minister held a first-ever news conference on the HIV/AIDS problem in China. The 2007 WHO/UNAIDS report estimated that 600,000 Chinese are HIV infected.

The first AIDS case in China was in an IDU discovered in the Yunnan province near the Burmese border in 1985. Since then HIV has spread rapidly among IDUs across China. Currently about 70% of China's IDUs are HIV positive. Eighty percent of reported AIDS cases are among IDUs and prostitutes. However, among new HIV infections (2006 through 2008), injection drug use accounted for about 50%, and sexual contact about 48%. Approximately 2% occurred via mother-to-child transmission. Women make up 28% of the infected population. Although data relating to HIV transmission among gay men is limited, once HIV becomes established in this population the HIV problem in China will become much more serious, because there are an estimated 5 million to 10 million gay men in China.

HIV/AIDS: China's Titanic Peril—A current survey[1] finds that most of China's population does not know what causes AIDS or how to prevent it—and 17% or 1 in 6 respondents had never heard of HIV or

---

SNAPSHOT 10.4

A TOUCHING MOMENT IN THE STRUGGLE AGAINST AIDS IN INDIA

Told by an AIDS physician—Some weeks ago, an HIV-infected girl came to me with her fiancé. Both were highly educated and had in fact studied together. The boy was healthy and didn't know the girl was infected when he proposed marriage. Since the girl didn't want to keep him in the dark, she brought him to my clinic. When I told him, he became absolutely silent and after some time walked out of the room. I could see the girl was devastated so I took her to our canteen for a cup of coffee. We came back into the room after ten minutes and found the boy had returned and was sitting with a huge bouquet of roses. He said that his love and respect for his girlfriend had gone up because she had not hidden the disease from him. He said he didn't want to know how she acquired the infection but only how he could take care of her. Both the girl and I started crying and that was one day that I didn't bother to hide the tears rolling down my face. I really wish there would be more such men.

---

[1](The survey, "Current HIV/AIDS-Related Knowledge, Attitudes, and Practices Among the General Population in China: Implications for Action," was published on AIDScience.org (http://www.aidscience.org/articles/aidscience028.asp), a website run by the journal *Science*.)

DEATH IN SUB-SAHARAN AFRICA: A GROWING INDUSTRY

BURIAL CHANGES BECAUSE OF TOO MANY AIDS DEATHS IN ZAMBIA

AIDS has changed the way people live. Now it is changing the way they are buried. As the AIDS toll rises, Zambia's local government authorities complain that burial ground is being filled up almost as soon as it is designated. Zambians are being encouraged to look at cremation as a burial option. This has elicited serious debate. Zambians are by nature a very superstitious people who fear changes in cultural practices. University of Zambia's Department of History Professor Yizenge Chondoka says to shift peoples' thinking from burial to cremation will be hard. There are certain rites that can only be performed at graveyards to complete the burial process and ensure that the spirit of the buried is at peace. Chondoka says Zambians have shrines at burial sites where they consult the spirits of the dead in times of need. "If we begin to cremate and throw or keep ashes in small clusters in our houses, where will the shrines be put up?" Lusaka has three designated cemeteries (besides unofficial ones), which can take about 10,000 graves, but these are already full and people are now squeezing their dead on what used to be thoroughfares.

BURIAL ECONOMICS

Then there is the problem of economics. A teacher at the Zambian School of Education asks, "Do we really want valuable land to be taken up by graves?" Death in Africa is a very public affair. Funerals are big social events at which grief is expressed openly and lavishly. Families take large spaces in newspapers to announce the death of a loved one, complete with a picture, lists of achievements, and names of children. Now, about half the faces staring out of the public death notices are young. They have died of AIDS. But in contrast to the public rites of death, this increasingly frequent cause goes whispered or unmentioned. AIDS is a taboo subject in Africa. At the rate they are dying from AIDS, three-quarters of Zambia will be a graveyard. There must be another way of disposing of their dead.

FUNERALS ARE BANKRUPTING FAMILIES IN AFRICA

A 2004 study by the Joint Economics, AIDS and Poverty Program of the University of KwaZulu-Natal in Durban stated that the average cost of a traditional funeral in South Africa is about $4900,

while the annual household income in South Africa is $3630. The Health Economics and AIDS Research Division of the university estimates that people in Swaziland spend up to $980 on funerals, even though two-thirds of the population live below the poverty line. In Botswana, families typically spend $740 to $920 on funerals, while the average monthly salary for a working class person is $55.

THE FUNERAL INDUSTRY—SOUTH AFRICA

Rising death rates in South Africa due to HIV/AIDS have led to the creation of a makeshift funeral industry. Many fly-by-night undertakers, who are unlicensed and operate out of storefronts, compete to make funeral arrangements and leave bodies to decompose while they search for the cheapest means of disposal, creating a health hazard and raising costs to the government. The problem is greatest in Durban, capital of the hard-hit KwaZulu-Natal province. Morgues and cemeteries have run out of room and the unlicensed undertakers are tempted to cut corners by mishandling bodies—burying them in mass graves or abandoning them in mortuaries. The government has not regulated the new undertakers (who are mainly black) because they were previously disadvantaged, but established funeral directors (mostly white and Indian) complain that the new undertakers should be subject to the same regulations. The newcomers said they are subcontractors for licensed morticians—they sell coffins and transport the body for burial while a licensed mortician washes, dresses, and stores the body. Sometimes licensed morticians front for the newcomers by picking up bodies at morgues for a fee, a violation of health regulations. This corpse shell game often results in bodies being moved several times or left to decompose. As AIDS deaths rise, the problem will only worsen. But talk of the rising death rate is all but taboo among government officials who, taking their cue from President Thabo Mbeki, barely acknowledge the extent of the HIV/AIDS epidemic or the rising death toll. What to do with bodies in Africa is becoming a massive problem!

THE CASKET/BURIAL PLOT INDUSTRY—ZIMBABWE

Griffin Shea reported on the demand for caskets and burial plots in Zimbabwe. Deep in the shadow of Harare's office high-rises, Luck Street is mostly islands of pavement in a river of mud and potholes. Despite its name, this side street in Zimbabwe's capital is where the city's least fortunate residents make their most-lasting purchases, a casket or coffin. With an economy in free fall and over 3000 people dying of AIDS every week, coffin-making has become one of the country's few reliable sources of income. In outlying townships, vendors line up caskets for sale next to tables of fruits and vegetables on the dusty roadside. But if you're on a budget—and almost everyone in Zimbabwe is—Luck Street is where you go for a bargain. At Sunshine Funeral Service, a darkened room behind a motorcycle repair shop, the owner and salesperson shows off his company's entire line of caskets, from a pressed-wood model that sells for about $15 to polished hardwood with shiny brass handles, $130. For about 30 cents per mile, the enterprising owners of Sunshine Funeral will send corpses back to their hometowns for burial.

According to Harare's director of cemeteries, 8 of the city's 10 cemeteries are full. So the city is clearing 5 square miles of land to expand one of its cemeteries on the outskirts, where most of the graves will be dusty plots in the bare earth.

THE COFFIN INDUSTRY IN MALAWI

Coffin and casket shops line a quarter-mile-long stretch of road like a funeral train waiting for Malawians to die from a brew of poverty, infectious diseases, and AIDS, especially AIDS—60,000 AIDS deaths a year. The name of the street is Lubani Road but it is better known as Coffin Road. Life expectancy has now fallen below age 38. Twelve million people live in Malawi with one million being HIV infected. It is one of the poorest countries in the world.

AIDS! Of respondents who had heard of HIV and AIDS, 73% did not know it was a virus, and 89% did not know how it can be detected. Of those respondents who knew that HIV can be transmitted, 22% could not identify a single route of transmission. Over 77% did not know that condoms offer protection, and 83% did not know infection could be avoided by not sharing injection needles. Among those least likely to be knowledgeable about HIV/AIDS were the poorest and least educated, women and farmers.

Zeng Yi, chief scientist with the sexually transmitted infection and AIDS Prevention Center of the Ministry of Health said in mid-2006 that HIV/AIDS is expected to cost China's economy nearly $40 billion over the next five years, mostly because of lost labor as people become sick of AIDS-related illnesses.

Over the past three years (2006–2008), China's government has reacted to its HIV/AIDS challenge by providing routine HIV testing of at-risk groups, free antiretroviral drugs, and safer sex campaigns and needle exchange centers for injection drug users. In 2008, there were about 50,000 new HIV infections and about 20,000 AIDS-related deaths.

Russia

Russia now has the largest HIV epidemic in Europe and accounts for about 66% of HIV/AIDS cases in Eastern Europe and Central Asia. HIV quietly crept into Russia in 1987 through sex between gay men— a practice that was then illegal, making the disease

unspeakable. But even as the numbers grew rapidly in the mid-1990s, primarily through intravenous-drug use, few people paid attention. In his January 2002 address to the nation, Russian former President Vladimir Putin spoke about the nation's overall health crisis but made no specific mention of HIV or AIDS. Peter Piot, executive director of the United Nations AIDS Programs (UNAIDS) said in April 2002 that "Russia now has the fastest growing epidemic in the world, and I believe that the situation in Russia and the CIS (group of 12 ex-Soviet republics) is rapidly getting out of control." If the current rate of infection continues, estimates are that about over 1.7 million Russians will be infected ending 2009. By 2025 between 4 million and 8 million will have died of AIDS. The major route of HIV transmission in Russia is through IDU and sex workers. Beginning 2005, about half of all new HIV infections resulted from heterosexual intercourse. Victor Molotilov and colleagues reported in 2006 that about 2% of Russia's population injects drugs, and an estimated 5% to 8% of all men under age 30 have injected drugs. The age group most affected, as it is globally, is between ages 15 and 30. Half are under age 20. A major problem for Russia is that with this pandemic affecting the younger generations, Russia's shrinking population of 140 million people will continue to fall.

In late 2006, Russia formed a National Advisory Council on AIDS. Former President Putin referred to the issue for the first time in his annual state-of-the-nation address in the spring of 2007! By then, Vadim Pokhrovsky, Russia's head of the federal AIDS center, said about 1.3 million Russians were HIV infected. And of the estimated 40,000 newly infected, 44% are women. On average, one in every 50 males is HIV positive. The worst affected areas are St. Petersburg followed by the Sverdlovsk region, then the Samara region of Moscow.

Summary

In 1981, the CDC reported the first case of AIDS in the United States, and, from that time onward, has constantly tracked the prevalence of AIDS cases in different geographical areas and within different behavioral risk groups. In all behavioral risk groups, the common denominator is the exchange of body fluids, in particular blood or semen. The heterosexual population at large is considered to be at low risk for HIV infection in the United States. By 1993, all states and the District of Columbia, Puerto Rico, and the Virgin Islands have reported AIDS cases in people who have had heterosexual contact with an at-risk partner.

A major problem exists in attempting to determine the number of HIV-infected people. Several different approaches have been used by the CDC to estimate the total number of HIV infections. These estimates can be evaluated by examining their compatibility with available prevalence data.

With respect to race and ethnicity, the cumulative incidence of AIDS cases is disproportionately higher in blacks and Hispanics than in whites. The ratio of black to white case incidence is 3.2:1 and the Hispanic to white ratio 2.8:1. This racial/ethnic disproportion is also observed in HIV-positive blood donors and in applicants for military service. Even among homosexual and bisexual men and IDUs, where race/ethnicity-specific data are available, blacks appear to have higher seroprevalence rates than whites.

With regard to prostitution, in a large multi-center study of female prostitutes, black and Hispanic prostitutes had a higher rate of HIV infection than white and other prostitutes. This disproportion existed for both prostitutes who used injection drugs and for those who did not acknowledge injection-drug use.

The risk of new HIV infections in hemophiliacs and in people who receive blood transfusions has declined dramatically from 1985 because of the screening of donated blood and heat treatment of clotting factor concentrates. Evidence also indicates an appreciable decline in the incidence of new infections in homosexual men. However, the risk of new infections appears to remain high in IDUs and in their heterosexual partners.

There are some 5.3 million healthcare workers in the United States. Even though they are supposed to adhere to Universal Protection Guidelines set down by the CDC for their protection, a significant number are exposed to HIV annually. A relatively small number of those infected have progressed to AIDS.

Estimating the number of HIV-infected people in the United States continues to be a numbers game. Various agencies and private industries have, for different reasons, attempted to determine the number of HIV-infected people. The numbers from the different groups vary widely. However, the 2007 estimated numbers of 1 to 1.5 million HIV-infected people may be too low.

Ending year 2008, with over 1.2 million people living with HIV infection in the United States and with over 56,000 new infections occurring each year from 2002 through the year 2008, the face of AIDS in America is changing. It's a younger and older face than it used to be. It's more likely to be a face of color than it used to be. And it is more likely to be female than it used to be. More people with HIV and AIDS are from areas outside major cities. Overall, the number of new AIDS cases appears to be leveling. But the HIV epidemic should be viewed as many different epidemics in different stages that vary according to age, race, gender, and locality. Although gay and bisexual men continue to make up the largest portion of new HIV infections, the epidemic is increasing more rapidly among people who become infected through heterosexual contact and through sharing injection-drug equipment.

Review Questions

(Answers to the Review Questions are on page 429.)

1. Looking back, in what year was "AIDS" first recognized?

   A. 1972

   B. 1959

   C. 1982

   D. 1995

   E. 1981

2. Why are people placed in potential HIV risk groups?

3. True or False: The time it takes for HIV-infected people to become AIDS patients is different for each ethnic group, risk group, and exposure route. Explain.

4. What percentage of all U.S. HIV-infected IDUs are in the New York–New Jersey region?

5. What is the rate of college students currently HIV-infected? Is this more or less than the rate for military personnel? Explain.

6. Compare the college student rate of HIV infection with the rate of HIV infection for the general U.S. population.

7. What is the risk of a healthcare worker converting to seropositivity after exposure to HIV-contaminated blood?

8. What single job-related event causes the greatest risk of HIV infection among healthcare workers?

9. Are healthcare workers more apt to become infected with the hepatitis B virus or the AIDS virus?

10. Worldwide, it is estimated that _____ AIDS patients will die by the end of 2009? In the United States?

11. Data on AIDS deaths indicated that of AIDS patients diagnosed between 1981 through 2008, in the United States, _____ % had died.

12. Ending 2009, how many people in the world are estimated to be living with HIV?

13. About how many people were newly infected with HIV in 2008?

14. Does the drop in the global annual number of AIDS cases mean that AIDS is under control?

Prevalence of HIV Infection and AIDS Cases Among Women and Children

CHAPTER CONCEPTS

- Annual International Women's Day—March 8.
- A global estimate of HIV-positive women is presented.
- In proportion there are significantly more black and Hispanic women with HIV/AIDS than white women.
- Injection-drug use is a major route of HIV infection for women.
- From 1994 through 2008 at least 38% of women infected in the United States contracted HIV from men through sexual intercourse.
- Injection-drug use and prostitution are strongly associated with HIV infection.
- AIDS is the leading cause of death for black women ages 25 to 34 and the sixth for all women in this age group.
- The only disease killing more women than AIDS are cancer and heart disease.
- First 100,000 AIDS cases in women in the United States were documented in December 1997.
- About 24% of all HIV-infected adults/adolescents in the United States are women.
- About 30% of all new HIV infections in the United States are in women.
- Women make up about 24% of all U.S. AIDS cases and about 25% of new AIDS diagnoses.
- Black American women make up 13% of the female population but made up about 68% of HIV infections and 67% of AIDS cases in 2002 through 2008.
- In the United States, about 70% of new AIDS cases among women now occur among those ages 30 to 49, 18% among those ages 20 to 29, and 12% among women over age 50.
- Questions that every HIV-postive woman should ask her physician.
- Women now make up about 50% of worldwide HIV positives and about 50% of those living with HIV/AIDS.
- It is estimated that 98% of HIV-infected women live in developing countries. Seventy-eight percent live in sub-Saharan Africa.
- An estimated 12 million women will have died of AIDS and about 17.5 million will be living with HIV/AIDS ending 2009.
- Worldwide women account for 58% of AIDS cases among people ages 13 to 19.
- Of an estimated 2 million adult/adolescent AIDS deaths worldwide in 2008, about 850,000 were women.
- Pediatric means under age 13 in the United States and under age 15 in Canada and most underdeveloped nations.
- About 99% of new pediatric AIDS cases received the virus from their HIV-infected mothers.
- In proportion there are significantly more black and Hispanic pediatric AIDS cases than whites.
- Perinatal HIV infection without anti-HIV drug intervention in the United States is about 25%; with drug intervention it is about 8%. With drugs and cesarean section it is less than 2%.
- Not all newborns who test HIV positive are HIV infected.
- About 300,000 children under age 15 became HIV infected in 2002 worldwide and in each year through 2008.

- It is estimated that about 90% of HIV-infected children live in sub-Saharan Africa.
- By year 2020, there will be an estimated 35 million HIV/AIDS-related orphans under age 15 in 23 underdeveloped countries.

It is a little-remembered fact that the first cases of AIDS occurring in women were reported within months of the often-cited initial 1981 publication detailing the presentation of *Pneumocystis jiroveci* pneumonia in gay men residing in Los Angeles and New York City.

AIDS IS DEFINING THE LIVES OF MILLIONS OF WOMEN

The pandemic of HIV/AIDS is growing more rapidly in women than in men in almost every part of the world. The growing proportion of infected women reflects the cumulative effect of many risks. They include teenage girls, the inability of many women to require their partners to use condoms, the infidelity of husbands and the high-risk behavior of sexual partners, the exploitation of young women by older men, rape and other forms of sexual coercion. Ending 2009, there will be about 17.5 million women over the age of 15 living with HIV/AIDS in the world, of whom only a fraction have access to antiretroviral drug therapy. And each year, since 1999, about 1 million of these women have died of AIDS.

In the nine most heavily infected countries in Africa, 59% of adult women and nearly 75% of young women are infected with HIV. In some African countries, young women are four to 13 times more likely to be HIV infected than young men. These figures represent the feminization of the epidemic. In hard-hit areas, it is undoing developmental gains for women. Among other things, this feminization reflects the reality that the HIV-related needs of women are not being addressed in national responses to HIV. It also reflects the fact that age-old, widespread discrimination and violence against women makes them extremely vulnerable to HIV infection and to the impact of AIDS.

FEMALE VULNERABILITY

A woman's vulnerability to HIV infection is in direct proportion to her lack of control over the risk of infection. Globally, the vast majority of women with HIV/AIDS became infected through heterosexual in-tercourse, frequently in settings where saying no to sex or insisting on condom use is not an option because of cultural factors, lack of financial independence, and even the threat of violence. These issues compel science and society to develop HIV prevention tools that women can use in situations when negotiating with sexual partners is difficult or impossible. Further, there has never been a prevention message for women. Instructions to abstain or to be faithful or to wear a condom don't work in the growing number of places where the single greatest risk of HIV infection is to be a married, monogamous woman. These instructions speak to the realities of most men's lives and, in fact, require their consent. There is virtually nowhere on the planet that a woman's right to safe sex and autonomous decision-making over sexuality are as respected as those of men.

Of the people who live in abject poverty, nearly 70% are women. Women perform two-thirds of the world's work, earn less than 5% of its income, and own less than 1% of its property. Three of every four illiterate adults are women, and two-thirds of children denied primary education are girls.

EVERY DAY A TRAGEDY

Every single day HIV-infected women somewhere in the world are thrown out of their homes, beaten, cheated, lied to, deceived, stoned, scorned, or attempt suicide to escape the stigma associated with being HIV positive. In one recent case, in South Africa, a 25-year-old woman was arrested for allegedly hacking her nine-month-old son to death with an axe and attempting suicide after they both tested HIV positive. She was frightened of what her husband and neighbors would say or do. In Zambia, a man said, "I might transmit the disease to my wife, then tell my wife to go for an AIDS checkup. If she is found positive, I blame it on her and tell the whole community that she has infected me."

TRIPLE JEOPARDY

In the face of the AIDS pandemic, women worldwide face a triple jeopardy. They are at risk as individuals, as mothers, and as family caretakers. They

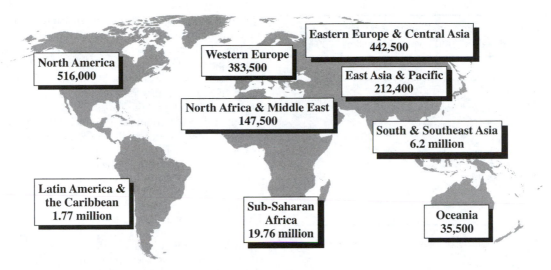

FIGURE 11-1 Estimated Global Total: 29.5 Million HIV-Positive Women Ending 2009. At the end of 1993, women made up an estimated 8 million HIV cases. Ending year 2009, 50% of all HIV positives worldwide will be women. And about 12 million will have died. About 17.5 million women over age 15 will be living with HIV/AIDS.

face violence, discrimination, and abandonment. Of all HIV-infected women, about 61% live in sub-Saharan Africa.

ANNUAL INTERNATIONAL WOMEN'S DAY—MARCH 8

The world is also starting to grasp that there is no policy more effective in promoting development, health, and education than the empowerment of women and girls.

Kofi Annan, Former U.N. Secretary General

Women and Society

Women play a central role in society and the benefits are apparent: families are healthier and better fed, savings and income rise, and a supportive environment is created. Take away women's ability to fulfill these roles and the entire societies fall apart. March 8 marks the annual celebration of International Women's Day. The Charter of the United Nations, signed in San Francisco in 1945, was the first international agreement to proclaim gender equality as a fundamental human right. Since then, International Women's Day has assumed a global dimension for women in developed and developing countries alike. International Women's Day is used as a time to reflect on progress made, to call for change, and to celebrate acts of courage and determination by ordinary

women who have played extraordinary roles in the history of women's rights.

The global AIDS pandemic will be 28 years old in mid-2009. Ending 2009 there will be an estimated 59 million HIV-infected people, about 50% of whom will be women (Figure 11-1). The face of AIDS has changed rapidly over this time span such that some say there has been a feminization of AIDS. It has been said that "a woman's work is invisible until it is not done." In 2008 over a million families realized the truth of this quotation after losing a female relative to AIDS. How many more women will be lost and families traumatized into 2010 and beyond?

WOMEN: AIDS AND HIV INFECTIONS WORLDWIDE

The Growing Gender Disparity of HIV/AIDS

In 1999 it was estimated that worldwide half of AIDS cases are women.

Globally through 2009, women, children, and teenagers are in the middle of the HIV/ AIDS pandemic (Table 11-1).

In sub-Saharan Africa, 61% of the HIV-positive adults are women. In parts of Latin America and the Caribbean, the proportion has reached as high as 43%, and this figure is on the rise. This alarming development must be recognized by concerned parties

Table 11-1 Estimated: Women as Percent of Adults Living with HIV/AIDS by Region, End of 2009

Region	Percent
Global	51%
Sub-Saharan Africa	61%
Caribbean	43%
North Africa/Middle East	40%
Latin America	28%
Eastern Europe/Central Asia	28%
South/Southeast Asia	34%
North America	28%
Western Europe	30%
Asia	29%
Oceania	47%

(*Source:* WHO/UNAIDS AIDS Epidemic Update 2007-updated)

as an absolutely central consideration in the design of strategies to halt the spread of the disease worldwide.

Figures from UNAIDS show that the risk of infection is increasing for women everywhere—in developed and developing countries alike.

In sub-Saharan Africa, the **ratio of women to men** infected with HIV/AIDS is currently 10:6. In Rakai and Masaka, rural districts of Uganda, of women ages 15 to 25, 70% were HIV infected. When compared with HIV-infected young men of the same villages and age group, there was a female-to-male ratio of 6:1. In Rwanda and Tanzania, women under age 25 to men under 25 is 2:1. The female-to-male ratio of AIDS cases among Ethiopian teenagers is 3:1; in Zimbabwe, it is 5:1. In Brazil, the ratio of female-to-male infection in Sao Paulo changed from 1:42 in 1985 to 1.8 to 1 in 2002. In Northern Thailand, 72% of sex workers are HIV infected. By the year 2004, about 90% of HIV transmission worldwide was associated with heterosexual intercourse.

Women are Biologically More Vulnerable to HIV Infection

Women are biologically more vulnerable to HIV infection than men because HIV in semen is in higher concentration than in vaginal and cervical secretions and because the vaginal area has a much larger mucosal area for exposure to HIV than the penis.

Gender Transmission of HIV

Transmission of HIV from male to female is about three times more effective than from female to male

(World Health Organization, 1994). Paradoxically, since time immemorial women have been blamed for the spread of sexually transmitted diseases. Among certain peoples in Thailand and Uganda, STDs are known as "women's diseases." In Swahili, the language of much of East Africa, the word for STD means, literally, "disease of woman." Also, it is not coincidental that the countries in which HIV is now spreading fastest heterosexually are generally those in which women's status is low.

The World Health Organization reported that globally, during 2002 through 2008 there were about 1.7 million AIDS deaths annually; on average 850,000 of these deaths each year were women. That is about two female deaths per minute, and two women become HIV infected every minute. According to the World Health Organization, in 2006, 30% of women ages 15 to 17 in Lesotho were HIV positive. In Swaziland about 53% of pregnant women ages 25 to 29 were HIV positive. The prevalence of HIV infection in Swaziland's population is at 26%. Stephen Lewis, former UN Special Envoy for AIDS in Africa, said, "Lesotho and Swaziland are but symbols of the greater whole: that we are losing millions of young women in Africa. If there was a powerful international force for women, we would not be in this galling predicament."

WOMEN: HIV-POSITIVE AND AIDS CASES—UNITED STATES

March 10, 2009 marks the fourth National Women and Girls HIV/AIDS Awareness Day. This day of recognition serves to raise awareness of the increasing impact of HIV/AIDS on women and girls in the United States and throughout the world. In the early days of the pandemic, relatively few women were infected with HIV. Today, however, women and girls represent one of the fastest-growing groups affected by HIV/AIDS.

Women most at risk are ethnic minorities and the economically disadvantaged. Among sexually active teenagers, college students, and healthcare workers nationwide, nearly 60% of the heterosexual spread of HIV is among women (Pfeiffer, 1991).

HIV/AIDS in women is a tragedy, but in addition, women are the major source of infection in infants. From 1993 through 2008, over 97% of HIV-infected children aged 0 to 4 years got the virus from their mothers.

At the end of 1988, women made up 6964 or 9% of the total adult AIDS cases in the United States. By

AFRICA: POVERTY AND RITUALS LEAD TO THE SPREAD OF HIV BECAUSE OF DRY SEX

SEXUAL RIGHTS AND POVERTY

A woman from Zimbabwe explained her use of dry sex to please her man, but it is not by choice. She used herbs from the Mugugudhu tree. After grinding the stem and leaf, she mixed a pinch of the powder with water, wrapped it in a bit of nylon stocking, and inserted it into her vagina for 10 to 15 minutes. The herbs swell the soft tissues of the vagina and dry it out. That makes sex very painful. But she adds, "Our African husbands enjoy sex with a dry vagina."

Many African women concur that dry sex hurts, but it is common throughout Southern Africa where the AIDS pandemic is out of control. Researchers who conducted a study in Zimbabwe had trouble finding a control group of women who did not engage in some form of the practice. Some women dry out their vaginas with *mutendo wegudo*—soil with baboon urine— that they obtain from traditional healers, while others use detergents, salt, cotton, or shredded newspaper. Research shows that dry sex causes vaginal lacerations and suppresses the vagina's natural bacteria, both of which increase the likelihood of HIV infection. Some AIDS workers believe the extra friction makes condoms tear more easily.

Africa contains thousands of cultures, some of which have strict sexual codes. But common to many sub-Saharan societies are the gender roles represented by dry sex: Women are unable to negotiate sex and so must risk infection to please the man. There are very few female checks and balances on male behavior. This stark inequality is part of the reason why HIV is spreading in countries with strict sexual codes, such as in Africa.

Lack of Authority

African women lack authority. Zimbabwe's Supreme Court ruled in 1999 that women have no more status of rights in the family than that of a "junior male"— usually an adolescent. In most sub-Saharan traditional cultures men pay for their wives, which gives them license to dominate the relationship. The very concept of marital rape doesn't exist in most of Africa and even the aunties, traditional marriage counselors for many young African wives, tell women that they cannot refuse sex with their husbands. Once a man has paid *lobola*—the word for dowry in several southern African languages—he is not forcing his wife to have sex. It's his right to have sex when he chooses.

Widow Inheritance

Many cultures especially in eastern and southern Africa provide **home guardianship/widow inheritance.** When a husband dies, one of his brothers or cousins marries the widow. This tradition guarantees that the children will remain in the late husband's clan and it also ensures that the widow and her children are provided for. When the guardian takes the widow, sexual intercourse is believed to cleanse her of the devils of death. A woman who refuses to take a guardian brings down *chira*—ill fortune on the entire clan. If her husband died of AIDS she might very well pass on the virus to her guardian. A Luo public health worker with the Red Cross said, "We have homes where all the males have died of AIDS because of this widow inheritance."

In some rural African villages, tradition holds that widows must sleep with the ritual "cleanser"—men who sleep with women after their husbands die—in order to be allowed to attend their husband's funerals or be inherited by their husband's brother or relative (a custom presented above). Unmarried women who lose a parent or child must also sleep with cleansers. Village elders in Gangre, Kenya, say the custom must be carried out or the community will be cursed with bad crops. Areas that still practice the tradition have the highest rates of HIV/AIDS. The cleansing job, held by hundreds of thousands of men across rural Africa, is seen as low class but essential to "purifying women." Cleansers are paid in cows and crops, as well as cash. They can be found in some rural parts of Uganda, Tanzania, and Congo. They are also a staple in Angola and across West Africa, specifically in Ghana, Senegal, Ivory Coast, and Nigeria. The tradition dates back centuries and is rooted in a belief that spirits haunt a woman after her husband dies. She is also thought to be unholy and "disturbed" if she is unmarried and abstains from sex.

POVERTY: BLACK, POOR, AND FEMALE

Poverty means a day-to-day struggle for life in which individuals may be unable to afford the luxury of worrying about HIV/AIDS. The greatest inequality for women is poverty. Poverty is not a uniquely African phenomenon. Of the world's 1.3 billion people living in abject poverty, 70% are women—and most of them face the same basic problems as African women. In developing countries women are trapped in their reproductive roles. In numerous studies on HIV, women from Latin America, Asia, and Africa report that they dare not insist on safer sex or object to painful sex for fear of being abandoned by their men. In a 19-country study, the International Center for Research on Women found that the lower a woman's status, the greater her chance of becoming HIV infected.

ZAMBIA—WOMEN AND THEIR INCOME-GENERATING PROJECT

This story was told by Stephen Lewis, former United Nations Special Envoy for HIV/AIDS in Africa.

Just weeks ago, I was in Zambia, visiting a district well outside of Lusaka. We were taken to a rural village to see an income-generating project run by a group of Women Living With AIDS. They were gathered under a large banner proclaiming their identity, some fifteen or twenty women, all living with the virus, all looking after orphans. They were standing proudly beside the income-generating project, a bountiful cabbage patch. After they have spoken about their needs and the needs of their children (as always, hunger led the litany), I asked about the cabbages. I assumed it supplemented their diet? Yes, they chorused. And you sell the surplus at the market? And energetic nodding of heads. And I take it you make a profit? Yes again. What do you do with the profit? And this time there was an almost quizzical response as if to say what kind of ridiculous question is that surely you knew the answer before you asked? "We buy coffins of course; we never have enough coffins." It's at moments like that when I feel the world has gone mad. That's no existential spasm on my part. I simply don't know how otherwise to characterize what we're doing to half of humankind.

I want to remind you that it took until the Bangkok AIDS conference in 2004—more than twenty years into the pandemic—before the definitive report from UNAIDS separated out the statistics and commented, extensively, upon the devastating vulnerability of women. The phrase "AIDS has a woman's face" actually gained currency at the AIDS conference in Barcelona two years earlier, in 2004, and even then it was years late. Perhaps we should stop using it now as though it was a new dimension. The women of Africa have always known whose face it is that's withered and aching from the virus. Female mutilation, the contagion of violence against women, sexual violence in particular, rape as a weapon of war—Rwanda, Darfur, Northern Uganda, Eastern Congo—marital rape, child defilement, as it is called in Zambia, sexual trafficking, maternal mortality, early marriage—I pause to point out that studies now show that in parts of Africa, the prevalence rates of HIV in marriage are often higher than they are for sexually active single women in the surrounding community; who would have thought that possible?

And because I believe that, and because I see the evidence month after month, week after week, day after day, in the unremitting carnage of women and AIDS—God it tears the heart from the body—I just don't know how to convey it—these young, young women, who crave so desperately to live, who suddenly face a pox, a scourge which tears their life from them before they have a life—who can't even get treatment because the men are first in line, or the treatment rolls out at such a paralytic snail's pace—who are part of the 90% of pregnant women who have no access to the prevention of Mother-to-Child Transmission and so their infants are born positive—who carry the entire burden of care even while they're sick, tending to the family, carrying the water, tilling the fields, looking after the orphans—the women who lose their property, and have no inheritance rights, and no legal or jurisprudential infrastructure which will guarantee those rights—no criminal code which will stop the violence—because I have observed all of that, and have observed it for four years, and am driven to distraction by the recognition that it will continue, I want a kind of revolution in the world's response, not another stab at institutional reform, but a virtual revolution.

I'm 67 years old. I'm a man. I've spent time in politics, diplomacy and multilateralism. I know a little of how this man's world works, but I still find much of it inexplicable. I don't really care anymore about whom I might offend or what line I cross: that's what's useful about inching into one's dotage. I know only that this world is off its rocker when it comes to women. I must admit that I live in such a state of perpetual rage at what I see happening to women in the pandemic, that I would like to throttle those responsible, those who've waited so unendurably long to act, those who can find infinite resources for war but never sufficient resources to ameliorate the human condition.

the end of 2009 it is estimated that women will account for about 289,000 AIDS cases or about 24% of all AIDS cases in the U.S. (Table 11-2). About 75% of all female AIDS cases will have been reported in the 14 years between 1995 and the end of 2008. They will have been reported from all 50 states and territories. About 67% of these females are between the ages of 13 and 39 (HIV/AIDS Surveillance, 1997 updated). Between 1989 and the end of 2009, female AIDS cases were and continue to be twice as frequent among black women as among white, and almost three times higher in black women than in

Hispanic women (Figure 11-2). Black and Hispanic women account for about 80% of U.S. AIDS cases among women but represent only about 30% of the U.S. female population over the age of 18. Ending 2009, at age 18 and over, there will be about 96 million white females, about 15.3 million black females, and about 15.6 million Hispanic or Latino females in the United States.

In the United States, ending 2009, about three-quarters of the estimated 289,000 women living with HIV and AIDS will be black or Hispanic.

Among the most alarming HIV/AIDS statistics to emerge is that of HIV transmission through heterosexual sexual contact. Of new HIV infections in women, acquired through heterosexual contact, in 2002 through 2009 in the United States about 30% will be women. Of AIDS cases and new HIV infections that occur in women ages 13 to 24, about 76% are due to heterosexual contact.

The median age for women reported with AIDS is 35 years, and women ages 25 to 44 account for 85% of female AIDS cases. Ending year 2009 women ages 55 years and older will account for about 18% of all female AIDS cases. Most of these women became infected through heterosexual sexual activities (Schable et al., 1996 updated). Figure 11-3 presents the cumulative **source** of U.S. female HIV cases through 2008.

Table 11-2 Reported and Estimated AIDS Cases for Women, United States Through 2009

Year	Number	Total
1981 (From June)	6	
1982	47	
1983	144	
1984	285	
1985	534	
1986	980	
1987	1701	
1988	3263	
1989	3639	
1990	4890	Through 1990 (15,489)
1991	5732	
1992	6571	
1993	16,824[a]	
1994	14,379	
1995	14,100	Through 1995 (73,095)
1996	13,820	
1997	11,651	
1998	10,500	
1999	10,800	
2000	11,000	Through 2000 (130,989)
2001	11,117	
2002	11,300	
2003	12,000	
2004	12,900	
2005	13,000	
2006	13,200	
2007	13,200	
2008	13,200	Through 2009 (estimated) (290,000)
2009	13,200	
Men	950,000	
Total:[c]	**1.24 million**[b]	

[a]The large increase in women's AIDS cases for 1993, over previous years was due to the January 1, 1993, implementation of the new definition of AIDS. Ending 2009 about 437,000 women will have been HIV infected. Of these about 290,000 will be diagnosed with AIDS and about 141,000 of these will have died of AIDS.

[b]Total AIDS cases include 9936 pediatric.

[c]End of year 2009.

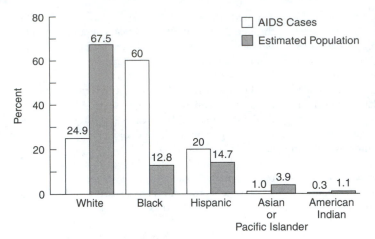

FIGURE 11-2 Incidence of AIDS Cases Among Women of Different Ethnic Groups, United States. Worldwide, every minute two women become HIV infected, and every minute two women die of AIDS. *(Source: WHO/UNAIDS AIDS Epidemic Update 2007-updated)*

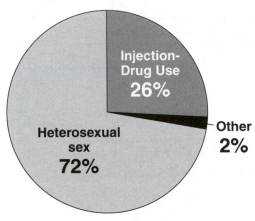

FIGURE 11-3 Cumulative Major Sources of HIV Infections in U.S. Women Through 2008. *(Adapted from U.S. Centers for Disease Control and Prevention, Surveillance Report Year 2006 updated)*

Location, Location, Location

Beginning in 2001, the South accounted for the largest percentage of AIDS cases reported among women (46%), followed by the Northeast (36%), West (8%), Midwest (6%), and Puerto Rico and U.S. territories (4%). In the Northeast, 1.4% of women with AIDS resided outside metropolitan areas compared with 10.2% of women who resided outside metropolitan areas in the South.

In July 1982, the first female AIDS case was reported to the CDC. Currently, women in 10 states make up about 70% of their cumulative AIDS cases (Table 11-3). With respect to **new HIV infections,** the South with about 30% of the female population has about 76% of newly infected females.

Of all new female AIDS cases, over 50% are associated with heterosexual transmission. The second most frequent cause was injection-drug use at about 26%. The AIDS rate for Hispanic women was eight times higher than for white women. The AIDS rate for black women was four times higher than for Hispanic women and 23 times higher than for white women.

As the frequency of HIV/AIDS increases in women, the question of whether AIDS will explode in the heterosexual community of the United States becomes more a question of when will the number of female AIDS cases equal male cases. For the first time, in 1997 American women made up over 20% (22%) of AIDS cases for the year. For 2009 the estimate is between 25% and 30%.

Table 11-3 Ten States Reporting Highest Estimated Number of Women with AIDS Through 2008

State	% of Total (276,000)
New York	17.8
California	14.4
Florida	10.6
Texas	7
New Jersey	5
Illinois	3.4
Pennsylvania	3.4
Georgia	3.2
Maryland	3
Massachusetts	2
	69.8% of women's AIDS cases in these 10 states (192,648)

BLACK WOMEN AND HIV/AIDS

Los Angeles (FinalCall.com)—"I'm 22 and I'm celebrating life each day. I continue to speak because when I was in high school, the number of kids that were having sex and the type of sex that they were having was amazing to me . . . so I continue to speak. I continue to speak because now I have a 14-year-old sister who is infected and I want her to have the same opportunities that I have, to be welcomed and loved by so many people. To my peers, as people we need to wake up. Parent, please talk to your child. How many times do you have to tell us to take out the trash, or do our homework? And don't just lecture us, speak to us. Have an open conversation. The reason why I do what I do is because I don't want anybody to go through what I've gone through. I'm so happy that we're finally taking this stand and raising our voices."

When she was three years old, doctors discovered that Hydeia Broadbent was infected with HIV, and they told her new adoptive parents that she would not live to be five. Tearfully speaking these words, the HIV/AIDS activist helped to convene the First Annual National Black Women and HIV/AIDS Conference in 2005.

It's All About M.E.E. !

The third (2008) national black women's AIDS conference was held in Los Angeles, California. The conference was called, "It's All About M.E.E.! (Mobilization, Education, Empowerment) Sistahs Getting Real About HIV." Congresswoman Maxine Waters (Figure 11–4) noted that a 6% reduction in HIV/AIDS infections among black women is hopeful, but it is not enough. "African Americans, in general, still account for almost half of all the new AIDS cases, although we're only 13% of the population. African American women still represent nearly 70% of all the new AIDS cases among women, and African American teenagers represent 65% of all the new AIDS cases among teenagers."

Despite growing beliefs that AIDS is no longer a lethal disease, black American women are dying from AIDS-related illnesses every year in ever-increasing numbers. Black women who test HIV positive are seven times more likely to die from it than whites. AIDS remains the leading cause of death for black women between the ages of 25 and 34 and ranks among the leading causes of death for all black women. Far too many black women do not realize that they are at risk or don't believe they are at risk.

Among women, black women account for an estimated 68% of new HIV infections, about 67% of women's AIDS cases, and 13% of the U.S. female population.

HIV TRANSMISSION IN BLACK WOMEN THROUGH 2008

Heterosexual sex is by far the most common route of HIV transmission for black women (78%), followed by injection-drug use.

Deaths

Black women account for about 68% of all women who have died from AIDS, white about 18%, and Hispanic about 14%. Of black women, about 41% of deaths occur in ages 35–44; ages 45–54, about 25%; ages 25–34, 21%; ages 15–24, 3%; and over age 55, 10%.

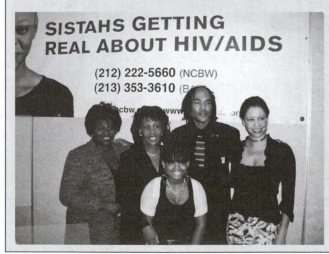

FIGURE 11–4 Grazelle Howard, J.D. (The Libra Group), Congresswoman Maxine Waters (D–Calif.), Hydeia Broadbent (22-year-old AIDS activist), Phil Wilson (The Black AIDS Institute), and Gloria Reuben (actress/ songstress) pose after convening "It's all About M.E.E.! Sistahs Getting Real About HIV" first National Black Women and HIV/AIDS Conference December 1, 2006. *(Courtesy of Charlene Muhammad).*

BOX 11.1

THE FEMALE GENDER AND THE IMPACT OF HIV/AIDS

AIDS NOW HAS A WOMAN'S FACE

In the early 1990s women were on the periphery of the HIV/AIDS pandemic. From 2003 through 2008 women have been at the epicenter. Across the world, more women than men are now becoming HIV infected and dying of this disease. The biggest factor appears to be how HIV is transmitted. Women are most at risk in countries where heterosexual sex is the main mode of transmission. This is the case in Africa, the Middle East, and the Caribbean. A new United Nations report stated that 80% of new HIV infections in women worldwide occur in marriages or long-term relationships with primary partners. By comparison, HIV is mostly transmitted by men who have sex with men and injection-drug users in Western Europe, Australia, New Zealand, and in North America.

QUESTIONS ABOUT THE FEMALE FACE OF AIDS

In 2002 it became clear that women equaled men in the global number of HIV/AIDS cases. But this alarming finding did not just happen overnight. The phenomenon of women and HIV/AIDS has grown relentlessly over the 27 years of this pandemic. What shocks our senses is how long it has taken to focus the world on the fact that this was happening. Why wasn't the trend identified much earlier? Why, when it emerged in cold statistical print, did emergency alarm bells not ring out? Why has the continuing pattern of sexual carnage among young women, so grave as to lose an entire generation of women, gone on unrecognized? And why did it take until 2003 for the UN to form a task force on the plight of women in Africa or until 2004 to put in place a Global Coalition on Women and AIDS?

HETEROSEXUAL TRANSMISSION

Why does heterosexual transmission strike more women than men? The answer has to do with physiology, economics, and culture. Women are physiologically more vulnerable to infection: If an HIV-positive man has unprotected sex just once with an HIV-negative woman, her chance of infection is around 1 in 300. Reverse the gender and the odds fall to around 1 in 1000. This means women have more incentive to insist on safer sex than men. But here's where economics comes in: In many cultures worldwide, women are denied equal access to education, income, ownership of land or other productive assets, even to credit. Too many women are left heavily dependent on men, and on exchanging sexual access to their bodies for the means of survival—both for themselves and their children. This situation makes negotiation of safer sex very difficult. Women are vulnerable for many reasons: They face domestic violence, at times worsened by conflict or insecurity; girls are the first to be pulled from school and put to work when HIV/AIDS strikes home; women lack the power and economic independence to negotiate sexual safety; women face the full brunt of the stigma and discrimination associated with HIV, which fuels their fear of getting tested and prevents them from seeking care if they are infected; and there are inequalities between the sexes and women have a lack of power to challenge these inequalities.

Global Impact: The Gender Imbalance Grows

It has been said that men are driving the HIV pandemic, but that women will ultimately be its main victims. According to Peter Piot, executive director of UNAIDS, higher deaths among young women due to HIV will lead to a hole in the age pyramid that has only been seen before in times of war, when more men die. According to UNAIDS, the situation is so badly tilted against women that they are now two to three times more likely to contract HIV than men. For example, so many more women will die from AIDS in the next 10 years than men that it will culminate in an unprecedented gender imbalance and will change reproductive choices dramatically in years to come.

SUMMARY: Peter Piot said, "Women may be vulnerable, but we must distinguish between vulnerability and weakness. Women have shown great courage and resourcefulness in facing the epidemic. They have practiced safer sex when it was dangerous to do so; they have successfully pushed through legal reforms protecting their rights; they have consistently provided care, both at home and in healthcare settings. Wherever we look, we see the hope women have generated by their actions."

PROFILE: WOMEN WITH HIV/AIDS IN THE UNITED STATES

At the end of 2009, there will be over 150 million American women in the United States.

The majority of women with AIDS in the United States reside in the Northeast and the South, are un-employed, and 83% live in households with income less than $10,000 per year. Only 14% are currently married, compared to 50% of all women in the United States ages 15 to 44 years. Twenty-three percent of HIV-infected women live alone, 2% live in various fa-cilities, and 1% are homeless. Approximately 50% have at least one child younger than 15 years old. Sim-ilar to other population groups with AIDS in the United States, the majority of women with AIDS are from mi-nority racial and ethnic groups, with 64% of all AIDS cases diagnosed in blacks, 19% in Latinos, and 15% in whites (HIV/AIDS Surveillance, 1998 updated).

AIDS IN OLDER WOMEN

According to the CDC, ending year 2009, an esti-mated 18% or about 52,000 AIDS cases will have oc-curred in women ages 55 and older: white 18,200, black 23,900, Hispanic 8840, all others about 1000.

TWO TYPICAL SENIOR HIV/AIDS ANECDOTES

A soft-spoken, 63-year-old, self-described "churchy" woman from rural South Dakota, who has been living with HIV since her late 50s, said, "I got very sick. I kept going to the doctor and he kept giving me antibiotics, and he would just kind of hit-and-run. He thought it was menopause, arthritis, high blood pres-sure, possibly a heart problem. Suddenly I found my-self in the emergency room after two years of misdiagnosed infections, monthly visits to my pri-mary care doctor, and an allergic reaction to daily doses of penicillin. That's where I was tested for HIV. When the doctor came into my room, I pulled on his sleeve and told him to sit down a minute. He said, 'What you have is really nasty, and you don't want to know.'"

In a second case, a 66-year-old woman said, "He was 10 years older than I was and he said, 'I've never worn a condom in my life and I'm not going to start now.'" Most older men say that. Older women won't insist that the man wear a condom. They don't ask where he's been. Older women especially don't pry. They can no longer have children, so why bother with condoms? Usually they tend not to be very assertive until they get HIV or an STD. Most seniors are first di-agnosed with HIV in the hospital after they've already progressed to AIDS.

These two stories are typical of HIV-positive older women. The majority become infected through sexual contact with a husband or boyfriend. After months and sometimes years of being sick, they're tested for HIV as a last resort. Healthcare providers rou-tinely fail these women by not readily screening them for HIV and other sexually transmitted dis-eases. They also neglect to ask about their sexual and drug-using behaviors. Ailments that accom-pany HIV often masquerade as signs of aging, throwing physicians even further off track. Fevers, night sweats, tuberculosis, chronic fungal infec-tions, shingles, decreased vision, *Pneumocystis jiroveci* pneumonia, and cervical cancer can signal HIV, AIDS, or aging.

Women, Drug Use, and HIV Infection

Until recently, most drug users have been men, and their non-drug-using female partners have func-tioned as the glue that kept their families together, sheltering as best they could the next generation, often suffering abuse in the process. Today, 60% of crack users are women, the majority of whom are mothers of small children and the heads of single-parent households. It is estimated that more than half of all drug-using women in the major epicenters of the eastern United States are HIV infected, and drug use among women is correlated to unprotected sex, injection-drug use, and needle sharing.

Artificial Insemination

To date there are six cases of transmission through **artificial insemination** reported in the United States, and six other cases are known to have occurred (Joseph, 1993 updated). Four of eight Australian women who received semen from a single infected donor became infected. HIV-contaminated semen had been injected into the uterus through a catheter. In 2003, a woman in Tokyo became infected after being artificially insemi-nated with sperm from her HIV-positive husband. According to the report, several procedures involved in obtaining HIV-free sperm were not performed. Chil-dren have been born free of HIV when the procedure for stripping HIV from sperm was used properly. For other cases of men infecting women see Box 8.7.

Prostitutes

The term **"prostitute"** is used here in preference to the more recently coined **"sex worker."** No single term can adequately encompass the range of sex for money/drugs/friendship/accommodation transactions that undoubtedly occurs worldwide. However, the term prostitute is at least relatively clear in referring to those who are directly involved in trading sex for money or drugs. In the United States, prostitutes represent a diverse group of people with various lifestyles. About 31% of female IDUs admit to engaging in prostitution. They need money to support their drug habit, pay rent, and eat. Cities with large numbers of IDUs subsequently have large numbers of prostitutes. Evidence is overwhelming—IDU, prostitution, and HIV infection are strongly associated.

However, non-injection-drug-using prostitutes in the United States play a small role in HIV transmission. This is believed to be because of the low incidence of HIV infection among their male clients

and on the insistence by many prostitutes that their clients use condoms. In Africa, Asia, and other underdeveloped nations where the "Customer is King," prostitution plays a major role in HIV transmission (Figure 11-6).

Women Who Have Sex with Women (Lesbians)

Research on female-to-female transmission remains inconclusive. But the large numbers of HIV-positive

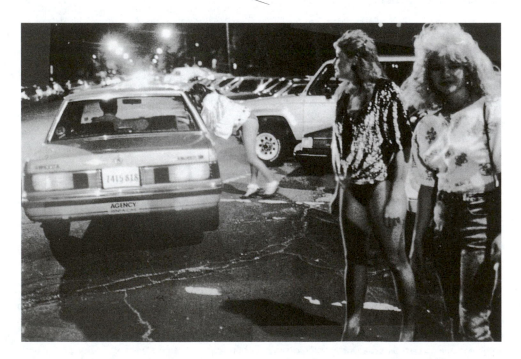

FIGURE 11-5 Street scene, sex workers plying their trade, any major city. *(Courtesy of The Centers for Disease Control and Prevention, Atlanta, GA)*

REBEKKA'S STORY

At the young age of eighteen, Rebekka aspired to become a Playboy Playmate like she had seen in the magazines found under her grandfather's bed. Her pictures were sent to Hugh Hefner, and against all odds Rebekka was chosen to become a Playboy centerfold, Miss September '86. Rebekka's sunny disposition and enthusiastic spirit brought her all she could desire. It seemed a time when nothing could harm her. Rebekka said, "I led an exciting life as a Playmate. Traveling, meeting tons of people, parties, etc. However as time passed, I began to suspect something was wrong. I became fatigued easily and was plagued with a general feeling of malaise." She went to her doctor for tests and, as an afterthought, asked to be tested for HIV. It came back positive. Rebekka said, "Surprisingly I did not become infected living the wildlife in the light of Hollywood; no, it happened years earlier, as a teenager having unprotected sex with a young man I met on a summer beach vacation." She was diagnosed positive in 1989.

When her doctor called with her results, she became confused. "I thought my doctor was telling me I was pregnant, but I was positive for HIV, and the only thing I knew about HIV was death." Attempting to mask her anguish, she began using speed and partying heavily, and began taking 18 anti-HIV pills a day in hopes of curing her illness. Her hands and feet began tingling with the sensations of pins and needles. She had drug toxicity from the medication and was diagnosed with neuropathy, which is a severe form of nerve damage. She was rushed to the emergency room in Los Angeles and had seven spinal taps in four days and was diagnosed with two brain infections. She was given a second set of new medications for everything the doctors could find wrong. She began regaining her strength and she began partying again and her drugs failed again.

When placed on a third set of new HIV medications her pancreas ruptured. Broke and about homeless she thought about suicide. She mixed numerous pain pills with tequila and drove into a brick wall. She was in a coma for three and a half days. When she awoke she was transferred to the psychiatric ward of the hospital. After being released she decided to reveal her HIV infection. She went public with her illness in 1994 by speaking to family, friends, and the media. She was put on a fourth set of drugs, this time a three-drug combination. It caused severe diarrhea. She had to wear diapers for 18 months. For the fourth time, her drugs failed. Her doctor prescribed a new drug regime, which she said

was "pure evil." She did not have a bowel movement for eight days, and realized the medications were ruining her digestive system. Her medications were switched yet again, but this time it worked. She takes about 10 pills a day and is now into her 24th year of HIV infection. About five years ago Rebekka found her way into nutrition and bodybuilding (Figure 11-5). Her coach, now her husband and also HIV positive, trained her intensely. On May 31, 2004, Rebekka won first place in her first attempt in a women's bodybuilding competition.

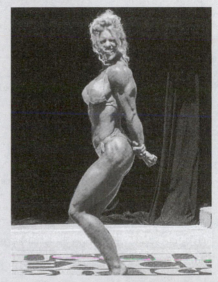

FIGURE 11-6 Rebekka Armstrong: 24 years HIV positive and counting. After suffering antiretroviral failures, wasting and near death at 90 pounds, she switched her lifestyle to accept better nutrition, new anti-HIV drugs, exercise, weight lifting and bodybuilding. *(Photograph by Joanne Greenstone, used with permission)*

Rebekka currently lives in Los Angeles with her trainer husband Oliver. Although infected with HIV for 24 years and diagnosed with AIDS, she is in excellent health. Medications and a super healthy lifestyle that includes mornings of cardio and weight training have helped Rebekka to maintain a normal T cell count (over 500) and undetectable viral load. She says she has never felt better.

Rebekka has dedicated herself to increasing AIDS awareness. She has toured across the U.S. educating others about HIV prevention.

women and women with AIDS should alert women who have sex with women that they cannot assume their partners are uninfected because they are lesbians. It has been reported that 80% of lesbian women have had sex with men during their lifetimes. Also, certain sexual behaviors common among lesbians probably put them at risk for transmitting and receiving HIV through vaginal fluid, menstrual blood, sex toys, and cuts in the vagina, mouth, and on the hands.

The evidence is clear: HIV infection is present among lesbians, and lesbians engage in behaviors that put them at risk for HIV infection. Whether or not lesbians put their female sexual partners at risk is less clear. In fact, there is a great deal of controversy about this question. Some HIV/AIDS investigators believe the risk of sexual transmission increases as the number of HIV-positive lesbian partners increases. Others believe that lesbians are not getting infected through lesbian sex, but only through unsafe behaviors like IDU. Female-to-female transmission has been reported in one case and suggested in another (Curran et al., 1988; Chu et al., 1994).

In 2003 Helena Kwakwa and colleagues reported that based on genetic evidence of the strain of HIV found in two women, sexual contact between the two resulted in the transmission of HIV.

A 20-year-old female had exclusive sexual activity with an openly bisexual HIV-infected woman for two years before testing HIV positive. Their sexual relations involved oral contact and the use of sex toys. The investigators ruled out other possible means of HIV transmission in this case (Kwakwa et al., 2003).

Special Concerns of HIV/AIDS Women

First, HIV/AIDS has a profound impact on women, both as an illness and as a social and economic challenge. Women play a crucial role in preventing infection by insisting on safer sexual practices and caring for people with HIV disease and people with AIDS. The stigma attached to HIV/AIDS can subject women to discrimination, social rejection, and other violations of their rights. A study by Sally Zierler and colleagues (2000) estimates that about 21% of HIV-infected American women were assaulted by a partner or another relation after becoming HIV positive. The percentage of women receiving physical harm after receiving an HIV diagnosis in a developing nation is at least twice that found in America. In South Africa, for example, Gugu Dlamini was stoned to death by her neighbors after she revealed that she was HIV positive on World AIDS Day, 1999.

POINT OF INFORMATION 11.3

HIV INFECTION AMONG WOMEN

There are over 6 million women ages 18 to 40 in the United States who are unmarried and having sexual relationships. Those most at risk for HIV infection are: (1) those who have multiple sexual partners (defined as having more than four different partners/year), and (2) those women who do not insist on the use of a condom.

Three of the nation's top five metropolitan areas with the highest incidence of AIDS in women are located in Florida within a 70-mile radius of each other (West Palm Beach, Ft. Lauderdale, and Miami). This area is an epicenter of HIV infection for Florida women. The other areas of highest incidence of AIDS in women are Puerto Rico, followed by New Jersey, New York, the District of Columbia, Florida, Connecticut, Maryland, Delaware, Massachusetts, Rhode Island, Georgia, and South Carolina. In Florida's Palm Beach County the rate is 24%; in Broward and Dade Counties, 18%. The epidemiologist for the state of Florida stated that what is happening in Florida is happening in inner cities nationwide. What may distinguish the AIDS epidemic in women is that it hinges on the low self-esteem and lack of personal power experienced by women in many walks of life.

Most of Florida's women with AIDS are poor and receive their medical care through the public health system. Among women in South Florida, HIV transmission is associated with crack cocaine. Pam Whittington, director of the Boynton Community Life Center, a family support facility in southern Palm Beach County, said, "If you have 10 women on crack, probably 8 of them are HIV infected."

Crack cocaine is cheap and readily available. Its use contributes to anonymous, high-risk sex with multiple partners. Those who cannot afford crack exchange sex for it. In isolated communities of crack users, there is a high degree of sharing sex partners, many of whom are HIV positive.

QUESTIONS THAT EVERY HIV-POSITIVE WOMAN SHOULD ASK HER PHYSICIAN

1. What is my CD4 count and viral load?

2. If on antiretroviral drugs, are they working? If not, when should I start?

3. Do I have any sexually transmitted diseases?

4. Is my Pap smear normal? How often do I need one?

5. What can I do to improve my overall health?

6. Do you know of any local, county, or state support groups for HIV-positive women?

7. What can I do if I am depressed, using drugs, or drinking a lot?

8. What other issues might be affecting my health?

And three more to ask if you are having a baby:

1. How can I prevent HIV transmission to my child?

2. Are my current HIV antiretroviral drugs safe during pregnancy?

3. Should I have a vaginal delivery or a C-section?

These questions are of particular importance because most HIV-infected women are in their years of child-bearing potential. Therefore, issues of fertility and mother-to-child transmission are particularly important to them. In a recent French study (reported in January 2007), one-third of HIV-infected women intended to have children. Twenty percent of HIV infected men intended to father a child. Similar data came from a Canadian study.

Women need to know that they can protect themselves against HIV infection. Women have a traditionally passive role in sexual decision making in many countries. They need knowledge about HIV and AIDS, self-confidence, the skills necessary to insist that partners use safer sex methods, and good medical care.

Efforts to influence women to practice safer sex must also be joined by efforts to address men and their responsibility in practicing safer sex.

Second, women become pregnant. Women who are ill and discover they are pregnant need information about both the potential impact of pregnancy on their own health and maternal-fetal HIV transmission.

Third, women have the role of mothering. From this role come two important consequences. First, when a woman becomes ill with HIV disease or AIDS, her role as caretaker of the child or children or other adults in the household is immediately affected. The family is severely disrupted and each family member has to make adjustments. Second, the mother must cope with her own life-threatening illness while she also deals with the impact of the disease on her family. Demographic studies show that many women who are HIV infected or have AIDS have young children; and these women are often the sole support of these children.

Fourth, a woman's illness may be complicated further by incarceration and the threat of foster care proceedings. If the mother is healthy enough to care for her child, she must still cope with the complex issues of medical and home care, school access, friends, and family stress.

Biology and the Clinical Course of AIDS Among Women and Men

According to Birgit van Benthem and colleagues (2002), sex differences with respect to response to HIV infection do exist. CD4 cell counts are higher in women than in men throughout infection and viral loads are lower initially in women than in men, although this difference eventually disappears. Despite these disparities, women have not been found to have a more rapid clinical progression to AIDS than men.

According to Arlene Bardeguez (1995) and other similar reports (Cohen, 1995), biology does not influence the prevalence of AIDS-defining illnesses, with the exception of invasive carcinoma of the cervix and possibly Kaposi's sarcoma. Access to HIV-related care and therapies is the dominant factor influencing the prevalence of AIDS-defining illnesses among women. Injection-drug use in HIV-infected women leads to a higher incidence of certain diseases, particularly esophageal candidiasis, herpes simplex virus, and cytomegalovirus. Once an initial diagnosis of AIDS has been made, several major AIDS-defining illnesses appear more frequently in women: toxoplasmosis, herpes genital ulcerations, and esophageal candidiasis.

The currently proposed female-specific markers of **HIV disease** include **cervical dysplasia** and

WOMEN + SEXUAL PARTNERS + DECEPTION = AIDS

Across the world, women in support groups or with a close friend have been telling their stories of trusting their sexual partners and ending up with AIDS. Their trust was violated—their lives forfeited. Here are a few examples of the thousands of similar cases worldwide.

1. She is 48 years old with curly red hair and bags beneath her eyes. She slouches slightly in the office chair, stretching out her feet. From her eye shadow to her sneakers, everything is blue. Married to one husband for 28 years, she has children and grandchildren. She also has AIDS. She did not use drugs or have multiple sexual partners. She did have sex with her husband without a condom!

2. One 23-year-old had a boyfriend with hemophilia; he never used condoms and never mentioned HIV, even though he had already infected another woman.

3. A divorced man with two children did not tell his 46-year-old girlfriend he had AIDS, even when he was hospitalized with an AIDS-related infection.

4. A seven-year live-in partner of a woman denied infecting her, even though he tested positive for HIV; she did not know he was having sex outside their relationship.

5. Because she had only two boyfriends, because "we were perfectly ordinary," they did not use condoms.

6. This woman with a baby did not know "my man was shooting up drugs and sharing needles." Not until he died of AIDS.

7. She never dreamed her partner had used a needle. When the doctor said she had AIDS, she replied, "You have made a mistake. I cannot have AIDS. How could I have that?"

All these women discovered their HIV status only after they became seriously ill with infections they should not have had. Heterosexual transmission is rising dramatically. A seldom-mentioned fact is that a large percentage of infected women are married or in committed relationships.

---

neoplasia (tumor), **vulvovaginal candidiasis,** and **pelvic inflammatory disease** (PID).

No biology-related differences in the survival of HIV-positive persons have been documented when equal access to medical care is considered. The shorter observed survival of women in some studies is thought to occur because of the lack of access to physicians who are knowledgeable about HIV-related care and therapies. Shannon Hader and colleagues (2001) found no differences between women and men infected with the virus in terms of natural history, progression, survival, and HIV-associated illnesses. Drug use, high-risk sexual behaviors, depression, and unmet social needs among infected women contributed to their underuse of HIV resources. Also in 2001, Timothy Sterling and colleagues reported that although viral loads were lower in women than men, the rates of progression to AIDS were similar.

Female HIV/AIDS Deaths

Women's deaths in the United States rose from 18 cases in 1981 to an estimate 142,000 ending year 2009. That is, about 50% of all women with AIDS will have died. AIDS is the sixth leading cause of death for all

women between the ages of 25 and 34, the fifth leading cause of death for all women between the ages of 35 and 44, and the eighth-leading cause of death in white women. It is the second-leading cause of death for black women and the third-leading cause of death for Hispanic women between the ages of 25 and 44 (*MMWR,* 1996b updated).

Identifying and Preventing HIV Infection

Currently, women make up 61% of adult/adolescent HIV infections in sub-Saharan Africa, 30% in Southeast Asia, and about 23% in Europe and the United States.

Identification of HIV-Positive Women—At age 26, a woman and her physicians were baffled when she began suffering from a variety of strange medical conditions: fevers, throat sores, unexplained vaginal bleeding, and fatigue. **It took a variety of doctors and seven years to find out what was wrong. She tested HIV positive!**

This woman's difficulty in getting diagnosed points out the extent to which women still are invisible when it comes to AIDS. After more than 27 years into the epidemic, the message still hasn't reached primary care physicians: Their female patients may be at

BOX 11.2

TWO WOMEN'S COMMENTS ON THEIR HIV DISEASE TREATMENTS

CASE I

"I was fired from my job when they found out I was HIV positive. The boss said, 'You have a modern problem—and this is an old-fashioned business.'"

This woman, in 1995, was 29 years old and HIV positive since age 22. When her T4 cell count dropped to 250, her doctor put her on zidovudine (ZDV, also called AZT). She was not given any literature or verbal explanation of how this drug would affect her. In 12 months she became anemic; she could not sleep or hold down food, and her menstrual cycle became erratic. Without explanation, she next received two other HIV replication inhibitors, ddI and ddC.

The side effects were very bad: persistent premenstrual symptoms; mood swings; increased cravings for certain foods, alcohol, or drugs; breast tenderness; and bloating. But there was no literature for her to read and her doctor said, "I knew how the drugs affected men, but I knew nothing of what to expect when I gave these drugs to women." "I stopped taking these drugs—they were killing me faster than the virus! I have severe yeast infections, shingles, sinus infections, and a host of other infections. My doctor is dealing with me like I'm some kind of experiment."

CASE II: PERSONAL STORY BY CHRISTINA ROCK

I forgot to take my meds right before the Los Angeles AIDS Walk. Pretty ironic, huh? You'd think that since I've been HIV positive for all of my 23 years and on meds for 17, I wouldn't screw up—especially before walking six miles to raise awareness for the disease. What rattled me most, however, was the memories it revived from high school, when I battled with med adherence—and lost big time. I skipped so many doses that I'm resistant to the whole class of NRTI meds. Luckily, I've found another regimen, and I'm very healthy, but I can't risk my safety again.

In the fall of 1998, I moved from Key West, Florida to live with my aunt and uncle in suburban Boston. They enrolled me in a large public school and told the administration and my teachers about my status. The students weren't told—except for a few I disclosed to. I found my niche: I joined the drama club, the choir, and the color guard and made cool friends. Still, taking 14 to 20 pills two times a day, with all the food requirements were really tough in that environment. There's so much else to adhere to: being cool, fitting in, and keeping my

grades up. I felt that taking my pills made me different, even though hardly any of my classmates knew I was positive. While other students struggled with the pressure to take drugs they shouldn't take, I felt pressured to skip drugs I had to take.

The pills were huge and swallowing them was hard. I hated starting my school day with 19 pills rolling around inside me. As a result, by the end of my sophomore year, my room had become a minefield of missed doses. I hoarded them in plastic baggies and socks, behind books and clothes. When I started fainting and getting weird rashes, fevers, and swollen glands, I lied to my doctors and said I'd taken the meds. My aunt and uncle, meanwhile, weren't monitoring me closely. I would always take meds when they were in the room but they made the mistake of trusting me at other times.

Though my body was falling apart, I was doing well in school. Our color guard was asked to perform at a Red Sox game (a dream for a fan like me). A few weeks before the event, my aunt confronted me with some baggies she'd found. I fessed up and pulled out my stockpiles of missed doses. The next day, she and my doctors admitted me to the psych ward at Children's Hospital Boston for passive suicide. A part of me is grateful for that intervention though I'd never thought about killing myself. I just didn't want to take all those pills that made me feel sick.

The Red Sox performance took place while I was in the hospital so my doctors gave me a day pass. I surprised my classmates and we had a great time. Afterward, my aunt and uncle were supposed to pick me up and return me to the hospital but got stuck in traffic. When the chaperones couldn't wait any longer, the whole busload drove me back to the psych ward. Talk about embarrassing.

The hospital staff helped me through my pill anxiety—developing side-effect strategies too—and I was released after three weeks. That began a process of self-acceptance and more disclosure. Once I was out about everything, the wall that I let HIV build between me and normal people crumbled. My medication is no longer a reminder of my difference, just something that helps me maintain a busy, happy life. I guess it's all just a part of growing—and growing up—with HIV.

(From *POZ Magazine*, January 2007. Reprinted with permission. Copyright 2007 CDM Publishing, L.L.C.)

risk. This young woman said, **"I went into doctors' offices and all they saw was a white, middle-class woman, not someone at risk for HIV."**

Early identification of women with HIV infection is a pressing problem. Risk-based screening at a Johns Hopkins perinatal clinic showed that 43% of HIV-positive women were not identified as at risk on the basis of such screening, with infection being found in 20 (9.5%) of 211 women admitting to at-risk behaviors and in 15 (1.6%) of 949 who were not at risk according to their response to screening questions (Garcia, 1995).

Prevention: United States—To prevent HIV infection, women have been told to reduce their number of sexual partners, to be monogamous, and to protect themselves by using condoms. **But these goals, generally speaking, do not fit the realities of women's lives or may not be under their control.**

Women do not wear the condom. (A female condom is now available but not yet in heavy demand. See Chapter 9.) For women to protect themselves from HIV infection, they must not only rely on their own skills, attitudes, and behaviors regarding condom use, but also on their ability to convince their partner to use a condom. Gender, culture, and power may be barriers to maintaining safer sex practices.

Women who have more than one sexual partner in their lifetime often practice serial monogamy, remaining with one partner at a time. People living as couples reduce the number of their sexual partners. Still, in many phases of life, sex is practiced with new partners in new relationships. American women, on average, are single for many years before their first marriage; they might be single again after a divorce; they might marry again; and, in later phases especially, they might be widowed. For some women, multiple partners throughout life is an economic necessity; urging them to reduce the number of partners is meaningless unless the economic situation for these women is improved (Ehrhardt, 1992). In addition, public health strategies, not necessarily targeted to women, can also play an important role for women. Syringe exchange and drug treatment are important strategies because almost half of all HIV infections in women are due to injection-drug use. Because women are now more likely to be infected by men through heterosexual contact, programs that specifically target men, especially IDUs, will have a beneficial impact on women's programs.

Prevention: Africa

Although they are exceptionally vulnerable to the epidemic, millions of young African women are dangerously uninformed about HIV/AIDS. According to UNICEF, over 70% of adolescent girls (ages 15–19) in Somalia and more than 40% in Guinea Bissau and Sierra Leone have never heard of HIV or AIDS. In countries such as Kenya and the United Republic of Tanzania, more than 40% of adolescent girls harbor serious misconceptions about how the virus is transmitted. One of the targets fixed at the UN General Assembly Special Session on HIV/AIDS in June 2001 was to ensure that at least 90% of young men and women should, by 2005, have the information, education, and services they need in order to defend themselves against HIV infection. Beginning 2009 this goal still has not been achieved! The vast majority of African women living with HIV still do not know they have been infected. One study found that 50% of adult Tanzanian women know where they could be tested for HIV, yet only 66% of these have been tested. In Zimbabwe, only 11% of adult women have been tested for the virus. Moreover, many people who agree to be tested prefer not to return and learn the outcome of those tests. An additional problem is that in many African countries where pregnant women agree to undergo HIV testing, most have no access to drug therapy to prevent mother-to-child transmission of HIV. Over half the HIV-infected women who were surveyed by Kenya's Population Council said they had not disclosed their HIV status to their partners because they feared it would expose them to violence or abandonment. Not only are voluntary counseling and testing services in short supply across the region, but stigma and discrimination continue to discourage people from discovering or disclosing their HIV status.

The Bottom Line

More women are becoming infected with HIV. With early testing and treatment, women with HIV can live as long as men. Women need to know more about how they can be infected, and they should get tested for HIV if they think there is any chance they have been exposed. This is especially true for pregnant women. If they test positive for HIV, they can take steps to reduce the risk of infecting their babies. The best way to prevent infection in heterosexual sex is by using the male condom. Other birth control methods do not protect against HIV. Women who use intravenous drugs should not share equipment. Women should discuss vaginal problems with their doctors, especially yeast infections that don't go away or vaginal ulcers (sores). These could be signs of HIV infections.

CHILDBEARING WOMEN

The extent of HIV infection among pregnant women is often used as an indicator of HIV penetration into the population at large. By this yardstick, several Asian countries have serious epidemics. In some of India's HIV/AIDS surveillance sites, more than 2% of pregnant women are infected, with some sites as high as 6%. Myanmar recorded prevalence rates of up to 5% among pregnant women in some areas of the country. In Thailand, HIV infection prevalence among pregnant women peaked at 2% nationally.

Worldwide each year, of an estimated 200 million women who became pregnant, about 1.6 million become HIV positive. Annually, from 1999 through 2008, about 400,000 children were born HIV positive, and 300,000 died before their first birthday. Of the 4 million women who become pregnant each year in the United States, 6000 are estimated to be HIV infected. These pregnancies now result in less than 100 HIV-infected children each year, a 95% reduction from the 1990s high of 1700 cases. The difference is that in underdeveloped nations, only 25% of pregnant women or less receive antiretroviral drugs.

Women, in general, have two children before they find out they are infected (Thomas, 1989 updated). The birth of an infected child may serve as a **miner's canary**—in some cases it is the first indication of HIV infection in the mother.

Pregnancy and HIV Disease

Early findings in pregnant women indicated that those with T4 or CD4+ cell counts of less than $300/\mu L$ of blood were more likely to experience HIV-associated illness during pregnancy. Pregnant HIV-infected women exhibit a greater T4 or CD4+ cell count decline during pregnancy than do women without HIV infection. T4 cell counts in the HIV infected do not return to prepregnancy levels. However, the overall declines in HIV-infected women likely represent declines that would have occurred in the absence of pregnancy and suggest that pregnancy does not accelerate disease progression (Newell et al., 1997; Bessinger et al., 1997).

Over the last dozen years, HIV-positive pregnant women have been attracting more attention from the medical establishment, **first,** because there are better medications for the HIV-positive mother and fetus, and **second,** because of the relatively high incidence of HIV births.

As an aside, it should be mentioned that protease inhibitors reduce blood levels of the estrogen component in oral contraceptive pills so women taking both the pill and PIs may need to use back-up methods of contraception.

BOX 11.3

HIV-INFECTED WOMEN: DIFFICULT CHOICES DURING PREGNANCY

She was 19-years-old, a nursing student, pregnant, and HIV positive. She spent 4½ months of pregnancy in constant fear for herself and for her baby. She waited, her health began to falter, then she decided to have an abortion.

Several studies have reported that HIV-positive women who perceived their risk of infecting their fetus to be greater than 50% were more likely to abort than those who perceived a lower risk. HIV-positive women who chose to continue their pregnancy cited the desire to have a child, strong religious beliefs, and family pressure (Selwyn et al., 1989).

For women who are HIV positive, pregnancy poses difficult choices. First, pregnancy may mask the presence of HIV disease symptoms and having a child poses other questions such as: Can the mother cope with a normal or infected child? Who will care for the child if the mother becomes too ill or dies? Such questions bring up a number of moral issues.

DISCUSSION QUESTION: Do couples have a right to have children when one of the partners is known to be HIV positive? If the woman is HIV positive? If both are HIV positive? Is there any stage of HIV disease/AIDS when you think a woman should lose the right to become pregnant? (See Chapter 7 for the four stages of HIV disease.)

DISCUSSION QUESTION: Nationwide, approximately 2 of 1000 pregnant women are HIV infected, an incidence much higher than that of fetal neural tube defects, for which pregnant women are screened routinely. Should all pregnancies be screened for HIV?

INTERNET

Among the hundreds of websites containing information on HIV, there are key addresses that provide comprehensive information, including links to a vast array of other resources. The key sites listed here include special areas focused on **women and HIV.**

AIDS Community Research Initiative of America (ACRIA): www.criany.org/treatment/treatment_edu_women.html

American Medical Association home page: http://www.ama-assn.org

The Body: www.thebody.com/women.html

Centers for Disease Control and Prevention (CDC) Home Page: http://www.cdc.gov

HIV Insite: Gateway to AIDS Knowledge: http://hivinsite.ucsf.edu

National Women's Health Information Center: www.4woman.gov/

Women Organized to Respond to Life-Threatening Disease (WORLD): www.womenhiv.org

PEDIATRIC HIV-POSITIVE AND AIDS CASES—UNITED STATES: A FIGHT WE CAN WIN!

The Pediatric HIV Conundrum

One of the biggest puzzles in understanding mother-to-child transmission of HIV is why the majority of babies born to HIV-infected women remain uninfected in utero, at birth, and—perhaps most remarkably—during breast-feeding. It's even more remarkable in view of studies suggesting that cell-free viral load in breast milk can vary from undetectable to more than 200,000 copies per mL, meaning that a breast-feeding infant may ingest up to millions of viral copies each day.

Table 11–4 Ten States Reporting Highest Estimated Number of Pediatric AIDS Cases Through 2008

State	% of Total (9900)
New York	25
Florida	16.2
New Jersey	8.2
California	7
Texas	4.1
Pennsylvania	3.8
Maryland	3.4
Illinois	3
Georgia	2.4
Massachusetts	2.2

75.3% of pediatric cases from these 10 states (7455)

This apparent resistance to infection puts infants in the category of exposed, seronegative individuals who can repel or effectively control HIV despite repeated exposures. Katharine Lazuriaga and Sarah Rowland-Jones have both documented cases of infants apparently clearing a transient HIV infection. It is these immune defenses that vaccine researchers seek to boost, or mimic, with a neonatal vaccine. But there are little hard data on just what they are and how this apparent protection works.

Pediatric AIDS in the United States

Pediatric AIDS in the United States affects two age groups: (1) infants and young children who became infected through perinatal (vertical) transmission, and (2) school-age children, the majority of whom acquired HIV through blood transfusions (mostly hemophiliacs).

Ending 2009, over 21,000 pediatric AIDS cases will be reported and about 13,000 (60%) will have died from AIDS. Pediatric AIDS cases represent about 1% of the total number of AIDS cases to date. Of the pediatric AIDS cases, 3% were/are hemophilic children who received HIV-contaminated blood transfusions or blood products (pooled and concentrated blood factor VIII injections). About 5% of pediatric AIDS cases occurred in non-hemophilic children who were transfused with HIV-contaminated blood. From 1995 on, virtually all HIV-infected newborns contracted HIV from their mothers (vertical transmission). The Pediatric AIDS Foundation reported in April 1995 that hospital costs for each HIV-infected newborn were $35,000 per year. Worldwide ending year 2009 about

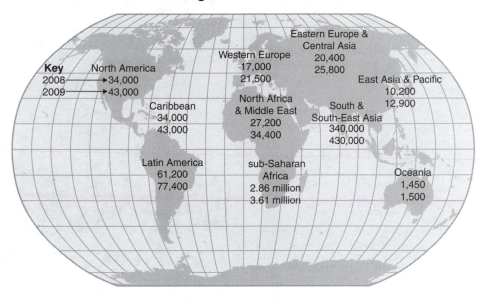

Year End Estimates: Children Living With HIV Infection

Key
2008 ——▶ 34,000
2009 ——▶ 43,000

North America
34,000
43,000

Western Europe
17,000
21,500

Eastern Europe &
Central Asia
20,400
25,800

East Asia & Pacific
10,200
12,900

Caribbean
34,000
43,000

North Africa
& Middle East
27,200
34,400

South &
South-East Asia
340,000
430,000

Latin America
61,200
77,400

sub-Saharan
Africa
2.86 million
3.61 million

Oceania
1,450
1,500

Totals are estimates for the entire globe.
Total: 2008—3.4 million
2009—4.3 million

FIGURE 11-7   Year 2008 and 2009 Global Estimates of Children Living With HIV Infection. Note that sub-Saharan Africa and South and Southeast Asia have the highest burden of HIV-infected children. Sub-Saharan Africa has about 90% of children living with HIV/AIDS. (*Courtesy of UNAIDS updated*)

2.7 million children will be living with HIV disease and about 4.5 million will have died from AIDS (Figures 11-7).

Ethnic Prevalence of Pediatric AIDS Cases

Children of color make up 14% of all children in the United States but account for 57% of pediatric AIDS cases. Whites make up 70% of children and account for 18% of pediatric AIDS cases. Hispanics make up 12% of children and account for 23% of pediatric AIDS cases.

ORPHANED CHILDREN DUE TO HIV INFECTION AND AIDS

World AIDS Orphans Day is held on May 7. "Orphan" is an English word that does not have an exact translation in many languages. The concept of orphan is a social construct, so the meaning assigned to it varies from one society to another. In the United States and Africa, typically the term is understood to mean a child who has lost either or both parents. UNAIDS reports orphans as children who have lost their mothers or both parents. They limit their estimates to children below age 15. The UN Convention on the Rights of the Child defines children as being below age 18, unless the age of majority (adulthood) is reached under national law. Who is a child and who is an adult is defined differently in different countries and among different cultures. This further complicates the meaning of the word because orphans are generally considered to be children.

Children: The Missing Face of AIDS

Children are missing not only from global and national policy discussions on HIV/AIDS, but they also lack access to even the most basic care and prevention services. Millions of children are missing parents, siblings, schooling, health care, basic protection, and many of the other fundamentals of childhood because of the toll the disease is taking. Nearly 28 years into the pandemic, help is reaching less than 10% of the children affected by HIV/AIDS, leaving too many children to grow up alone, grow up too fast, or not grow up at all. Every minute of every day a child dies of AIDS-related illness and another is HIV infected.

Orphaned Children: Unheard Voices, Hidden Lives

Ending year 2009, of the estimated 14 million AIDS-related orphans, 90% live or have lived in Africa. The problem of AIDS-related orphans will become much greater over the next 10 to 15 years.

AIDS orphans present a chilling illustration of the far-reaching effects of the AIDS pandemic.

Orphans in the United States

His mother was young, single, and HIV positive. When she went to the hospital to give birth, she checked in under a false name and address and then slipped out of the hospital leaving her baby who was only a few hours old.

An increasing number of HIV-infected children are being left in hospitals because their HIV-infected mothers and fathers are unable to care for them and no one else wants them. The hospital becomes their home.

As HIV continues to spread across the United States and HIV-infected women continue to become pregnant, the question is: What will happen to their HIV-infected babies? For one young woman who passed the HIV to her baby two years ago, the decision has been made. The baby has AIDS and is in foster care. The mother is very ill. The courts are now deciding whether her six other children should also be put in foster care.

Unless the course of the epidemic changes drastically, through the year 2009, the cumulative number of U.S. children, teens, and young adults left motherless due to AIDS will exceed 150,000. About 80,000 children under age 15 have already lost their mother or both parents to AIDS. The great majority of these children, uninfected by the virus, will begin to affect already burdened social services in major American cities. Things will get immediately worse in such places, where children already spend years going from foster home to foster home and caseworkers are overwhelmed by long lists of families needing everything from housing to medical care (Figure 11-8).

The Silent Legacy

Orphans are often referred to as the silent legacy of AIDS. It is expected that about a third of the

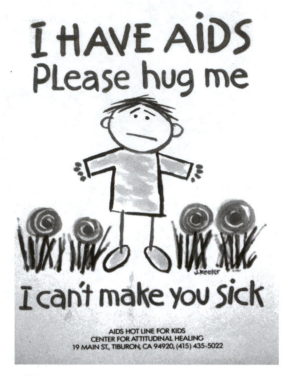

FIGURE 11-8 I Have AIDS—Please Hug Me. (*Permission granted and copyrighted by The International Center for Attitudinal Healing, 33 Buchanan Drive, Sausalito, CA 94965.*)

children orphaned in America will be from New York City, which has the nation's largest number of AIDS cases. Other cities expected to be hit hard are Miami, Los Angeles, Washington, Newark, and San Juan, Puerto Rico. Most of these orphans will be the children of poor black or Hispanic women whose families are already dealing with stresses like drug addiction, inadequate housing, and health care. Relatives who might in other circumstances be called upon to care for the children often shun them because of the stigma attached to AIDS.

THE PHENOMENON OF AIDS ORPHANS

Sub-Saharan Africa

The HIV/AIDS orphan crisis is one of the greatest humanitarian and development challenges facing the global community. The orphan epidemic is still in its infancy. In the years and decades ahead, the impacts of HIV/AIDS on children, their families, and their communities will grow far worse—expanding to dimensions difficult to imagine at present. During 1995 through 2008, on average, 400,000 children were born with HIV infection annually (about 1100 per day); of these children, about 90% were in sub-Saharan Africa, 8% in Southeast Asia, 2% in Latin America and the Caribbean.

In Lesotho, Malawi, Mozambique, Swaziland, Zambia, and Zimbabwe, people are battling a lethal mix of food shortages and HIV/AIDS. About one in four to one in five adults in the six countries now live with HIV or AIDS; increasing deaths and sickness have ground social safety nets way below the reach of poor households. The outlook for children is particularly bleak: The six countries are home to about 3 million children who have lost one or both parents to AIDS (Figure 11-9).

In April 2004, the International AIDS Trust and Children Affected by AIDS Foundation released a report stating that worldwide, every 14 seconds a child is orphaned by AIDS, and that by 2010 worldwide, there will be about 15 million AIDS orphans (lost one or both parents to AIDS-related illness).

Of the current 34 million people living with HIV/AIDS, about 3 million are less than age 15 and 11 million are between ages 15 and 24.

Mother-to-Child Transmission (MTCT) or Vertical HIV Transmission

Vertical transmission means that HIV passes directly from the infected mother into the fetus, newborn, or infant. Data released in mid-2003 on 5000 mother-infant pairs showed that 40% of all HIV transmission within this group occured during breast-feeding, at least four weeks after delivery. (Also see Gray et al., 2008)

Stigma—Stigma is particularly strong surrounding mother-to-child transmission. The very phrase "mother-to-child" itself may be stigmatizing as it puts all the responsibility of transmission on the mother and none on the father of the child. Stigma stops women coming forward to get themselves tested. It reduces their choices when it comes to health care and family life once they are diagnosed as HIV positive and

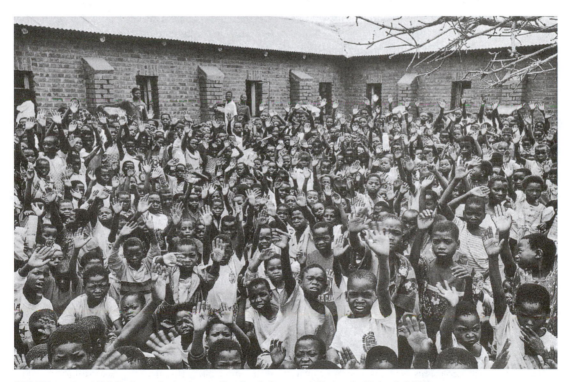

FIGURE 11-9 AIDS Orphans Gathering to Get Food, Care, and Shelter in Malawi, Africa. (*Photograph courtesy of Ellen McCurley—The Pendulum Project*)

has a negative effect on their quality of life. Equally troubling is the lack of sympathy or respect given to pregnant women with HIV, especially in the developing nations where they are open to blame, ridicule, and rejection. For example, in rural Zambia a man stated, "If a pregnant woman is sick and has a sick and premature baby who dies before 3 months, then we know she is affected [infected with HIV] and turn away from her. This is our [HIV] test!"

Timing of HIV Transmission—The exact time of HIV transmission to the fetus during pregnancy is unknown. It has been shown to occur as early as the fifteenth week of gestation, at or near the time of delivery and through breast-feeding.

Breast-feeding by mothers with HIV infection established *before* pregnancy increases the risk of vertical transmission by 16%. When a mother develops primary HIV infection while breast-feeding, the risk of transmission rises to 29%. In general, it is believed that 50% of HIV-positive babies are infected during the last two months of pregnancy and about 50% are infected during the birthing process or through the early months of breast-feeding (Miotti et al., 1999).

A working definition of the timing of maternal HIV transmission has been established to differentiate infants infected **in utero (in the uterus)** from those infected near the time of or **during delivery (perinatally).** In utero infection occurs in approximately 30% of HIV-infected infants. Children who are infected in utero have a more rapid progression to AIDS and generally become symptomatic during the first year of life. Those infected perinatally have no detectable HIV at birth but demonstrate HIV in the blood by 4 to 6 months of age. These children constitute the majority of HIV-infected infants and have a slower progression to AIDS, about 8% per year (Zijenah et al., 2004).

Rate of Mother-to-Child Transmission (MTCT)— The worldwide rate of HIV transmission from mother, without drug therapy, to child varies geographically. In Africa, maternal transmission is as high as 50%. In Europe and the United States, without the use of antiretroviral drugs the overall rate is 25% to 30%, producing less than 500 infected babies a year. The use of antiretroviral drugs in the United States along with cesarean section, has lowered the MTCT to about 1.5%. This is about a 95% drop in the incidence of MTCT. Claire Townsend and colleagues (2008) reported that in the United Kingdom

and Ireland, the use of antiretroviral therapy to lower viral loads to less than 50 copies per milliliter of blood dropped MTCT to 0.1%. **This drop in maternal HIV transmission to their children remains the single greatest achievement in HIV/AIDS prevention methodology.**

The U.S. Public Health Service and 16 other national health organizations have recommended that HIV testing be offered to all women at risk prior to or at the time of pregnancy. Through year 2008, five states—New York, Vermont, Connecticut, Oregon, and Illinois—mandate HIV testing for pregnant women, and nine states—Texas, New Mexico, New Jersey, Tennessee, Michigan, Arkansas, Florida, Georgia, and Vermont use an "opt out" program where pregnant women sign a test refusal form if they do not want an HIV test. The United Kingdom offers all pregnant women an Opt-Out HIV test. Over 90% take the test. The rate of vertical HIV transmission in New York state has decreased dramatically from 25% to about 2% since September 2003, when New York state mandated that all babies born to mothers not tested will be tested within 12 hours after birth.

Viral RNA Load Associated with Perinatal HIV Transmission—Although the close association between stage of HIV infection in a pregnant woman and likelihood of perinatal transmission has been established, there are no precise numerical criteria for pregnancies at high and low risk of transmission. Viral load measurements are now helping to quantitate this risk.

Through 2008, data continued to accumulate that suggest that the use of HAART and achievement of optimal viral load suppression is associated with the greatest reduction of vertical transmission. The identification of HIV infection in pregnant women is the biggest hurdle in reducing vertical transmission.

States and Territories Most Affected by Pediatric Cases

There is evidence that HIV was present in female IDUs as early as 1977 because their babies developed AIDS (Thomas, 1988). As the number of HIV-infected women of childbearing age rises, so does the number of HIV-infected babies.

In the United States pediatric AIDS is most widespread among blacks, Hispanics, and the poor of the inner cities (Figure 11-10). Ending year 2009, New York will continue to have the highest incidence of pediatric AIDS cases, followed by Florida,

A GLIMPSE AT THE ORPHAN PROBLEM IN SOUTH AFRICA

To comprehend the AIDS pandemic ravaging Southern Africa/South Africa, one needs only to visit the village of Ingwavuma. Ingwavuma, a hilly community of eucalyptus trees and blooming orange aloe plants, is quietly suffering the same social meltdown that has devastated towns across KwaZulu-Natal, the South African province hardest hit by AIDS. Between 35% and 40% of Ingwavuma's population carries the virus. Many of the schools around Ingwavuma are struggling as teachers die and students miss classes to attend funerals of relatives. Annual school fees of about $5 a year have been slashed in half in many districts. Enrollment has nonetheless fallen by 30% over the last three years, and 75% of the kids are behind on their payments. The explosion in orphans around Ingwavuma is closing avenues to a better life even for the students who do manage to finish school.

Sthembile Nyawo, a 21-year-old recent graduate of Mthembu's school, had always hoped to find a job so she could help her family, particularly after her father's death from AIDS in 1998. In June, however, her mother died of AIDS. Now Nyawo spends her days looking after six of her younger brothers and sisters and trying to scrape together enough food with the help of her grandmother, whose $60 a month government pension is the only source of income for 16 family members.

Of the children playing in the dust outside Busisiwe Nhleko's hut, perched on a parched hillside near town, three are her brother's kids, orphaned after he and his wife died of AIDS last year. Another four were dropped off by her dying sister. Four more arrived in the arms of various ill cousins, and her neighbors left another four when they died of AIDS; one baby has since died.

Nhleko, age 38, who has 10 children of her own, now struggles to feed, bathe, and care for 24 kids each day, and without much help; her younger brother, her parents, and her husband have died of AIDS. "I don't have much time to tend to all of them. I've accepted all of this and tried to move on, but I still cry when the youngest ones call the older kids 'father' because they have no one else to call that."

Nhleko won't take time away from the 24 children she is raising to have an HIV test. "I've seen the dying and the pain of not being able to cure them. I couldn't stand to know. What would I do? What would they do?" she says, sweeping a hand toward the kids sitting in the dirt. "Life is not what it used to be," covering her face with her sleeve to hide the tears. "Every single person is a terrible loss," she said.

New Jersey, California, Puerto Rico, and Texas. Combined, these cases accounted for 66% of all AIDS cases reported among children.

AIDS Cases Among Children Declining

There are many reasons to believe that with continued HIV counseling of HIV-positive pregnant women and the use of AIDS drug cocktails that lower viral loads, fewer children will become infected and this will translate into a continued decrease in children with AIDS.

This possibility was inconceivable to many clinicians, families, and patients not too long ago. The rapid decline has many physicians suggesting that a goal of eliminating perinatal transmission may be attainable in the United States.

Breast-Feeding, Drug Therapy, and HIV Transmission

In reviewing the recent literature on breast-feeding, a variety of conflicting data have been reported by the respected authorities in this field of HIV/AIDS research. For example, it is not understood how AZT, nevirapine, or other drugs lower the vertical HIV transmission rate, except to say that these drugs inhibit HIV replication (Figure 11.11).

The World Health Organization and the United Nations continue to recommend the following: "When replacement feeding is acceptable, feasible, affordable, sustainable, and safe, avoidance of all breastfeeding by HIV-infected mothers is recommended. Otherwise, exclusive breast-feeding is recommended during the first 24 months of life." (Newton et al. 2008; Kuhn et al. 2008)

Life Span of Untreated HIV-Infected Newborns in Sub-Saharan Africa

According to Taha Taha and colleagues of Johns Hopkins University (2000) over 50% of HIV-infected newborns die within 12 months. Eighty-nine percent of HIV-infected children alive at 6 months died by age 3 years. In comparison, the authors note that in Europe and the United States, only 18% of HIV-infected children died by age 3 years, and 75% lived to age 5 years and older.

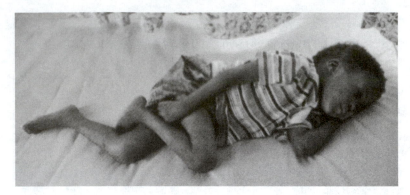

FIGURE 11-10 Josh, Age 3, Has Advanced-Stage AIDS. His older brother died from AIDS. Their mother died of AIDS, leaving them as AIDS orphans. (*Photo by Mike Stocker/South Florida* Sun-Sentinel)

HIV-Infected Newborns Now Having Children—a Third Generation of HIV/AIDS in America

Michelle McConnell of the CDC said, "It's a landmark in the HIV epidemic at least in the United States. Survival has increased to such an extent that not only are HIV-infected babies surviving but they're healthy enough to reach their teen years, get pregnant, and have healthy kids." McConnell was referring to the eight women living in Puerto Rico who contracted HIV from their mothers and who reported 10 pregnancies between August 1998 and May 2002. Five of the eight became pregnant accidentally; only two reported using condoms when they conceived. None of the babies born to the women, all of whom were teenagers when they conceived, were infected with the virus. All the mothers had received antiretroviral AIDS drugs consistently during pregnancy. The data showed that some women in the study reported becoming sexually active at around the same age that they learned of their HIV-positive status. That finding could indicate that teens and young adults infected with HIV at birth are just as likely to engage in risky sex later in life as their peers who were not infected with the virus. It may also mean that the decision by many parents to shield their children from knowledge of HIV disease until later in adolescence may be too late. Since this report at least 15 similar cases have been reported by the CDC. In addition to these 23 cases, one has to consider the relatively large number of HIV-positive babies who have reached their teenage years and have become sexually active. As these numbers increase, the means of heterosexual/homosexual transmission increases among the young. Clearly, the use of highly active antiretroviral therapy is allowing an increasing number of young women who were born with HIV

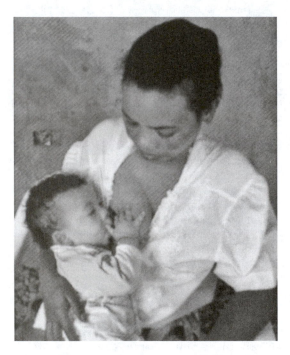

FIGURE 11-11 Drops of Danger. This woman nurses her 4-month-old son. She, her husband, and three other children have been diagnosed with AIDS. She did not know she could pass HIV to her newborn via breast-feeding. She said that her husband was her only sexual partner. After her health began to decline and she tested HIV positive, her husband refused to be tested and he abandoned the family for another woman. (*Photo by Hilda M. Perez/South Florida* Sun-Sentinel)

DISTURBING THOUGHTS

Much has been said over the past year, by politicians and the press, about getting cheap antiretroviral drugs into developing countries in order to extend lives and reduce the transmission of HIV from the HIV-infected mother into her infant. However, Karen Beckerman of San Francisco General Hospital (2002) says that treatment programs that use antiretrovirals to prevent mother-to-child transmission are likely to succeed only in creating a generation of orphans and ruining the treatment chances of mothers. Beckerman raised the question "Is it justifiable to visit the antiretroviral mistakes of the industrialized world on regions that have been devastated by the HIV epidemic but are at least antiretrovirally naïve?" She states that active deployment of AZT/3TC during delivery for millions of pregnancies may prevent hundreds of thousands of pediatric infections per year. However, these same women and their infected children exposed to short-course zidovudine plus lamivudine or single-dose nevirapine will be at substantial risk of treatment failure when antiretroviral therapy becomes available. Instead of inducing resistance to AIDS drug therapies, prophylaxis against mother-to-child transmission must be linked to preventing the creation of orphans.

SAVING THE ORPHANS, FOR WHAT?

On average, about 400,000 HIV-infected babies have been born each year over the past eight years. But, save these children for what? To become orphans who then become street urchins who are poorly fed, undisciplined, unsheltered, and uncared for? These children form gangs and add to the growing crime wave in all orphan-populated cities. About 30% of these orphans are HIV positive and require care they cannot get. They are left in already crowded hospitals and homes that offer little more than a place to die. Regardless of the town, city, or country's economic plight, the growing mass of orphans tends to further decrease the economy and care available to healthy adults and school-age children. It is not universally agreed that saving an infant born to an HIV-infected mother is a sensible use of public funds in poor countries. It has been written that President Mbeki of South Africa follows this reasoning. He believes the cost of drugs and care would ruin the economy of South Africa. He is not alone in his beliefs. The infant will be born into extremely difficult circumstances. Death is predicted at least for its mother and probably for its father. Should public dollars be invested in preventing infant deaths—an investment that will translate into a rising tide of orphans? In hard-hit countries such as Zimbabwe, Botswana, Malawi, Namibia, Swaziland, and South Africa, it is predicted that ending 2008, one in three children younger than 15 years will be orphaned. Currently, about 40% of South Africa's population of 47 million people are under the age of 15. A report from the 2002 International AIDS Conference from UNAIDS states that 50% of South African new mothers could die because of HIV, and that mortality among 15- to 34-year-olds will be 17 times higher because of AIDS.

African children infected and affected by HIV/AIDS are the ultimate development nightmare for a continent grappling with major socioeconomic problems. According to UNAIDS, every day about 1100 infants contract HIV through their mothers throughout the world. At least 95% of these infants are born in Africa. Every day, worldwide, 6000 children lose one or both parents to AIDS. More than 90% of these children are Africans. Today in Africa, 95% of pregnant mothers do not have access to health programs that can significantly reduce the incidence of mother-to-child transmission of HIV. But, the worst is yet to come. According to UNAIDS, UNICEF, and USAID, by 2010 at least 20 million of the global 25 million AIDS orphans will live in Africa. This is in a continent where children face the deadly combination of high rates of infant deaths, vaccine-preventable deaths, under 5 mortality, diarrhea-related deaths, and death from malaria. It is also a continent where children face major challenges of going to school, staying in school, eating nutritious meals, and having access to adequate sanitation.

DISCUSSION QUESTION: Take a stand, for or against saving the lives of some 40 million AIDS orphans who will populate the underdeveloped nations by year 2020. Support your presentation with facts, not just emotions. Answer the question, "Is the social cost of so many young people being raised without parental or adult guidance too high to tolerate?"

infection to live long enough to become sexually active and become pregnant.

Entering 2009, because of early access to care in the United States and advances in anti-HIV drug treatment, approximately half of all HIV-infected children will live to enter and graduate from high school and beyond. However, globally, less than 15% of the 2.5 million children in need of antiretroviral drugs are getting them. Without treatment, most of these children will die before their 5th birthday. Ninety percent of HIV children live in sub-Saharan Africa.

Summary

For over the past 27 years, HIV infection and its consequent disease, acquired immunodeficiency syndrome (AIDS), have affected more women worldwide than any other life-threatening infectious disease. Women account for about 50% of the 34 million people living with HIV. In sub-Saharan Africa, females now constitute 60% of those infected with HIV. Women make up half of the adults living with HIV in the Caribbean and one-third in Latin America. In addition to the direct impact that HIV infection has on these women, there is also the known high risk of HIV transmission to their infants and a resulting plethora of consequences for the family. In the United States, the annual number of estimated AIDS cases increased 18% among women and only 1% among men from 1999 to 2008. The major burden of disease was in young women and women of color, particularly black American and Hispanic women, who often have reduced access to health care. The rate of AIDS diagnoses for black American women is approximately 25 times the rate for white women and four times the rate for Hispanic women. The majority of infections were due to heterosexual transmission or to injecting-drug use. These same risk factors, especially injecting-drug use, have led to a 50% increase in infections in women in Asia and eastern Europe during the past four years. This growing feminization of the HIV pandemic reflects women's greater social and biological vulnerability.

The predominance of heterosexually acquired HIV infection in women of reproductive age has important implications for vertical HIV transmission to their offspring: Nearly 30% of children with AIDS were infected by mothers who acquired infection through heterosexual contact. One of the greatest tragedies of the AIDS pandemic is orphaned children. They are left in hospitals because (1) their parents have died of AIDS or cannot care for them, or (2) no one wants them.

The magnitude of the problems of children affected by HIV/AIDS dwarfs the scale of the existing response. Children and adolescents around the globe are increasingly at risk of infection, and many of those infected by HIV/AIDS are being left to grow up alone, grow up too soon, or to not grow up at all.

Review Questions

(Answers to the Review Questions are on pg. 429.)

1. By the end of year 2009 how many women are expected to be HIV positive worldwide?

2. Globally, what percent of *new* HIV infections occur in women?

3. What are the major routes of HIV transmission into women?

4. What is the most likely way a female prostitute in the United States becomes HIV infected?

5. During year 2009, how many women worldwide will have become HIV positive and how many will have died from AIDS?

6. AIDS is now the _____ cause of death for all women between ages _____ and _____. It is the _____ leading cause of death in _____ women between the ages of _____ and _____ and the _____ cause of death for black women ages _____ to _____.

7. Of the 4 million women who become pregnant each year in the United States, how many are estimated to be HIV positive?

8. Through year 2008, how many states have not reported a pediatric AIDS case?

9. Since 1995, what percentage per year of HIV-infected newborns received HIV from their mothers?

10. List three major factors that are associated with perinatal HIV transmission.

11. Where do most of the orphaned AIDS children come from? Why are they called AIDS orphans?

12. Globally, ending 2009, how many people are living with HIV/AIDS?

   A. 34 million
   B. 77 million
   C. 24 million
   D. 10 million

13. Of those living with AIDS, how many are women?

   A. 14 million
   B. 5 million
   C. 3 million
   D. 10 million

14. Women are about _____ as likely as men to contract an HIV infection from a single act of unprotected sex.

   A. half
   B. equally
   C. about twice
   D. three times

15. Studies have shown that in many parts of the world, including India, Kenya, Colombia, Zambia, and all of sub-Saharan Africa, _____ women are more at risk than are their _____ counterparts.

   A. married, unmarried
   B. unmarried, married

16. True or false: If you are HIV positive and pregnant, there are antiretroviral drugs you can take that can greatly decrease the chances of your baby becoming infected.

17. True or false: Women will not become HIV infected if they properly use birth control pills and/or diaphragm.

12 Prevalence of HIV Infection and AIDS Among Young Adults, Ages 13 to 24

CHAPTER CONCEPTS

- United States and global statistics on HIV infection in young adults.
- Over half of all new HIV infections globally occur in young adults.
- Only a fraction of HIV-infected young adults know they are infected.
- The vast majority of young adults have no access to the information, skills, and services needed to protect themselves from HIV infection.
- Seven of ten people are sexually active by age 19.
- The total number of HIV-infected teenagers/young adults is unknown.
- Black and Hispanic young adults account for a disproportionate number of AIDS cases compared to whites.
- Young adults are being exposed to quality HIV prevention but they choose to ignore it.
- Sex thrills but AIDS kills.
- HIV babies reaching adulthood.
- Abstinence education: Saying no over and over again.
- Worldwide, people ages 13 to 24 account for about 50% of all new HIV infections.
- In the 20 highest HIV-prevalence countries, less than one-third of young adults have sufficient knowledge to prevent HIV infection.
- Young adults make up about 23% of the U.S. population and about 4% of AIDS cases.
- Heterosexual sexual transmission is the leading cause of HIV infection in young adults.
- Young adult-specific behaviors and biologic factors make them particularly vulnerable to unsafe sexual practices.
- In the U.S. about 3 young adults per hour become HIV infected.
- Substance abuse is a risk factor for HIV infection in young adults.
- About 60% of new HIV infections among U.S. women occurs in those between ages 13 to 24.

GLOBAL HIV INFECTIONS IN YOUNG ADULTS

Global Youth AIDS Day, February 26. A Movement By Youth to Bring an End to AIDS

Over the summer of 1999, especially in the United States, young people ages 13 to 24, flocked to theaters to experience the **Dark Side of the Force.** Many thousands saw the STAR WARS movie repeatedly. But the real **Dark Side** of their lives is the threat of HIV infection and the **Force** should be their education to prevent their infection.

Over half of all new HIV infections worldwide are occurring in this age group. Hopefully, reading this chapter will encourage the young to stay on the **Light Side with the Force.**

The Spread of HIV in Young Adults (Ages 13 to 24)

There is no shortage of statistics indicating that young adults continue to be the most vulnerable group of individuals to HIV infection. Every year since 2002, about 50% of all new infections in the United States occurred among young adults. In the United States it comes to about 27,000 new infections, or three infections every hour. About two-thirds contracted HIV sexually, and in the U.S. three-quarters of them occurred in racial and ethnic minorities. Some global statistics on young adults and HIV/AIDS are:

- Of 35 million people living with HIV/AIDS ending year 2009, over a third will be young adults (11.7 million).
- Every day about 3600 young adults become infected with HIV, or about 1.3 million a year.
- Only a fraction of HIV-infected young adults are aware of their infection, and even a smaller number are linked to proper medical care or social services.
- Of young adults who become HIV infected, most are infected by age 24 and usually die of AIDS by age 35.
- In the United States, young adults make up about 20% of all HIV infections (about 380,000 infections through 2009).
- Most young people with HIV/AIDS were infected sexually.
- Only 19% of teens ages 15 to 19 report that they have ever been tested for HIV, versus 44% of young adults ages 20 to 24.
- Many young people do not know some basic facts about HIV risk, prevention, and treatment. Over one-third (37%) of 18- to 25-year olds incorrectly believe at least one of the following, or do not know that they are all false: transmission of HIV is possible by sharing a glass, kissing, or touching a toilet seat.
- The median age at first intercourse is 16.9 years for boys and 17.4 years for girls. There are differences in age of initiation by race and ethnicity, with 27% of African American high school boys, 11% of Latino boys, and 5% of white boys initiating sex before age 13.
- Over half of males (55%) and females (54%) ages 15 to 19 report having had oral sex with someone of the opposite sex. Approximately one in ten males and females ages 15 to 19 had engaged in anal sex with someone of the opposite sex; 3% of males ages 15 to 19 have had anal sex.

ADDRESSING THE AIDS PANDEMIC AMONG YOUNG ADULTS

Young adults are central to any discussion of HIV/AIDS because there are so many! There are about 2 billion people ages 13 to 24 in the world. Young adults are and will continue to be the sector of the population most affected by HIV/AIDS. As today's children grow up, the proportion of 13- to 24-year-olds will continue to increase, particularly in developing countries (Table 12-1 and Figure 12-1).

United Nations Commitment to Young Adults

In order to reduce the size and impact of the AIDS pandemic on young adults worldwide, in 2004 the United Nations General Assembly Special Session on

Table 12-1 Young People, Ages 13–24, Living with HIV/AIDS by Region, End of 2009

Region	Number	Percent of Global Total
Global Total	**11,700,000**	**100%**
Sub-Saharan Africa	7,254,000	62%
South/Southeast Asia	2,106,000	18%
Eastern Europe/Central Asia	737,100	6.3%
Latin America	713,700	6.1%
East Asia	397,800	3.4%
Caribbean	152,100	1.3%
North America	152,100	1.3%
North Africa/Middle East	140,400	1.2%
Western Europe	46,800	0.4%
Oceania	9,360	0.08%

(Source: UNAIDS 2005 Updated)

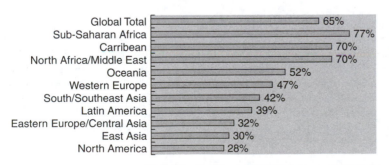

Region	Percentage
Global Total	65%
Sub-Saharan Africa	77%
Carribean	70%
North Africa/Middle East	70%
Oceania	52%
Western Europe	47%
South/Southeast Asia	42%
Latin America	39%
Eastern Europe/Central Asia	32%
East Asia	30%
North America	28%

FIGURE 12-1 Estimated Young Adult Women as a Percentage of All Ages 13–24 with HIV/AIDS Ending Year 2009. *(Source: UNAIDS 2005 Updated)*

HIV/AIDS produced a "Declaration of Commitment on HIV/AIDS: Global Targets & Principles for Young People." This declaration is as follows:
By 2005—

1. Reduce HIV prevalence among youth ages 15 to 25 in the most affected countries by 25%; by 2010, reduce global HIV prevalence among this age group by 25% (Article 47).

2. Ensure that at least 90% of youth ages 15 to 24 have access to the information, education, including peer education and youth-specific HIV education, and services necessary to develop the life skills required to reduce their vulnerability to HIV infection; ensure at least 95% access by 2010 (Article 53).

3. Ensure access of both girls and boys to primary and secondary education, including HIV/AIDS education (Article 63).

4. Ensure safe and secure environments, especially for young girls (Article 63).

5. Expand good quality youth-friendly information and sexual health education and counseling service (Article 63).

6. Involve young people in planning, implementing, and evaluating HIV/AIDS prevention and care programs (Article 63).

RESULTS—Steps 1–4 failed and steps 5–6 were marginally implemented.

Why the High HIV Infection Rates Among Young Adults?

Of the world's young adults, 85% live in developing countries, and this is where over 90% of the pandemic is now concentrated. But population percentages tell only part of the story. There are special reasons why young people are exposed to infection. Remember that above all HIV is a sexually transmitted virus. Being a young adult is a time of discovery, emerging feelings of independence, and the explo-

ration of new behavior and relationships. It is also a time of examination, rebellion, and change. By definition young people take risks and experiment. Sexual behavior, an important part of this, can involve risks; the same is true of experimentation with drugs. During this time, young people get mixed messages. They are often faced with double standards calling for virginity in girls but early and active sexual behavior in boys. They have been told **"Just say no"** since the early 1980s, yet risk taking continues, perhaps because they are confronted with hundreds of millions of dollars worth of media images of sex, smoking, and drinking as glamorous and risk-free. They are told to be abstinent, but exposed to a barrage of advertisements using sex to sell goods. Compounding the challenge, in the name of morality, culture, or religion, young people are often denied their right to education about the health risks of sexual behavior, and to important tools and services for protection. Among the world's young adults, some are more exposed to HIV than others. Those living in what UNICEF terms "especially difficult circumstances" include young people who are out of school, who live on the streets, who share needles with other injecting-drug users, engage in commercial sex, or are sexually and physically abused. Young men who have sex with men are disadvantaged by the lack of information and services available to them and directed to their needs.

As the HIV/AIDS pandemic spreads, even younger age groups are becoming exposed to the risk of HIV. Infection spreads to younger age groups as men choose increasingly younger sexual partners. Many men believe, perhaps correctly, that younger girls are less likely to be infected with HIV, while others hold the mistaken belief that having sex with a virgin can cure AIDS.

HOW LARGE IS THE YOUNG ADULT POPULATION IN THE UNITED STATES?

In the United States there are about 43 million young adults (73% white, 11% black, 16% Hispanic), and about 22 million between the ages of 25 and 29. That's 65 million or about 21% of the population between the ages of 13 and 29. Over 86 percent of all STDs occur in this age group. It has been estimated that about 40% of all heterosexual adults with AIDS were infected with HIV as young adults.

Young Adult Women at Greatest Risk for HIV/AIDS in the United States

In the United States, 50% of all new HIV infections occur in young people between the ages of 13 and 24. While more research needs to be done on this topic, several factors associated with young women are clear: (1) they tend to be partnered with **older men** who have had more sexual partners and have a greater chance of being infected with HIV and other sexually transmitted diseases; (2) their risk of HIV infection is greater because of their immature cervix and relatively low vaginal mucous production presents less of a barrier to HIV; (3) many lack the education, social status, economic resources, and power in sexual partner relationships to make informed choices; (4) A 2003 Kaiser Family Foundation study of young adults showed that one in four contract a sexually transmitted disease annually. And 70% of women ages 13 to 24 consider forms of contraception other than condoms, such as birth control pills, to be a form of "safer sex."

Lets Talk About Sex: Safer Sex: Sex Thrills but AIDS Kills

There was a time when safer sex meant not getting caught by your parents. With time, sexually transmitted diseases and in particular HIV/AIDS have changed the meaning of safer sex. Today, over half of teenagers (ages 13 to 19) in the United States have had sex by the time they reach 16, and 7 in 10 are sexually active by 19. Many enter the sexual arena unprepared for the responsibility of their actions. About 1 million teenage women become pregnant outside of marriage each year.

Whether or not society openly discusses it, young adults are having sex. Many women—and most men—have their first sexual relations prior to marriage, usually during their teens, and most often those first encounters are unprotected. Research in family planning has revealed that the quality of reproductive health information is generally low among young adults. This is a reflection in part of the lack of social acceptance of providing sex education and contraceptive services to teens in many countries. In the developing world, contraceptive services are often available only to married women, and in some situations, only to women who have already borne one or more children.

The guiding philosophy in dealing with sexuality in many cultures is **"If you don't talk about sex they won't do it."** This logic, however, is critically flawed. Young adults are sexual beings at varying stages of self-awareness and understanding. Many teenagers continue to engage in sexual intercourse despite lack of access to any accurate information about sex and, in most cases, they engage in unsafe sex. **Safer sex requires an ability to distinguish between risky and nonrisky sexual activities and the emotional security to choose safer sex.**

Young Adults, Sexual Partners, and Sexually Transmitted Diseases and HIV/AIDS

In a CDC nationwide survey reported on in 2008, 19% of high school students have had four or more sex partners by their junior year and 29% had four or more by their senior year (*MMWR,* 1992). They are experiencing skyrocketing rates of sexually transmitted diseases. The CDC survey, released in March 2008, reported that half of black women ages 13 to 19 had an STD, compared to 20% of Hispanics and 20% of whites. Every minute about 21 young adults somewhere in the United States become infected with an STD. People under age 25 account for 66% of all new STDs every year. One in four young adults will contract an STD before finishing high school. Experts fear that if these diseases are being transmitted, then HIV is too. Entering 2009, among ages 13 to 24 or young adults, heterosexual transmission accounted for about half of all HIV infections in the United States. Among males, about 60% of infections occurred among men having sex with men (MSM).

AIDS cases are relatively rare among 13- to 19-year-olds. This is because of the 11-year time average from HIV infection to AIDS diagnosis. In 1981, there was one reported teenage AIDS case; by 1991 there were 789 reported AIDS cases. Ending 2009, there will be an estimated 26000 (2% of the total AIDS cases). (See Snapshot 8.2 for insight on young adults' view of oral sex.)

HIV/AIDS WON'T AFFECT US!

It is estimated that at least two young adults per hour become HIV infected. Regardless of available information on prevention, meaning that they do know how HIV is transmitted, there has been a

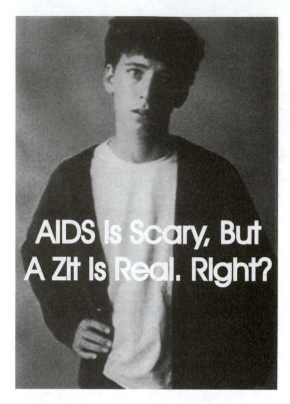

FIGURE 12–2 In the Life of a Young Adult, Items of Importance May Change Rapidly. *(Courtesy of the Center for Disease Control and Prevention, Atlanta)*

continuing increase in HIV infections. They continue to engage in sexual intercourse without condoms (Figure 12-2).

Two groups, young adult gay men and young adult women infected via heterosexual sex, account for about 75% of young adult HIV infections. Race is an important factor with regard to who becomes infected. Sixty-one percent of AIDS cases that occur in people ages 20 to 24 occur in blacks and Latinos, but they were HIV infected in their teens (Collins et al., 1997).

ESTIMATE OF HIV-INFECTED AND AIDS CASES AMONG YOUNG ADULTS IN THE UNITED STATES

The total number of HIV-infected young adults is unknown. **Federal health agencies estimate that they make up about 20% or 380,000 of the HIV-infected population.** They are a silent pool for eventual cases of AIDS. About 50% of HIV-infected young adults come from seven locations: New York, New Jersey, Texas, California, Florida, Washington D.C., and Puerto Rico. The male-to-female ratio of AIDS cases in the United States among 13- to 19-year-olds is about 1:1.

Sixty percent of new HIV infections in women now occur between ages 13 and 24.

Young Adults: Is the Fear of HIV/AIDS Being Lost?

This generation of young adults has not been subjected to AIDS activists' marches, disruptions, newspaper headlines and TV programs showing the earlier years of people with AIDS and their ghostly appearances. In addition, because of the success of antiretroviral drug therapy, this generation of young adults has been spared the many gruesome details of AIDS patients and their stories. Together this may mean young adults are losing their fear of HIV/AIDS. Here are some recent comments made by some young adults in the United States:

1. We call it "three to six sex." This means having sex after school and before our parents come home. Question: Are condoms being used? Answer: No, duh, not really! Are you worried about HIV? Who cares?
2. A 16-year-old said, "I'm, like, terrified of getting pregnant. But I don't think anybody thinks about AIDS."
3. From a 15-year-old, "I've only had sex with one person so I don't have to worry about AIDS."
4. A 15-year-old boy who doesn't use protection says he's not afraid of getting infected with the deadly virus because "most people get it from drugs. And I don't use heroin."

The bottom line is health officials and activists say that lots of kids are having lots of sex and might not be hearing the safe sex message because it isn't stressed in school.

Young Adults and Incidence of AIDS Cases and HIV by Gender and Color

Entering 1999, for the first time, more females than males ages 13 to 19 were reported as AIDS cases. Ending 2009, of about 56,000 AIDS cases among ages 13 to 24 years, about 65% were black, 20% were Hispanic and 15% were white. About 30,000 are living with AIDS.

TEACH YOUR CHILDREN WELL
BY REGAN HOFMANN—HIV POSITIVE (FIGURE 12-3)

I never had proper sex ed. There was some reference to genitalia in my eighth grade health class: our teacher brandished rubber devices that showed, in 3-D, where children grew inside women's bellies and how liquids were transported from the inside to the outside of a man. But the creepy crash test-dummy-pink models hardly addressed what we really needed to know, like how to ask partners about their health status or how to put on—and take off—a condom. I left the classroom more confused than I had entered it. I wonder if that wasn't the idea—to scare us off sex altogether. Those frightening rubbery forms were as effective a form of birth control as a screaming baby.

I had perfunctory conversations with my mom and dad years after I first needed to know the ins and

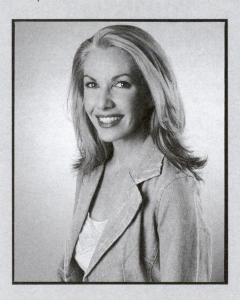

FIGURE 12-3   Regan Hofmann. She lived with her HIV-positive status for almost 10 years. She broke her silence and released that fear in April of 2006. On announcing her HIV status, she became editor-in-chief of *POZ magazine*.* Regan said that her "desire to remain silent was huge. I liked the feeling of being treated like a perfectly healthy person. As with many difficult things, it's easier to turn away from the truth of HIV than it is to face it. But looking it square in the eye is the first step in beating it. I took that first, large, step." Since her HIV diagnosis in 1996 she has taken over 50,000 pills.

POZ magazine's mission is to educate people with HIV to take responsibility for their health. Founded in 1994 by people living with AIDS (PLWA) to promote the vision that surviving AIDS is possible.

outs of my body and how to protect it. I didn't want to admit that I wasn't a virgin; they didn't want to hear it. As for my younger sister, I tried to be a role model and discourage her from having sex for as long as possible. Which meant that the first real conversation we had about it was after her child was born. And my friends? Our conversations have always lacked sufficient specifics to be of any help. It's always, "Did you or didn't you?" and never, "How did you and were you safe?"

In America, for all our obsession with lascivious, prurient pleasures, we are terrified to talk frankly and specifically about sex. It is not a topic of polite conversation and if you ask people even basic questions they squirm and sidestep. We let ourselves and our kids watch—on TV and the internet—people having all sorts of sex but we can't seem to talk about having safer sex. Why are we in denial?

I admit that it makes me a little uncomfortable to think of a 12- or 13-year-old having sex, as nearly 10% of that age group does. But if they're going to do it, shouldn't we teach them how to do it without life-long or life-threatening consequences? I'm not against abstinence; it's a great form of birth control and disease prevention—if you can keep people from having sex. But apparently, we can't. In fact, the less we talk about sex directly and the more we pretend that we don't have it, the more we elevate what is otherwise a simple fact of life into a forbidden fruit that hangs so heavy and juicy on the tree that no one can resist trying it.

I had what many would consider a really good education. Yet when I graduated from college, I couldn't cook, change a tire, or keep myself from contracting a sexual disease that might kill me. I am astounded that as HIV infection rates continue to rise among teenagers, our educational system, our government and our families continue to let our kids learn lessons the hard way. It's obvious that abstinence-only sex ed isn't working and that we desperately need to talk to America's youth openly and truthfully about an epidemic they know little about. I'm not into scare tactics, but today's kids are not afraid enough of HIV—too many of them perceive it as a manageable chronic illness that can be combated with a couple of pills a day. Maybe we've done too good a job educating them about how HIV can be treated and not a good enough job educating them about the difficulties of living with HIV. Maybe it's time to bust out those rubber forms again—and have a little talk.

(Reprinted with permission from *POZ Magazine*, January 2007. Copyright 2007 CDM Publishing, L.L.C.)

SHORT-TERM YOUNG ADULT RELATIONSHIPS AND HIV EXPOSURE RISK

Hey! We are celebrating our second anniversary. Yeah? Yeah, we've been together for two weeks. Let's have sex. Sure, they're monogamous, but only for the six weeks that the relationship lasts! Then they move on to others. In some cases such behavior can create a chain of relationships wherein each sexual partner exposes the other to whatever previous sexual partners may have had. For example, sociologists at Ohio State University have created the first "map" of young adult sexual behavior, outlining a sexual network of 288 one-to-one sexual relationships among high school students. While the teen at the end of the chain may have had contact with only one person, he or she had indirect contact with 286 others. Even so, despite reputations and popularity, most of the young adults were not promiscuous. They might know that their partner had a previous partner. But they don't think about the fact that this partner had a previous partner, who had a partner, and so on. This study suggests that young people need a different approach to sexual education and especially on HIV and STD prevention. The study was conducted at a high school in a mid-size town in the U.S. Midwest. The exact location was not given (Figure 12-4).

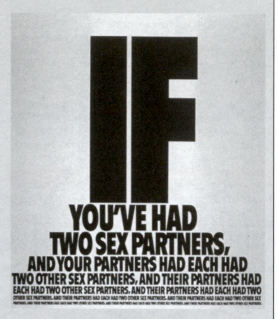

FIGURE 12-4 (*Courtesy of the Texas Department of State Health Services*)

Among males, whites account for 38% of reported AIDS cases, followed by blacks (39%) and Hispanics (21%). Among females, blacks account for 66%, white for 17%, and Hispanic for 17%. These females, unlike their adult counterparts, are more likely to become infected with HIV through sexual exposure than through injection-drug use. A program that followed a large group of HIV-infected young adults found that although 85% of females contracted HIV infection through heterosexual intercourse, very few were aware that their male partners had HIV infection at the time of their exposure (Futterman et al., 1992).

Runaway Young Adults

Each year since 1993, an estimated 3.4 million young adults dropped out of high school. These dropouts have higher frequencies of behaviors that put them at risk for HIV/STDs, and are less accessible to prevention efforts.

If you are a young adult or know of one who needs help or has HIV/AIDS questions, call:

National Teenagers AIDS Hotline: 1-800-234-8336.

Adolescent AIDS Program: Montefiore Medical Center, 111 E. 210th St., Bronx, NY 10467; 1-718-882-0023.

AIDS Community Alliance: Works with HIV-positive and HIV-affected individuals. 44 North Queens St., Lancaster, PA 17603; 1-717-394-3380.

Bay Area Young Positive: Youth-run, offers counseling, resources, newsletter. 518 Waller St., San Francisco, CA 94117; 1-415-487-1616; email: BAYPOZ@aol.com.

HIV-INFECTED CHILDREN: LIVING LONGER—PAYING A PRICE

HIV Babies Reaching Adulthood—Many Have To Live With Their Secret

AIDS, in America, is the seventh-leading cause of death in 15- to 24-year-olds.

Adolescents infected with HIV since birth are a new population in the ever-changing HIV/AIDS pandemic. Data from the CDC show that before 1996, HIV-infected children lived to an average age of 9. After 1996, with the use of antiretroviral drugs, the average age has risen to 18 and continues to climb.

Six years ago, an estimated three children died each week of AIDS at Detroit's Children's Hospital. Today, that rate has dropped to about one child per year. But as the children's life expectancy increases, so do the number of complex social issues they must face, especially as young adults. One mother of an HIV-positive child said she dreads the issue of dating because it's going to be emotionally crippling. "Unless current attitudes about those infected with HIV change, my daughter will not be very popular and that will hurt. It will just crush her." The parents have had their car tires flattened and parents of classmates forbade their children from playing with her. In response to these issues and new issues such as dating, the hospital has hired social workers and psychologists to hold support groups for these children, bringing them together to help them understand they aren't alone.

COMING OUT FOR AN "AIDS BABY": A SHORT STORY

If ever there was a time to tell her big secret, this was it, the seventh-grader thought. She and a few friends at a sleepover birthday party have sequestered themselves in a storage closet under a basement stairwell. They sat in a circle and talked for hours, promising, "Whatever we say here stays here." One girl shared her fear that her parents were on the verge of divorce. Another said she felt pressure to live up to her brother's example. There was a silence for a moment. Then the girl who had kept quiet for so many years took a deep breath and blurted a few quick words: "I have something to say. I'm HIV positive." Her friends took the news in stride. Until then, her friends had simply known her as their fun-loving buddy, the honors student, the girl with sarcastic wit who was as likely to use a big word they didn't understand as to address her friends as "dude." Now her friends knew something more: she was born an "AIDS baby," a term only vaguely familiar to most people her age. Three years after her disclosure, she reflects and strongly feels that she did the right thing. Coming out for these children is a complicated and terrifying task.

FEDERAL PUBLIC HEALTH POLICY SUPPORTS ABSTINENCE-ONLY PROGRAM: SEX EDUCATION

Abstinence is but one of the three approaches offered to lower the rate of HIV infection. The three approaches are A—abstinence, B—be faithful and C—if not operating in the A or B mode, use a condom.

ABC Is Not as Simple as It Sounds

One only has to look in African villages and communities to understand how these "ABC" prescriptions confuse people. One is talking ABC to about 54 countries in Africa, with different prevalence of HIV infection, different numbers of cases, and different religious beliefs. Obviously there will be thousands of understandings and interpretations of ABC. The health minister of Uganda said, "Even in the same individual, in the morning you are in mode A, by evening in mode B, and by night, after a drink, in mode C." Some religious groups believe the C is for those condemned for not being A.

In addition, proponents of ABC offer many one-liner slogans at people pretending to solve very com-plicated, deeply personal and sensitive issues in a way that is, to many, offensive.

DISCUSSION QUESTION: Do you believe that A, B campaigns protect women? Married women? Your position and reasons are:

Getting the right balance between each of the ABCs has led to unproductive disputes, which is why abstinence may be the hottest topic in HIV prevention. It raises temperatures among personal responsibility advocates and religious conservatives on the one hand, who believe people can and should just say no, and among sex-positive activists on the other, who believe any discussion of abstinence, even as an individual choice, is sex-negative.

Defining Abstinence Is Difficult!

One difficulty in measuring the efficacy or effectiveness of sex education programs lies in the conflicting definitions of the term abstinence. For example, some studies define abstinence as totally refraining from all sexual acts outside of marriage (including masturbation) and some link it to moral or religious beliefs. Other studies define abstinence as refraining from vaginal, anal, and oral sex. By some definitions, young adults who have experienced their first sexual encounter can become abstinent by refraining from further sexual activity; but by other definitions they cannot alternate back and forth. Everyone involved in this debate agrees on one fact: delaying the onset of a sexual experience in young adults is a good idea, at least in theory. Abstaining from sexual activity, that is, vaginal, anal, and oral sex, is 100% effective as a means for preventing sexually transmitted diseases (STDs), including HIV. For most people, however, abstinence is a temporary goal that may reflect current life circumstances, including being young, being between relationships, or waiting for an STD to heal. It remains effective in preventing HIV, STDs, and pregnancy only if it is applied consistently.

Abstinence Education: Saying No Over and Over Again

Abstinence education seems to reflect an all-or-nothing ideology; in the same way that a person cannot be a little pregnant or partially HIV positive, he or she cannot be sometimes abstinent. Although most parents are not eager for their children to become sexually active, there is much disagreement about how exactly to persuade young people to wait. Asking people to stop having sex may sound good, à la abstinence, but has it ever worked? It is not working now!

IN ONE LESSON—NO SEX!

When it comes to young adults and sex, abstinence forces say the message is simple—don't do it. The other side says give them all the facts—including how to use a condom. No wonder parents and their children are confused.

Imagine This! Jenny, a cartoon teenage virgin, is about to give in to her boyfriend and climb into the backseat of his car. Suddenly, the emergency brake gives out and his car rolls until it teeters from a cliff off lover's lane. Their lives hang in the balance. That is when Windy, the good witch in hightops, leaps to the rescue. "Paul loves me," Jenny protests. Windy asks, "Oh. Is that why he asked you to do something that could mess up your life forever?" Using her time machine, Windy shows Jenny how she would have awakened pregnant. Had the car's brake not failed her boyfriend's condom would have. The cartoon, shown to sixth-graders at Burbank Elementary School, is one weapon in an arsenal of films, celebrity rallies, and school classes pushing a message of chastity in classrooms around the nation.

Federal and State Dollars for Abstinence-Only Education

Federal support for abstinence-only education began in 1982 with an allocation of $4 million per year through 1996. In 1996, Congress passed the Welfare Reform Act, which set aside $50 million a year for abstinence education to begin in fiscal year 1998. The $50 million per year ran with updated legislation through 2007. States had to provide three matching dollars for every four federal dollars received. This boosted the total funding to $87.5 million per year. States had to assure that the abstinence funded programs "did not promote contraception and/or condom use." Through year 2006, the money was provided to promote abstinence for those ages 12 through 18. In 2007, the targeted population was redefined to include adolescents and/or adults ages 12 through 29. In 2008, 28 states and three U.S. territories accepted abstinence funding. For 2008 and 2009, former President Bush asked for but was denied an additional $27.7 million increase for each year in federal/state funding. To date, over $1.5 billion in federal and state funding has been spent on abstinence-only education.

This federal program specifically requires funded programs to teach the social, psychological, and health gains to be realized by abstaining from sex; that abstaining from sexual activity outside marriage is the expected standard for all school-age adolescents; that a mutually faithful monogamous relationship in the context of marriage is the expected standard of human sexual activity; and that **abstaining from sexual activity is the only certain way to avoid pregnancy, STDs, and other associated health problems.**

Abstinence or Safer Sex

Clearly there are numerous health, economic, and social benefits in delaying sexual onset in young adults, like disease prevention, but scientists say they **cannot** identify a long-term advantage to abstinence programs relative to safer sex programs.

Prevention Messages on Sexual Activity That Young Adults Should Hear?

Perhaps young people should receive two messages: one, promoting abstinence and the delay of sexual activity, the other, warning against high-risk behaviors and teaching them how to protect themselves. These messages are not contradictory, but they are complex. "Don't drink, but if you drink, don't drive" is a similar complex message that has saved many people from death on highways. Prevention scientists offer significant evidence that safer-sex interventions work. But there is no clear and compelling evidence that abstinence-only programs work (DiClemente, 1998).

The work of John Jemmott and colleagues (1998) and Douglas Kirby and colleagues (1997) demonstrate that for those adolescents that were sexually experienced at the beginning of their study, there was no difference in the proportion of the adolescents in the abstinence program relative to those in a safer-sex program with regard to having sexual intercourse. For those not sexually experienced, abstinence education was effective for a short time (three months). After 12 months the adolescents in the two groups were each as likely to become sexually active and were similar in their pregnancy and sexually transmitted disease rates.

The Risk of Abstinence-Only Education

Many critics of abstinence-only education agree that abstinence would be an ideal solution to the increase of new HIV infections among young adults. However, abstinence-only education does not seem to achieve the goal of reducing unsafe sexual activity and may actually lead to increased risk for HIV transmission. Surveys of sexuality conclude that with or without abstinence education, most young adults will be sexually active prior to the age of 18 and prior to marriage. A Harvard University study report (2006) found that 52% of surveyed young adults had sex within of one year of signing a virginity pledge. Of 14,000 surveyed, ages 12 to 18, 73% denied having taken the pledge. Researchers at Columbia University found that while a number of virginity pledge programs did help delay the onset of sexual activity for some, those who broke the pledge were less likely to use contraceptives once they became sexually active (Witkin et al., 2003).

The danger of abstinence-only education is revealed when youth begin engaging in sexual activity without the knowledge of safer sex choices to guide their behaviors. Surveys conducted by the Kaiser Family Foundation found that students who have received sex education feel better prepared and better informed to handle sexual situations than do those who do not receive sex education (Marks, 2003).

Young Adults' Perception of Abstinence

A 2001 Alan Guttmacher Institute survey revealed that young adults ages 15 to 19 considered oral sex to be a substitute for sex. They believe that oral sex is risk-free! In addition to this survey are the data from other public healthcare workers who have found that young people believe that neither anal nor oral sex places them at risk and that these activities maintain their virginity! In 2002 the Henry J. Kaiser Family Foundation with *Seventeen* magazine published the results of a teen survey on oral sexual behavior. The results were 23% of students questioned in 7th through 12th grade said they have had oral sex. In 11th and 12th grade the num-

ber increased to 42%. Thirty percent didn't know that a boy or girl could become infected with HIV by having oral sex. In a 2003 survey at Northern Kentucky University, of 600 young adults who took the abstinence pledge, 61% broke that pledge within a year. Of the 39% who did not break that pledge, over half had oral sex! One in three public schools nationwide teaches an abstinence-only curriculum that forbids talking about oral sex or safer sex. Clearly some of the students who are getting the abstinence-only message believe that they are engaging in abstinent behavior when they are having oral sex. In defense of these young people it can be said that health educators themselves are no more clear. And why not? In 1998, President Clinton, in testimony about an affair with a White House intern said, with great sincerity, that he had not had "sexual relations" but had engaged only in oral sex!

There are now about 1000 abstinence-only sex education programs in the United States. About 5000 school districts out of 17,468 teach abstinence as a part of their sex education programs.

In their April 2007 report written by independent researchers (Mathematica Policy Research, under contract to the Department of Health and Human Services), they state that there is no evidence that abstinence-only programs prevent young adult sex, pregnancy, or disease. The Mathematica Policy Research firm found, following 2000 elementary and middle school students, that in four communities that received abstinence instruction—sometimes on a daily basis—they were just as likely to have sex in the following years as students who did not get such instruction. Those who became sexually active—about half of each group—started at the same age (14.9 years on average) and had the same number of sexual partners. Of those who were sexually active, almost half said they used condoms only "sometimes" or "never." Less than a quarter of teens in both groups reported using a condom every time they had sex. Students in both groups were knowledgeable about the risks of having sex without using a condom or other means of protection. More than a third of all of the sexually active teens reported having had two or more partners. Despite claims by advocates, no reliable evidence exists on whether the programs work. Most studies of abstinence education programs have methodological flaws that prevent them from generating reliable estimates of program impacts.

ARE THE FEDERAL GUIDELINES GOVERNING ABSTINENCE-ONLY PROGRAMS IN TOUCH WITH REALITY?

In the ideal world, abstinence could be 100% effective in preventing STDs including HIV infection. The problem is in the practicing, not in the preaching! (See comments from the Mathematica Policy information.) In the April 2007 report, 95% of the U.S. population have premarital sex. James Wagoner, president of the Washington-based sex education group Advocates for Youth said, "To be preaching abstinence when 90% of people are having sex is in essence to lose touch with reality. It's an ideological campaign. It has nothing to do with public health. They've stepped over the line of common sense." Wade Horn, assistant secretary for the Administration for Children and Families at the Department of Health and Human Services said, "The guidelines merely clarify that people ages 12-29 can be targeted by abstinence-only programs. In addition, the move is a response to government data released last year showing 998,262 births to unmarried women ages 19-29. The message is "It's better to wait until you're married to bear or father children. The only 100% effective way of getting there is abstinence."

Clearly, abstinence is a topic fraught with dueling statistics and conflicting evidence as to whether abstinence education works in America. However, President George Bush's Emergency Program for AIDS Relief (PEPFAR, see Chapter 14 for further details on this program), which now gives $50 billion over the next five years, most of it to 15 developing nations, stipulates that 33% of that money must go to pro-abstinence programs that teach abstinence before marriage and fidelity.

In the 15 PEPFAR nations, as well as in most, if not all, developing nations, abstinence may only be feasible for those who can afford the practice. For example, abstinence is meaningless to many millions of women who are coerced into sex. Faithfulness offers little protection to millions of wives whose husbands have several partners or were infected before marriage. And condoms require the cooperation of men! Perhaps the answer to making abstinence work anywhere lies in the economic and cultural empowerment of women.

DISCUSSION QUESTION: Is it good science, poor politics, or poor science and good politics, or some other combination of events that made it logical for the federal government to earmark tax dollars specifically for abstinence-only educational programs? Do you sense a religious involvement in the government policy? Explain.

DISCUSSION QUESTION: In his book, "At the Center of the Storm," former director of the CIA, George Tenet, said, "Policymakers are entitled to their own opinions—but not to their own sets of facts." Do you see a relationship between this quote and the ongoing debate on abstinence? Explain.

SIDEBAR 12.1

CAN LIFE GET WORSE THAN BEING YOUNG, HOMELESS, AND DYING OF AIDS?

Survival Is Their Freedom?
Regardless of cause, to have AIDS and nowhere to go, no one to help, and no one who cares about you means that one has hit the bottom rung of life. Many young people are there now! There are 15,000 to 20,000 young homeless people just in New York City. About 40% of them sell themselves in order to survive. Too many are becoming HIV infected because of the demands of their lifestyle.

Case 1. In the 10th grade he was kicked out of his home—over time he meandered to San Francisco's tenderloin area. He began working as a street prostitute and injecting drugs. **He wanted to become HIV infected.** He said he actually cried when he tested HIV negative. At age 19 he tested positive. This time he cried because he now recognized the mistakes he made along the way. He had no money, no job skills, and no friends. Once, near death he said he had an epiphany (a sudden realization). He went to a clinic, received job training, gave up drugs, got a job and said, "I really want to live!"

Case 2. Her history begins in a North Carolina group home. She left and drifted to Georgia where she believes she became infected from a man who gave her $300 to have unprotected sex. She said she was a night child— she went to night clubs and adult bookstores to pick up her tricks. By her twenty-first birthday she said she was ready to jump off the Golden Gate Bridge—if she could find it. After finding help at a clinic she is now preparing to take her GED (graduate equivalence degree).

Case 3. He was raped by the son of his foster parents. His life was spent in a series of Milwaukee foster homes. He became HIV positive at age 13. He found his way to San Francisco. He said "I felt I would be accepted there, it's a city that understood AIDS and the people that have it." He goes to a clinic that services 3000 other young homeless people. He believes he has been sentenced to death. He has not been able to become comfortable with his HIV status. (Adapted from Russell Sabin, *San Francisco Chronicle*, Oct. 18, 1998.)

Homeless and on the Street in Russia
St. Petersburg is the second-largest city in Russia. Of the young people ages 15 to 19 living on St. Petersburg streets, 37% are HIV positive! About 70% of them are male. About 66% of these young people have lost both parents to AIDS and are themselves HIV positive. These numbers exceed the prevalence of HIV infection in Africa!

THOUGHTS AND COMMENTS FROM A GENERATION AT RISK

"I was only 13 when I started having sex. I knew what AIDS was, and how you get it, but I was more worried about something else: getting pregnant. In fact, it was a visit to the health department to get birth control injections in January 2002 that I discovered I had HIV. I couldn't believe it, the disease I read about in health class and heard about on television and in movies was now a part of my life. I never thought it would happen to me. Now at age 16, I am back in school and take anti-AIDS drugs twice daily. I still have sex, I don't tell my boyfriends, but I make them use a condom.—**From Virginia**

I became HIV infected at the same time I lost my virginity—at age 16. My 28-year-old boyfriend was an injection-drug user. He knew he was HIV positive but did not tell me. He has since died of AIDS. At 16 my only concern was pregnancy, so I took the pill and had unsafe sex. Living in Spain does not help either as the HIV infected are discriminated against—so be careful out there.—**A message from Spain**

"If you're going to educate kids about AIDS, you have to educate them about drugs as well. If you're a youth, you're going to experiment with drugs, especially if you live in a metropolitan area. Even though you get stupid with drugs, you still think about things you don't want to do, but you do it anyhow."—**16-year-old HIV-positive youth from San Francisco**

"We grow up hating ourselves like society teaches us to. If someone had been 'out' about their sexuality. If the teachers hadn't been afraid to stop the 'fag' and 'dyke' jokes. If my human sexuality class had even mentioned homosexuality. If the school counselors would have been open to a discussion of gay and lesbian issues. If any of those possibilities had existed, perhaps I would not have grown up hating what I was. And, just perhaps, I wouldn't have attempted suicide."—**Kyallee, 19**

"People say HIV is this or that group's problem, not mine. But for HIV, it's a matter of risk behaviors, not risk groups. Because if you say it's a risk group thing, I don't identify with that group, so I'm not at risk. That makes people feel invincible to HIV."—**HIV-positive youth**

"I was infected with HIV by my first partner when I was 16-years-old. Now at 20 I have this virus that's taking my life because everything I heard when I was younger was sugar-coated. We need more complete information than what we are being given. Even the pamphlets concerning HIV/AIDS prevention are too basic and bland. We need to know real stuff."—**Ryan, age 20**

"We, the young people of this country, need a place where we can go to ask our questions, where we won't be teased or ridiculed. We need a place where we can ask about our mixed-up feelings, about sex, and about AIDS."—**15-year-old high school student from Concord, N.H.**

"If I could talk to the president, or a senator, or anyone in the federal government who can make a difference, I'd tell them to take a look, learn a lesson from the youth that are currently dealing with the disease. Listen to them, hear their stories and then see that they have a future. If they don't have that future, then we don't have an America."—**Allan, San Francisco**

(Adapted and updated from a *Report to the President,* March 1996)

Comments: Unlike young adults who were infected by their mother perinatally and have grown up with the virus, the newly infected young adults, have daunting issues dumped on them virtually overnight. Do they tell anyone? How do they handle dating? How do they tackle the emotions clouding future relationships? And more immediately, how do they take on a life-saving medical regimen when they have the willpower of a teenager? Teens also have characteristics that work against treatment. They lead chaotic lives. Shun authority. Keep secrets. Feel invincible. And wear defiance like a badge of courage. That "you can't tell me what to do" attitude can be deadly. Some teens may not even know they have the virus. Years can pass before their viral loads are high enough to produce symptoms.

DISCUSSION QUESTION: If you were an HIV-positive young adult, would you tell others? Choose one and discuss.

A. Yes

B. Only with family and close friends

C. Only once I reached adulthood

D. Only if I planned to have sex

E. No

F. An option not listed

Summary

For the time being, abstaining from sex, mutual monogamy between uninfected partners, and the correct and consistent use of condoms are the only options that can be presented to young people for avoiding the sexual transmission of HIV. In order to decrease their risk of HIV infection today, it is essential that young adults receive education about HIV and have access to health and rehabilitative services.

Internet

1. **The Coalition for Positive Sexuality (CPS) website (http://www.positive.org/cps),** which provides information and advice on sexuality, is produced by and targets adolescents. The coalition is a grassroots volunteer group based in Chicago. Their self-described mission is "to give teens the information they need to take care of themselves and in doing so, affirm their decisions about sex, sexuality, and reproductive control; second, to facilitate dialogue, in and out of the public schools, on condom availability and sex education." Included among the topics is information about safe sex, birth control, STDs, pregnancy, and being gay. Homosexual relations are discussed in the same manner as heterosexual relations.

2. Although CPS is aimed at youth in general, **Oasis (http://www.oasismag.com)** targets and is written primarily by gay youth. Most of the columns written by contributors, who range in age from 14 to 22, read a lot like personal high school journals, an approach that undoubtedly makes readers feel comfortable—like hearing from a friend. A monthly advice column on sexual health is written by a physician and an epidemiologist, who are based in the San Francisco area.

Other Useful Sources

National Runaway Switchboard: 1-800-621-4000

National Network Runaway Youth Service: 1-202-783-7949

American Institute for Teen AIDS Prevention: 1-817-237-0230

Teen AIDS Student Coalition on AIDS, Washington, D.C.: 1-202-986-4310

Teen AIDS CDC: 1-800-342-2437

Teen AIDS Hotline: 1-800-440-8336

National Gay/Lesbian Youth Hotline: 1-800-347-8336

Review Questions

(Answers to the Review Questions are on page 429.)

1. There are _____ billion people ages 13 to 24 in the world.

2. What percentage of new HIV infections now occur among young adults?

3. Ending 2009, of the 35 million people living with HIV/AIDS globally, how many will be young adults?

4. Of those HIV-infected by age 24, how many will die by age 35?

5. Ending 2009, what percentage of young adult women with HIV/AIDS will be living in sub-Saharan Africa _____, Latin America _____, North America _____ and the Caribbean _____?

6. What percentage of young adult women believe birth control pills are a form of safer sex?

7. Young adult "3 to 6" means _____.

8. One danger of abstinence-only education is _____.

9. Entering year 2009, how many federal and state dollars have been spent on abstinence education in the United States?

10. What percentage of young adults live in developing countries?

11. How many young adults live in the United States?

12. What percentage of HIV-infected adults were infected as young adults?

13. Young adults are defined as ages _____ to _____.

14. Young adults make up _____ percent of the total HIV-infected population in the United States.

15. True or False: Young adults in general do not believe oral sex is sex.

Testing for Human Immunodeficiency Virus

13

CHAPTER CONCEPTS

- ELISA means **e**nzyme **l**inked **i**mmuno**s**orbent **a**ssay; it is a large-scale screening test for HIV infection.
- Western Blot is a confirmatory HIV test. It confirms the results of ELISA.
- The ELISA test has been used to screen all blood supplies in the United States since March 1985.
- HIV screening tests can produce both false positives and false negatives.
- A positive ELISA test only predicts that a confirmatory test will also be positive.
- False-positive readings result from a test's lack of specificity.
- There is a relationship between the incidence of HIV in the population being tested and the number of false positives reported. The higher the incidence, the fewer the false positives.
- Several new screening and confirmatory HIV tests are now available.
- June 27 is national HIV Testing Day.
- Screening should be repeated at least annually in persons with known risk.
- Screening of the nation's blood supply has improved.
- Saliva and urine HIV antibody tests are FDA-approved.
- The polymerase chain reaction test is the most sensitive HIV RNA test currently available.
- Other HIV RNA tests available are Amplicor and the branched DNA test.
- Currently there are six FDA-approved rapid tests requiring 20 minutes or less available in the United States.
- In pregnancy one test can save two lives.
- AIDS cases have been reported in all 50 states.
- All states now have a name or coded HIV reporting system.
- Percent reported being HIV tested by age and ethnic group.
- Competency and informed consent are necessary for most HIV testing.
- Mandatory HIV testing does not mean people can be forced to undergo testing.
- HIV testing, for the most part, is on a voluntary basis.
- Compulsory HIV testing is used in the military, prisons, and in certain federal agencies.
- FDA has approved two home HIV test kits; one remains on the market.
- U.S. Public Health Service guidelines for annual prenatal HIV counseling and voluntary HIV testing of all pregnant American women.
- New York is the first state to legislate mandatory HIV testing and disclosure of newborn HIV status to mother and physicians.
- American Medical Association endorses mandatory HIV testing of all pregnant women and newborns.
- CDC is recommending routine HIV testing in all U.S. residents ages 13–64.
- The United States policy on HIV and immigration revealed.

Let's begin this chapter by asking, **WHY DOES TESTING MATTER? ANSWER:** Basic epidemiology holds that early knowledge of where a virus is moving—into which populations—is essential to slowing its spread. Even if a disease cannot be cured, knowing who the infected people are may help prevent the transmission of the disease to other people. People who are unaware they are HIV positive account for an estimated 20,000 new HIV infections annually (Wolf et al. 2007). People often do not test for HIV because they do not perceive themselves at risk for infection. HIV testing is integral to HIV prevention, treatment, and care efforts. Knowledge of one's HIV status is important for preventing the spread of the disease. Studies show that those who learn they are HIV positive modify their behavior to reduce the risk of HIV transmission. Early knowledge of HIV status is also important for linking those with HIV to medical care and services that can reduce morbidity and mortality and improve the quality of life.

By the end of 2009, of the estimated 35 million living HIV-infected people worldwide, at least **half** will have become infected **before age 25.** About 10% will know they are HIV positive. HIV testing is not readily available in many places in developing nations. This chapter presents HIV testing information and describes some of the important problems connected with whom, how, and where to test.

Availability of HIV Testing in the United States

Commercial HIV antibody testing has been available since 1985. Testing technology has evolved considerably over the years, with a variety of new and improved tests coming into use in daily practice. Because determining one's HIV status is the first step in prevention and treatment decisions, it is important to understand the tests being used today, including their limitations.

How Do HIV Tests Work?

Once HIV enters the body, the immune system starts to produce antibodies, chemicals that are part of the immune system that recognize invaders like bacteria and viruses and mobilize the body's attempt to fight infection. In the case of HIV, these antibodies cannot fight off the infection, but their presence is used to tell whether a person has HIV in his or her body. In other words, most HIV tests look for the HIV antibodies rather than looking for HIV itself. There are

tests that do look for HIV's genetic material directly, but these are not in widespread use. These tests will also be presented below.

DETERMINING THE PRESENCE OF ANTIBODY PRODUCED WHEN HIV IS PRESENT

HIV antibody testing is a readily available, inexpensive, reliable, and accurate method to identify whether a person is infected with HIV. HIV antibodies are found in the blood and in other body fluids. When properly performed, HIV antibody testing is highly sensitive and specific.

Currently there are at least nine tests that detect HIV antibodies, antigens, or the nucleic acid of HIV in a person's body fluids. They are the enzyme linked immunosorbent assay (ELISA), Western Blot, polymerase chain reaction (PCR), saliva and urine tests, Aplicor's branched DNA test, immunofluorescent antibody assay, rapid HIV test kits, and at-home HIV test kits. They are discussed in the following pages.

REQUESTS FOR HIV TESTING

HIV testing is offered at some 11,600 CDC-publicly funded sites and in other public and private settings. These testing sites are becoming overwhelmed with requests for HIV testing. But, most of the requests are repeats. The majority of those people at risk who have not been tested includes most hardcore IDUs and sexual partners of IDUs and people who are image sensitive. Currently, about 100 million blood and plasma samples are HIV tested annually worldwide. In the United States about 16 million to 22 million blood and plasma samples are HIV tested annually.

In the developing world, where the greatest number of HIV-infected people are concentrated, HIV testing is done mostly for purposes of surveillance, which involves very small population samples and is done anonymously. Few people have any hope of treatment, so they feel little incentive to get tested. But even those who would want to know may not be able to find out. In many countries, there are no voluntary testing and counseling facilities; people have no acceptable way of learning if they are HIV infected. An ongoing study at a rural hospital in South Africa suggests that only 2% of people who are HIV positive know their status. The situation in the rest of sub-Saharan Africa is equally poor.

REASONS FOR HIV TESTING

HIV testing is done to monitor the pandemic—to determine how many people are infected, how many are becoming infected in a given time period (incidence), and their location. Testing is used to determine the impact of prevention efforts to slow the spread of HIV, to prompt behavior change, and to provide entry into clinical care. Also, if necessary, to provide a starting point for partner notification, education, and to protect the nation's blood supply.

Take the Test: Take Control

There is an immediate need to change perceptions about being HIV positive so that people feel good about taking the test to protect themselves and others, rather than the discrimination that now exists against those who have taken the test.

The Need for Routine HIV Testing

After 28 years of educating people about HIV/AIDS, about 42% of adults ages 18 to 64 in the United States have never been tested for HIV (Figure 13-1). Sixty-one percent of adults say their reason for not being tested is that they do not consider themselves to be at risk (Figure 13-2). Unless people are tested in greater numbers, it may be impossible to break the cycle of HIV transmission in America or anywhere else. The failure of educational programs to stem the rates of over 56,000 new HIV infections annually may need to be replaced by new policies on HIV testing. Joseph Inungu, a Central Michigan health science professor, is recommending an HIV test as part of the routine tests performed on office patients. Inungu analyzed

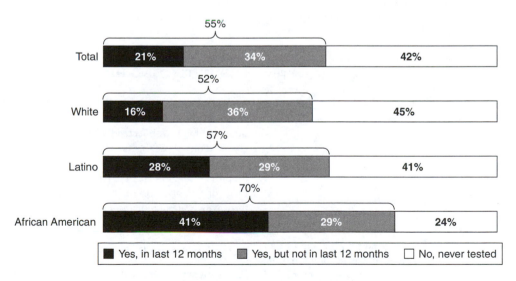

FIGURE 13-1 Percent, Ages 18 to 64, Who Report Being Tested by Race/Ethnicity, 2006. Not all numbers may add up due to rounding. *(Source: Adapted from Kaiser Family Foundation Survey of Americans on HIV/AIDS conducted March 24–April 18, 2006).*

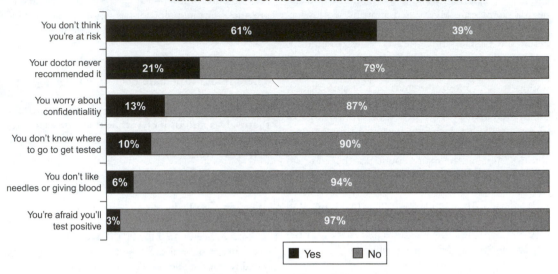

Asked of the 50% of those who have never been tested for HIV.

	Yes	No
You don't think you're at risk	61%	39%
Your doctor never recommended it	21%	79%
You worry about confidentialitiy	13%	87%
You don't know where to go to get tested	10%	90%
You don't like needles or giving blood	6%	94%
You're afraid you'll test positive	3%	97%

FIGURE 13-2 Reported Reasons for Adults Not Being HIV Tested. Note: "Don't know" responses not shown. *(Source: Adapted from Kaiser Family Foundation Survey of Americans on HIV/AIDS conducted March 24–April 18 2006).*

data on people ages 18 to 80 who participated in a national health interview survey conducted by the National Center for Health Statistics. He found the groups least likely to be tested for HIV were men, people over the age of 50 or between age 18 and 19, people with a low level of education, people in rural areas, and people in the Northeast or Midwest. While young adult groups are among the fastest-growing populations with HIV infection, few are tested for HIV unless they come to a physician for a sexually transmitted disease. Populations over the age of 50 feel they were not at risk but their numbers of HIV infected continue to increase. The groups most likely to get tested include blacks, people with higher educational levels, and people who are separated, divorced, or widowed.

**Misunderstanding Leads
to Lack of HIV Testing**

Misunderstanding surrounds HIV testing. For example, one of the pastors in a black church told about a conversation he had with a young man. He asked the young man if he had been tested for HIV and he said yes, and that he was negative. He asked him when he was tested, and he said four years ago. The pastor asked him if he had been at risk in that time and needed to get tested again. The young man seemed puzzled and asked, "Why should I be tested again?" There's such an

emphasis on "get tested, get tested" but in many cases the understanding as to why one gets tested is not there! It's not just testing, but an ongoing risk assessment and ongoing testing and ongoing awareness. It's a commitment to being aware and being open to discussing risks. People can openly talk about anything but sex. Yet men, women, and young adults are having sex. There is a need for counseling about having an HIV test.

LABORATORY METHODS
FOR DETECTING HIV

An arsenal of laboratory methods is available to screen blood, diagnose infection, and monitor disease progression in individuals infected by HIV. These tests can be classified into those that (a) detect antibody, (b) identify antigen, (c) detect or monitor viral nucleic acids, and (d) provide an estimate of T lymphocyte numbers. The focus of this discussion is on antibody detection, the most widely used and, in most situations, the most effective and least expensive way to identify HIV.

Detecting Antibodies to HIV

Refinements in the field of immunological testing, serology, and the study of antigen–antibody reactions have produced test names that reflect the component parts of the test being used. In most cases, tests are based on the detection of antibodies present in the serum, in this case antibodies to HIV. One immunological test uses antibodies, which if present in the person's serum, form a complex with a given antigen. An enzyme is then connected to the antibody. The presence of the antibody can be determined by adding a reagent that will form a colored solution if an antibody to HIV is present. This is called the **enzyme linked immunosorbent assay** (ELISA). The ELISA (E–liz–a) test was first used in 1983 to detect antibodies against HIV.

Because the ELISA test detects the presence of antibodies made against HIV, it is called an **indirect test.** This test suggests that HIV is or was present. The Western Blot test, presented next, is also an indirect test for the same reason. Indirect tests stand in contrast to those tests that directly test for the presence of HIV's nucleic acid—a **direct test.** These tests say that HIV is currently present in the system. They are also presented.

ELISA HIV ANTIBODY TEST

A Fable for the HIV/AIDS Era

It was a medieval mystery. Somehow, needles were finding their way into some of the kingdom's haystacks. Cows were eating the needles: not a good thing. The king sent out a proclamation offering a sack of gold to the first person able to find a needle in a haystack. After 20 days, the contestants were still trying to locate the needles hidden among 10 haystacks placed in the palace courtyard. The king was despondent. From his tower he could see thousands of haystacks in fields across the kingdom. "This is terrible," he said. "Either our cows go hungry while we look for the needles, or we let them eat the hay along with some needles. Either way it's not good for the cows. We need a way to tell which haystacks have the needles; then we can feed our cows the good hay while we figure out how to get the needles out of the bad haystacks." He was a logical king. In 1981 the needle had no name but its presence was known. The search for this needle—like those in the haystacks—was intense and even after the needle was found to be HIV, investigators had to find a way to distinguish between those who carried and did not carry HIV—which haystacks carried the needles. Because HIV was in human blood it was essential to protect the nation's blood supply, thereby preventing people from receiving contaminated blood and blood products. But, like the good king, it took time to find the means to find the needle in the blood supply—HIV.

It was not until 1985—nearly four years after the first cases of AIDS were announced—that an antibody test was developed that could indicate whether a person was infected with HIV. Even after this discovery, the fact that there were no effective treatments for those who tested HIV positive, coupled with the widespread perception of stigma associated with HIV infection, left many questioning the value of HIV testing. That equation shifted markedly with the availability of potent combination antiretroviral drug therapy, which significantly delays the progression of HIV disease in many people. There is now widespread consensus among public health officials and community leaders regarding the importance of HIV testing and counseling in order to link individuals who test positive with medical care and to counsel them on how to reduce the risk of further transmission.

Screening the Nation's Blood Supply

The initial application of the ELISA test outside the research laboratory was used primarily in large-scale screening of the nation's blood supply. **ELISA testing of the existing blood supply and all newly donated blood began in the United States in March 1985.** Very quickly testing also became an important aspect of HIV prevention. In recent years, the discovery of treatments for HIV and associated opportunistic infections has further increased the benefits of early detection.

The ELISA test is used as a screening test because of its low cost, standardized procedures, high reproducibility, and rapid results.

Whole viruses are disrupted into subunit antigens for use. The subunits of HIV are then bound to a solid support system.

Two different solid support systems are used in the five ELISA screening test kits licensed in the United States. Some attach or fix the antigens onto small glass beads (Figure 13-3), while others fix the antigens onto the sides and bottoms of small wells (microwells) in a glass or plastic microtiter plate. The serum to be tested is separated from the blood and is diluted and applied to the HIV-coated solid support systems (Figure 13-4). The ELISA test takes from 2.5 to 4 hours to perform and costs between about $8 in state-sponsored virology laboratories and about $60 to $75 in private laboratories.

In accordance with FDA recommendations, effective June 1992, blood collection centers in the United States began HIV-2 testing on all donated blood and blood components. Because of its rare occurrence in the United States, the CDC does not recommend routine testing for HIV-2 other than at blood collection centers.

Understanding the ELISA Test

The ELISA test determines if a person's serum contains antibodies to one or more HIV antigens. Although there are some minor differences among the FDA-licensed kits, test procedures are similar.

Problems with the ELISA Test

Any HIV screening test must be able to distinguish those individuals who are infected from those who are not. **The underlying assumption of an ELISA test is that all HIV-infected people will produce detectable HIV antibodies.** There are, however, problems with this assumption. **First,** although rare, there are documented cases of individuals who are infected but remain antibody negative. (See Point of Information 13.1.) **Second,** the HIV-infected population in general does not produce detectable antibodies for six weeks to one or more years after HIV infection. This is called the **window period.** Most often, HIV antibody is detectable within 6 to 18 weeks. Thus, HIV-infected peo-

ple can test HIV negative. This is a **false negative result.** In some HIV-infected persons, the virus ties up the available antibody as their disease progresses. Testing at this time may also produce false negative results.

An Unusual Case—At the VA Medical Center in Salt Lake City in 1997, a man tested HIV negative 35 times over a four-year period. Because his wife was HIV positive and because he demonstrated symptoms of HIV disease, tests other than the ELISA showed that he was HIV positive. (See Point of Information 13.1.) This case is unusual because (1) he was falsely negative almost four years beyond the window period; (2) the strain of HIV is typical of that found in the United States; and (3) the strain of HIV is closely related to the strain infecting his wife (Reimer et al., 1997).

False positive reactions may also occur. This means that the person's serum does not contain antibodies to HIV but the test results indicate that it does. Christine Johnson (2000) has compiled a list of 66 conditions taken from HIV/AIDS scientific literature that can cause false positive results.

People may test false positive who have an underlying liver disease, have received a blood transfusion or gamma globulin within six weeks of the test, have had several children, have had rheumatological diseases, malaria, alcoholic hepatitis, autoimmune disorders, various cancers, acute cytomegalovirus infection, or DNA viral infections; are injection-drug users; or have received vaccines for influenza or hepatitis B (Fang et al., 1989; MacKenzie et al., 1992). In each case, the person may have antibodies that will cross-react with the HIV antigens to give a false positive reaction. Other reasons for false positives are laboratory errors and mistakes made in reagent preparations for use in the test kits.

Why Is the ELISA Test Sensitivity and Specificity Set High?

Because the original purpose of the ELISA test was to screen blood, the sensitivity (ability to detect low-level color formation; see Figure 13-3) of the test was purposely set high. It was reasoned that it was better to have some false positives and throw away good blood rather than to take in any HIV-contaminated blood. Thus the ELISA test is a **positive predictive value** test. It only predicts that the serum tested will continue to test positive when a test with greater specificity, called a **confirmatory test,** is done.

In 1985, during the first month of donor screening, 1% of all blood tested HIV-antibody positive. On ELISA

Solid Supports

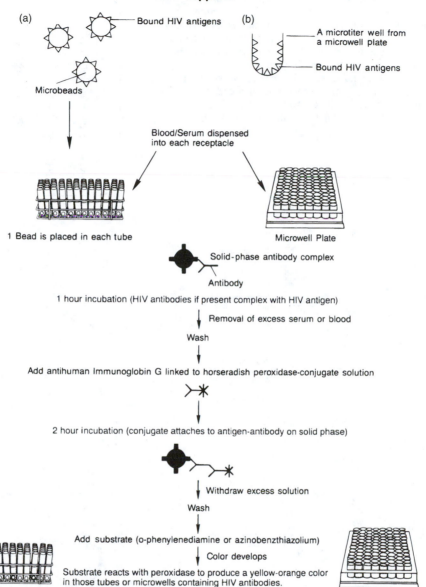

(a)

Bound HIV antigens

Microbeads

(b)

A microtiter well from a microwell plate

Bound HIV antigens

Blood/Serum dispensed into each receptacle

1 Bead is placed in each tube

Microwell Plate

Solid-phase antibody complex

Antibody

1 hour incubation (HIV antibodies if present complex with HIV antigen)

Removal of excess serum or blood

Wash

Add antihuman Immunoglobin G linked to horseradish peroxidase-conjugate solution

2 hour incubation (conjugate attaches to antigen-antibody on solid phase)

Withdraw excess solution

Wash

Add substrate (o-phenylenediamine or azinobenzthiazolium)

Color develops

Substrate reacts with peroxidase to produce a yellow-orange color in those tubes or microwells containing HIV antibodies.
The intensity of the color is proportional to the amount of antibody present in the serum.

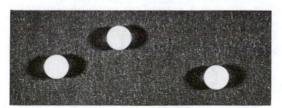

FIGURE 13-3 The ELISA Test. (a) Microbeads with attached antigen in test tubes. (b) Antigens bound to walls and bottom of microtiter wells. (c) Microbeads are 7 mm in diameter. The test takes between 2.5 and 4 hours to perform.

(c)

FIGURE 13-3 (Continued) (d) Specimens positive for HIV antibody have a deeper color in this microwell tray. Serum specimens from 15 patients were tested for antibodies to HIV. Two negative and three positive control specimens are provided in the first column. In wells 7, 9, 11, and 14, the dark yellow color change, matching the color in the three positive control wells, indicates that the specimens are positive. Well 3 shows a weakly reactive result. The remaining specimens showed no color change and were interpreted as negative for HIV antibodies. (*Adapted from Fang et al., 1989*). (e) Use of the (a) direct and (b) indirect ELISA Assay (test).

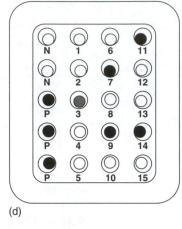

(d)

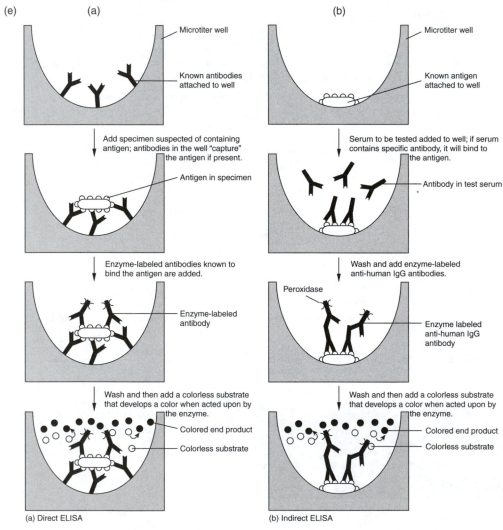

(a) Direct ELISA

(b) Indirect ELISA

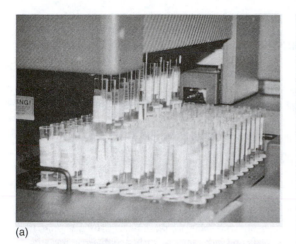

(a)

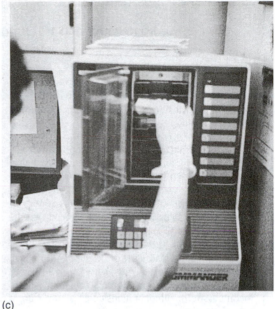

(c)

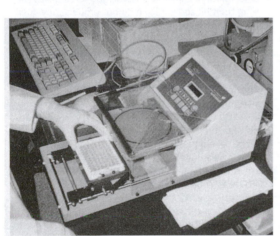

(b)

FIGURE 13-4 Semi-Automated ELISA Test. (a) Serum samples are individually machine diluted with a special solution 1 to 400 to achieve a balance between the amount of antibody to the amount of antigen. Antibodies, if present in the individual sera, attach to the HIV antigens in each well. (b) Excess serum is withdrawn from each sample and the beads are washed. The antihuman immunoglobulin-horseradish enzyme conjugate is added to each prepared sample. (c) The samples are incubated. (d) Each sample receives the chromogen or substrate (o-phenylenediamine or azinobenzthiazolium). A yellow-orange color appears in samples that contain antibodies to HIV. In mid-2006, the FDA approved Bayer's Automated HIV test. It detects HIV-1/2 in serum plasma. This first automated screening test eliminates manual labor and is more accurate than other HIV screening systems. *(Courtesy of Florida Department of Health, Retrovirology Unit, Jacksonville; photos by Gerald Stine)*

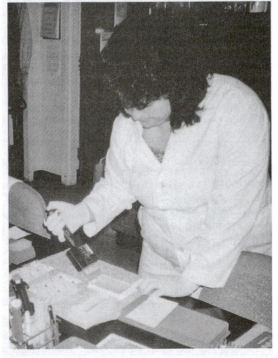

(d)

BOX 13.1

AN ASSUMPTION OF AIDS WITHOUT THE HIV TEST: IT SHATTERS LIVES

Case 1

San Francisco—For six years, a 53-year-old gay male lived in the world of AIDS. He stopped working, suffered the painful side effects of experimental drugs, and waited to die.

Now his doctors say he never had the disease.

His health shattered by AIDS treatment, his livelihood lost, he filed a $2 million claim against Kaiser Permanente health maintenance organization. He claims he underwent sustained treatment for full-fledged AIDS without receiving an HIV test.

His attorney said, "For six years he thought that the most he had was six months to live. So every day he'd wake up and think 'Is this the last day of my life?'"

To begin, this male says he checked into a San Jose hospital affiliated with Kaiser in 1986 with respiratory problems and doctors told him he had Pneumocystic pneumonia, considered a sure sign of AIDS at the time.

He underwent tests but *was not* given one to determine the presence of HIV, the virus associated with AIDS.

In 1986, he began taking the drug zidovudine in high doses, which gave him a chronic headache, high blood pressure, and peripheral neuropathy—permanent pins and needles pains from his calves to his feet. He is battling an addiction to Darvon and other prescription drugs.

Under doctors' orders, he quit his job as a skin care technician and lives on government welfare and disability benefits of $600 a month. (Associated Press, 1992)

Case 2

Every day, four times each day, for six years Mark swallowed his antiretroviral drugs. Mark was told by a "fine physician" that he was HIV positive in July 1990. Regardless of the drugs, Mark felt sick and suffered further physical effects and depression. For reasons not given, Mark moved from Chicago to Ohio. His new physician was puzzled that Mark did not demonstrate signs or symptoms of HIV infection. His tests on Mark came back HIV negative. On investigation, the Chicago clinic could not produce any documents showing that Mark was ever HIV tested!

Case 3

Boston—In December 2007, a jury awarded $2.5 million in damages to a woman who for almost nine years took a combination of antiretroviral drugs but was never actually tested for HIV. The ART triggered a variety of ailments including depression, chronic fatigue, weight loss, and intestinal inflammation. She filed a suit against her physician after her HIV test came back—HIV negative. The initial diagnosis, made by her physician, was based on her lifestyle.

---

retesting of these samples, only 0.17% (17/10,000) were HIV-antibody positive. On subjecting these samples to a confirmatory test, only 0.038% (4/10,000) were actually HIV positive. These early tests produced about 24 false positives for every true positive result. The main reason for such a high false positive rate or **lack of specificity** was that something other than HIV produced an antibody or other substance that reacted with HIV antigen causing the HIV test to appear positive.

Although high sensitivity tests eliminate HIV-contaminated blood from the blood supply, there is a downside to high sensitivity testing when proper procedure is *not* used. People told that they have tested positive have become emotionally distraught. Former Senator Lawton Chiles of Florida, at an AIDS conference in 1987, told of a tragic example from the early days of blood screening in Florida. Of 22 blood donors who were told they were HIV positive by the ELISA test, seven committed suicide. In 2006, the CDC reported that, over time, about 30% of HIV-infected Koreans commit suicide.

There continue to be false positive reactions among blood donors and low-level risk populations because of a low prevalence of HIV infection in such populations. The American Red Cross Blood Services laboratories report that using current ELISA methodology, a specificity of 99.8% can be achieved.

Positive Predictive Value—The positive predictive value of the ELISA test indicates the percentage of true positives among total positives in a given population. To determine a positive predictive value:

Number of true positives ÷ (Number of true positives + false positives) × 100 = %

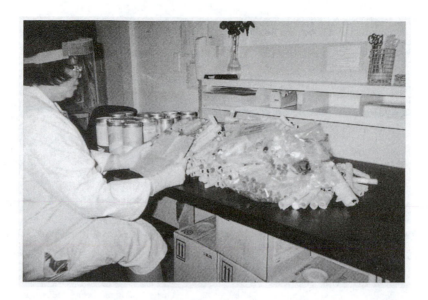

FIGURE 13-5 Incoming Specimens. About 900 to 1000 blood specimens are received each day and are prepared for testing. From those samples, those testing negative are reported in 8 to 10 hours. Positive samples are reported in 3 to 4 days. (*Courtesy of Florida Department of Health, Retrovirology Unit, Jacksonville; photo by Gerald Stine*)

There is also a negative predictive test. A negative predictive value refers to the percentage of individuals who test truly negative; they *do not* have HIV. It is determined by:

Number of true negatives ÷ (Number of true negatives + false negatives) × 100 = %

To safeguard against false-positive tests, the CDC recommends that serum that tests positive be retested twice (in duplicate). If both tests are negative, the serum is considered HIV-antibody negative and further tests will only be done should signs or symptoms of HIV infection occur (Figure 13-5). If one or both of the tests is positive, the serum is subjected to a confirmatory test, usually a Western Blot (WB). At blood banks, if the initial ELISA test is positive, the blood is discarded. If an individual's serum subjected to a confirmatory test is positive, the person is considered to be HIV infected.

Although confirmatory tests can be used to determine true-positive results, they are too labor intensive and expensive to be used in screening a large population. Thus the positive predictive value of an ELISA test is an important first step in large-scale screening. Recall, however, that **the predictive value depends on the prevalence of HIV infection in the population tested.** The higher the prevalence or number of HIV infection in a given population, the more likely a positive ELISA test is to be a true positive; and conversely, the lower the prevalence of infection, the less likely a positive ELISA test is to be a true positive.

Levels of Sensitivity and Specificity in Testing for HIV—A test's **sensitivity** is its capacity to identify all specimens that have HIV antibodies in them. A test's **specificity** is its capacity to identify all specimens that do not have HIV antibodies in them.

Sensitivity is determined as follows:

Number of true positives ÷ (Number of true positives + the false negatives) × 100 = %

If 100 persons are actually HIV infected and the test identifies only 90 of them, then the test has 90% sensitivity.

Specificity is determined as follows:

Number of true negatives ÷ (Number of true negatives + false positives) × 100 = %

Assume that, in a group of 500 people being tested for HIV antibodies, 100 individuals are actually not infected. If test results show that only 90 out of the 100 are identified as not having the virus, then the test has 90% specificity.

Table 13-1 The Meaning of Antibody Test Results

A Positive Results	B Negative Results
If you test positive, it does mean: 1. Your blood sample has been tested more than once and the tests indicate that it contained antibodies to HIV. 2. You have been infected with HIV and your body has produced antibodies. **If you test positive, it does not mean:** 1. That you have AIDS. 2. That you necessarily will get AIDS, but the probability is high. You can reduce your chance of progressing to AIDS by avoiding further contact with the virus, beginning antiretroviral therapy if recommended, and living a healthy lifestyle. 3. That you are immune to the virus. **Therefore, if you test positive, you should do the following:** 1. Protect yourself from any further infection. 2. Protect others from the virus by following HIV/AIDS precautions in sex, drug use, and general hygiene. 3. Consider seeing a physician for a complete evaluation and advice on health maintenance. 4. Avoid drugs and heavy alcohol use, maintain good nutrition, and avoid fatigue and stress. Such action may improve your chances of staying healthy. **If you test negative, it does mean:** 1. No antibodies to HIV have been found in your serum at the time of the test.	**Two possible explanations for a negative test result exist:** 1. You have not been infected with HIV. 2. You have been infected with HIV but have not yet produced antibodies. Research indicates that most people will produce antibodies within 6 to 18 weeks after infection. Some people will not produce antibodies for at least 3 years. A very small number of people may never produce antibodies. **If you test negative, it does not mean:** 1. That you have nothing to worry about. You may become infected; be careful. 2. That you are immune to HIV. 3. That you have not been infected with the virus. You may have been infected and not yet produced antibodies. **If You Test Negative, Does It Mean that Your Sexual Partner Is HIV Negative?** No. Your HIV test results reveal only your HIV status. Your negative results do not tell you whether your partner has HIV. HIV is not necessarily transmitted every time there is an exposure. Therefore, your taking an HIV test should not be seen as a method to find out if your partner is infected. Testing should never take the place of protecting yourself from HIV infection. If your behaviors are putting you at risk for exposure to HIV, it is important to reduce your risks.

(Adapted from the San Francisco AIDS Foundation)

WESTERN BLOT ASSAY

The gold standard for determining a true positive HIV-antibody test is the **Western Blot** (WB). This test is a method in which individual HIV proteins are used to react with HIV antibody in a person's serum. It should be understood that the WB test is not a true gold standard because it is not 100% certain, but it can come close to 100% if properly used.

Cells in which HIV is being cultured are lysed or broken open, and the mixture of cell components and HIV components (proteins) are separated from each other. The viral proteins are placed on a polyacrylamide gel, which then gets an electrical charge. The electrical current separates the viral proteins within the gel. This is called **gel electrophoresis.** The smallest HIV proteins will move quickly through the gel, separating from the next larger size, and so on.

Each different protein will arrive at a separate position on the gel. After proteins of similar molecular weight collect at a given site, they form a band; these bands are identified based on the distance they have run in the gel. Because each band is a protein produced as a product of a different HIV gene, the gel band patterns give a picture of the HIV genes that were functioning and the location of each gene's products on the gel. The protein or antigen bands within the gel are "blotted," that is, transferred directly, band for band and position for position, onto strips of nitrocellulose paper (Figure 13-6).

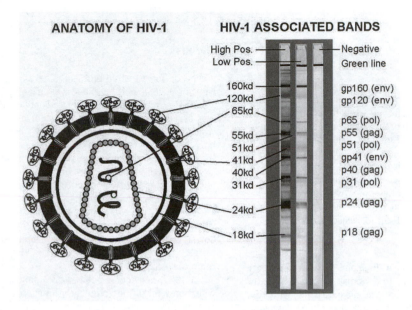

FIGURE 13-6 Western Blot. A Western Blot (WB) strip contains 10 separate antigenic proteins of HIV. Human serum or blood is applied directly to the strips. Because false positives can sometimes occur with the ELISA test, additional testing is needed to evaluate specimens that are repeatedly reactive by ELISA. The WB is more specific but less sensitive than the ELISA and is recommended for blood banks and organ donor centers. Its clinical usefulness in trials to aid in evaluating specimens that are questionably positive by other methods has been proven. It is not a screening test because it lacks a high level of sensitivity and is expensive. This line art drawing shows the immediate relationship between the gel bands, after electrophoresis and blotting onto nitrocellulose paper. The figure shows the gel bands as related to their constituent parts of the virus. (Permission to use the Bio-Rad HIV-1 Western Blot Illustration has been granted by Bio-Rad Laboratories, Inc. This permission is solely for inclusion in the AIDS update 2009.)

Once the antigen bands have been formed, serum believed to carry HIV antibodies is placed directly on them. That is, a test serum is added directly to antigen bands located on the nitrocellulose strip. If antibodies are present in the serum, they will form an antigen–antibody complex directly on the antigen band areas. Positive test strips are then compared to two control test strips, one that has been reacted with known positive serum and one that has been reacted with known negative serum.

In contrast to the ELISA test, which indicates only the presence or absence of HIV antibodies, the WB strip qualitatively identifies which of the HIV antigens the antibodies are directed against. **The greatest disadvantage of the WB test is that reagents, testing methods, and test-interpretation criteria are not standardized.** The National Institutes of Health (NIH), the American Red Cross, DuPont company, the Association of State and Territorial Health Officers (ASTHO), and the Department of Defense (DoD) each define a positive WB differently.

The WB procedure is labor intensive, takes longer to run (12 to 24 hours), and is therefore more costly than the ELISA test. **The WB is less sensitive than the ELISA but more specific.**

Because the WB lacks the sensitivity of the ELISA test, it is not used as a screening test. Despite the high specificity of the WB, false positives do occur, but they occur less frequently than with ELISA tests because the WB is only run on serum, blood, oral fluid, and urine already suspected of containing HIV antibodies.

Indeterminate WB

Western Blots may also turn out to be **indeterminate** in HIV infections—meaning, a person can be infected, but the blot is not conclusive—it may be positive but it may not be, it is too poor to tell. The

A FALSE POSITIVE HIV REPORT

Case 1

In January 2002, a man in Oklahoma City was awarded $1.4 million because he was wrongfully told he was HIV positive. At age 40 he received the news from a Health Maintenance Clinic. During the following four years, he became depressed, despondent, abused alcohol, and attempted suicide twice. Thinking he was HIV positive, he had unprotected sex with known HIV-positive partners. Reviewing his file to determine when he became infected he learned that his test four years earlier was HIV negative. He filed suit for negligence and won.

Case 2

In November 2002, a Richland County, S.C., jury awarded $1.1 million to a woman who said Palmetto Health Richland Hospital misdiagnosed her with HIV. She said the diagnosis wrecked her life. "I was so depressed thinking I was going to die a horrible death. I gave up hope. Now I'm trying to get my life back together. I have lost so much of my life. I thank God everyday for helping me find the mistake." In her lawsuit, the hospital—then, called Richland Memorial Hospital—diagnosed her as HIV-positive in February 1994. For several years she took anti-HIV medications, including the drug zidovudine. She said she never had symptoms of the disease and that another test in 1998 by a different laboratory confirmed she had been misdiagnosed. The lawsuit said she suffered extreme depression, emotional distress, anxiety, fear, side effects from the drugs, and other related trauma because of the misdiagnosis.

Case 3

In 1980, she received a blood transfusion during surgery at a hospital in a Southeast Georgia town. During a checkup for a thyroid problem, a decade later, at a clinic in Hialeah, Fla., her blood was taken for testing.

On November 13, 1990, her telephone rang. She was asked to come down to the local health clinic where she was told she had AIDS. They were not sure how long she had to live. She was 45-years-old. Her three sons were then teenagers; their father had died.

She kept the television on continually in a usually unsuccessful effort to block out the thought of AIDS.

The nights were the worst.

"I'd go to bed every night thinking about dying. What color do you want the casket to be? What dress do you want to be buried in? How are your kids going to take it? How will people treat them? I was afraid to go to sleep."

In 1992, her doctor put her on didanosine, (ddI), which brought on side effects that included vomiting and fatigue.

"I had put my kids through hell. They were scared for me."

When she joined a local hospice group for AIDS patients, counselors heard her story and noted that her T cell counts had remained consistently high. At their suggestion, she was retested.

In November 1992, nearly two years to the day she was told she was HIV positive, another call came. She was greeted at the clinic with these words: **"Guess what? Your HIV test came out negative!"**

She sued the Florida Department of Health and Rehabilitative Services—the agency that performed the test—and the clinic and doctor who treated her.

A jury awarded her $600,000 for pain and suffering but cleared the clinic and said the bulk must be paid by the agency.

REPEATEDLY ANTIBODY NEGATIVE PEOPLE WITH VERY ADVANCED HIV DISEASE

In early 2008, Raul Ortiz de Lejarazy and colleagues reported that there were 11 unknown cases of hidden or "occult" HIV infections. In the latest case, a 28-year-old man was hospitalized with a severe chest infection and a four-month history of thrush. Kaposi's sarcoma was also diagnosed, and tests showed the man's chest infection was caused by *pneumocystis jiroveci* pneumonia. But his HIV antibody tests were repeatedly negative, although his viral load test revealed 122,000 copies/ml of blood and he was infected with a sub-type-B, CCR5-topic strain of HIV. Antiretroviral therapy was initiated, and after three weeks the patient's viral load fell to 12,000 copies/ml. But his Kaposi's sarcoma progressed rapidly, and the patient developed significant lung disease, leading to his death two weeks later (de Lejarazy et al. 2008). The investigators noted that in all 17 cases, the people had extremely weak immune systems and high viral loads.

indeterminate WB results can occur either during the window period for HIV seroconversion or during end-stage HIV disease. Indeterminate WBs have occurred in uninfected individuals because of cross-reacting autoantibodies related to recent immunization, prior blood transfusion, organ transplantation, autoimmune disorders, malignancy, infection with other retroviruses (for example, HIV-2), or pregnancy. Some patients have a persistent pattern of indeterminate reactivity that remains stable over several years in the absence of true HIV infection.

In general, most persons with an initial indeterminate Western Blot result who are infected with HIV will develop detectable HIV antibody within one month. Thus, clients with an initial indeterminate result should be retested for HIV infection after one month.

NEW ELISA ANTIBODY TESTING AND VIRAL LOAD PROCEDURES REVEAL EARLY VERSUS LATE HIV INFECTION

STARHS—A Sensitive/Less Sensitive HIV Test

The best data for understanding recent changes in HIV transmission are measurements of the number of new infections in a defined time period (incidence of infection). But this has been difficult because ELISA testing simply gave a positive or negative response to the presence of HIV antibody without regard to the actual time of infection. However, in mid-1998 (Janssen et al.) through 1999 (McFarland et al.) a new testing strategy provided a means to detect new or early HIV infections versus older HIV infections. The new testing technique is called **STARHS (the Serologic Testing Algorithm for Recent HIV Seroconversions).** The test uses two different ELISAs to test a single blood sample to tell if an infection is old or new. By more accurately pinpointing the time of infection, STARHS may help patients identify when and from whom infection took place. Because people can live symptom-free with HIV for over a decade, there was no way previously to tell when they might have become infected. But the new technology changes that. For example, while it's hard for many sexually active people to recall the names and addresses of all their partners, spanning years of activity, it is typically a simple matter to make a list for the past four months. Armed with this new information, public health authorities can track down individuals who appear to be spreading HIV, and—for the first time—interrupt the chain of transmission on a large-scale basis.

How It Works

The standard ELISA blood test is very sensitive and measures the presence of antibodies against HIV. The very sensitive or **standard ELISA tests** can pick up even minute numbers of antibodies present in the first days of infection before the immune system has mounted a full response to the virus. Conversely, a less sensitive B E and D test (tests only for antibodies to HIV types B,E, and D of the M group) **does the reverse.** It detects only the presence of antibodies at higher levels that typically appear three to six months after infection. By administering both ELISA tests, technicians, by comparing the results of both tests, can tell an individual's stage of infection. In brief, if someone tests positive on the sensitive test and negative on the detuned test, they likely have a recent infection. Positive results on both tests indicate the infection is more than four to six months old.

Viral Load Related to Stage of Infection

As described in Chapter 4, a viral load test measures the number of viral RNA strands in the blood. Before the immune system produces antibodies to fight HIV, it multiplies rapidly. Therefore, this test will show a high viral load during the acute stage of HIV infection. Thus, a negative HIV antibody test and a high viral load indicates a recent HIV infection, most likely within the past two months. If both tests are positive, then HIV infection probably occurred a few months or more before the tests.

In May 2007, the FDA approved two new viral load tests. One is Abbot's RealTime HIV-1 viral load test for use on the company's m2000™ automated instrument system. The Abbott RealTime HIV-1 assay is designed to detect and precisely measure levels of HIV circulating in a patient's blood (viral load), including the three major groups of HIV-1 M, N, and O as well as non-B subtypes. The test is intended for use as a marker of disease prognosis and an aid in assessing viral response to antiretroviral treatment. The test can detect as few as 40 RNA molecules (strands) per milliliter (mL) of blood plasma and as many as 10 million molecules per mL. A second new viral load test is the COBAS AmpliPrep test by Roche Diagnostics; it is similar in use to the Abbot's test.

Immunofluorescent Antibody Assay

The **immunofluorescent antibody assay (IFA)** uses a known preparation of antibodies labeled with a fluorescent dye such as fluorescein isothiocyanate

(FITC) to detect antigen or antibody. In the direct fluorescent antibody test, fluorescent antibodies detect specific antigens in cultures or smears. In the indirect fluorescent antibody test, specific antibody from serum is bound to antigen on a glass slide.

The indirect procedure is modified for use in detecting antibodies to HIV. Cells that are HIV infected will have HIV antigens on their cell membranes and will later fluoresce when the antihuman fluorescent conjugate is added.

In late 1992, the FDA-approved Fluorognost for marketing, the first assay for HIV-IFA confirmation and screening.

The assay allows doctors to do in-office tests for antibodies to HIV in human serum or plasma. Fluorognost posts almost no indeterminate test results. In addition, the test takes only 90 minutes to complete, while the Western Blot takes from 12 to 24 hours to process. This FDA-approved test allows smaller healthcare facilities, emergency rooms, and doctors' offices to conduct in-office HIV screening and confirmation with accuracy, ease, and low overhead.

Urine-Based Tests—A urine sample, collected in a cup, is used for the ELISA/Western blot tests. The results of this noninvasive and nontechnical method can be obtained at a return visit, typically in one to two weeks. It's commonly used in community-based and outreach settings, adolescent, school, and university-based settings. Anyone with a positive urine result must have a confirmatory test.

Screening for p24 Antigen Looks Directly for Key Pieces of HIV—In August 1995, the FDA mandated that all blood and plasma collection centers screen all blood for p24 antigen (Figure 13-6). The FDA recommended p24 screening as an additional safety measure because recent studies indicated that p24 screening reduces the infectious window period (the FDA-approved Coulter p24 antigen blood test detects HIV as early as 16 days after infection). Among the 12 million-plus annual blood donations in the United States, p24-antigen screening is expected to detect four to six infectious donations that would not be identified by other screening tests. FDA regards donor screening for p24 antigen as an interim measure pending the availability of technology that would further reduce the risk for HIV transmission from blood donated during the infectious window period (*MMWR,* 1996 updated).

Nucleic Acid Testing—Beginning Spring 1999, the American Red Cross and 16 member laboratories of the America's Blood Centers began testing donor blood pools for the Human Immunodeficiency Virus (HIV) type 1 and the hepatitis C virus with a new research testing method known as **nucleic acid amplification testing (NAT).** The test was FDA-approved in June 2004. The power of NAT is its ability to detect the presence of infection by directly testing for viral nucleic acids, RNA, rather than by indirectly testing for the presence of antibodies. **NAT provides a *yes* or *no* answer as to whether HIV is present.**

Pitfalls to the Use of NAT—There are some serious drawbacks to the use of NAT. The requirement of specially trained lab technicians, space constraints, a minimum 12 hours required to perform NAT, and the cost of a NAT test kit, which is currently 10 times higher than the ELISA test kit, will be difficult to overcome. Also, as NAT currently exists there is a 1% chance of obtaining false-negative results. Regardless, NAT continues at Red Cross blood collection centers. The NAT was approved in October 2006 and became available for general diagnostic testing nationwide in 2007. Since then, the NAT has been used to determine the presence of HIV infection in newborns aged one month and older from HIV-positive mothers. It can also be used to identify HIV present during the window period. (HIV is present but is not detectable using the ELISA HIV screening test.) NAT costs about $25 to $30 per test. The commercial test name is Aptiva HIV-1 RNA.

SNAPSHOT 13.2

Just the Facts

The CDC estimates that 25% to 30% or about 320,000 people infected with HIV don't know they have it. The decision to get tested for HIV is the first step in taking responsibility for your health and the health of those you care about. Indeed, the only way to know if you are infected is to be tested for HIV infection. You cannot rely on symptoms alone because many people who are infected with HIV do not have any symptoms for 10 or more years. Someone can look and feel perfectly healthy and still be infected, which means he or she can infect others.

HIV screening can bring life-saving information and therapy to infected people earlier, when it is most beneficial in helping them to protect themselves and their sexual partners. Previous large-scale screening programs for syphilis and tuberculosis have been very successful.

RAPID HIV TESTING

A rapid test for detecting antibody to HIV is defined as a screening test that reveals the presence or absence of antibodies for HIV during the length of the patient's visit to the clinic, which is usually between 10 and 30 minutes. In the United States, 10% to 20% of pregnant women do not know their HIV status at the time of delivery. In Africa and Asian countries, it is estimated that over 90% of pregnant women do not know their HIV status at delivery. But the HIV status of pregnant women is essential to prevent mother-to-child HIV transmission.

Rapid HIV test results are also necessary for deciding whether to initiate treatment for healthcare workers after accidental exposures to patient body fluids, and there is a need for rapid HIV tests to assist with diagnosis and appropriate treatment of persons who may have opportunistic infections due to AIDS in urban emergency departments, which have been shown to have high rates of undiagnosed HIV infection among their patient populations. In short, the value of rapid HIV tests in public health has been well established.

There are over 30 different rapid HIV tests currently marketed worldwide. The first FDA-approved rapid HIV antibody test appeared in 1992. It is called the Single Use Diagnostic System (SUDS). Because of an unacceptable level of false positive results, it is no longer used.

Rapid Tests Now In Use

Each year about 750,000 or 30% of 2.5 million tested do not return to receive their test results. Using a rapid test, in less than 20 minutes, they can learn preliminary information about their HIV status (Table 13-2). Unlike other antibody tests for HIV, this test can be stored at room temperature, requires no specialized equipment, and can be used outside of traditional laboratory or clinical settings. In early 2008, New York City hospitals began offering rapid HIV testing. Under the new program, the hospitals hope to test 150,000 people in 2008 and another 160,000 in 2009. This program will reduce the large number of people (about 33%) who don't return for their ELISA test results.

The collection of oral fluids to look for HIV antibodies using the OraQuick Rapid HIV Antibody Test may not be as accurate as the other rapid assays that use blood samples. At present, the OraQuick test is only approved for use by medical professionals. It is very important to understand that these new tests do not change the length of time you have to wait after a possible exposure to HIV to get a reliable result. You still need to wait three months (13 weeks) to allow time for antibodies to become detectable in the blood for an accurate result. (See Table 13-3.)

The 3-Minute Test—On April 17, 2003, the FDA-approved the MedMira's Reveal Rapid HIV-1 Antibody Test, the first FDA-approved, rapid, point-of-care test designed to detect HIV-1 antibodies within three minutes. With the FDA-approval, MedMira can market the test for the detection of HIV-1 antibodies in serum or plasma. It is designed for point-of-care diagnostic purposes in medical settings such as hospitals and clinics.

The 1-Minute Test—In March 2004, Hedley Technologies delivered their Ultra Rapid 60 Second HIV Test Kit to the Uganda AIDS Commission. At this time only trained healthcare workers will be able to administer the test.

POINT OF VIEW 13.1

SOME RELATIVE DRAWBACKS TO THE CURRENT HIV SCREENING TEST— ELISA/WESTERN BLOT

Regardless of the high sensitivity and high specificity or overall test performance, there are a few test-related problems. For example, although only 24 hours are required to complete the ELISA/Western Blot testing procedures, most labs batch specimens for processing, causing a one- to two-week wait for definitive results. The results of several studies have shown that at least 35% of those who test positive and 42% of those who test negative never returned for their test results. Perhaps because of concern about maintaining anonymity or other factors, many individuals with HIV are not tested until they develop symptoms. Up to one-third of patients receive their HIV diagnosis within two months of an AIDS diagnosis.

Cost and time invested in the two-step process (pre- and post-test counseling) have also impeded testing. Even when tested without charge at a publicly funded clinic, clients must take time out of work or caring for children for waiting time, counseling, or travel. The true cost of this process has been estimated at $41 per test. And individuals tested in private offices may incur not only the cost of the test by commercial or hospital labs, but also the physician's office fee (Sax et al., 1997).

TABLE 13-2 Rapid HIV Test Kits Currently Available in the United States

Test Kit Name	Manufacturer	Specimen Type
1. OraQuick* Advance Rapid HIV-1/2 Antibody Test	Orasure Technologies, Inc. 20 minutes	Whole blood Oral fluid Plasma
2. Reveal G3* Rapid HIV-1 Antibody Test	MedMira, Inc. 20 minutes	Serum Plasma
3. Uni-Gold Recombigen HIV Test	Trinity Bio Tech 10 minutes	Whole blood Serum Plasma
4. Multispot HIV-1/ HIV-2 Rapid Test	Bio-Rad Laboratories 10 minutes	Serum Plasma
5. Clearview* Stat-Pak Assay	ChemBio Diagnostic Systems, Inc. 15 minutes	Whole blood Serum Plasma
6. Clearview Complete Assay	ChemBio Diagnostic Systems, Inc. 15 minutes	Whole blood Serum Plasma

*OraQuick, Reveal, and Clearview's Stat-Pak rapid tests are available for use in clinics and physician's offices nationwide (see Figures 13-7 and 13-8).

New Twist to the Dating Game

The two young single women, attractive and confident, were sitting at the bar of a popular after-hours tavern when they were asked how a relatively quick do-it-yourself HIV test might affect their dating life. One of them, age 23, laughed. "I would definitely make someone take it, hopefully before the sex." She said she would not be embarrassed to insist that a man submit to the test. "I really think we've got what they want. And if they want it, they can have it on our terms." Her friend, age 25, agreed and added, "Especially if you're getting serious with someone." Their comments were not idle speculation: a rapid at-home HIV test could be available on pharmacy shelves within the next year. Encouraged by a federal drug advisory committee early in 2006, OraSure Technologies in Bethlehem, Pa. has applied to the Food and Drug Administration for permission to start selling its HIV test over the counter. Currently it's available only in clinics.

Problem—Both women thought there would be a lot more unprotected sex if there was a 20-minute test that people could take. In a gay bar, the men said, "We're sick of hearing about condoms and prevention and safer sex. If a test could allow us to skip such prevention efforts, many would. An easily available HIV test could quickly reassure us of a prospective partner's health; it would allow a couple to jump into bed faster than they might have before." Then there is the fact that an HIV test also addresses an issue that more and more singles face—knowing next to nothing about their next date. The popularity of the Internet dating and group setups has led many singles to participate in blind dates, no references included (Figure 13-9).

Conclusion—An over-the-counter rapid HIV test will most likely lead to more casual encounters among most sexually active people. It is possible that a rapid at-home HIV test could help lower a stubbornly high rate of HIV infections that has not fallen since 1989.

Summary

Through 2008 the FDA has approved at least six rapid HIV screen tests for use in the United States.

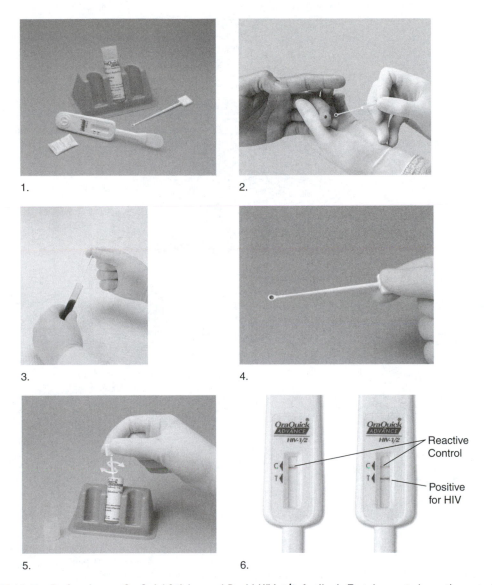

FIGURE 13-7 **Performing an OraQuick® Advanced Rapid HIV-1/2 Antibody Test.** Image 1 shows the materials required for this test. To collect a specimen for the test, either touch the collection loop to a fingerstick blood droplet (image 2) or use standard blood collection procedures for whole blood and dip the collection loop into the test tube (image 3). Five microliters of whole blood should adhere to and fill a single collection loop (image 4). Next, insert the loop and stir the specimen in the vial of developer solution (image 5). The OraQuick® device is inserted into the developer vial where it remains until the results are read (image 6). Test results must be read no sooner than 20 minutes but no later than 40 minutes after the device is added to the developer solution (image 6). (*Photographs© OraSure Technologies, Inc., 2006*)

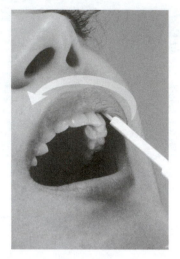

1.

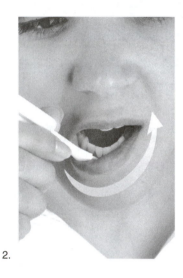

2.

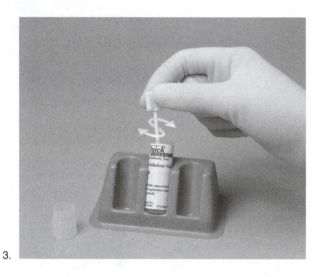

3.

FIGURE 13-8 **(a) OraQuick® oral fluid collection.** After the gums are swabbed with the paddle, the paddle is placed into a developer vial. **(b) Images, their readings and interpretations after a minimum of 20 minutes.** Possible results using the OraQuick® Advanced Rapid HIV-1/2 Antibody Tests are as follows: A nonreactive test will yield a line in the control **(C)** area and no line present in the test (T) area (Image 1). A nonreactive test result should be interpreted as negative for HIV-1/2 antibodies. A reactive test will yield a line in the control area and a line in the test area (Image 2). A reactive result should be interpreted as a preliminary positive for HIV-1/2 antibodies and must be confirmed. Also shown here are two samples of invalid test responses (Images 4–5), which required that a second test be performed. A weakly reactive test will yield a line in the control area and a weak line in the test area (Image 3). Follow-up testing is recommended to confirm an initial weakly active result. (*Photographs© OraSure Technologies, Inc. 2006*)

(b)

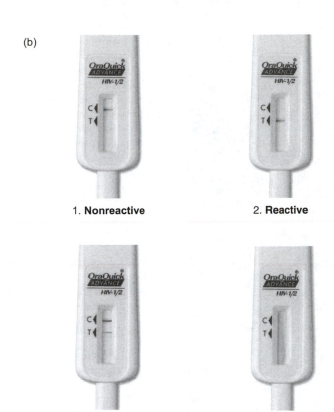

1. **Nonreactive**

2. **Reactive**

3. **Weakly reactive**

4. **Invalid**

FIGURE 13-8 (*Continued*)

All have at least a year-long shelf life when stored at room temperature and have sensitivity and specificity values equal to the ELISA test. In 2004, New York City, and the state of California, Washington, D.C., by law, made an HIV rapid test available to anyone who wanted to take it.

FDA APPROVES TWO HOME HIV ANTIBODY TEST KITS

On May 14, 1996, the FDA, which for years opposed home-based HIV testing kits because of the lack of face-to-face counseling, reversed its stance by saying

Table 13-3 Comparison of Conventional and Rapid HIV Testing

Specimen Required	Conventional Blood (Phlebotomy)	Rapid Oral swab or blood (finger stick)
Time to Result	3–10 days	20 minutes
Sensitivity	99.9%	99.3–99.6%
Specificity	99.9%	99.8–100.0%
Cost	ELISA $20	Test kits $14
Tested Persons Who Receive Their Test Results	Approximately 70%	99.3%

(*Source: Adapted from* PRN Notebook, *May, 2006*)

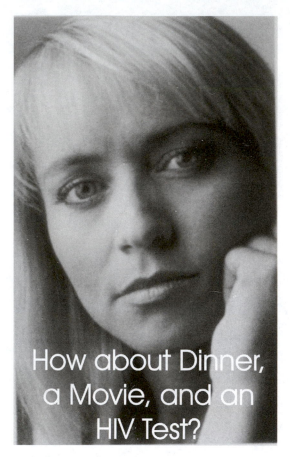

How about Dinner, a Movie, and an HIV Test?

FIGURE 13-9   A Woman Who Cares About Herself and Her Sexual Partner Becoming HIV Infected. (*Courtesy of the Centers for Disease Control and Prevention, Atlanta*)

the benefits of early detection of HIV infection outweigh any risks posed by the test. FDA Commissioner David Kessler said, "We are confident that this new home system can provide accurate results while assuring patient anonymity and appropriate counseling."

The FDA-approved the home test because in a 1994 study by the CDC of people at increased risk of infection, like injection-drug users and sexually active homosexual men, 42% indicated that they would use a home test (Figure 13-10).

Test Kit Operation

A person who buys the kit uses an enclosed lancet to prick his or her finger and places three drops of blood on a test card with an identification number. The card is mailed to a laboratory for HIV testing, and samples

that test positive are retested to ensure reliability. People who use the home system do not submit names, addresses, or phone numbers with the specimen sent in on filter paper. Therefore, the HIV test results are anonymous. To get results, the individual calls three days later and punches into the phone his or her identification number.

If the caller's test results are positive or inconclusive, he or she will be connected to a counselor who will explain the results, urge medical treatment, and, if necessary, make a referral to a local doctor or health clinic. If the person's results are negative, he or she will be connected to a recording that will note that it is possible to be infected with HIV and still test negative if the antibodies to HIV haven't yet developed. A counselor is available for anyone who tests negative and wants to discuss the results.

The FDA said the kit is as reliable as tests conducted in doctors' offices and clinics.

Test Kit Availability

The first FDA-approved HIV test kit, called Confide HIV Testing Service, was made available in June 1996. It was withdrawn from the marketplace in June 1997 due to poor sales. A second FDA-approved HIV home test kit went on sale nationwide in July 1996. This kit, called **Home Access Express HIV Test** (Figure 13-10) (1-800-448-8378), lets people take a blood sample at home, mail it to a laboratory, and, three days to a month later, learn by phone their results. The two tests are very similar to each other with regard to use and performance.

In 2006, the administrators at Home Access reported they had processed over 500,000 HIV tests since FDA-approval. The overall HIV-positive rate for these tests was 0.08% (8 of 10,000 were positive). The general population rate in America is about 0.03%. These data suggest that this form of testing appeals to an at-risk population.

SOME SCREENING AND CONFIRMATORY TESTS FOR HIV

There are a variety of HIV antigen detection tests now on the market, and others are on their way. A few of these tests have been singled out because they are currently in use or because of their potential to make a contribution in the field of HIV antibody–antigen testing methodology.

It should be emphasized that these tests identify parts of the virus. These are not antibody-related tests.

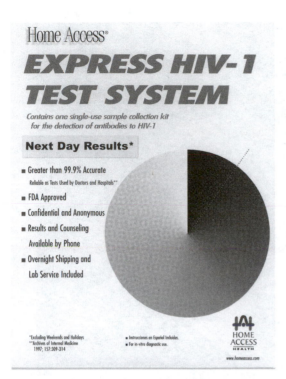

Home Access®

EXPRESS HIV-1 TEST SYSTEM

Contains one single-use sample collection kit for the detection of antibodies to HIV-1

Next Day Results*

- Greater than 99.9% Accurate
  Reliable as Tests Used by Doctors and Hospitals**
- FDA Approved
- Confidential and Anonymous
- Results and Counseling
  Available by Phone
- Overnight Shipping and
  Lab Service Included

*Excluding Weekends and Holidays
**Archives of Internal Medicine
1997; 157:309-314

■ Instrucciones en Español incluidas.
■ For in-vitro diagnostic use.

HOME ACCESS HEALTH

www.homeaccess.com

FIGURE 13-10 Home Access Anonymous HIV Test Kit. This kit was FDA-approved in July 1996 and provides access to professional counseling and medical/social service referrals 24 hours a day, 7 days a week. (*Photograph courtesy of Home Access Health Corp., Illinois*)

Polymerase Chain Reaction

Interactions between HIV and its host cell extend across a wide spectrum, from latent to productive infection. The virus can persist in cells as unintegrated DNA, as integrated DNA with alternative states of viral gene expression, or as a defective DNA molecule. Determining the fraction of cells in the blood that are latently (inactive) or productively infected is important for the understanding of viral pathogenesis and in the design and testing of effective therapies. Determining the number of infected cells in a heterogeneous cell population and the proportion of those cells that are carrying the virus but not producing new viruses requires the identification of the proviral DNA and viral mRNA in single cells.

The polymerase chain reaction (PCR) is a technique by which any DNA fragment from a single cell can be exponentially multiplied to an amount large enough to be measured. Thus PCR could be an ideal diagnostic test for HIV

infection, since it directly amplifies or increases the amount of proviral HIV DNA and does not require antibody formation by the host. It is already used in settings where antibody production is unpredictable or difficult to interpret, such as in acute HIV infection or in the perinatal/postnatal period. The PCR is so sensitive that it can detect and amplify as few as 6 molecules of proviral DNA in 150,000 cells or 1 molecule of viral DNA in 10 µL of blood.

Now that there are some good anti-HIV therapies available to help slow the onset of AIDS, the diagnosis of individuals who carry the provirus is critical because they may benefit from early treatment. The PCR test will become even more important with the advent of an HIV vaccine. Vaccinated people will become HIV-antibody positive. The PCR test will be used to identify those who are truly HIV infected. In addition, PCR is now used to detect HIV-DNA in spots of dried blood taken from infants as early as six weeks of age and shipped to testing centers without refrigeration. Recall that an ELISA (antibody) test cannot accurately diagnose infants until about the age of 18 months.

Two types of PCR tests are used to detect parts of HIV:

1. **Quantitative Polymerase Chain Reaction (PCR):** The quantitative PCR, also known as the viral load test, is considered to be highly reliable for someone who may have recently been exposed to the virus, particularly in a high-risk situation. If the virus is present, the quantitative PCR will reveal how much virus is in a person's bloodstream (the viral load). In most cases, a quantitative PCR is highly accurate within 48 to 72 hours. However, a small number of people don't have viral loads that are high enough to confirm a diagnosis until 28 days after exposure. The most widely available quantitative PCR test, **Amplicor version 1.5,** can detect subtypes A through G, which account for 99.96% of HIV infections in the United States. It can measure down to about 50 copies of HIV RNA/mL of sample.

2. **Qualitative PCR:** The qualitative PCR, also known as the PCR-DNA test, looks for DNA in cells that suggest that HIV infection has taken place. It is not a viral load test, meaning that it will only determine if the virus is present, not how much virus is present. This test is frequently used to determine if an infant born to an HIV-positive mother is infected with the virus, given that it can detect virus before viral load becomes detectable. However, it's not at all clear if the qualitative PCR test has any advantages over the quantitative PCR test, which appears to be just as reliable, more widely available, and cheaper to perform.

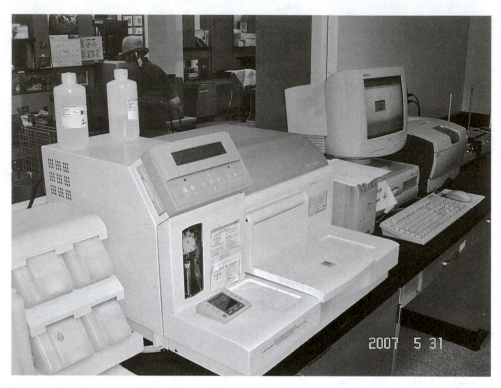

FIGURE 13-11 This FDA-approved instrument is used solely for branched DNA testing. It is capable of detecting/measuring RNA quantitatively from 75 to 500,000 RNA copies per milliliter of blood. It functions as an automated probe hybridization and signal amplification instrument used to quantify the amount of HIV RNA within the peripheral blood of an HIV-infected person. It is used in the long-term clinical management of an HIV-infected person. *(Courtesy of Florida Bureau of Laboratories, Retrovirology Unit, Jacksonville; photo by Berry Bennett, MPH.)*

Branched DNA Testing

Like the quantitative PCR test, the branched DNA (bDNA) assay can determine how much virus is present in someone who has been infected with the virus. The results of bDNA testing are comparable to those of quantitative PCR testing, and there are no known advantages of using bDNA testing over quantitative PCR testing for diagnostic purposes. This test is known as the Versant HIV RNA Assay and is available through most commercial laboratories. (See Figure 13-11.) This test can measure down to about 75 HIV RNA/mL of sample.

HIV Gene Probes

Gene probes or genetic probes are an idea borrowed from methodologies used in recombinant DNA research. The idea is to isolate a DNA segment, make many copies of it, and label these copies with a radioisotope or other tag compound. If the DNA sequence copied is contained in any of the HIV genes, the labeled copies of this DNA sequence can be used to hybridize or attach to DNA of cells that contain HIV DNA. This method of DNA probe analysis eliminates the need to search for HIV gene products or antibodies to these products to prove that a person is HIV infected.

At least two HIV-specific probes are on the market. One uses a radioactive sulfur label on the DNA for detection (^{35}S). This probe hybridizes to about 50% of the entire HIV genome and most specifically hybridizes to the HIV polymerase region. A second probe, also using ^{35}S, is an **RNA probe.** It is being used to detect HIV RNA in peripheral blood or tissue samples. **RNA probe hybridization** allows detection of 1 HIV-infected cell out of 400,000 uninfected cells. Specifically, the assay detects the presence of HIV in whole white blood cells as soon as the virus begins to replicate. The ^{35}S-labeled probes enter the white blood cells and combine with HIV; the procedure does not require DNA extraction and results are obtained in just over one day (Kramer et al., 1989).

DECIDING WHO SHOULD GET AN HIV TEST AND WHEN

Who Should Get Tested?

The following are behaviors that increase your chances of getting HIV. If you answer yes to any of them, you should definitely get an HIV test. If you continue with any of these behaviors, you should be tested every year. Talk to a healthcare provider about an HIV testing schedule that is right for you.

- Have you injected drugs or steroids or shared equipment (such as needles, syringes, works) with others?
- Have you had unprotected vaginal, anal, or oral sex with men who have sex with men, multiple partners, or anonymous partners?
- Have you exchanged sex for drugs or money?
- Have you been diagnosed with or treated for hepatitis, tuberculosis (TB), or a sexually transmitted disease (STD), like syphilis?

- Have you had unprotected sex with someone who could answer yes to any of the above questions?
- Have you been incarcerated in a prison?

If you have had sex with someone whose history of sexual partners and/or drug use is unknown to you or if you or your partner has had many sex partners, then you have more of a chance of being infected with HIV. Both you and your new partner should get tested for HIV and learn the results before having sex for the first time. For women who plan to become pregnant, testing is even more important. If a woman is infected with HIV, medical care and certain drugs given during pregnancy can lower the chance of passing HIV TO HER BABY. All women who are pregnant should be tested during each pregnancy. **One Test Can Save Two Lives**.

When Should You Get Tested?

Get the test if, for any reason (such as those listed above) you or your physician believes you might have been exposed to HIV. Most HIV tests are antibody tests that measure the antibodies your body makes against HIV. It can take some time for the immune system to produce enough antibodies for the antibody test to detect and this time period can vary from person to person. This time period is commonly referred to as the "window period." Most people will

---

SIDEBAR 13.2

BEST POLICY FOR PRENATAL TESTING?

Given the efficacy of antiretroviral drugs to reduce perinatal HIV transmission if administered to the mother while the fetus is in the womb or to the baby within 48 hours after birth, it has become a priority to maximize the number of pregnant women who consent to prenatal HIV testing. Three distinct approaches to obtaining consent for prenatal HIV testing are used: (1) the "opt-in" or voluntary policy (the test, after counseling, is offered to the woman, and she may refuse); (2) the "opt-out" policy (the woman is not counseled about HIV/AIDS but is informed that the HIV test is part of a battery of prenatal tests, which are automatic but she may refuse HIV testing by signing a form rejecting the test); and (3) the mandatory newborn HIV testing approach (the mother is informed that the newborn will be tested, with or without her consent, if her HIV status is unknown at delivery). Currently 10 states

mandate HIV testing of the newborn. Connecticut also mandates HIV testing of all pregnant women. Thirty-two states use the "opt out" policy and 29 states have the "opt in" policy. The CDC recently evaluated the efficacy of these three approaches in obtaining prenatal HIV tests in the United States and Canada. As a result of these evaluations, the CDC in April 2003 unveiled their HIV testing strategy for pregnant women. These guidelines were updated in 2006. The new strategy specifically urges the testing of all pregnant women rather than relying upon patients to volunteer for testing. The guidelines also make HIV testing a routine part of care in doctors' offices and clinics, rather than waiting for patients to specifically request it. The strategy is advisory but has some authority: CDC will ask state and local governments to adhere to it in exchange for federal funding.

develop detectable antibodies within two to eight weeks (the average is 25 days). Even so, there is a chance that some individuals will take longer to develop detectable antibodies. Therefore, if the initial negative HIV test was conducted within the first three months after possible exposure, repeat testing should be considered three months after the first test to account for the possibility of a false-negative result. Ninety-seven percent will develop antibodies in the first three months following the time of their infection. In very rare cases, it can take up to six months or longer to develop antibodies to HIV.

Addressing Barriers to HIV Testing

Knowledge of HIV infection status can benefit the health of individual persons and the community. Thus, HIV testing should be as convenient as possible to promote client knowledge of HIV infection status. Efforts should be made to remove or lower barriers to HIV testing by ensuring that:

- Testing is accessible, available, and responsive to client and community needs and priorities;

- Anonymous and confidential HIV testing is available;

- The testing process considers the client's culture, language, sex, sexual orientation, age, and developmental level; and

- Confidentiality is maintained. (In some places, like rural communities, **confidentiality** can't be assured, so people may decide not to get tested.)

WHY IS HIV TEST INFORMATION NECESSARY?

Thirty percent of adults who seek HIV testing do so to find out their HIV status; 12% are tested because of hospitalization or surgery; 16% for application for insurance; and 7% to enter the military. Another 1% are referred by their doctor, the health department, or sexual partner, and 4% are tested for HIV for immigration reasons (see Tables 13-4 and 13-5).

IMMIGRATION INTO THE UNITED STATES

Having HIV can make it very difficult to immigrate into the United States. Everyone 15 years of age and older who applies for a green card has to take an HIV test. If you test positive you cannot get a green card unless you get an HIV waiver. An HIV waiver is a

Table 13-4 Percentage of Adults Aged 18 Years and Over Who Had Been Tested for Human Immunodeficiency Virus, by Age Group and Sex: United States, January–March 2006[1, 2]

Ages and Sex[3]	Percent
18–24 years	
Total	35.3
Male	29.5
Female	41.1
25–34 years	
Total	53.5
Male	42.1
Female	64.8
35–44 years	
Total	49.3
Male	44.9
Female	53.5
45–64 years	
Total	28.7
Male	30.9
Female	26.6
65 years and over	
Total	11.8
Male	14.7
Female	9.7

[1] In early 2006 the percentage of U.S. adults (age 18 and over) who had ever been tested for HIV was 35.4%, which is the same percentage of adults found in 2003.

[2] For both sexes combined, the percentage of persons who ever had an HIV test was highest among adults aged 25–34 years (53.5%) and lowest among adults aged 65 years and over (11.8%).

[3] For age groups 18–24 years, 25–34 years, and 35–44 years, women were more likely than men to have ever had an HIV test. For adults aged 65 years and over, women were less likely than men to have ever had an HIV test.

Data Source: CDC; National Health Interview Survey, 2006. Data are based on household interviews of a sample of the civilian noninstitutionalized population.

special permission from the Immigration and Naturalization Service (INS) that allows an HIV-positive person to obtain permanent residency. A green card applicant who is the spouse, unmarried child, or parent of a U.S. citizen or legal permanent resident may be able to get a waiver if he or she meets the other requirements. Before you can get a waiver, you must show the INS that you are able to pay your medical expenses if you get sick. In other words, you must show that you will not need government benefits such as Medicare or free county services. You must also show that you are not a danger to the public health—that is, you must demonstrate knowledge of how HIV is spread and what you can do to minimize the chances of transmission.

Table 13-5 Age-Sex-Adjusted Percentage of Adults Aged 18 Years and Over Who Had Been Tested for Human Immunodeficiency Virus, by Race/Ethnicity: United States, January–March 2006

Race/Ethnicity[2]	Percent[1]
Hispanic or Latino	37.9
Not Hispanic or Latino:	
White, Single race	33.2
Black, Single race	49.4

[1] *Estimates are age-sex-adjusted using the projected 2000 U.S. population as the standard population using five age groups: 18–24 years, 25–34 years, 35–44 years, 45–64 years, and 65 years and over. Data Source: CDC; National Health Interview Survey, 2006. Data are based on household interview of a sample of the civilian noninstitutionalized population.*

[2] *The age-sex-adjusted percentages of persons who ever had an HIV test were 37.9% for Hispanic persons, 33.2% for non-Hispanic white persons, and 49.4% for non-Hispanic black persons. Of the three races/ethnicity groups, non-Hispanic black persons were most likely to have ever had an HIV test.*

In 2008, the United States partly lifted a ban on incoming travel across its borders by HIV-positive people. The 12 other countries that continue to ban are Iraq, China, Saudi Arabia, Libya, Sudan, Qatar, Brunei, Oman, Moldova, Russia, Armenia, and South Korea. Because of U.S. immigration policy, the International AIDS Society has not held the International AIDS Conferences in the United States since 1990, or in any country with an HIV-restrictive immigration policy.

HIV Legislation: United States

The U.S. Congress in 1993 enacted legislation, Section 212 (a) (1) (A) (I) of the Immigration and Nationality Act, that prevents HIV-positive foreigners from obtaining visas or citizenship. According to the U.S. Department of State, if any foreigners traveling to the United States including people from countries not requiring visas, reveal that they have a communicable disease of public health significance, they are prevented from entering the country. The same rules apply to green card applicants.

However, in view of humanitarian and family unity concerns, the law also provides waivers to inadmissibility, which are discretionary and granted on a case-by-case basis. Two specific waiver policies have been implemented for applicants seeking admission as **nonimmigrants** (for a temporary period of time) who are inadmissible due to HIV infection:

Routine HIV Waiver Policy—Nonimmigrants may be granted a waiver for admission to the United States for 30 days or less to attend conferences, receive medical treatment, visit close family members, or conduct business. The applicant must demonstrate that he or she is not currently afflicted with symptoms of the disease.

The Designated Event Policy—This policy facilitates the admission of HIV-positive persons to attend certain designated events, which are considered to be in the public interest, such as academic and educational conferences and international sports events.

If the INS discovers a noncitizen is HIV positive, he or she can be prevented from entering the country even if they have a green card. The INS does not require an HIV test to reenter. However, they are allowed to ask you if you have HIV. If you reenter the United States with AIDS-related materials such as pamphlets or medicine such as AZT in your luggage, or if you are clearly sick, the INS may ask you if you are HIV positive and detain you for medical examination. However, tourists and other nonimmigrants such as business people, temporary workers, or those seeking medical treatment are generally not asked to take an HIV test. There is no HIV test when applying for citizenship. Only persons applying for permanent residency are required to be tested by the INS. Always consult with an immigration/naturalization attorney.

Illegal Immigrants and HIV

According to immigration authorities, an unknown number of the 12 to 20 million undocumented immigrants in the United States are infected with HIV, and the secretive existence they live out of fear of deportation is adding to their health risks, according to medical experts. In the worst cases, immigrants are dying because they cannot access health care or they are spreading the disease because they do not know they are infected. Undocumented persons with HIV may be getting a patchwork of inconsistent care, turning to emergency rooms for treatment of opportunistic infections and then returning to the shadows, afraid that deportation to a homeland without medicines or health care is a certain death sentence.

Immigration and Entry into Foreign Countries

An increasing number of foreign countries require that foreigners be tested for HIV prior to entry. This have no restrictions. Before traveling abroad, check with the embassy of the country to be visited to learn entry requirements and specifically whether or not HIV testing is a requirement. If the foreign country indicates that U.S. test results are acceptable "under certain conditions," prospective travelers should inquire at the embassy of that country for details (which laboratories in the United States may perform tests and where to have results certified and authenticated) before departing the United States. For a copy of HIV Testing Requirements for Entry into Foreign Countries, send a self-addressed, stamped, business-size envelope to: Bureau of Consular Affairs, Room 5807, Department of State, Washington, D.C. 20520.

TESTING, COMPETENCY, AND INFORMED CONSENT

Competency is often used interchangeably with capacity; it refers to a person's ability to make an

is particularly true for students or long-term visitors. Information available from 168 countries at the beginning of 2009 reveals that 62 countries require an HIV test prior to entry, on arrival, or on application for residency. Entering 2009, a total of 105 countries had entry or residence restrictions against HIV-infected people. There are 89 countries that

UNITED KINGDOM DEPORTS HIV–POSITIVE PEOPLE

In May 2005, a House of Lords ruling ('N'[2005] UKHL31) concluded that the deportation of a person living with HIV to a country where he or she was unlikely to receive adequate HIV treatment was not incompatible with their right to be free of inhuman treatment under Article 3 of the European Convention on Human Rights. The decision essentially authorized the deportation to their countries of origin of hundreds of HIV-positive people living in the UK whose applications for asylum have been rejected, regardless of whether HIV treatment is accessible or affordable. In mid-2007, the African HIV Policy Network (AHPN) launched a campaign calling on the UK government to stop the deportation of people living with HIV to countries where access to HIV treatment is not readily available or affordable. The campaign, Destination Unknown, is also asking MPs to sign a House of Commons Early Day Motion, which "notes that there is a clear contradiction between the UK's policy aim of universal access to treatment for all those who need it by 2010 and the deportation of people living with HIV who are on treatment to countries where treatment is not readily available or affordable."

informed decision. For example, to consent to medical treatment, a person must be mentally capable of comprehending the risks and benefits of a proposed procedure and its alternatives. While a healthcare provider can assess competence, a legal finding of competency is often required based on the testimony of a mental health professional. Mental illness by itself does not indicate that a person is incompetent to make medical decisions. Various degrees of mental incapacity may occur with HIV infection, requiring an assessment of competency. AIDS Dementia Complex (ADC) occurs in approximately 70% of HIV-infected patients at some point in HIV disease/AIDS and may interfere with the patient's capacity to provide an informed consent.

Informed Consent

Informed consent is not just signing a form but is a process of education and the opportunity to have questions answered. The concept of informed consent includes the following components: full disclosure of information, patient competency, patient understand-

ing, voluntariness, and decision making. The process of obtaining informed consent involves appropriate facts being provided to a competent patient who understands the information and voluntarily makes a choice to accept or refuse the recommended procedure or treatment.

When the concept of informed consent is applied clinically, complexities arise regarding both the content and the process. The concept contains ambiguous requisites such as "appropriate" facts, "full" disclosure, and "substantial" understanding. The process is affected by many variables including the communication skill and range of practice style of the physician; the maturity, intelligence, and coping strategies of the patient; and the interaction between the physician and the patient (Hartlaub et al., 1993).

Testing Without Consent

Entering 2009, at least 35 states had laws that allowed HIV testing without informed consent under certain conditions. The required conditions vary and include:

1. Patient or other authorized person is unable to give or withhold consent.
2. Test result will help determine treatment.
3. Patient is unable to give consent, and physician can document that a medical emergency exists and that the test is needed for diagnosis and treatment.
4. Test is needed to protect the health of other patients, health workers, or emergency or law enforcement personnel.
5. Several states require post-test counseling.
6. Minors ages 12 to 14, depending on the state, can consent to HIV testing and treatment.

Generally, HIV antibody testing without consent is legally considered battery. Legal liability for "unlawful touching" may result from performing an HIV antibody test without consent. Such a procedure may also constitute an illegal search.

DISCUSSION QUESTION: Are federal and state governments overemphasizing personal privacy at the expense of prevention? (Defend your answer with examples/situations.)

Voluntary Named HIV Testing

In **voluntary named** HIV testing, the individual freely provides his or her name. In this type of testing, an individual voluntarily seeks to learn his or her HIV status and receives a result that is known both to the individual and the test provider/testing agency.

An advantage to named testing is that healthcare providers can contact the person tested if he or she does not return for the results.

Voluntary Unnamed or Anonymous HIV Testing

HIV testing is voluntary, and the identity of the person being tested is not placed on the blood sample or the testing form. As a result, the only person who can link the test result with an individual is the person being tested. This form of testing may encourage people concerned about HIV infection status to obtain testing as it eliminates risk of discrimination or stigmatization. However, it places the exclusive responsibility for seeking counseling, support, and preventive measures on the individual who is infected. Unnamed testing permits reporting of test data to public health authorities without the risk of breaching confidentiality.

The Downside to Voluntary, Voluntary Anonymous Testing

Testing that is voluntary may miss populations that disproportionately need to be reached. The people least likely to have the virus, it appears, are the most likely to say yes to a test, and the people most likely to be infected are the most likely to say no. In one study, infection rates were 5.3 times as high among people who refused HIV testing as among people who consented to it. In voluntary anonymous, the downside is that such testing reduces the probability that they will return for post-test counseling and linkage to follow-up services, and a substantial reduction in partner notifications (Moser, 1998).

Mandatory HIV Testing

HIV testing is mandatory if it is required to participate in a process or activity that is not itself required. For example, if an HIV test is required for travel to some foreign countries, or to donate blood, this is considered mandatory testing because, while the test is required, one is not required to travel or donate blood. In mandatory testing, care must be taken to ensure that people are not in fact forced to undergo testing. At least in theory, mandatory testing is a form of voluntary testing: People can decide not to participate in the process or activity for which testing is required. In practice, however, the degree of voluntary consent is in some cases questionable. For example, in a situation where employment is not possible unless

one agrees to be tested, and one needs that job, the voluntary nature of the test appears to have vanished (*AIDS, Health and Human Rights,* 1995).

Why Mandatory Testing?

Mandatory testing is for the protection of a certain group or the public at large. Although it is not anonymous, results are kept confidential on a need-to-know basis. Mandatory testing for HIV continues to be angrily debated primarily because of the possibility of error when running large numbers of test samples, inadvertent loss of confidentiality, and lack of overall benefit to those who are found to be HIV positive. Mandatory HIV testing is routine for blood donors and military and Job Corps personnel.

Mandatory HIV Testing of Newborns and Disclosure of Test Results to Mothers and Physicians

Perhaps no call for mandatory HIV testing has caused as much recent controversy as those requiring all pregnant women to take the test or their newborns will be tested. On June 26, 1996, New York became the first state in the nation to mandate and disclose the HIV status of newborns to mothers and physicians. Governor George E. Pataki signed into law legislation known as the **"Baby AIDS" Bill,** which authorizes the state health commissioner to establish a comprehensive program of HIV testing of newborns. Over the next eight years, there was an 80% decline in HIV-infected babies born to infected mothers.

The passage of this bill was immediately followed by the American Medical Association announcement endorsing mandatory testing of all pregnant women and newborns for the AIDS virus. (See Sidebar 13.2.)

Compulsory HIV Testing

In **compulsory testing,** a person cannot refuse to be tested. Compulsory testing may be forced onto an individual, groups, communities, or even entire populations. A court may order an individual to be tested, or a government may decree or legislate that, for example, commercial sex workers, homosexuals, prisoners, hospital patients, or persons seeking immigration must be tested.

In Colorado, Florida, Georgia, Illinois, Kentucky, Michigan, Nevada, Rhode Island, Utah, and West

THE TIME FOR ROUTINE HIV TESTING IS NOW?

The editorial of the March 5, 2005 edition of the *British Medical Journal* and the March 20, 2006 editorial in the *New England Journal of Medicine* state that both the United Kingdom and the United States are ready for routine voluntary HIV testing of all their people. Health experts across the United States are recommending such action, similar to the testing for various cancers and other diseases. The experts argue that HAART has made HIV like any other serious illness. And testing for HIV can take place without counseling. Patients for other serious diseases do not receive counseling. Times have changed. HIV testing should not be accorded any special status. The CDC estimated that beginning in the early 1990s through 2007, about 19 million people per year received an HIV test.

STIGMA AND ITS IMPACT ON HIV TESTING

To this point in time stigma has kept many people away from testing centers. After over 60 years of this disease (the first HIV infection is suggested to have occurred in the 1940s and to have given rise to the first confirmed AIDS case in 1959—see Chapter 2, Point of Information 2.1 for details) and billions of prevention education dollars spent, stigma still reigns. Routine HIV testing of all people should, at least, reduce such behavior and make AIDS a socially acceptable disease as has occurred during the history of cancer in the United States.

PRESSURE FOR UNIVERSAL HIV TESTING U.S.A.

At the 13th Conference on Retroviruses and Opportunistic Infections (Denver 2006), it became clear that the issue of HIV testing's role in prevention can no longer be ignored. Timothy Mastro said that a CDC study showed that HIV-positive people reduced the amount of unprotected serodiscordant sex (only one of the sexual partners being HIV positive) they had by 68% after diagnosis. This led them to believe that the 25% to 30% of people who do not know their HIV status contributed to about 50% of infections. He cited the startlingly high prevalence and incidence figures among gay men and particularly black gay men in cities other than San Francisco. In a large sample of gay men in five U.S. cities, 25% of gay men had HIV and 48% were unaware of their infection. In another city, 46% of black gay men were positive and 67% did not know it. Late testing was also common: 45% of AIDS diagnosis were among people who had been diagnosed HIV positive less than 12 months before.

Mastro said that HIV testing in the U.S.A. has not been increasing in recent years despite the fact that the CDC had launched its Advancing HIV Prevention strategy in 2003 to make voluntary HIV testing a routine part of medical care. For example, only about one in 500 visits to hospital emergency departments involved an HIV test despite the fact that, when tested, rates of previously undiagnosed HIV among accident and emergency patients varied from 1% to 3%. Taking it upon themselves, one STD clinic in Dallas, Texas shows a notice which says that "All patients seen in this clinic will be tested for gonorrhea, syphilis, chlamydia and HIV."

WIDESPREAD HIV SCREENING IS BENEFICIAL

Two studies conclude that routine testing of most Americans for the AIDS-causing virus would reduce new infections (see Table 13-4).

Table 13-4 Finding the HIV Infected[1]

Current Practice vs. More Testing	Current Practice	Testing Once	Every Five Years	Testing Annually
Percentage of cases not detected before symptoms appear[2]	37%	35%	21%	8%
Percentage currently detected	63%	61%	44%	19%
Percentage that would be detected in proposed testing	–	3%	34%	73%

[1]The CDC Surveillance system identifies only those who choose to be HIV tested. In 20% of patients AIDS is diagnosed at the time of HIV testing and 40% are diagnosed in the same test year. Up to 70% of HIV infections in the U.S. are associated with persons who have undiagnosed HIV infections.

[2]For high-risk groups including IV-drug users, gay men and residents of major cities.

Source: Adapted from *New England Journal of Medicine* February 10, 2005, 352:570–586.

Cost-Effectiveness of Voluntary Routine HIV Testing?

Two studies in the *New England Journal of Medicine* (Paltiel et al., 2005 and Saunders et al., 2005) showed that routine HIV screening is both cost-effective and life extending with today's available antiretroviral therapy. Testing of all Americans ages 13–64 would cost over $100 million. Identifying the HIV infected early gets them to treatment early and costs less for therapy overall, and the patients live longer. The benefits of widespread HIV screening can be seen in Table 13-4. A study by researchers at Duke and Stanford Universities and the Veterans Affairs Palo Alto Health Care System estimated that routine one-time testing for everyone would cut new infections each year by just over 20%, and that every HIV-infected patient identified would gain an average of 1-1/2 years of life.

CENTERS FOR DISEASE CONTROL AND PREVENTION'S RESPONSE TO CURRENT FINDINGS

After the two studies were published in the *New England Journal of Medicine* last year, the CDC determined in September 2006 that routine screening would be cost-effective and decided to revise its HIV screening guidelines and would be recommending routine, voluntary or "OPT-OUT" screening for all persons ages 13 to 64 in healthcare settings, without regard to risk, and annual HIV testing for people with risk behavior. Pretest counseling and written consent would not be required (currently 10 states still require written consent for HIV tests). Healthcare settings include all hospital in-patient and out-patient departments and community clinics as well as STD clinics. An exception would be made for prisons, where it was recognized that receiving an HIV diagnosis created profound difficulties both for inmate and institution.

The new CDC guidelines will urge that HIV testing become an opt-out process in all healthcare settings—meaning, all patients should automatically be tested unless they specifically ask not to be. In other words, it will no longer be necessary to obtain written consent to conduct an HIV test. The test will also become a standard part of the bevy of prenatal tests given to pregnant women. The CDC's recommendations are not legally binding upon state and local laws and regulations, but they heavily influence how local officials design their rules, in part because of the implicit threat of jeopardizing federal funding by failing to comply. Two years after the CDC call for routine HIV testing, at least 30 states still have laws that prevent physicians from adopting the CDC recommendations.

QUESTION: IS THE TIME RIGHT FOR NATIONAL ROUTINE TESTING?

The CDC's suggestion that the time is right, the time is now, has raised very serious issues both pro and con. A pro/con debate on this question will reveal many issues about the HIV/AIDS pandemic, such as why have the political, medical, and scientific establishments, up to now, placed this disease in an exceptional category, never allowing routine testing of the HIV infected when, in fact, no other disease in history has held such status!

David Holtgrave, an epidemiologist with the Johns Hopkins Bloomberg Public School of Health, writes in his research article in the June 12 issue of *PLoS Medicine* that targeting HIV testing at high-risk groups and populations might be a more effective method of identifying people who are unaware of their HIV-positive status than conducting routine testing among all U.S. residents ages 13 to 64. According to Holtgrave, who headed CDC's Division of HIV/AIDS Prevention in the late 1990s, the U.S. healthcare system would spend about $864 million in one year to diagnose nearly 57,000 new HIV cases using the routine testing system. The data is based on the assumption that 1% of people tested are HIV positive. However, the healthcare system could identify up to 188,170 new HIV cases for the same cost by targeting drug treatment facilities, prisons, and community health centers in high-risk neighborhoods. Targeted testing also would focus on people known to have drug habits or to engage in high-risk sexual activities regardless of where they live.

The CDC does recognize that universal HIV testing could encroach heavily on doctors' workloads, so the agency dropped the requirements for written consent and pretest counseling. (In June of 2007 the state of Illinois became the first state to drop the requirement of written consent prior to an HIV test and in September 2007 California became the second state to drop the requirement). However, Holtgrave says that pretest counseling is an essential way to educate patients about HIV prevention. He also estimates that targeted testing and counseling would prevent more than 14,000 new HIV cases annually at a cost of $59,000 per case prevented, compared with 3600 cases at a cost of $237,000 each using CDC's guidelines.

Holtgrave said, "I don't want to make it seem that I'm anti-testing—the question is whether there are better ways to do this. Under CDC recommendations, there would be a lot of testing and not much in the way of diagnosis and if we don't do the counseling of people at risk we're not going to do much in the way of prevention." Timothy Mastro, deputy director of the CDC's Division of HIV/AIDS Prevention, said that the federal government has focused on reaching high-risk populations. The CDC's new recommendations seek to broaden testing by reducing missed opportunities in physicians' offices, emergency departments, and elsewhere. Mastro said, "There's a role for targeted testing of people perceived to be at risk. It's brought us a long way on HIV prevention but not far enough."

United Nations Program on AIDS (UNAIDS) and the World Health Organization (WHO) Release New HIV Testing Guidelines

In mid-2007, UNAIDS and the WHO released new HIV testing guidelines that advise healthcare workers in countries with an HIV prevalence greater than 1% to routinely offer confidential, voluntary HIV tests to all patients seeking treatment at clinics or hospitals regardless of why they initially sought care. Earlier WHO and UNAIDS guidelines advised health workers to offer HIV tests only if treatment was available, and health workers often administered the tests only when re-

quested. According to the new guidelines, people would be allowed to decline testing or OPT OUT. In addition, the guidelines require that everyone who receives an HIV test also receive counseling.

The guidelines also advise physicians worldwide to offer testing to patients who show signs of HIV infection. The guidelines also suggest HIV testing for anyone whose medical history suggests possible HIV infection, including children of HIV-positive women and people with tuberculosis. Botswana, Kenya, Malawi, and Uganda already have implemented testing policies similar to the new guidelines.

DISCUSSION QUESTION: Do you think that targeting HIV testing at high-risk groups might be a more effective way of identifying people who are unaware of their HIV status than conducting routine testing among all U.S. residents ages 13 to 64? Do you think that perhaps the CDC should just consider what changes they can implement to make it easier for people to learn their HIV status and go with that?

Virginia, HIV testing is compulsory for people convicted of prostitution. However, many prostitutes are back on the streets before their test results are in. In many cases, the prostitutes could not be found for follow-up counseling. In Duval County, Fla., county judges agreed to impose a 30-day jail term for convicted prostitutes, a time period long enough to get their test results and provide counseling. Prostitutes have to sign the test results sheet. They are released as soon as they do.

Under Florida law, a prostitute who knows he or she is carrying HIV but continues to offer sexual favors can be jailed for one year.

In June 1999, the state of Oregon passed legislation that allows a judge to order a person accused of a crime to be tested for HIV. The person also would be tested for other communicable diseases if he or she transmitted bodily fluids to a victim. The results do not become public record.

In mid-2004, the governor of Wisconsin signed into law a bill that allows teachers to require students to be tested if a teacher is exposed to students' blood. The teachers in this state were added to a list of professionals who are permitted to require HIV tests on people whose blood they are exposed to. The list includes firefighters, police, emergency medical technicians, and other healthcare workers.

At least 45 states and the District of Columbia authorize HIV testing for charged or convicted sex offenders.

Fear of Compulsory Testing—If a massive compulsory screening test program were implemented, would it be possible to keep results confidential? What would be done with the information? For example, would the state prevent an uninfected person from marrying an infected one? Officials fear that mandatory testing will drive many people who might have volunteered for anonymous testing underground and away from health care. These people will be lost to the counseling and education that would benefit them and others. The reason for going underground would be fear of discrimination and social ostracism if found to be HIV infected.

A case can be made that a compulsory program could maintain strict confidentiality even with large numbers of people being tested. But, it would appear that the political powers and public in general are not ready for broad-scale compulsory testing in the United States.

Confidential, Anonymous, and Blinded Testing

Both confidential and anonymous testing involve the use of informed consent forms that are, to date, with the exception of the U.S. military, Job Corps workers, and certain criminals, done on a voluntary basis. Blinded testing does not, because of procedure, require informed consent.

Confidential HIV Testing—The person's name and test results are recorded. If their test is positive the

CONFIDENTIALITY AND SEXUAL PARTNER BETRAYAL

This story took place in an HIV/AIDS clinic in the South. A husband and wife came into the clinic for an HIV test. They said the *only* reason for requesting the test was that they wanted to begin a family and hoped that nothing in their past would have led to either of them being HIV positive. The tests were completed.

The husband came in on a Monday; the wife came in that Friday.

Monday A.M.

Counselor: Mr. X, your test came back HIV positive.

Reactions and counseling were similar to those presented in this chapter. Then Mr. X said he wanted to be the one to tell his wife; *he insisted on it.* The counselor agreed, Mr. X left the clinic agreeing to come back for a follow-up counseling session.

Friday A.M.

Counselor: Mrs. X, your HIV test was negative.

Mrs. X: That's wonderful news. I can't wait to tell my husband. We've been waiting for my results. I want to get pregnant immediately.

Mrs. X received HIV-negative counseling and left the clinic very happy.

Clearly, the husband did not tell his wife the truth about his test results. A follow-up phone call to the husband went unanswered; so did a letter from the clinic. Several months later, Mrs. X called the counselor to tell her that she was pregnant!

What do you think the counselor should do now?

1. Inform the woman about her husband.
2. Take no action.
3. Call the husband and discuss the situation.
4. Threaten the husband with legal action if he does not tell his wife.
5. Your position?

Discuss the moral, ethical, and legal responsibilities of each participant.

---

results are reported to the state health department. A consent to HIV testing must be given freely and without coercion. The volunteer does not have to provide any information unless he or she wants to.

The following example demonstrates one of the problems with confidential testing: A young homosexual male with signs of oral thrush agreed to an HIV test. Later that day, he called and asked that his blood *not* be sent to the lab. He was a teacher in a parochial school and feared the results would be revealed. His sample was set aside, but the laboratory courier mistakenly took it for testing. The result was positive, yet no one could tell the patient. A malpractice attorney said to make certain all records of the test were deleted and to send the patient a letter urging him to return for a blood test. He never appeared (Wake, 1989).

Because in any given year, only 20% of U.S. residents at high risk for HIV are tested, many national public health agencies and committees favor a confidential screening and counseling program that includes all individuals whose behavior places them at high risk of HIV exposure. These agencies recommend that the following eight groups seriously consider volunteering for HIV antibody testing at least twice annually:

1. Homosexual and bisexual men
2. Present or past injection-drug users
3. People with signs or symptoms of HIV infection
4. Male and female prostitutes
5. Sexual partners of people either known to be HIV infected or at increased risk of HIV infection
6. Hemophiliacs who received blood clotting products prior to 1985
7. Newborn children of HIV-infected mothers
8. Immigrants from Haiti and Central Africa since 1977

Anonymous HIV Testing—No name is ever given. And, no one can ever learn of your test results. This is also a form of voluntary testing. It differs from confidential testing only in that those who request anonymity receive a bar-coded identification number. They provide no personal information and they come back at a predetermined time to find out if their test number is positive or negative. No follow-up occurs. All states have anonymous test sites providing over 2.5 million tests a year (Nash et al., 1998 updated). Things change when the individual seeks treatment: If one goes to a doctor and the doctor does a viral load test, he reports the person and their viral load test to the health department. There is no way to keep treatment for HIV anonymous.

Blinded HIV Testing—This occurs when blood or serum is available for HIV testing as a result of another medical procedure wherein the patient's blood has been drawn for analysis. In this case, the demographic data have been recorded and can be used for epidemiological studies even if the name of the individual is withheld and a bar code is used. In 1988, the CDC asked for a blinded study of all 1989 newborn blood samples taken in certain cities in 45 states for metabolic studies. The name and other demographics of each newborn were recorded on the label of each tube. After the metabolic tests were completed, the name was changed into a bar code and leftover blood was sent to a state HIV testing center.

DISCUSSION QUESTION: What are reasons for and against blinded testing?

Where Can One Get Tested for HIV Infection?

Many places provide testing for HIV infection. Common testing locations include local health departments, clinics, offices of private doctors, hospitals, and other sites set up specifically to provide HIV testing. You can also ask your healthcare provider about getting tested, or for information on where to find an HIV testing site, visit the National HIV Testing Resources Web site at http://www.hivtest.org or call CD-INFO 24 hours a day at 1–800–232–4636; 1–888–232–6348 (TTY), in English, en Español. Between the time of a possible exposure and the receipt of test results, individuals should consider abstaining from sexual contact with others or use condoms and/or dental dams during all sexual encounters.

Summary

HIV infection can be detected in three ways: first, by HIV-antibody or antigen testing prior to the appearance of signs and symptoms of AIDS; second, by detecting the presence of HIV nucleic acid; and third, by physical examination after symptoms occur.

The test most often used to screen donor blood at blood banks and individuals referred to testing centers is the ELISA test. ELISA (enzyme linked immunosorbent assay) is a highly sensitive and specific test that determines the presence of HIV antibodies in a person's blood or serum. The ELISA test was first used in 1985 to reduce the number of HIV-infected blood units for blood transfusions.

Because the ELISA test is only a predictive test that gives the percentage chance that a person is truly positive or truly negative, serum from those who test positive is retested in duplicate. If still positive, the serum is then subjected to a Western Blot (WB) test. The WB is a confirmatory test. If it is also positive, the person is said to be HIV infected.

Other screening and confirmatory tests are available. The indirect immunofluorescent antibody assay (IFA) is relatively quick and easy to perform. Although it can be used as a screening test, it is generally used as a confirmatory test. The test is similar to the ELISA test except that the analysis is made by looking for a fluorescent color, indicating the presence of HIV antibodies, with a dark field light microscope. The FDA, through 2008, has approved six rapid tests for use in the United States.

The polymerase chain reaction (PCR) is a process wherein a few molecules of HIV proviral DNA can be amplified into a sufficient mass of DNA to be detected by current testing methods. It can determine if newborns of HIV-infected mothers are truly HIV positive.

Gene probes are also being used to detect small HIV proviral DNA sequences in cells of people who are HIV infected but not yet making antibodies. The CDC is recommending that everyone be HIV tested.

The availability of oral fluid, urine, and finger prick testing, along with rapid tests, has made it easier to provide HIV testing in a wide range of clinical and nontraditional settings and has led to new strategies for

---

SNAPSHOT 13.3

Just Devastated—I was tested last week and my doctor called and said that I was HIV positive. I went into shock, I was devastated. Here I was a straight male with no history of drug use and a relatively short list of female sexual partners, and I have HIV. I've only told two people, the girl that I think who gave it to me and a close friend. I am clueless as to what my next move should be. I'm losing my mind trying to figure out what and when I should tell my parents and my close friends. I really don't want to tell anyone yet. At this point, however, I feel that I am going to die a slow and lonely death.

reaching more persons with undiagnosed HIV infection. Rapid tests produce results in 20 minutes or less and make it possible to give HIV-seronegative and provisional HIV-seropositive test results in a single visit to more than 95% in many testing programs. The CDC is developing recommendations to make HIV screening a routine part of medical care, to remove barriers that hamper early HIV diagnosis and treatment, and to demonstrate and disseminate effective models for testing in clinical and nontraditional settings.

Free confidential HIV testing is available. To find a testing center in your area, call the CDC National AIDS Hotline (24 hours/7 days, 365 days a year) 1-800-342-2437 (AIDS); 1-800-344-7432 (SIDA); or call your local health department. Additional resources: www.hivtest.org.

Review Questions

(Answers to the Review Questions are on page 429.)

1. What is the acronym for the most commonly used HIV-antibody test, and what does each letter stand for?

2. What basic immunological assumption is this test based on?

3. Does a single positive HIV antibody result mean the person is HIV infected? Explain.

4. Is there a specific test for AIDS? Explain.

5. What is currently the most frequently used HIV confirmatory test in the United States?

6. What is the name of one additional confirmatory test in use in the United States?

7. How is HIV antibody detected in the ELISA test?

8. True or False: All newborns who are antibody positive are HIV infected and all go on to develop AIDS.

9. What is the greatest shortcoming of the ELISA and WB tests?

10. What are the two major problems in interpreting ELISA test results?

11. What two factors may account for false-positive and false-negative results?

12. What is the relationship between false-positive results and prevalence of HIV in the population?

13. In an HIV screening test, what is a positive predictive value? Why is it called a predictive value?

14. What is the current gold standard of confirmatory tests in the United States?

15. What is the major problem in using this test?

16. Why is the polymerase chain reaction (PCR) considered so useful in HIV testing? Name two situations when PCR can be significant in HIV testing.

17. How quickly can one get reliable HIV test results using the OraQuick HIV test?

18. How quickly can one get reliable HIV test results using the MedMira HIV test?

19. True or False: Two home-use HIV antibody test kits are now available in the United States.

20. Using the ELISA test, when are HIV antibodies first detectable?

21. How early are HIV antigens detectable in human serum?

22. What are three benefits of early identification of HIV-infected people?

23. Name the four kinds of testing privacy available to people who want to take an HIV test.

24. What is the major difference between an anonymous and a blind HIV test?

25. Why would someone want an anonymous test?

26. True or False: The ELISA serological test is adequate to confirm HIV infection.

27. True or False: Pre- and post-HIV-antibody test counseling is recommended any time an HIV antibody test is performed.

AIDS and Society: Knowledge, Attitudes, and Behavior

14

In the end, they will say, we died not at the hands of our enemies, but in the silence of our friends.

Martin Luther King

CHAPTER CONCEPTS

- HIV infections keep on going and going . . .
- HIV/AIDS is here to stay.
- The HIV/AIDS devastation is now.
- Inaccurate journalism leads to public hysteria.
- Vignettes on AIDS.
- It's 27 years later, and what do we know about HIV/AIDS?
- Use of explicit sexual language on TV and in journalism.
- Goal of sex education: to interrupt HIV transmission.
- Education, Just Say Know.
- An education about HIV/AIDS is an education for and about life.
- What does the red ribbon mean?
- Education is not stopping HIV transmission.
- Students still have misconceptions about HIV transmission.
- The general public, homophobia, and HIV transmission.
- Employees are not well informed and fear working with HIV/AIDS-infected coworkers.
- Educating employees about HIV/AIDS.
- Teenagers are not changing sexual behaviors that place them at risk for HIV infection.
- Physician–patient relationships in the HIV/AIDS era.
- U.S. Supreme Court renders its first ever ruling in the HIV/AIDS pandemic.
- Placing the risk of HIV infection in perspective.
- Federal response to the AIDS pandemic—create an AIDS industry.
- Global AIDS, Tuberculosis, and Malaria Fund began June 2001.
- President's Emergency Plan for AIDS Relief (PEPFAR), January 2003-2008, renewed for $48 billion through 2013.

Too many times the litany of broken promises to reverse the spread and impact of HIV/AIDS rings hollow against the unrelenting advance of the epidemic throughout the world. In this context, knowledge, attitudes, and behavior underline our understanding of what the various statements on commitments and declarations on HIV/AIDS actually mean and are essential first steps toward greater and more authentic accountability of global leadership against this pandemic.

HIV/AIDS IS A STORY IN OUR LIFETIME

AIDS is a story about the way the world is. A world that is home to a deadly but preventable disease that thrives in the human family, infecting or killing some 59 million of its members over 28 years. It's a world where every 15 seconds a man, woman, or child dies of AIDS. It's a world where every day about 6850 people become HIV infected. It's a world in which the human right to health does not exist for most people. It is a world in which respect for life itself seems to be lost. AIDS in the world? It is a story about ourselves. About humankind. What kind of people are we? How did we get to this point? This disease is preventable! Where are we going? And, what social changes are occurring because of this pandemic? It is said that we must crawl before we can walk, but we are still crawling, albeit at an ever-increasing pace—when will we walk through a world of HIV-free people? Can we find a way to compassion, humanity, and dignity for all men, women, and children? AIDS is becoming the worst plague in human history. Soon it will have killed more people than all the wars in the 20th century, but too few seem to know or even care about it. Humankind is paying a steep price for its ignorance, arrogance, and apathy toward each other. Many, for instance, believe AIDS is an African disease, and they blame Africans for its spread. Africans are not responsible for AIDS or spreading HIV, humankind is. The virus happens to be in our world. HIV and AIDS, like so many other epidemics, will thrive in the human family for generations to come, and as before, the cost is in human lives. We can only overcome AIDS if we accept that HIV has become a part of the human condition and that HIV and AIDS exist because we exist. We as a human species have to integrate that in all aspects of our lives. That is the nature of the world, that is the price of life. AIDS is but one ticket to the show on planet earth.

LOOKING BACK 14.1

AIDS COALITION TO UNLEASH POWER: ACT UP

The gay, lesbian, and transgender communities and their heterosexual supporters must be acknowledged for their immediate, aggressive, and humanitarian response to AIDS. Years before government was ready to accept its rightful role, these communities were caring for the sick, fighting for treatment and research, and making remarkable changes in personal and organizational behavior to curb the risk of AIDS. Their efforts and accomplishments are without precedent in modern medical history. In years past, an AIDS action group called ACT UP (AIDS to Unleash Power) under its mantra, "Silence = Death," urged people to get out there and raise hell because nobody else was doing anything about this disease. In order to promote prevention, they draped a 35-foot condom over Republican Jesse Helms's house, scattered the ashes of people who died of AIDS on the White House lawn, and tossed a coffin in front of a San Francisco hospital after an AIDS patient was denied a liver transplant. And these were some of the milder forms of protest. But it took these actions to get the attention of mainstream America and its politicians. Today's more recently infected people may not recognize the names of those who demonstrated in the streets, stopped meetings, defied government policies, and demanded adequate research funding and better medicines for AIDS, but they should know that without the efforts of these early warriors in the AIDS battle, the nationwide infrastructure of care, prevention, and treatment education would be much less than it is. The successes achieved by gay-empowered ACT UP later empowered women and heterosexuals to demand action for better drugs and a government commitment to finding an HIV vaccine, which served as a model for international AIDS activism that has recently achieved great price reductions in HIV/AIDS drugs for their countries. ACT UP has also served as a model for people with other diseases, like breast cancer, to form action groups to demand more from their government.

Whatever weakness and failings exist in the current structures, they do provide structures to build and improve upon. Those who have died have left a legacy that can serve as a guide in the future as the epidemic cuts its way around the world.

Anthony Fauci, director of the National Institute of Allergy and Infectious Diseases (NIAID) said that modern medicine can be divided into two periods: before ACT UP and after ACT UP started. These people put medicine back in the hands of the patients, which is where it belongs.

THE NEW MILLENNIUM
AND HIV/AIDS

September 11 and June 27, 2001—The first is the date of the terrorist attack on the United States in New York. The second is the date on which 189 nations signed a UN Declaration of Commitment on HIV/AIDS in the same city. September 11 changed the world, June 27 apparently changed very little.

HIV/AIDS is becoming more of a global disaster with each passing year of the new millennium. This disaster will be with us for many years to come, perhaps lifetimes or generations to come—like smallpox, the bubonic plague, cholera, and other diseases from ancient times. It does not appear that there are any new surprises that scientists are about to spring on this virus—but this virus continues to surprise our best scientists. HIV just keeps spinning its genetic building blocks looking for its next jackpot—how to overcome the next onslaught of antiretroviral drugs. Those jackpots keep coming up and the virus is winning the drug war. In developed nations, too many people think the AIDS crisis is over—they have been fooled by erroneous television and press coverage. Globally in 2002 through 2009, between 2 million and 3 million people will have died of AIDS annually and in each year about 2 million new infections will have occurred. But estimated numbers of AIDS deaths and new infections for 2010 into 2015 are even higher!

AIDS in the new millennium is like a train heading toward a horrific wreck. As the train gains speed, the global rate of HIV infections increases. As T4 or CD4+ cells drop, the distance to the wreck becomes shorter; on impact millions more will have died of AIDS. Like the **Energizer bunny,** HIV infections keep on going and going and . . .

The impact of AIDS is so monumental on societies as a whole, and on communities and families in particular, that there is no precedent in human history. There's nothing from the Black Death (a European plague in the fourteenth century) to the world wars of the twentieth century that even approximates it. That we've never had such numbers or seen the focus on a single gender, or ever had so many orphans, so many social breakdowns in various sectors, has became an overwhelming linkage of events for which there are no modern parallels, and therefore, we have to respond in ways that are unprecedented. AIDS is going to leave a fossil-like imprint on civilization that we can't yet begin to imagine.

Peter Piot, head of the United Nations campaign to combat AIDS (UNAIDS) said in June 2005 that "it is no longer realistic to hope that the world will meet its goal of halving and reversing the spread of the AIDS pandemic by 2015." Piot believes that the world is faced with multiple HIV/AIDS epidemics with an expanding pandemic. He said, **"we are still moving into the globalization of the AIDS pandemic."**

This pandemic is unfolding in waves that span human generations, and societies are making incremental adjustments along the way as they try to cope with the horrible impact AIDS is taking, not only in terms of human lives lost, but in the devastation of families, clans, civil society, social organizations, business structures, armed forces, and political leadership. Further, the HIV/AIDS pandemic is occurring primarily in regions that are hard hit by a range of other devastating diseases, acute and ever-rising poverty, political instability, and many other conditions that may mask or worsen the various impacts of AIDS. Of the 35 million people living with HIV/AIDS ending 2009, most will die between 2015 and 2020. And many millions more will have become HIV infected (Figure 14-1).

HIV/AIDS IS AN UNUSUAL
SOCIAL DISEASE

AIDS, like other severe epidemics in America, has a powerful social force that has allowed it to become established and that has promoted its rapid spread. But this disease is unique in the sense that it seems to track the fault lines in our society and profits from the social flaws and weaknesses inherent in societies in transition. The spread of AIDS is determined by very powerful social and economic factors.

HIV is mainly sexually transmitted and therefore closely associated with and intertwined in people's relationships.

DISCRIMINATION VS. COMPASSION
AND SUPPORT

AIDS is a schizophrenic condition. It is a pandemic worldwide, but it has not yet fully emerged. It often promotes stigma and rejection at the very time when people need comfort, compassion, and support. Stigma and discrimination further serve to propagate the disease because in this climate individuals do not feel confident or free to disclose their status, often not

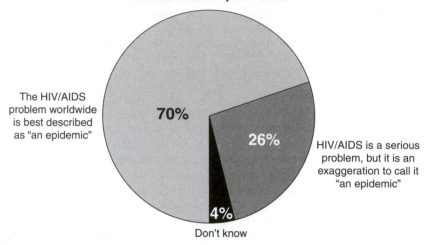

Now thinking about the issue of HIV/AIDS in countries outside the United States and the AIDS problem worldwide... Which ONE of the following two statements comes CLOSER to your views...

The HIV/AIDS problem worldwide is best described as "an epidemic"

70%

26%

HIV/AIDS is a serious problem, but it is an exaggeration to call it "an epidemic"

4%

Don't know

FIGURE 14-1 Is HIV/AIDS a Global Epidemic? *"Kaiser Family Foundation Survey of Americans on HIV/AIDS, Part Three— Experiences and Opinions by Race/Ethnicity and Age," (#7140), The Henry J. Kaiser Family Foundation, August 2004. The information was reprinted with permission from the Henry J. Kaiser Family Foundation. The Kaiser Family Foundation, based in Menlo Park, California, is a nonprofit, independent national healthcare philanthropy and is not associated with Kaiser Permanente or Kaiser Industries. (Conducted March 15–May 11, 2004.) National random sample of 2902 respondents age 18 and older.*

even to their sexual partners or their spouses. The disease remains silent and spreads relentlessly. HIV is transmitted through our most creative and spiritual potential, our ability to create life. It is also passed in the breast milk of mothers to their newborn infants; the very food of life can sow seeds of death. These spiritual connections can trigger negative and harmful perceptions and thoughts, promoting the concept that this epidemic is God's punishment to the wicked and to the sexually immoral. These can easily be translated into negative actions, blame, and rejection, further serving to keep the epidemic hidden and invisible, and fostering continued denial of the problem and its spread. Unlike most other terminal or life-threatening diseases, this one affects mainly the young and middle-aged adults, the adults on whom we all depend; they drive the economy, they parent and teach the children, they care for the sick, and keep the planes and trains running on time.

HIV/AIDS IS HERE TO STAY

The past 27 years of the global AIDS pandemic have taught us that HIV disease is a permanent part of life

on planet earth. HIV is simultaneously a virus and a phenomenon. When it is viewed only as a virus, it is hard to see why HIV prevention is a problem. People normally want to avoid harming themselves and others. When viewed as a phenomenon, HIV points to the many personal and societal causes of disease transmission. It points to the difficulties people have in making their intentions match their behavior. It points to the inequalities in relationships, which help to spread HIV. It points to societies' reluctance to prepare young people to manage their intimate relations, to admit to sexual diversity, to responsibly manage complex health and social problems such as drug abuse, and to provide access to health care. It points to the world's failure to care about improving living conditions in poor countries.

These are indeed the dark days of the global AIDS pandemic. About ninety percent of people who need treatment are dying without it. Necessary prevention and vaccine programs go underfunded. By the time you read this, another 2 million men, women, and children have died since summer 2008. About 24 million people will have died of AIDS ending 2009. And yet, the darkest days of this global pandemic are ahead. Many millions more will become HIV infected and many millions more will die from AIDS. Nicholas Everstadt, a fellow at the American Enterprise Institute, a neoconservative think tank, estimated that up to 155 million people could become HIV infected in just three countries (China, Russia, and India) between 2000 and 2025.

AIDS

HIV/AIDS was first described in the United States in 1981. Who would have thought then that almost 28 years later about 59 million people or about 1 in every 100 people on earth would be infected with the virus that causes AIDS? And that this virus, regardless of the involvement of the world's governments, the best scientists, and the expenditure of over $420 billion just in the United States, continues to spread out of control in many nations of the world. There is no way at the present time to prevent the 2 million to 3 million new HIV infections each year. No drugs offer a cure, and most of the 35 million living with HIV, ending 2009 cannot afford and will not receive those drugs that offer some temporary improved quality of life. An HIV-preventative vaccine now is wishful thinking. But, there is one commodity in plentiful supply—blame—enough for everyone, everywhere.

BLAME SOMEONE, DÉJÀ VU

The greater **hostility** and greatest **stigma** tends to be assigned to diseases in which individuals are seen as responsible for having the disease; in which the disease's course is fatal; in which fear of transmission is a major issue; and in which the disease leads to highly visible and frightening physical expressions. All these conditions are associated with HIV disease and AIDS. With AIDS more than any other disease in history, people have found verbal mechanisms for distancing themselves from thoughts of personal infection. Worldwide, from the onset of this pandemic, people have learned in a relatively short time to **categorize, rationalize, stigmatize,** and **persecutize** those with HIV disease and AIDS. AIDS statistics are published in categories to identify how many gay or bisexual men, injection-drug users, persons with hemophilia, and so on, have developed AIDS. Also listed are the countries, states, and cities with the highest incidence of the disease, along with which racial and ethnic groups are highest among reported HIV and AIDS cases. **By focusing on categories of people, have we made it possible for society to rationalize that AIDS belongs to somebody else? Have we made the thought of HIV/AIDS somewhat impersonal? HAVE WE FOUND A WAY TO BLAME SOMEONE ELSE?**

Placing blame does not always require reason and tends to focus on people who are not considered normal by the majority. Thus, minorities and foreigners are often singled out to blame for something, sometimes anything. Epidemics of plague, smallpox, leprosy, syphilis, cholera, tuberculosis, and influenza have historically focused social blame onto specific groups of people for spreading the diseases by their "deviant" behavior. Blaming others leads to their stigmatization and persecution.

While the Black Death, a pandemic of bubonic plague, swept across Europe in the fourteenth century, blame was variously attached to Jews and witches, followed by the massacre and burning of the alleged culprits. In Massachusetts between 1692 and 1693, some 20 people were hanged or burned at the stake after being accused of having the powers of the devil. Eighty percent of those accused were women. When Hitler blamed Jews, communists, homosexuals, and other undesirables for the economic stagnation of Germany in the 1930s, the result was death camps and ultimately World War II. Now there is a new plague—HIV/AIDS. What blame comes packaged with this new disease?

Jonathan Mann, former head of the World Health Organization's Global Program on AIDS, said in 1998 that there are really three HIV/AIDS epidemics,

---

SIDEBAR 14.1

A MOTHER'S NIGHTMARE

Recently, at a bus stop, a woman saw a man walking toward her. The man was so thin she could see his face, leg, and arm bones. His eyes were sunken and sad. As he got closer, she recognized it was her son! He was living in the streets, an injection-drug user; he told her he was dying of AIDS. She was too stunned to be hurt, she just put her arms around him and let him cry.

There are some things mothers can fix—this wasn't one of them. But she set out trying to find him a place to live and a doctor to care for him. At age 35, her son is watching himself shrink into an old man. His mother, age 61, wonders how she will pay for his burial.

which are phases in the invasion of a community by the AIDS virus.

First is the epidemic of silent infection by HIV, often completely unnoticed. **Second,** after a period of incubation/clinical latency that may last for years, is the epidemic of the disease itself.

Third, and perhaps equally important as the disease itself, is the epidemic of social, cultural, economic, and political reaction to HIV/AIDS. The willingness of each generation to place blame on others when believable explanations are not readily available simply recycles history. We have been there before; we have placed blame on others and it will continue. With respect to the HIV/AIDS pandemic, blame has been disseminated among nations. There is no shortage of political, economic, social, or ethical issues associated with this new disease.

AIDS needs no translation. In New York, California, Paris, Nairobi, Calcutta, Moscow, or in any other large city across the globe, those four letters provoke a universal reaction: fear, panic, and, too often, revulsion.

FEAR: PANIC AND HYSTERIA OVER THE SPREAD OF HIV/AIDS IN THE UNITED STATES

With the 1981 announcement by the U.S. Public Health Service and the CDC that there was a new disease, AIDS quickly became a symbol for our darkest fears. Responsible public officials gave out conflicting messages: **reassurance** on one hand and **alarm** on the other. **Public panic and hysteria began.** People fear what they do not understand and can not control.

People with HIV disease and AIDS are still abused, ridiculed, and maligned. Some people believe that AIDS is divine retribution for immoral lifestyles. People who have not indulged in high-risk lifestyles (for example, newborns and recipients of blood products) continue to be labeled as **innocent victims,** implying perhaps that other HIV-infected individuals are guilty for their behavior that led to their infection and therefore deserve their illness.

Families and communities continue to be divided on their beliefs and acceptance of HIV/AIDS patients. Federal and state agencies stand accused of a lack of commitment and compassion in the war against AIDS. The bottom line is that **value judgments** are associated with HIV/AIDS because the disease involves the most private areas of people's lives—**sex, pregnancy, drug use, and finances.**

The Fear Factor

Worldwide, the political, medical, and legal communities used the media or vice-versa, to scare people about a new disease called AIDS. The result has been to scare people into fearing other people rather than the disease. For example, a recent survey of 1000 black American church members in five cities found that more than one-third of them believed the AIDS virus was produced in a germ warfare laboratory as a form of genocide against blacks.

Another third said they were unsure whether the virus was created to kill blacks. That left only one-third who did not criticize the theory that HIV crossed into humans from chimpanzees.

Frightening Messages from the Media

Soon after young homosexual men began dying in large numbers, a barrage of frightening rhetoric began filling the airwaves, television, the popular press, and even the most reputable scientific journals. The AIDS disaster was here. One healthcare administrator stated, "We have not seen anything of this magnitude that we can't control except nuclear bombs."

Myron Essex of the Department of Cancer Biology at the Harvard School of Public Health noted,

> The Centers for Disease Control and Prevention (CDC) has been trying to inform the public without overly alarming them, but we outside the government are freer to speak. The fact is that the dire predictions of those who have cried doom ever since AIDS appeared haven't been far off the mark . . . The effects of the virus are far wider than most people realize. It has shown up not just in blood and semen but in brain tissue, vaginal secretions, and even saliva and tears, although there's no evidence that it's transmitted by the last two.

Columnist Jack Anderson reported that the Central Intelligence Agency (CIA) concluded that in just a few years heterosexual AIDS cases would *outnumber* homosexual cases in the United States. Otis Bowen, former secretary of Health and Human Services, said AIDS would make the Black Death that wiped out one-third of Europe's population in the Middle Ages pale by comparison. And sex researchers William Masters, Virginia Johnson, and Robert Kolodny stated in their book, *New Directions in the AIDS Crisis: The Heterosexual Community,* that there was a possibility of HIV infection via casual transmission—from toilet seats, handling of contact lenses from an AIDS patient, eating a salad in a restaurant prepared by a person with AIDS, or from instruments in a physician's office used to examine AIDS patients.

In contrast to these reports is the article by Robert Gould in *Cosmopolitan* reassuring women that there is practically no risk of becoming HIV infected through ordinary vaginal or oral sex even with an HIV infected male. According to Gould, the vaginal secretions produced during sexual arousal keep the virus from penetrating the vaginal walls. His explanation was: "Nature has arranged this so that sex will feel good and be good for you."

Reaction Based on Fear

In December 1997, a male entered a bar and held a syringe full of blood against a female patron's throat. He said the blood contained HIV. He demanded money. He was caught and was charged with robbery and attempted murder, pending the outcome of HIV tests of the blood from the syringe. The man thought the fear of AIDS would be sufficient to rob the bar.

In Taiwan, people with HIV have been hired to work as debt collectors. The widespread fear of HIV/AIDS is being used to force people to pay their debts. The HIV infected need a job and the loan agency needed a clever way to get their money back. The loan agency believes it's a proper business agreement.

In June 2007, the results from the China Youth University for Political Science survey showed that of 1089 students from 12 universities in Beijing, 23% were unwilling to have an HIV-positive classmate. Seven percent said that HIV-positive people should not be admitted to universities, and 31% said they should be admitted but "with certain restrictions." Four percent of respondents said that the HIV positives should not be allowed to find employment, and 43% said they should be allowed employment "with certain restrictions."

In rural Zimbabwe to be a widow and old is very dangerous. Self-appointed witch hunters backed by community leaders are accusing widows of bewitching people with AIDS. If the widow is lucky, she is banished from the village. If not, she undergoes a brutal cleansing ritual. Witchcraft dates back to the communities' forefathers and continues. Elderly women and widows are often referred to as witches. The prevalent belief is that HIV/AIDS can only attack a person if he or she has been bewitched or made unfortunate with the use of charms. One woman whose husband and two children died of AIDS was given one hour to leave the village and was not allowed to take her possessions—she lost everything. In another case, in an exorcism ceremony, the woman was made to crouch over a large bucket of boiling water with a blanket over her head. After 10 minutes the blanket was removed—her face and arms were scalded and disfigured.

While causing physical and mental suffering to those widows identified as witches, witch hunters are profiteering by cheating villagers in exorcising ceremonies. For one to be exorcised of witchcraft, one has to pay a large price. Some families have had to give their livestock in order to pay the witch hunters. When a village calls in witch hunters it also has to pay for their keep.

Fear of AIDS is understandable, given that AIDS is fatal and its cause, HIV, is communicable. AIDS appeared suddenly and spread quickly—it took a number of years to identify the virus that causes it and the mechanisms for spread. Yet, today the routes of transmission are well established and widely known, as are the precautionary measures that can be taken to prevent its spread. Early on, fear of AIDS took an unhealthy turn, anxieties were projected onto those who were hit the hardest by the disease, and the fear of AIDS became an irrational fear of *people* with AIDS.

WHOM IS THE GENERAL PUBLIC TO BELIEVE?

Because of the complexity of HIV disease, a great deal of press coverage of AIDS issues reflects what scientists say to journalists. A journalist's responsibility is to check that the facts are accurate, but not necessarily to judge their overall merit. Why should a good story be spiked just because other scientists disagree with the data interpretation? When scientists say contradictory things to the public, how can the public assess whom to believe? Science has a duty to inform and educate the public, but it must neither frighten people unnecessarily nor give them unjustified expectations. Claims of **"AIDS cures"** in the popular press need to be based on much more than just test tube data or rumors! Whatever the need to attract research funding, is five minutes of fame ever worth a day of fear or weeks of false hopes for many? The popular press has provided HIV-infected persons with a roller coaster ride between hopelessness and fantasies of imminent cure.

As a result of journalistic promises, there was and still is a range of emotions that run from real hope of a cure to public panic and hysteria. In at least five states, children with AIDS were barred from attending local public schools. The case of 12-year-old Ryan White of Kokomo, Ind., was made into a TV movie, *The Ryan White Story,* in 1989. (See Box 14-1.)

In some localities, police officers and healthcare workers put rubber gloves on before apprehending a drug user or wear full cover protective suits when called to the scene of an accident. In other communities, church members, out of fear of HIV infection, have declined communion wine from the common cup.

Significant Percentages of Americans Distrust Information About HIV/AIDS

Although most Americans believe they are receiving accurate information about the AIDS pandemic, significant percentages doubt what the government and media are telling:

- 34% do not believe the government is telling the whole truth about AIDS; and
- 25% do not believe the media is telling the whole truth about AIDS.

In addition, fewer, but still some Americans question the origins of the epidemic:

- 18% believe there is some truth to reports that the HIV was produced in a germ-warfare laboratory; and
- 12% believe that AIDS came from God to punish homosexual behavior.

AIDS Polarized the Attitudes of Millions of People into Stances of Love and Compassion and Hate and Rejection

Since the epic announcement in 1981, HIV/AIDS has refashioned America. HIV/AIDS is a disease molded to the times, one that strikes hardest at the

---

SIDEBAR 14.2

THE PROMOTION OF FEAR AND ITS AFTERMATH: AN ANALOGY TO HOW FEAR SPREAD WHEN AIDS ENTERED THE WORLD

Once there was a peaceful village and its lovely village green with small shops encircling the green. On any given day, villagers stopped and chatted and exchanged pleasantries and told each other stories about their children, their lives. All was well in this village until one day, **two large bears** walked out of the woods and stood at the edge of town with their heads turned toward each other—the people watching the bears **thought** the bears were whispering to each other. At first nobody paid much attention, then little by little the people stopped what they were doing and tried to hear what the bears were saying. But nobody could. That night the bears went back into the forest. And the townspeople stood around and one woman said she knew what they were whispering about—**they were making fun of the people in the village.** And then everybody started noticing how everybody else walked funny or talked funny or looked weird and they all ended up laughing at each other, and everybody got mad and there were all kinds of fights in town that evening.

The next day the bears came out of the forest again and started whispering, ya-da, ya-da, ya-da, and again the townspeople watched, and all were suspicious. That night the bears again returned to the woods. And this time an older man said he knew what they were talking about. **They were gossiping about the people in town.** And so everybody figured, if the

bears knew then everybody else must know all their secrets, and so they went home and closed all their windows and doors and they became angry and afraid to go out in public.

On the third day the bears again returned to the edge of the woods. Once again the same thing happened—the bears were talking to each other. But, this time the mayor of the village said, **"I know what they're saying! They're making plans to attack the village."** And he ordered the villagers to get torches to scare away the bears, but one of the villagers accidentally set his house on fire and the fire spread rapidly around the village and the whole town burned down!

In short, many lives became ruined for no reason. **Bears can't talk!** The town was destroyed and lives changed forever because people projected their own pettiness, and jealousy, and aggression on some innocent creatures. Much like the lives of so many millions of HIV/AIDS people have been changed forever because of petty fears, jealousies, and hatred for those who need compassion and understanding. Yes, sadly, there exist a rather large village of people who judge others harshly before knowing the facts.

(A favorite fairy story of the author, who in this case adopted the anecdote to make a point about discrimination. From "Speaking In Tongues" by Jeffery Deaver.)

---

outcasts—gay men, injection-drug users, prostitutes, and impoverished whites, blacks, and Hispanics. HIV/AIDS has brought forth uncomfortable questions about sex, sex education, homosexuality, the poor, and minorities. The disease has inevitably polarized the people, accentuating both the best and worst worldwide. Many churches, schools, and communities have responded to the new disease with compassion and tolerance; others have displayed hate and reprisals of the worst kind.

As Camus wrote in *The Plague,* "The first thing (the epidemic) brought . . . was exile." Anyone who carried the disease could inspire terror. They became pariahs in society.

People with hate in their hearts torched the house of the Ray family and their three HIV-positive hemophilic children in Arcadia, Fla. Someone shot a bullet through the window of Ryan White's home to let the teenager know he should not attend the local high school. After he died, his 6-foot, 8-inch gravestone was overturned four times, and a car ran over his grave! (See Box 14-1.)

Misconceptions About HIV/AIDS Linger

Despite widespread reports that casual contact does not spread the virus, families have walked out of restaurants that employed gay waiters and hospital workers have quit rather than treat HIV/AIDS patients.

Each example points out that regardless of education, the public assumes the virus can be casually transmitted. **FEAR IS BEING TRANSMITTED BY CASUAL CONTACT—NOT THE VIRUS.** How would you react if a good friend, classmate, or coworker told you he or she was HIV positive? What if you found out that your child's schoolmate, a hemophiliac, had AIDS? What if you were told this child had emotional problems or a biting habit? What if your work put you in direct physical contact with people who might be HIV positive?

An AIDS diagnosis for one person resulted in his physician's refusal to treat him, his roommate left him, his friends no longer visited him, his attorney advised him to find another attorney, and his clergyman failed to support him. They were all afraid of "catching" AIDS. In another case, a mother whose young son has AIDS sent cupcakes to his classmates on his birthday. School officials would not permit the children to eat the cupcakes. The elementary school principal said the school had a policy against homemade food because it could spread diseases such as AIDS.

In Hinton, WV, one woman was killed by three bullets and her body dumped along a remote road. Another was beaten to death, run over by a car, and left in the gutter. And each, authorities say, was killed because she had AIDS.

In Calcutta, India, October 2000, the body of a 45-year-old male who died of AIDS laid in the morgue of a hospital for 45 days because undertakers refused to take it for cremation. The "doms"—low-caste Hindus who take bodies for cremation—refused to remove the corpse after learning that he died from AIDS. Some of the doms threatened to stop work unless the body was removed immediately by someone else. India accounts for 60% of HIV cases in Asia and 20% of the world's HIV infections. But AIDS awareness is still extremely limited and the HIV infected are more often than not ostracized by their families and local communities. The fear and stigma associated with HIV/AIDS has no boundaries.

What Do We Know?—Ending year 2009 and 28 years of the AIDS pandemic, it is clear that the scare headlines and tactics lack substance. From what has been learned about the biology of HIV, it appears the virus is not casually nor easily spread but it has reached the magnitude of the great plagues and a vaccine has not yet been found!

However, a survey of 3500 American adults was conducted by the National Institute of Allergy and Infectious Diseases on their state of knowledge concerning the availability of an HIV/AIDS vaccine. One in five white Americans, or 20%, believe that an HIV vaccine already exists but is being kept secret from patients and the general public. Twenty-eight percent of Hispanics and 48% of blacks held this belief. Also, 42% of those surveyed did not know that vaccines require testing on human volunteers before being made available to the public. About 33% believe that vaccines in study could cause an HIV infection in humans receiving a test vaccine.

What Is So Different About HIV/AIDS that Leads to Such Discrimination?

The biggest difference between HIV/AIDS and other diseases is the larger amount of social discrimination. For example, if someone is known to be HIV positive, most people think they know that the person got the virus through sex, that they are possibly gay, or are

UNIVERSITY STUDENTS' EXPERIENCES

University students taking a senior semester course on HIV/AIDS in 2006 and 2007 experienced firsthand the fear-related ignorance that still exists.

FALL SEMESTER 2006

On this particular Monday afternoon, as I was reading my assigned chapter in the book *AIDS Update 2005,* a lady walked into my nail salon wanting to get her nails done. I asked her to come sit at my nail booth and I put the AIDS book down next to me on the nail table. When she sat down, I took her hand and begin to file her nails. Unexpectedly she quickly pulled her hand back and demanded another person to do her nails. I asked her, "Why can't I do your nails?" She said, "You're nasty and I do not want you to touch me." That comment got me angry. I replied, "How am I nasty, you don't even know me." Meanwhile, her eyes kept glancing from my AIDS book back to me with this disgusting look on her face. At that point I just knew that she thought I have AIDS or have something to do with AIDS. My parents, who were in the back room, quickly came out to see what was going on. She quickly asked my dad to do her nails. I told her that my dad would not do her nails and told her to "get the hell out of my nail salon." As she was leaving she squeezed in her last comment calling me a "Dirty Chink with AIDS." She then flicked me her middle finger and left. I said, "So much for education on nontransmission of HIV by casual contact!"

FALL SEMESTER 2007

A group of college friends and I decided to go out to dinner one night to hang out, relax, and get our minds off midterms for a while. It was to be an ordinary night of jokes, laughter, and catching up. The only thing out of the ordinary was taking my textbook along. I took my *AIDS Update* book with me to help the class explore still-existing discrimination, a voluntary class assignment. After being seated our waitress came to take our drink order. I had my textbook lying face up on the table. She looked at the book and then looked at me. For a moment our eyes met but then she averted her eyes quickly as if she was perhaps uncomfortable. That was the last time she would look at me. She then brought out our drinks and passed them out accordingly. When she got to me she handed me a plastic take-home cup with a plastic lid while everyone else had their drinks in a glass. She then took our dinner orders, avoiding eye contact with me, and left. That was the last time she appeared at our table for the evening. Another waitress presented herself to us and refilled our drinks. The second or third time around of checking up on our table I asked the waitress what had happened to the other girl, to which she replied that she had to go on break. When she left I looked over to the right and saw our original waitress waiting another table. So much for break time. The new waitress then delivered our dinners. She placed each plate and then handed out regular silverware to my friends and gave me plastic silverware, you know the type, enclosed in a little plastic baggie. I shook my head in disbelief. I mean I knew that AIDS was a highly stigmatized disease but, come on, this is year 2007 for God's sake, how can people still be so closed minded and act in such an uneducated manner? Regardless, my friends and I carried on in a regular fashion, just having a good time and enjoying one another's presence until it got late and we decided to call it quits. I paid using my credit card, and on the restaurant's copy I wrote a friendly little note declaring their ignorance and chastising their false assumptions. The only regret that I had that night was not reporting the incident to the manager, but then again why embarrass the man or woman about the staff of rude and ignorant employees that he or she hired? If education is the only hope, short of a vaccine, to cure AIDS then we are all in some very serious trouble.

Since reporting the first event in this book, students in each of my HIV/AIDS courses ending 2007 have reported similar experiences of discrimination while reading their AIDS textbook in a beauty salon and in the office waiting rooms of a physician, veterinarian, optometrist, and a car wash.

---

possibly an injection drug user or both. And, if they contracted HIV through sex, then it must have been with someone they shouldn't have had sex with, or with someone who had sex with someone they shouldn't have had sex with, like an injection drug user or bisexual, etc. That is, being HIV positive suggests a questionable background, lifestyle, or history.

Society does not reject those with a variety of sexually transmitted diseases or with cancer, diabetes, heart disease, or any other health problems to the degree that it rejects people with HIV disease or AIDS.

The AIDS pandemic has taught people about risk behavioral groups, homosexuals in particular. In some, this has promoted tolerance and understanding; in others, it has reinforced feelings of hatred. Information on HIV disease and AIDS, how it is spread, and how to avoid becoming infected, has, over the past 27 years, become a part of TV talk shows, movies, TV advertisements, and newspaper and magazine articles.

Phil Donahue, host of a former popular TV show, said in 1990, "On *Donahue,* we're discussing body cavities and membranes and anal sex and vaginal lesions. We've discussed the consequences of a woman's swallowing her partner's semen. No way would we have brought that up five years ago. It's the kind of thing that makes a lot of people gag."

The language, photography, and artwork used by the media are explicit and have upset certain religious groups. They believe that open use of language about condoms, homosexuality, anal sex, oral sex, vaginal sex, and so on promotes promiscuity.

It would appear that although biotechnology has provided methods of HIV detection, new drugs, and hope for a vaccine, human emotional responses have not changed much from those demonstrated during previous epidemics (Figure 14-2).

DISCUSSION QUESTION: How can people learn to prevent HIV infection and AIDS without talking about sexual behavior and injection-drug use? Does it seem at times as if opponents of sex education would rather have people suffer with AIDS than have them learn about sex?

Regardless of who is correct, few could have predicted in 1980 the casualness with which these topics are now presented in the media. If the AIDS pandemic has done nothing else, it surely has affected the nature of public discourse. In 1987, prior to the TV broadcast of the **National AIDS Awareness Test,** viewers were warned of objectionable material. By 1990, few if any such viewer warnings were given.

Former Presidents Ronald Reagan and George H. W. Bush: Their Policies on AIDS

Early on, the federal government and its public health apparatus showed little interest in the HIV/AIDS epidemic. Former President Ronald Reagan never once met with former Surgeon General C. Everett Koop to talk about AIDS despite Koop's pleas. Koop said, "If AIDS had struck legionnaires or Boy Scouts, there's no question the response would have been very different."

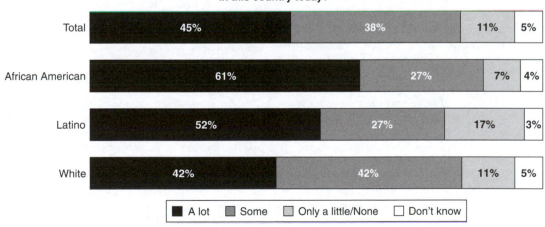

How much prejudice and discrimination do you think there is against people living with HIV and AIDS in this country today?

FIGURE 14-2   Perceptions of Prejudice and Discrimination Against People Living with HIV and AIDS in the U.S. *"Kaiser Family Foundation Survey of Americans on HIV/AIDS, Part Three—Experiences and Opinions by Race/Ethnicity and Age," (#7140), The Henry J. Kaiser Family Foundation, August 2004. The information was reprinted with permission from the Henry J. Kaiser Family Foundation. The Kaiser Family Foundation, based in Menlo Park, California, is a nonprofit, independent national healthcare philanthropy and is not associated with Kaiser Permanente or Kaiser Industries. (Conducted March 15–May 11, 2004). National random sample of 2902 respondents age 18 and older.*

Recently released documents from the Reagan administration show that the president's delay in addressing the AIDS issue was based on the perceived "political risk" in doing so. It took 10 years and over 120,000 AIDS deaths before the Congress and former President George Bush enacted the nation's first comprehensive AIDS-care funding package—the Ryan White CARE Act (1990). (See Box 14-1.)

AIDS EDUCATION AND BEHAVIOR: DISSIPATING FEAR WITH EDUCATION

I said education was our **"basic weapon."** Actually it's our **only** weapon. We've got to educate everyone about the disease so that each person can take responsibility for seeing that it is spread no further.

—C. Everett Koop
Former U.S. Surgeon General

For some, the occurrence of the recently estimated 56,000 new HIV infections in the United States each year from 2002 through 2008 is evidence that HIV education and prevention efforts have failed. If HIV prevention programs are held to a standard of perfection and are expected to protect 100% of the people from disease 100% of the time, the efforts are by definition doomed to failure. No intervention aimed at changing behaviors to promote health has been or can be 100% successful, whether for smoking, diet, exercise, or drinking and driving. For example, even though warnings regarding the health effects of smoking were issued in 1964, warning labels on cigarettes were not mandated until 1984, and smoking-related illness still remains a major cause of death.

Because some of the behaviors and activities that need to change in order to avert HIV infection are pleasurable, it should be no surprise if short-term interventions do not lead to immediate and permanent behavior changes. An important difference between HIV infection and other life-threatening diseases is that HIV can be contracted by a single episode of risk-taking behavior. **Once HIV infected there is no second chance—no giving up the behavior, like drinking alcohol or smoking, that will make any difference;** HIV disease, except on rare occasions, progresses to AIDS.

After nearly 28 years of experience with HIV, it has demonstrated that lasting changes in behavior needed to avoid infection can occur as a result of carefully tailored, targeted, credible, and persistent HIV risk-education efforts. Given experience in other health behavior change endeavors, no interventions are likely to reduce the incidence of HIV infection to zero; indeed, insisting on too high a standard for HIV risk-reduction programs may actually undermine their effectiveness. A number of social, cultural, and attitudinal barriers continue to prevent the implementation of promising HIV risk-reduction programs. The remote prospects for a successful vaccine for HIV and the difficulty in finding long-lasting effective drug treatments have underscored the importance of sustained attention to HIV prevention and education.

The Solution to the AIDS Pandemic Is, Let's Just Educate Everyone?

This sounds so easy: Educate people and they will do the right thing. **Wrong.** Knowledge does not guarantee sufficient motivation to change sexual behavior or stop the biological urge to have sex. Education has not stopped teenage pregnancy, nor has the knowledge about cigarettes causing lung cancer stopped people from smoking.

Perhaps the reason education is not as effective as it could be is because the public receives its education by daily doses from the mass media. With so much going on in the world, people have become more or less dependent on the media for information essential to their well-being. Gordon Nary (1990) said, "The public wants to know what's right or wrong in five three-second images or 25 words or less. It wants simple problems with simple solutions. It wants *Star Wars* with good and evil absolutely defined. The media often respond to these demands."

Public AIDS Education Programs

Over the years billions of dollars have been spent by federal and state health departments and private industry to inform the public about cardiovascular risks, health risks associated with sexually transmitted diseases (STDs), smoking and lung cancer, chewing tobacco and oral cancer, drug addiction, alcohol consumption and driving drunk, and seat belt use to name just a few. In some cases these campaigns were eventually supported by specific state and federal legislation. Tobacco advertisements were outlawed on TV, and drivers in some states who are not buckled up must pay a fine. But even with laws to support these educational programs, many adults have failed to change established behavior patterns. In the larger cities, educators must combat the fear that

BOX 14.1

HOW SOME PEOPLE RESPONDED AFTER LEARNING THAT SOMEONE HAD AIDS

VIGNETTES ON COMMUNITY BEHAVIOR AND AIDS

In **Colorado Springs, CO.,** Scott Allen's wife, Lydia, had contracted HIV from a blood transfusion hours before their son Matthew was born. A second son, Bryan, was also born before Lydia learned of her HIV infection. Scott wasn't infected, but was dismissed as minister of education at First Christian Church in Colorado Springs when he sought his pastor's consolation. Matt was kicked out of the church's day care center and the family was told to find another church.

When the family moved to Dallas and moved in with Scott's father, Jimmy, and his wife, church after church refused to enroll Matt in Sunday school. Allen, a former president of the Southern Baptist Convention, wrote in his book, *Burden of a Secret: A Story of Truth and Mercy in the Face of AIDS,* "Good churches. Great churches. Wonderful people. Churches pastored by fine men of God, many of whom I had mentored. Nobody had room for a boy with AIDS" (Figure 14-3).

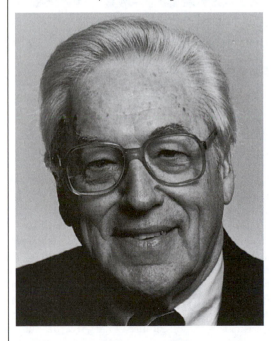

FIGURE 14-3 **Reverend Jim Allen.** Author of *Burden of a Secret: A Story of Truth and Mercy in the Face of AIDS.* "Jimmy," as he insists people address him, found peace for himself and family in a little village, Big Canoe, Georgia, where he is on staff at the Big Canoe Chapel.

Bryan, an infant, died in 1986, Lydia died in 1992, and Matt died in 1995.

In **Florida** in 1987, Mrs. Ray, the mother of three hemophilic HIV-infected sons (Ricky, 14; Robert, 13; and Randy, 12) turned to her pastor for confidential counseling. He responded by expelling the family from the congregation and announcing that the boys were infected. As a result, the boys were not allowed to go to church, school, stores, or restaurants. Barbers refused to cut their hair. Some townspeople interviewed said they were terrified at having the boys in the community. They had to move to another town. The Rays sued the DeSoto County School District. They agreed to pay a $1.1 million settlement in 1988. Ricky Ray died of AIDS on December 13, 1992, at age 15. Robert died at age 22 in 2000. Randy, age 28, was diagnosed with AIDS in May 1993 and is still living.

In **California,** a young man arrived home one evening to find that the locks had been changed. A few days later he discovered that everything he had ever touched had been thrown out—clothes, books, bed sheets, toothbrush, curtains, and carpeting. Even the wallpaper had been stripped from the walls and trashed. The day before, he had told his friends he had AIDS. "Overnight, I had no friends. I slept on park benches. I stole food. I passed bad checks. No one would come near me. I was told that I had 14 weeks to live."

Almost daily, similar senseless acts of violence and cruelty occur across the United States as a response to AIDS. Such episodes of panic, hysteria, and prejudice are perpetuated by the very people society uses as role models: clergy, physicians, teachers, lawyers, dentists, and so on. Philosopher Jonathan Moreno said, "Plagues and epidemics like AIDS bring out the best and worst of society. Face to face with disaster and death, people are stripped down to their basic human character, to good and evil. AIDS can be a litmus test of humanity."

THE LIFE OF RYAN WHITE

In Kokomo, IN, Ryan White was socially unacceptable. He was not gay, a drug user, black, or Hispanic. He was a hemophiliac; he had AIDS. His fight to become socially acceptable, to attend school, and to have the freedom to leave his home for a walk without ridicule made him a national hero (Figure 14-4).

Ryan's short life was a profile in courage and understanding. Like many other people with AIDS, Ryan tried to change the public's misconception of

BOX 14.1 (Continued)

how HIV is transmitted. Ryan suffered most from the indignities, lies, and meanness of his classmates and his classmates' parents. They accused him of being a "fag," of spitting on them to infect them with the virus, and other fabrications. Ryan said he understood that this discrimination was a response of fear and ignorance. Ryan got the virus from blood and blood products essential to his survival. Ryan's wish was to be treated like any other boy, to attend school, to study, to play, to laugh, to cry, and to live each day as fully as possible. But AIDS was an integral part of his life. AIDS may not have compromised the quality of his life as much as the residents of his community did. One day, at age 16, as Ryan talked about AIDS to students in Nebraska, another boy asked Ryan how it felt knowing he was going to die. Showing the maturity that endeared him to all, Ryan replied "It's how you live your life that counts." Ryan White died, a hero of the AIDS pandemic, at 7:11 A.M. on April 8, 1990. He was 18 years old.

In Honor of Ryan White: The Ryan White CARE Act Enacted by Congress in 1990

The Ryan White Comprehensive AIDS Resources Emergency (CARE) Act, the largest HIV-specific federal grant program in the United States, is the nation's care and treatment safety net for people living with HIV/AIDS who have no other source of coverage or have coverage limits. The CARE Act was due to be reauthorized for the third time in 2006, and will need to be renewed in December 2009.

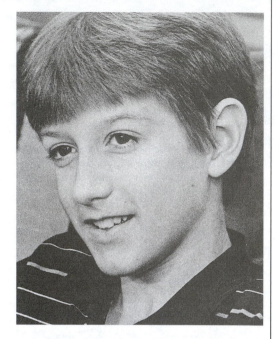

FIGURE 14-4 Ryan White Was Diagnosed with AIDS in 1984 and Died on April 8, 1990. This young male became another teenage AIDS tragedy. He gained the respect of millions across the United States before he died of an AIDS-related lung infection. (© *AP/Wide World Photos*)

AIDS is a government conspiracy to eliminate society's "undesirables"—minorities, drug addicts, and homosexuals. They must overcome cultural and religious barriers that prevent people from using condoms to protect themselves.

It might also be added that there have always been educational programs against crime, but from 1990 through 2008 more new jails were built in the United States than ever before. In short, educational programs on TV, radio, in newspapers, and in the popular press have achieved only limited success in changing peoples' behavior.

It is not that education is unimportant; it is essential for those who will use it. That is the catch. Although education must be available for those who will use it, too few, relatively speaking, are using the available education for their maximum benefit. In general, people, especially young adults, do not do what they know. They sometimes do what they see, but most often do what they feel. In short, knowledge in itself may be necessary but it is insufficient for behavioral change. A variety of studies have failed to show a consistent link between knowledge and preventive behaviors (Fisher, 1992; Phillips, 1993).

Costs Related to Education/Prevention—The assertion that spending more money on educational programs will ensure disease prevention for the masses, as the examples given suggest, may not be the case. In particular, peoples' behaviors regarding the prevention of HIV infection do not appear to be changing significantly despite the billions of dollars used to produce, distribute, and promote HIV/AIDS education. The major educational thrust is directed at how not to become HIV infected. Most of this information is being given out to people ages 13 and older.

The problem with AIDS education is that communicating the information is relatively easy but changing behavior, particularly addictive and/or pleasurable behavior, is quite difficult. The mass media have provided near saturation coverage of key AIDS issues and it is very unlikely that significant numbers of future HIV infections in the United States will occur in individuals who did not know the virus was transmitted through sexual contact and IV drug use. Yet new infections over the past six years occurred at an incidence of over 56,000 year.

Although humans are capable of dramatic behavioral changes, it is not known what really initiates the change or how to speed up the process.

Public School AIDS Education: Just Say Know

QUESTION: How Do Educators Communicate The Dangers Of HIV Without Stigmatizing Those Who Already Have It—And Without Scaring Youth Into Avoidance And Denial?

Some information relevant to AIDS education can be learned from educational programs that have been designed to reduce pregnancy and the spread of STDs among young adults. However, data from a variety of high school sex education classes offered across the country indicate that young adults are

learning the essential facts but they are not practicing what they learn.

Risky sexual behavior is widespread among young adults and has resulted in high rates of STDs. Over 25% of the 19 million STD cases per year occur among young adults. One in four have been infected with an STD. Over 50% of sexually active young adults (12 million) report having had two or more

Do you think, in general, the HIV/AIDS pandemic has made people more likely or less likely to practice safe sex, or hasn't it made much difference?

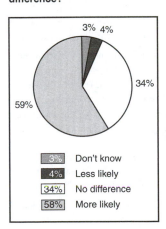

3%	Don't know
4%	Less likely
34%	No difference
58%	More likely

Do you think, in general, the HIV/AIDS pandemic has made people more likely or less likely to talk openly about safe sex, or hasn't it made much difference?

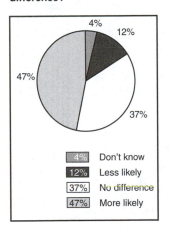

4%	Don't know
12%	Less likely
37%	No difference
47%	More likely

Do you think, in general, the HIV/AIDS pandemic has made people more likely or less likely to discriminate against gays and lesbians, or hasn't it made much difference?

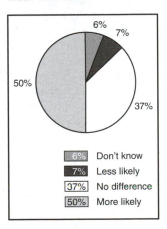

6%	Don't know
7%	Less likely
37%	No difference
50%	More likely

FIGURE 14-5 Perceived Impact of HIV Pandemic on Culture.
Source: Adapted from the Kaiser Family Foundation "Survey of Americans on HIV/AIDS" conducted March 24–April 18, 2006.

sexual partners; and fewer than half say they used a condom the first time they had intercourse.

Young Adult Perceptions About AIDS and HIV Infection in the United States—A recent survey by *People* magazine indicated that 96% of high school students and 99% of college students knew that HIV is spreading through the heterosexual population; but the majority of these students stated that they continued to practice unsafe sex and that 26% of American young adults practice anal intercourse. Data such as these have prompted a number of medical and research people to express concern for the next generation. If HIV becomes widespread among today's young adults, there is a real danger of losing tomorrow's older adults. Available data suggest that teenagers have not appreciably changed their sexual behaviors in response to HIV/AIDS information presented in their schools or from other sources.

Young adults at high risk include some 200,000 who become prostitutes each year and others who become IDUs. About 1% of high school seniors have used heroin and many from junior high on up have tried cocaine (Kirby, 1988). A large number of children ages 10 and up consume alcohol. Is it possible that too much hope is being placed on education to prevent the spread of HIV? Teenagers must be convinced that they are vulnerable to HIV infection and death. Until then, it only happens to someone else. The World Health Organization estimates that worldwide, ending 2009 there will be about 20 million HIV-infected young adults.

College Students—Everyone must know and act on the fact that a wrong decision about having sexual intercourse can take away the future. For example, a young college student had a three-year nonsexual friendship with a local bartender. She was bright, well-educated, and acutely aware of AIDS. After drinks one evening, as their friendship progressed toward sexual intercourse, she asked him if he was "straight" (a true heterosexual) and he said yes. But he was a bisexual. It was a single sexual encounter. She graduated and left town. She found out that the bartender died of AIDS three years later. She did not think much of it until she was diagnosed with AIDS five years after their affair. This young, talented, bright, and personable girl has since died, she lost her future. It is difficult to change something as complex as personal sexual behavior regardless of knowledge. It also brings up at least one other important point in personal relationships: **telling the truth** (Figure 14-6).

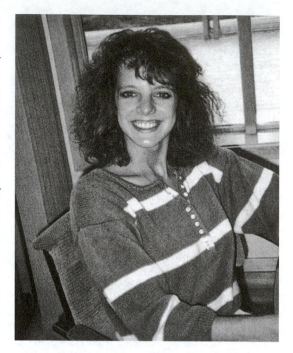

FIGURE 14-6 Dawn Beckhols at age 23, about the time of her infection. She believed that she became infected via one sexual encounter while on vacation. Dawn died of AIDS on July 13, 1997, at age 33. *(Photo courtesy of L. Schwitters)*

Nothing but the Truth, or Telling Lies?

During the 1988 American Psychological Association Convention, the following facts were presented with respect to telling the truth or lying in order to have sex. The data came from a survey of 482 sexually experienced southern California college students:

1. Thirty-five percent of the men and 10% of the women said they had lied in order to have sex.
2. Forty-seven percent of the men and 60% of the women reported they had been told a lie in order to have sex.
3. Twenty percent of the men and 4% of the women said they would say they had a negative HIV test in order to have sex.
4. Forty-two percent of the men and 33% of the women said they would never admit a one-time sexual affair to their long-term partner.

Researchers at the French National Research Institute reported that men and teenage boys are far less likely than females to tell their main sexual partners they have been diagnosed with HIV or other sexually transmitted diseases. Researchers found that 14% of

THE RED RIBBON

Frank Moore II, a Manhattan painter who was instrumental in launching the overlapping red ribbon as a symbol of AIDS awareness in 1991, he died April 22, 2002, from AIDS-related complications at the age of 48. Moore, who said that his paintings represented a journal of his long battle with HIV, was a board member of Visual AIDS, a Manhattan-based group that raises money to fund artists with HIV/AIDS and helps maintain the art of people with the disease. The red ribbon became an international symbol of AIDS awareness and has been used in other colors by groups to represent different causes.

The color red was chosen because the disease was a blood-borne disease. The shape of the ribbon was meant to signify the connectedness of all of us with or without the disease, who wanted to make a statement of visible support for those who were infected or had AIDS.

THE EVENT

We were sitting in a small Italian restaurant. I had just come back to town from a presentation on AIDS. The jacket I wore still had the red ribbon on the lapel. As we enjoyed our meal, I noticed a woman at the next table who appeared to be glaring at me and making statements to her companion. At one point her voice became loud enough for us to hear her say, "I am sick and tired of those people trying to push the lifestyle of homosexuals down our throats," as she was looking right at me. She then said, "That red ribbon is a sign of a sick person trying to make all of us sick too. That ribbon and all that it stands for ruins my day." With that she and her companion left the restaurant.

That outburst left my family and me embarrassed and confused. My children deserved an explanation. I don't think I have ever explained the idea of the red ribbon to anyone before. Like so many things we observe in life, after a while they become understood by each in his or her own way. This woman expressed her way rather forcefully. To my children I said that the ribbon is a symbol to call attention to a social problem that needs a solution. I went on to say, "Do you recall the song 'Tie A Yellow Ribbon Round the Old Oak Tree' in 1973 and what that meant? And, do you recall the ribbons tied around trees, on car antennas, mailboxes, and so on while our 56 servicemen were held captive in Iran in 1980 and again for our captives in the 1991 Persian Gulf War? Remember the first lady Nancy Reagan's campaign using red ribbons for 'just say no to drugs' and more recently the pink ribbons for women against breast cancer and most recently the purple ribbons for stopping violence in our schools? These are all symbolic gestures to show support for those enduring suffering and pain. All the ribbons then and now serve to connect people emotionally, to help unite people in a common cause, to help people feel less isolated in a crisis."

I explained to my children that the problem with the red ribbon now is similar to what occurred over the long time period our soldiers were in captivity—people begin to wear the ribbon as an accessory.

The Author

---

men diagnosed with an STD in the past five years had not told their main partners, compared with just 2% of women. Similarly, 51% of boys who had been diagnosed with an STD had not talked about it with their partner at the time, in contrast to 9% of girls. In a 2002 online poll Gay.com/PlanetOut.com Network wanted to know what people thought about the fact that a San Francisco court awarded $5 million in damages to a man who claims he was infected with HIV from his ex-lover, a former city health commissioner, who lied about his HIV status. When asked, "Should lying about one's HIV status to a sexual partner be a crime?" 69% of respondents said yes, 8% said no. Another 20% answered, "only if someone is infected as a result."

RECOMMENDED FILM: DAWN'S GIFT

She relates her story of becoming HIV infected. Running time, 38 minutes on DVD. Cost, $5.50 includes shipping.

Make check out to L. Schwitters—Dawn's Gift and send to:

L. Schwitters—Dawn's Gift
1745 Brookside Dr. SE
Issaquah, WA 98027
1-425-392-9161 fax 1-425-837-9971
email dawnsgift@hotmail.com
Purchase orders accepted

Adult Perceptions About HIV Infection and AIDS in the United States—One aspect about what adults now think about the AIDS pandemic has changed dramatically. The proportion of Americans naming HIV/AIDS as the nation's number one health problem has been steadily declining over time. In 1987, seven in ten Americans (70%) named HIV/AIDS as the most urgent health problem facing the nation. In 2006, 16% named HIV/AIDS as the nation's number one health problem. Some 56% of residents of Britain, France, and Germany* thought that AIDS was "the greatest risk to world health today" followed by heart disease (37%) and bird flu (7%). In 2004, the Kaiser Family Foundation surveyed people by age group to assess their concern about becoming HIV infected. Those age 18 to 24 were the most concerned (Figure 14-7). To, "do you personally know anyone who has died from AIDS or tested positive for HIV?": Yes, 39%; No, 61%. Fifty percent favored teaching safer sex as the major focus in prevention, while 40% favored teaching abstinence only.

The Workplace—If a person is not working near or beside someone who is HIV positive, they will be relatively soon. But they may not know it because a person's right to privacy prevails over an employee's right to know.

AIDS can have a variety of impacts in the workplace. The obvious one, of course, is on the employee who is diagnosed with HIV. The probability of sick-

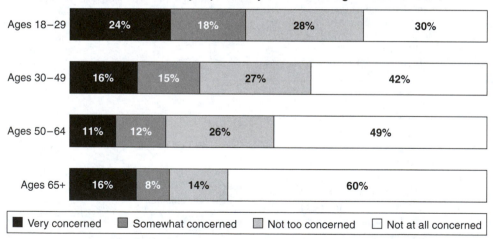

Bearing in mind the different ways people can be infected with HIV, the virus that causes AIDS—how concerned are you personally about becoming infected with HIV?

Age	Very concerned	Somewhat concerned	Not too concerned	Not at all concerned
Ages 18–29	24%	18%	28%	30%
Ages 30–49	16%	15%	27%	42%
Ages 50–64	11%	12%	26%	49%
Ages 65+	16%	8%	14%	60%

■ Very concerned   ■ Somewhat concerned   □ Not too concerned   □ Not at all concerned

FIGURE 14-7 Personal Concern About Becoming Infected by Age. *"Kaiser Family Foundation Survey of Americans on HIV/AIDS, Part Three—Experiences and Opinions by Race/Ethnicity and Age," (#7140), The Henry J. Kaiser Family Foundation, August 2004. The information was reprinted with permission from the Henry J. Kaiser Family Foundation. The Kaiser Family Foundation, based in Menlo Park, California, is a nonprofit, independent national healthcare philanthropy and is not associated with Kaiser Permanente or Kaiser Industries. (Conducted March 15–May 11, 2004). National random sample of 2902 respondents age 18 and older.*

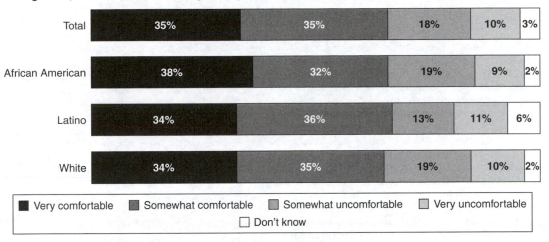

In general, how comfortable would you be, personally, working with someone who has HIV or AIDS?

	Very comfortable	Somewhat comfortable	Somewhat uncomfortable	Very uncomfortable	Don't know
Total	35%	35%	18%	10%	3%
African American	38%	32%	19%	9%	2%
Latino	34%	36%	13%	11%	6%
White	34%	35%	19%	10%	2%

■ Very comfortable ■ Somewhat comfortable ■ Somewhat uncomfortable ■ Very uncomfortable □ Don't know

FIGURE 14-8 Reported Comfort Level Working With Someone HIV+. *"Kaiser Family Foundation Survey of Americans on HIV/AIDS, Part Three—Experiences and Opinions by Race/Ethnicity and Age," (#7140), The Henry J. Kaiser Family Foundation, August 2004. The information was reprinted with permission from the Henry J. Kaiser Family Foundation. The Kaiser Family Foundation, based in Menlo Park, California, is a nonprofit, independent national healthcare philanthropy and is not associated with Kaiser Permanente or Kaiser Industries. (Conducted March 15–May 11, 2004.)*

ness and death obviously affects the individual and his or her ability to continue to contribute to the organization's activities and goals.

Employees' fear of AIDS can create a widespread loss of teamwork and productivity, and it can create an environment that is inhumane and insensitive toward the infected employee.

As the incidence of HIV and AIDS increases, the impact on organizations will obviously increase as well. While there are important logical and moral reasons for ensuring that infected people are not discriminated against, there are also practical reasons for addressing the employee HIV/AIDS problem.

An educated workforce, aware of the facts regarding diagnosis, testing, treatment, and transmission of HIV, can have a positive impact on the overall health of all employees. People are more inclined to openly acknowledge their HIV status and to seek treatment when assured of a supportive workplace environment. This increases productivity.

In 2004, the Kaiser Family Foundation surveyed black, Hispanic, and white Americans on their comfort level working with HIV-positive people (Figure 14-8).

THE CHARACTER OF SOCIETY

Rumors of Destruction

Today, friends are asked on street corners, at social gatherings, or over telephones: "Did you hear that he/she has AIDS?" Or: "Do you believe that he/she might be infected? You never know with the life they lead!" Some of the famous people rumored to have HIV/AIDS are Madonna, Elizabeth Taylor, Burt Reynolds, and Richard Pryor.

Rumors ruin lives. People suddenly subtly lose services; the lawn boy quits, no reason given. Quietly, job applications are turned down or car and homeowner insurance policies are canceled, and so on. In one case, after rumors of HIV infection spread in a small town, a man, if he was served in local bars at all, received his drinks in plastic cups. A health club refunded his membership dues. His apartment manager asked him to leave and when his toilet backed up the maintenance man came in wearing a hat over a World War II gas mask, deep water fishing boots, a raincoat, and rubber gloves. In frustration, he had an HIV test. The results were neg-

MAC AIDS FUND SURVEY: NOVEMBER 2007

In one of the first-ever global surveys of public perceptions and attitudes around HIV and AIDS, the MAC Fund has unveiled when opinion defies fact and where belief and education compete. The voices—spanning nine countries and five continents—provide a sense of the issue areas where more than 25 years of activism and funding have fallen short. (The MAC AIDS Fund is the philanthropic arm of Estée Lauder-owned MAC Cosmetics.) The survey involved 4,510 interviews with people from the United States, United Kingdom, Russia, France, China, India, Mexico, Brazil, and South Africa. A major find of the survey is that after 27 years of HIV/AIDS enveloping the world, nearly half of the respondents still do not view HIV/AIDS as a deadly affliction. Forty percent of the respondents do not understand that AIDS results in death! Other findings from the survey are:

- 86% of adults in the United States, United Kingdom, France, Russia, China, India, Brazil, Mexico, and South Africa believe stigma and shame to be a contributor to the spread of HIV. Seventy-six percent report lack of access to treatment to be a problem as well.

- In India, 59% of people polled believed a cure for HIV infection is available.
- Nearly half of all respondents believed most people with HIV are receiving treatment; in fact, 2007 data show only one patient in five is being treated.
- Almost half of respondents said they felt uncomfortable walking next to someone with HIV; 52% would not want to live in the same house as an HIV infected person; and 70% said they would not want to date someone with the virus.
- 73% of respondents said HIV is spreading, in part, because women are uncomfortable discussing safe sex practices with their partners.
- In the United States blacks are twice as likely as whites to believe there is a cure for HIV/AIDS.

Nancy Mahon, the MAC AIDS Fund's executive director, said, "The results of this survey, coupled with the recent failure of a promising AIDS vaccine trial, underscores that we are not going to vaccinate or cure our way out of this epidemic."

ative and he gave copies of the test to every "joint" in town, his physician, dentist, theater manager, grocery store manager . . . He felt this approach was better than running. Do you agree?

In another case in Brantly County, Ga., population 11,077, the 22-year-old mother of a 2-year-old son was the subject of a rumor that she was HIV infected. The rumor also stated that she had had intercourse with 200 men in the past year. To convince the townspeople, she took the HIV test and was not HIV infected. This young woman had to circulate the results of her blood test around town, but it was still not enough to stop the rumor. A newspaper in nearby Waycross, Ga., quoted an unnamed source saying that this woman was HIV positive.

There was the case of a compassionate person who opened a home for helping AIDS patients. Rumor quickly spread that the entire neighborhood was in danger, especially after the mail carrier refused to deliver mail and was ordered to wear rubber gloves and return to the post office for disinfection. To help the neighborhood understand AIDS and stop unfounded fears, a seminar was held at the AIDS home, but no one would enter the house.

A young person with AIDS reluctantly returned home—it meant revealing that he was gay to his family—and to the community. He said to his parents, "I have good news and bad. The bad is that I'm gay. The good is I have AIDS. I won't be around long enough to interfere with anyone." Once the word got out, a catering service refused to do the annual family Christmas party. They could not hire a practical nurse. Family and friends who used to drop in stayed away. People whispered that the son had gay cancer . . . that it was lethal . . . that it could be caught from dishes, linens, a handshake, and breathing in the same air he breathed out.

In Athens, Ala., the headline of the town's newspaper read, "Athens doctor: 'I don't have AIDS.'" This doctor, a prominent pediatrician in town for 18 years, had to produce a public defense to dispel the gossip that he had AIDS. The doctor offered a $2000 reward for any information about who began the rumor. To date no one has collected the money, but the townspeople did gather to support him.

In Nebraska, a man sued a prominent woman for starting a rumor that he had AIDS. The Nebraska Supreme Court upheld a lower court ruling that the man was slandered and he received $25,350 in damages.

In Atlanta, Georgia, the CDC said it had received many inquiries about reports that drug users infected with HIV had left contaminated needles in public places, on seats in movie theaters and under gas pump handles. Some reports have falsely indicated that CDC confirmed the presence of HIV in the needles. But the CDC said in a statement, "CDC has not tested such needles. Nor has the CDC confirmed the presence or absence of HIV in any samples related to these rumors. The majority of these reports and warnings appear to have no foundation in fact. CDC is not aware of any cases where HIV has been transmitted by a needle-stick injury outside a healthcare setting."

Good News, Bad News, and Late News

Good News—Good news is thinking and believing you're HIV infected and you're not. There must be a reason to think you're infected, so not being infected is, as some would say, a new lease on life. All too often that feeling is soon forgotten and many people continue lifestyles that place them at risk for infection.

Bad News—Bad news is thinking you're HIV infected and you are. It is difficult to predict what a person sees, hears, or does after being told he or she is HIV positive. For example, some have contemplated suicide, some have committed suicide, others have become completely fatalistic and proceeded to live a reckless and careless lifestyle that endangered others. Some have said it's like death before you're dead.

You are never prepared to hear the bad news regardless of how sure you are that you're infected. For example, one man who had suffered from night sweats, fevers, weight loss, and other classic symptoms knew he was infected. Yet when told of the positive test results he said "I got so angry, I ripped a shower out of the wall." Being told you are infected is totally devastating, said another infected person. "You feel that everyone is looking at you, everyone can tell you're dirty." Another person said, "The fact that I'm HIV positive completely dominates my life. There is not a waking hour that I do not think about it. I feel like a leper. I live between hope and despair." Still another said, "I did not leave the house for two days after being told I was HIV positive. The initial shock was that I was contaminated—unhealthy, soiled, unclean. I carried this burden in isolation for over

two years. After all, I had met people who had AIDS but never a person who said—I'm HIV infected."

The bad news is not confined to those hearing they are HIV infected; it touches everyone they know—lovers, family, friends, and employers. Nothing remains the same. The more symptomatic one becomes, the greater the social and human loss. One symptomatic mother said, "Whenever I tell my four-year-old I am going to the doctor, he screams because he knows I could be gone for weeks. I try to put him in another room playing with his sister when they come for me." This woman died. Relatives care for her children.

Late News—Late news is remaining **asymptomatic** after infection. Asymptomatic can be defined as when no clinically recognizable symptoms appear that would indicate HIV infection. During this time period, the virus can be transmitted to sexual partners. By the time either antibodies and/or clinical symptoms appear, the news is too late for those who might have been spared infection had their sexual partner tested positive or demonstrated clinical symptoms early on.

Munchausen's Syndrome: When People Pretend to be HIV Positive or to Have AIDS

As Hector Gavin wrote in 1843 in his 400-page history *Of Feigned and Factitious Diseases,* "The monarch, the mendicant, the unhappy slave, the proud warrior, the lofty statesman, even the minister of religion . . . have sought to disguise their purposes, or to obtain their desires, by feigning mental or bodily infirmities."

Donald Craven (1994) reported that a growing number of people may pretend to have AIDS either because of emotional disorders or because they want to gain access to free housing, medical care, and disability income. In one case, seven patients with self-reported HIV infection were treated for an average of 9.2 months in a clinical AIDS program before their seronegative status was discovered at the hospital (in general, hospitals in the United States do not require a written copy of the HIV test results proving that someone is HIV positive). Craven noted that "because patients with AIDS often have preferred access to drug treatment, prescription drugs, social security disability insurance, housing, and comprehensive medical care, the rate of malingering may increase and reach extremes."

Other doctors who have treated AIDS patients said that they have seen many patients who repeatedly

BOX 14.2

TELLING STORIES ABOUT AIDS-RELATED EVENTS

At the International AIDS Society-USA course in New York in March 2001, Mary Fisher, a mother, author, and AIDS activist who was diagnosed with AIDS in July 1991, reminded those in attendance of the importance of telling stories by and to the community of people affected by HIV and AIDS. She said that a community is defined by its stories; stories of victory and loss, of heroes and scapegoats, of tragedy and triumph. For the American AIDS community to become a community again, we must find ways to tell the stories again, to let others know that each story has a name, each with a purpose, each with a life. Here are two of her favorite HIV/AIDS stories.

During Bill Clinton's last run for the presidency—1996—I was invited to speak at an AIDS-related event in Little Rock, Arkansas. It was an awards night for regional folk who'd made significant contributions to the fight against HIV. The room was packed with social workers, people with AIDS, family members, religious leaders, a few politicians, and journalists—in other words, the room was packed with Democrats. Out of deference to me, every speaker had been very discreet never to mention politics or Republicans, until the community awards were being handed out, and the last recipient wanted to talk. She was a wonderful, elderly public health nurse: bright, quick, tiny, 77-years-old, and feisty. And you could hear every politically correct person in that room stop breathing when she reached up, grabbed the microphone and said, "I've had it with them dumb Republicans. For 15 years, I've talked to them dumb Republicans. Over and over, I've explained there ain't but three ways you can get AIDS: swap needles or blood, have sex, or get born with it. And, for 15 years them dumb Republicans been askin,' 'But can't you get it from mosquitoes?'" She paused for a moment, and then she said, "I'm telling y'all tonight that, from now on, I'm gonna tell 'em, 'Yep, you can get it from mosquitoes—but only in three states: Florida, Louisiana, and Arkansas. Cause them's the only places mosquitoes grow so big Republicans can have sex with 'em.'"

Her second story is taken from the book *I'll Go Quietly*.

Billy Cox came out of his hospital bed in Birmingham, Alabama, to bring me a hug in Montgomery. I'd first met him a year earlier at the University of Alabama at Birmingham where I was visiting Michael Saag (Michael is known for his work with antiretroviral drug therapies). Michael wanted me to meet Billy, to see his spunk and spirit. "Billy is the boxer in the ring," Michael once observed. "The doctors and nurses and medical staff, we're just the trainers in his corner. His friends and family are his fans, cheering him on." Now, a year later, I'd come to Montgomery to speak. But what I said there was not as eloquent as the events that soon played out in the life of Boxer Billy and Cousin Michael. Six weeks after he'd brought his hug to Montgomery—7 years, 4 months, and 3 days after testing positive of the AIDS virus—Billy Cox died on November 23, 1994. On Billy's last day, Michael Saag was leaving town for a few days and stopped in just to say good-bye. When he heard Billy's labored breathing, he called the family together and told them the end was near. And then—as nurses and old friends and Billy's family crowded into the room forming a remarkable community bound only by love for the boxer—Michael rested his head on Billy's chest and, unashamed, before the crowd, sobbed, "I'm sorry, I'm sorry." Science has limits. Even community has bounds. But no one will ever know what love might do.

Nkosi Johnson

Nkosi died at 6 A.M. on June 1st in his Melville, Johannesburg home with his foster mother, Gail Johnson, at his bedside. He had turned 12-years-old on February 4, 2001.

Danny Schechter, executive editor of Mediachannel .org writes of Nkosi. "I've met Nkosi and I love him, so can't profess any objectivity here. On the other hand, you probably haven't heard about him or, for that matter, heard much about the larger cause that he embodies and championed. It is not your fault if you don't know about Nkosi or the growing army of other Nkosis in Africa, because no one is telling you about them. Not with any regularity. Not with any context or explanation. Not in a way that will encourage you to care. Alas, when an issue like this is not on TV regularly in the United States, it doesn't exist for millions of us." Sadly, Schechter shows that it matters not who or where you are, violence is an everyday commodity available to all. On April 27, 2001, South African Freedom Day: Some armed robbers slipped into his Johannesburg home at one o'clock in the morning, pointing a gun at the woman named Grace who was taking care of him. They took the TV and the VCR and whatever else they could grab. She was traumatized. "Nkosi, who cannot speak, saw what happened and had seizures the next day." Nkosi lost

BOX 14.2 (*continued*)

his parents to AIDS, and now AIDS claimed his 12-year-old existence.

April 2004. Sister Priscilla Dlamini, a 55-year-old nurse of Gingindlovu, South Africa, clutched a corner of her billowing black wimple as she pointed down the muddy dirt road that runs past the Holy Cross AIDS Hospice, where she works. She tells this story: "The first house, there, the white one, you see it on the right," her thick finger tracing the path of the road to a thatched roof barely visible above the cane. "The father and the mother died of AIDS, so did the boy and two girls. That pink house over there, seven died. And there. All eight dead." Her hand swept toward the horizon to cloud-shrouded mountains. "Everywhere between here and there are empty houses. In the mountains, it is even worse. And where there are people in the houses, there are graves beside them." From one wardroom comes a shrill sound: a 7-year-old girl lets out a whooping cry, punctuated by a dry, congested cough; she is thirsty. Her hollow eyes are round with fear and overflow with tears. In Zulu she cries, "I want to go home. Why do you keep me? Why? Why?" Sister Priscilla offers water as she leans over and whispers a few words of comfort, but she does not tell her the truth. The girl will never go

home, even when she dies. Her father and mother are dead. There is no home to go to. Sister Priscilla opened the hospice because so many people dying from AIDS were being left in the sugar cane fields by their families for the clinic workers to find. She said, "People come home from Durban and the other cities to die. But relatives do not accept them. They chase them away or dump them on the edge of the sugar cane plantations and we go around picking them up and bring them here." Some of the dying children arrive at the hospice with nothing, not even identification documents. We give them a stone to hold before they die, and tell the children, "Your mother held this stone."

The Sister knows that death is never far away in the heart of what people here call the AIDS belt, a region in rural KwaZulu-Natal Province that stretches along the Indian Ocean from Richards Bay 80 miles southwest toward the port city of Durban. This is where South Africa faces the full fury of the AIDS pandemic and its social, economic and political devastation. It is also here that the South African government confronts an awful truth: There is too much to do and too little to do it with. Deaths from AIDS complications will continue to rise for many years to come.

come to their offices fearing that they have AIDS, even though multiple tests have shown that they do not (Zuger, 1995, Mileno, 2001).

An Oklahoma physician has written about the AIDS **Munchausen's syndrome**—an emotional disorder in which people pretend to have the disease simply to get attention from doctors. Confidentiality requirements make AIDS a perfect illness for people suffering from Munchausen syndrome because the laws shield them from being discovered.

Medical Moral Issues

HIV/AIDS represents a new era in medicine, one in which physicians are faced with complex moral issues. When the American Medical Association (AMA) issued a statement to the effect that it is unethical to refuse to treat HIV/AIDS patients, that statement reflected a deep concern in the medical community about the possibility of their becoming infected by treating patients with HIV/AIDS.

The AMA statement for an ethical call to arms is *unprecedented* in this century. It is the result of a spreading fear that HIV/AIDS is too contagious to tolerate in spite of the knowledge that the virus is

not transmitted via casual contact. Emotions, not education, are in control of those whose fears exceed reality. But these emotions are real and they are having an impact on the medical community.

There is an ongoing dilemma concerning the rights of the physician and other healthcare workers to practice medicine in a safe environment as opposed to the rights of HIV infected and AIDS patients to receive care and medical support. Although the risk of HIV transmission through medical occupational exposure appears to be quite low, the fact that it is possible at all, coupled with the uniformly fatal prognosis associated with AIDS, suggests that physicians, nurses, and other healthcare workers have legitimate concerns about health risks.

In a recent survey of U.S. doctors in residency training, 39% said that a surgeon or other specialist had refused to treat a patient with AIDS in the resident's care. In Canada, only 13% reported a specialist had refused to treat a patient with AIDS; in France, only 8% said a specialist had rejected care.

Further, 23% of U.S. doctors would not care for AIDS patients if they had a choice as compared with 14% of Canadian physicians and 4% of French doctors.

The survey results may be a disturbing indicator of how U.S. physicians view their work and a reflection of cultural and political attitudes here that view those with AIDS with veiled hostility.

To combat that fear, medical schools are now providing their students with disability insurance that covers AIDS. Hospitals have adopted policies that require physicians to treat AIDS patients or face dismissal.

DEALING WITH DISCRIMINATION: THE AMERICANS WITH DISABILITIES ACT

Although incidents of discrimination are disheartening, they are only a part of the story. Another part of the story is how discrimination has been fought and how courts, legislatures, and other social institutions have responded with attempts to reduce HIV/AIDS discrimination and to minimize its impact. To this end a brief synopsis of the Americans with Disabilities Act is presented along with the first U.S. Supreme Court ruling based on this act.

Americans with Disabilities Act

The primary federal nondiscrimination statute that prohibits discrimination on the basis of a person's disability or health status is the Americans with Disabilities Act (ADA) of 1990. The ADA provides that no individual "shall be discriminated against on the basis of disability in the full and equal enjoyment of the goods, services, facilities, privileges, advantages or accommodations of any place of public accommodation." The ADA's definition of "public accommodation" specifically includes hospitals and professional offices of healthcare providers. A critically important issue under the ADA is whether persons with **asymptomatic** HIV infection have a disability and thus are protected under the ADA. Disability is defined as a physical or mental impairment that substantially limits one or more of the major life activities of the individual, a record of such impairment, or being regarded as having an impairment. In the past, many courts have ruled or assumed as undisputed that HIV infection, as the underlying cause of a life-threatening illness, is a disability. However, several recent court decisions have held that HIV does not automatically qualify as a disability, and in each case there must be an individualized determination as to whether the infection actually

limits, in a substantial way, a major life activity. The ADA's legislative history, however, indicates that Congress intended to include HIV infection within the definition of disability, and the Equal Employment Opportunity Commission's regulations embody that view. In its first AIDS case ever, the Supreme Court had to decide whether and to what extent persons with HIV infection are protected under the ADA.

The Case of *Bragdon* v. *Abbott:* United States Supreme Court

1998—In the 17-year history of the HIV/AIDS pandemic, the U.S. Supreme Court had never considered a case directly involving HIV or AIDS until March 30, 1998, when oral arguments began in the case of *Bragdon* v. *Abbott*. The *Bragdon* case is also the first time the court has ever heard a case involving the ADA. On September 16, 1994, Sidney Abbott, age 37, went to her dentist in Bangor, Maine, to get a cavity filled. Dr. Randon Bragdon refused to fill a gum-line cavity in his office when he read on her medical form that she was HIV positive. He told her he could do the procedure in a hospital, a change of venue that would have added approximately $150 to the bill. According to a cover story about the case in the *American Bar Association Journal,* Dr. Bragdon did not have privileges to practice in any area hospitals, nor had he applied for them. Dr. Bragdon maintains that he could have sought and received permission to perform occasional procedures without having been granted full privileges.

Abbott's Lawsuit—Her lawsuit argues that in refusing to treat her in his office, Bragdon violated the ADA and the Maine Human Rights Act. Federal district and appeals courts both agreed with her.

United States Supreme Court Decision June 25, 1998—The Supreme Court ruled 5 to 4, upholding the District Court and the First Circuit Court of Appeals, finding that Bragdon violated Abbott's rights to treatment under the provisions of the ADA of 1990. Abbott's HIV infection constituted a disability under the ADA in that her HIV infection "substantially limits" a major life activity—her ability to reproduce and bear children (to have a child she places her husband at risk for HIV infection and risks infecting her child). Justice Kennedy, in delivering the opinion of the court, held that from the moment of infection and throughout every stage of the disease, HIV infection satisfies the statutory and regulatory definition of a "physical impairment." Applicable Rehabilitation Act regulations define "physical or mental impairment" to mean "any physiological disorder or condition affecting the body['s] hemic and lymphatic [systems]." HIV infection falls well within that definition. The medical literature reveals that the disease follows a predictable and unalterable course from infection to inevitable death. It causes immediate abnormalities in a person's blood, and the infected person's white cell count continues to drop throughout the course of the disease, even during the intermediate stage when its attack is concentrated in the lymph nodes. Thus, HIV infection must be regarded as a physiological disorder with an immediate, constant, and detrimental effect on the hemic and lymphatic systems.

Dissent in Part

Justice O'Connor stated that Abbott's claim of a disability should be evaluated on an individual basis and that she has not proven that her symptomatic HIV status substantially limited one or more of her major life activities. "In my view, the act of giving birth to a child, while a very important part of the lives of many women, is not generally the same as the representative major life activities of all persons—caring for one's self, performing manual tasks, walking, seeing, hearing, speaking, breathing, learning, and working"—listed in regulations relevant to the Americans with Disabilities Act. Based on that conclusion, there is no need to address whether other aspects of intimate or family relationships not raised in this case could constitute major life activities; nor is there reason to consider whether HIV status would impose a substantial limitation on one's ability to reproduce if reproduction were a major life activity.

U.S. Supreme Court Rules on Insurance Coverage Cap for HIV/AIDS Treatment

In January 2000, the U.S. Supreme Court let stand a ruling that allowed an insurance company to provide less coverage for AIDS-related illnesses than for other conditions under the same policy. The high court, without comment, refused to hear the appeal brought by two HIV-positive Chicago men who claimed that their insurance company's policies violate the Americans with Disabilities Act. The two policies in question were issued by Mutual of Omaha. One

policy set a $25,000 lifetime coverage limit for AIDS-related illnesses and the other contained a $100,000 cap, while both allowed a $1 million cap for other illnesses. Attorneys for Mutual of Omaha argued that the insurance company had not discriminated because it offered the men the same coverage offered to other customers. In 1998, the federal judge in Chicago ruled in favor of the two men, but the 7th U.S. Circuit Court of Appeals reversed that ruling. The Appeals Court said the ADA guarantees access to insurance but does not regulate the content of coverage.

DISCUSSION QUESTION: Clearly a 5 to 4 ruling is not an overwhelming mandate to support Abbott's lawsuit. Is a simple majority, 55% in this case, sufficient or because this case has vast implications, should it require a two-thirds majority, 6 in favor, 3 against (67%)? What are the legal and moral issues in accepting a simple majority versus a two-thirds ruling?

Bragdon raised a question for you to consider as you research the question above. Looking at **Magic Johnson**—he asks if it really makes sense to consider someone "disabled" who can earn millions of dollars playing professional basketball, or go to work, or otherwise perform the tasks of daily living. Your response is?

Patients' Right to Know If Their Physician Has HIV/AIDS—In a recent Gallup Poll, 86% of those polled felt that they had the right to know if a health-care worker treating them was HIV infected. Many lawyers also take this position. The courts appear to be moving toward an interpretation of the doctrine of informed patient consent as "what a reasonable patient would want to know," rather than "what a reasonable physician would disclose." Because it is so difficult for surgeons to avoid occasionally cutting themselves during surgery, it has been suggested that the best solution is not to have HIV-infected surgeons perform surgery at all.

Public anxiety on HIV/AIDS and medical care is becoming increasingly tinged with hysteria. A recent national Gallup Poll undertaken for *Newsweek* asked a representative sample of 618 adults, "Which of the following kinds of healthcare workers should be required to tell patients if they are infected with the AIDS virus?"

The answers were: surgeons 95%; all physicians 94%; dentists 94%; all healthcare workers 90%.

Clearly, people do not differentiate between doctors who perform invasive procedures and those who do not. However, the patient could ask what the probability is of a single dentist (Acer) infecting six of his patients (Bergalis, Web, and four others). Extremely low, yet it did happen! The lowest of probabilities and best of guidelines and precautions do not stop the fire of fear. It must also be mentioned that the same *Newsweek* poll found that 97% of those interviewed felt that HIV-infected patients should tell their healthcare workers that they are infected.

There is one important aspect related to this poll that needs to be addressed. That is, many of the people interviewed stated that if they knew their surgeon was HIV infected, they would "get another surgeon." This switching dilemma may, at some point, have the majority of the population needing surgery standing in line for the uninfected surgeons. Services provided by the reduced number of surgeons, it could be claimed, at some point, result in increased costs and diminished quality.

HIV-Infected Healthcare Professionals' Duty To Disclose—Several courts have held that healthcare professionals have a duty to disclose their HIV status to patients or health authorities, assuming that their professional activities pose a risk of transmission to patients. The Maryland Court of Appeals ruled that a surgeon has a duty to inform his patients of his infection; even if the patient has not actually been exposed and tests HIV negative, the contact with the surgeon may subsequently give rise to a claim for their infliction of mental distress due to fear of transmission. Courts justify orders to disclose based on a duty to protect patients and on the doctrine of informed consent. Requiring disclosure to patients, of course, can severely jeopardize a healthcare professional's career. To avoid this result, some states allow the professional to continue practicing, with appropriate restrictions and supervision, but without disclosing his or her HIV status (Gostin et al., 1998).

FEDERAL AND PRIVATE SECTOR FINANCING: CREATION OF AN AIDS INDUSTRY

About 27 years ago, when the public was just learning about a new disease that would be called AIDS, some scientists tracking down the cause were already thinking about how their research could be marketed. French and American groups eventually claimed to have codiscovered HIV independently and in different ways. In one respect their approach was the same: Shortly before announcing their discoveries, both rushed to file patents that described how to determine whether a person's blood harbored the virus. By doing this, they gave birth to the HIV/AIDS industry (Figure 14-9).

Financing the Multi-Billion Dollar AIDS Industry: A Quilt with Many Holes

Federal Government—In 1990, the U.S. Congress did something quite rare: It allocated money specifically for the treatment of one disease—HIV/AIDS. In some ways the increased commitment of federal and state government to cancer research and treatment in the early 1970s is similar to what happened in the war on AIDS in the 1980s. In both decades, there was a major funding surge to stimulate research, therapy, and prevention. A major difference, however, is that dollars for cancer came more slowly over a longer time period that began well before the 1970s. With AIDS, federal funding began in 1981 (Figure 14-10), and has increased at an unprecedented rate.

No Cheap Way Out: HIV/AIDS Is a Very Expensive Disease

During the 28 years from 1982 through 2009, federal spending on AIDS-related projects will have increased from $8 million in 1982 to $24.1 billion for 2009. The Presidential Advisory Council on HIV/AIDS provided the president with six AIDS goals that will be funded with the federal budget for AIDS. The

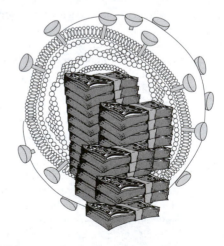

FIGURE 14-9 The Enormous Sum of Federal, State, and Private Sector Monies Spent on HIV/AIDS Has Made This Disease an Industry unto Itself.

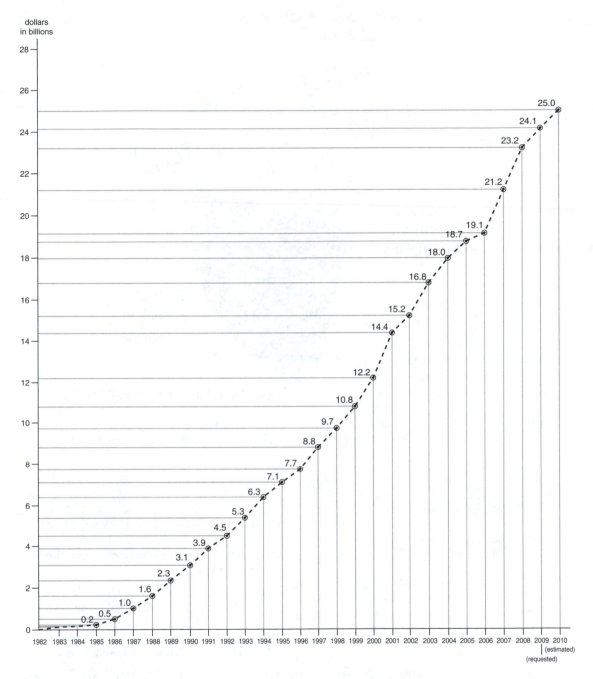

FIGURE 14-10 Federal Government AIDS Expenditures Through the Year 2009. Federal expenditures were $1 billion in 1987, and over $24 billion for 2008. Bernhard Schwartlander of UNAIDS said in 2002 that the United States is now spending over $20 billion a year on prevention, care, and research. By the end of 2009 the U.S. federal government will have spent about $262 billion over 28 years on this disease.

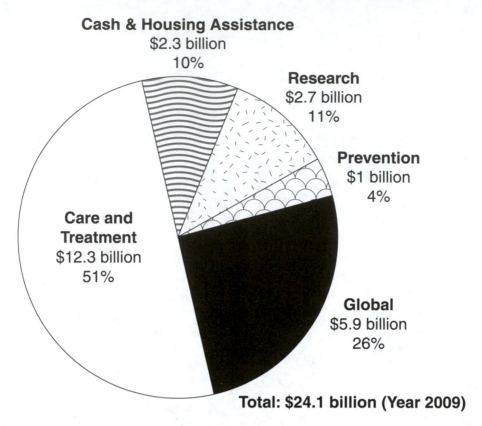

Cash & Housing Assistance
$2.3 billion
10%

Research
$2.7 billion
11%

Prevention
$1 billion
4%

Care and Treatment
$12.3 billion
51%

Global
$5.9 billion
26%

Total: $24.1 billion (Year 2009)

FIGURE 14-11 Total Federal HIV/AIDS Spending by Category FY 2009. Federal HIV/AIDS spending is divided generally into four categories: Care and Assistance, Research, Prevention, and Global and Housing. Numbers do not equal 100% due to rounding.

goals are to: (1) develop a cure, (2) reduce/eliminate new infections, (3) guarantee care/service for the HIV infected, (4) fight against HIV/AIDS discrimination, (5) quickly translate scientific advances into improved care/prevention, and (6) provide support for international AIDS efforts. (See Figure 14-11.)

Private Sector Funding: United States—In addition to the money spent by the federal government, collectively the states also spend between $6 billion and $8 billion each year. The private sector spends about $5 billion a year. By the end of 2009, the federal government and the states and private sector will have spent about the same. Adding in unspecified federal dollars that went to AIDS-related projects and the dollars spent in the state and private sector would most likely bring the total AIDS-related expenditures to over $440 billion. Yet, in spite of this massive expenditure on HIV/AIDS, the United States still does not have the underpinning of a uniform healthcare

system to provide an organized, controlled use of AIDS funds. The current funding is **heterogeneous** and provides **unequal access** to HIV/AIDS care. (See Box 14.3 and Figure 14-11; Figure 14-12.)

AIDS Costs as a Percentage of the National Federal Budget

The $24.1 billion for 2009 HIV/AIDS represents about 0.7% of the $3.1 trillion federal budget.

AIDS Expenditures per Death Compared to Other Major Diseases Causing Death

Federal spending for AIDS research, educational programs, counselor training, testing, and prevention programs has been compared with federal spending for other diseases. There is a discrepancy between the total federal dollars spent on certain diseases and the number of deaths they cause. In 2008, with about 13,000 deaths, HIV/AIDS received $23.2 billion.

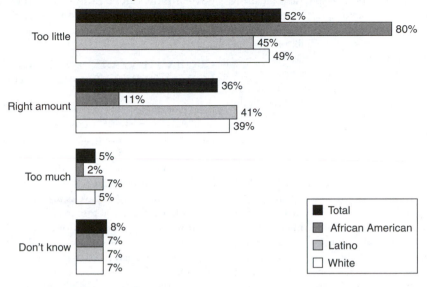

Thinking about the HIV/AIDS epidemic in the United States specifically, in general, do you think the federal government spends too much money on HIV/AIDS, too little money on HIV/AIDS, or about the right amount?

Too little
- 52%
- 80%
- 45%
- 49%

Right amount
- 36%
- 11%
- 41%
- 39%

Too much
- 5%
- 2%
- 7%
- 5%

Don't know
- 8%
- 7%
- 7%
- 7%

Legend:
- ■ Total
- ■ African American
- □ Latino
- □ White

FIGURE 14-12 Views of U.S. Spending on Domestic HIV/AIDS. *"Kaiser Family Foundation Survey of Americans on HIV/AIDS, Part Three—Experiences and Opinions by Race/Ethnicity and Age," (#7140), The Henry J. Kaiser Family Foundation, August 2004. The information was reprinted with permission from the Henry J. Kaiser Family Foundation. The Kaiser Family Foundation, based in Menlo Park, California, is a nonprofit, independent national healthcare philanthropy and is not associated with Kaiser Permanente or Kaiser Industries. (Conducted March 15–May 11, 2004.) National random sample of 2902 respondents age 18 and older.*

That's equivalent to about $1.8 million per AIDS-related death! In 2008, cancer caused about 566,000 deaths and received about $4 billion or about $7000/death. Heart disease, which caused about 700,000 deaths in 2008 (28% of all deaths for the year), received about $1.7 billion or about $2430/death. Some 2 million Americans require insulin injections for type I diabetes and perhaps as many as 19 million have type II diabetes (diet controlled). Diabetes, a severe progressive disorder, kills 75,000 people each year. This disease received $636 million, or about 2.2% of the AIDS budget or about $8480/death. Stroke, which affects millions of Americans and is involved in about 170,000 deaths per year, received $228 million or $1341/death. Overall, between 1981 and the beginning of 2009, while some 594,000 people died of AIDS, about 20 million died of heart disease and about 12 million died of cancer. HIV/AIDS is the most expensive disease in history relative to time, 1981 through 2008.

U.S. GOVERNMENT BELIEVES HIV/AIDS IS A THREAT TO NATIONAL SECURITY

A nation's national security interests will be defined as the protection of its people and the preservation of territorial integrity, national sovereignty, political, social, economic, and defense institutions against direct or indirect threats.

Today, more than ever before, threats are interrelated, and a threat to one is a threat to all. The mutual vulnerability of weak and strong has never been clearer—the security of the most affluent state can be held hostage to the ability of the poorest state to contain an emerging disease. Imagining the future shape of the HIV/AIDS pandemic, some two or three wavelengths (30 to 50 years) ahead, is exceedingly difficult. If no effective vaccine or cure is found within the next 20 years, areas of the world that are now witnessing explosive pandemics may well be more deeply altered than Europe was following the plague or Black Death. In Africa, for example, there are many features in place that mirror pre-plague Europe, including an enormous surplus of unskilled labor, lack of clear property rights for the bulk of the population, domination by tiny social elites, widespread warfare waged both by state and mercenary forces, and transition from dispersed agrarian to disastrously urbanized societies. Each of these factors was radically altered by the Black Death, and they could well be reshaped by HIV.

Security at Stake

The U.S. federal government declared in May 2000 that "AIDS is a threat to our national security." Past U.S. Secretary of Health and Human Services Donna Shalala said, "We know that infectious diseases know no borders, that they can affect this country, and in this case it is both in our economic interest and in our national security interest to work on infectious diseases abroad. The high rates of AIDS in Africa are putting security and stability at risk by disabling national armies, disrupting economies and killing off people who might become the next generation of leaders. Basically AIDS is uncoupling the economic gains in Africa as African countries are forced to shift more resources to their healthcare systems from their economic investments." Shalala also said that countries in other parts of the world face a growing HIV/AIDS crisis. "Eastern Europe has an AIDS problem, Russia has it, India has it, every country in the world that we do business with, but more importantly our need to be politically stable, is suffering from this huge onslaught of AIDS. And that makes the relationship economically and from the security point of view relevant to America's national security."

In a June 12, 2003 speech, then–U.S. Secretary of State Colin Powell placed the pandemic in a national security context by equating the virus to a terrorist. "The HIV virus, like terrorism, kills indiscriminately and without mercy," Powell asserted. "As cruel as any tyrant, the virus will crush the human spirit. It is an insidious and relentless foe, more destructive than any army, any conflict, and any weapon of mass destruction. It shatters families, tears the fabric of societies, and undermines government, undermines the very basis of democracy. It can destroy countries and, as we have seen, it can destabilize entire regions."

DISCUSSION QUESTION: Present reasons that agree or disagree with the federal government's declaration that HIV/AIDS is a threat to America's national security.

GLOBAL HIV/AIDS FUNDING FOR UNDERDEVELOPED NATIONS

Peter Piot (Figure I-2), executive director of UNAIDS, said, "AIDS is essentially a crisis of governance, of what governments do and do not do for their people. We have the drugs to treat HIV infection and we have the tools to confront the risks that drive HIV transmission and prevent infection itself. What we don't have is national political will. We have demanded too little from our leaders and excused too much."

In many ways, we are of one world. In the long run, Africa and Asia's destiny is our destiny. There is hope on the horizon, but that hope will only be realized if the developed nations take constructive action together. As South Africa's Archbishop Desmond Tutu said: "If we wage this holy war together—we will win."

The bottom line is this: There is no vaccine or cure for AIDS in sight, and the world is somewhere in the beginning of this global pandemic, not the end. What is happening in Africa now is just the tip of the iceberg. As goes Africa, so will go India and the Newly Independent States of the former Soviet Union. There must be a sense of urgency for the developed world to work together; to learn from their failures and successes, and to share their experience with those countries that now stand on the brink of disaster. Millions of lives—perhaps hundreds of millions of lives—hang in the balance. AIDS is a devastating human tragedy that requires global help.

HINDSIGHT Nineteen years ago, when the AIDS death toll in the United States crossed 100,000, few paid heed to a grim prediction by the World Health Organization (WHO) that "by the year 2000, 40 million persons may be infected with HIV." In the developed world, AIDS was seen as a serious but small disease, restricted to gay men, drug users, hemophiliacs, and their infants. In the developing world, just a few courageous voices were warning about the silent spread of a deadly new plague. Africa is in crisis. In some countries, about 40% of the adult population is infected. Many millions have died, and millions more will follow, leaving their societies trapped in poverty, burdened with a generation of orphans, and facing demographic catastrophe. The grim statistics are not confined to Africa. Asia and the Caribbean face explosive HIV epidemics, while the nations of the former Soviet empire are looking at an overwhelming increase of drug addiction, untreated sexual diseases, and the unchecked spread of HIV. Finally the world has begun to take notice.

The Beginning of UNAIDS and a Unified Attack Against HIV/AIDS

In January 1996, the United Nations took the innovative step of bringing six United Nations organizations together in a joint cosponsored program, UNAIDS. These six organizations were joined by four other organizations in the following years through 2007. In January 2000, the United Nations Security Council held a precedent-setting special session in which for the first time it identified a disease—AIDS—as a global security threat. A second UN HIV/AIDS special session of the General Assembly was held June 25–27, 2001. There have been no additional special sessions on HIV/AIDS.

Former United Nations Secretary-General Kofi Annan Calls for Large-Scale Mobilization in Fight Against AIDS, Tuberculosis, and Malaria

In mid-2001, calling the battle his personal priority, the secretary-general outlined five priority areas for the global campaign.

BOX 14.3

AIDS PROGRAMS: AN EPIDEMIC OF WASTE?

Through 2002 there has been constant pressure on politicians and leaders of private industry to contribute higher levels of money in the fight against HIV/AIDS. In 2002, AIDS activists marched in Washington in an attempt to get Congress to allocate $2.5 billion to the Global AIDS, Tuberculosis, and Malaria Fund. Their belief is that America is not spending enough money at home or globally on HIV/AIDS. Others, however, protest this notion and feel that if graft and corruption were eliminated there would be sufficient money such that yearly increases in the federal HIV/AIDS program would not be called for. To support this belief, a group called Citizens Against Government Waste (CAGW) released a report in February 2002 on **"AIDS Programs: An Epidemic of Waste"** (www.cagw.org). Citizens Against Government Waste is the nation's largest nonpartisan, nonprofit organization dedicated to eliminating waste, fraud, abuse, and mismanagement in government. Some of the fraud found by this group is listed exactly as it is presented in their report:

- CAGW has obtained a copy of a $20,000 grant from the Vermont Department of Public Health to the Twin State Women's Network (TSWN) to be used for a weekend retreat. Topics for the weekend included "Toys 4 Us" and "Self Loving/Self Healing: Discussing the Role of Masturbation as a Tool for Healing." TSWN also received: $1500 for long distance phone calls; $1000 for books, including "The New Good Vibrations for Sex" manual; and $250 for videos, choices of which included "Fire in the Valley: A Guide to Masturbation for Women" and "Fire in the Valley: A Guide to Masturbation for Men." Each participant received a welcome bag filled with mints and chocolate and each room was equipped with welcome packets containing condoms, lubricant, candles, massage lotion, and lip balm. TSWN received 86% of its funds from government sources, including the Centers for Disease Control (CDC).

- Positive Force in San Francisco receives $1 million a year from the CDC. The group offers flirting classes and, last July, hosted a workshop on how to have anal intercourse if you suffer from diarrhea. (Diarrhea is a common side effect of AIDS.)

- On February 28, 2002, the Stop AIDS Project of San Francisco, which received nearly $700,000 from the CDC in fiscal 2001, will sponsor "GUYWATCH: Blow by Blow." The advertisement for the seminar reads, in part: "What tricks do you want to share to make your man tremble with delight?"

- A Central Florida AIDS Unified Resources (CENTAUR) staffer spent $600,000 in Ryan White CARE Act money on tickets to Disney World, hotels, and restaurants.

- In April 2001, *The New York Post* revealed New York City was spending nearly $180,000 a week ($9 million a year) on hotel rooms for HIV and AIDS patients. That month, the city had reserved 20 rooms at the Sofitel Hotel in Midtown Manhattan at $329 apiece. Advocates say DASIS must use the expensive hotels because it has ruined its relationship with lower-cost hotels by not paying bills on time. New York City received $52.6 million in Housing Opportunities for People With AIDS (HOPWA) program funding in fiscal 2001.

- The University of California–San Francisco AIDS Health Project (AHP), which received a $633,765 grant from the CDC prevention in fiscal 2001 and continually receives nearly 85% of its funding from government sources, sponsored a workshop in November in physical intimacy, focusing on "holding, kissing, licking, sucking, and . . ."

- A doctor in Puerto Rico used $2.2 million in federal funds to buy luxury items like cars and jet skis, while severely neglecting the AIDS patients in his care.

- More than $20 million in grant money intended to help house AIDS patients was collected—but never spent—in Los Angeles.

- AID Atlanta, Inc., which received more than $3.5 million from the government in fiscal 2000 and only $1.2 million in private contributions, sponsors "Deeper Love: A Workshop for Gay and Bisexual Men of African Descent" that addresses such subjects as dating, relationships, and erotica. The program lists the following topics of discussion: "Dirty talk: what makes it good; Tossing salad; Strollin' in the park, through the trails; The art of latex; Safety versus trust." AID Atlanta, Inc. also sponsors "Slipping and Sliding" where men can explore their needs and desires and learn how to fulfill them.

- FBI investigation into the South Dallas Health Clinic revealed that more than $60,000 in the Title I funds had been spent on calls to psychic hotlines and on shopping trips to Neiman Marcus.

BOX 14.3 (*continued*)

- The nonprofit Tampa Hillsborough Action Plan (THAP) gives its top executives plenty of perks despite its financial woes. THAP boss and THAP chief executive officer rang up nearly $1000 in meal charges in a three-week period and were also afforded the use of sport utility vehicles. THAP boss received up to $45,000 a year annually for the maintenance of his vehicles. THAP's top executives also received four season tickets for Tampa Bay Buccaneers games and two season tickets for both the Tampa Bay Devil Rays and the Tampa Bay Lightning. Meanwhile, THAP owed nearly $25,000 in delinquent payroll taxes. THAP receives $450,000 a year from the federal government to provide housing to people with AIDS.

- In the CAGW investigation is the Los Angeles County Auditor Controller's Office report that states, "officials in the county's Office of AIDS Programs and Policy cannot account for $83 million it spent in 2001." That is more money than the budget for many American cities.

CONCLUSION OF CAGW

Before new resources are added to the $14 billion in federal money currently allotted for AIDS-related programs, the Departments of Health and Human Services and Housing and Urban Development should conduct extensive audits of the Ryan White CARE Act Title I and the HOPWA program. Such audits will give Congress more incentive to reform or eliminate these antiquated and duplicated social programs. Congress should redirect many CDC prevention grants to international AIDS relief efforts or increase funds for researching an AIDS cure. Many CARE Act programs, including all of Title I, should be phased out and incorporated into existing federal safety net programs such as Medicaid and Medicare. This would ensure necessary, life-saving medical care to those with HIV and AIDS who are low income or uninsured, while also eliminating nonessential AIDS services. It would also save money to bolster the AIDS Drug Assistance Program.

In May 2002, U.S. Treasury Secretary Paul O'Neill took a 10-day tour of Africa. On his return, he called for increased access to HIV/AIDS treatment and greater accountability for assistance programs. O'Neill went to Chris Hani Baragwanath Hospital in Soweto where he met with HIV-positive women whose children had been treated at birth with the antiretroviral drug nevirapine to reduce the risk of vertical HIV transmission. O'Neill, who has been critical of foreign aid in the past, asked why the South African government was not providing treatment to all HIV-positive pregnant women. O'Neill said, "This whole business about having so much money ... and it not going primarily to treatment is just a stunning revelation." In an interview with ABC's *This Week*, on May 26, O'Neill echoed his call for greater accountability. "My problem is that it isn't clear why we aren't getting better choices about the priority use of the money that is already there. For me, this is about getting real results on the ground."

Since the CAGW report in 2003, several hundred cases of financial fraud and corruption have been uncovered in the United States and worldwide—far too many to report here. One is the recent case of antiretroviral drugs provided, at cost, to various countries in Africa. The drugs were smuggled out of Africa into Britain, France, The Netherlands, Germany, and other developed countries and sold for millions of dollars in profit.

In 2005, Florida's Medicaid bureau chief and possibly others in the agency diverted $200,000 in federal AIDS funds to pay for treatments for a "politically connected" Broward County couple's adopted autistic child. Also in 2005, New York City's Human Resources Administration (HRA), which finds temporary shelter for people living with HIV/AIDS, paid $2.2 million in questionable payments over two-and-a-half years, which included paying $182,391 for hotel rooms assigned to 26 people for up to two years after they died. HRA also paid $1 million to vendors for clients who had not signed verification registration logs.

In 2006, according to U.S. senator Tom Coborn, the federal government did not act prudently, spending (wasting?) millions of dollars to subsidize six separate HIV/AIDS conferences in five months. The conferences were attended by hundreds of federal employees at taxpayers' expense. The attendees lived in plush oceanside hotel rooms, watched fashion shows, and enjoyed luxury spas. In 2006 and 2007, representatives of the FBI said that Medicare and Medicaid programs involving monies for HIV/AIDS patients were "rampant in fraud." For example, in 2007, ten Florida medical clinic owners were indicted for allegedly defrauding **Medicare** by improperly billing the program for HIV/AIDS treatments and medical equipment. According to a report conducted by the Governor's Office, Florida has far fewer HIV/AIDS cases than California or New York, but HIV/AIDS providers in the state submitted three times as many claims as providers in California and five times as many claims as providers in New York. According to authorities, the defendants submitted

BOX 14.3 (*continued*)

more than $12.5 million in false and fraudulent claims. Also in 2007, the president of Miami-based clinic Medlife Services was arrested for defrauding **Medicaid** out of $73,000 by improperly billing the program for the antiretroviral drug, WinRho, at a rate one hundred times higher than average. And so it continues . . .

DISCUSSION QUESTION: Do you think in other countries, there is at least an equal amount of fraud and corruption as found in America with regard to the allocation and spending of HIV/AIDS dollars donated for the prevention and treatment of HIV/AIDS? Support your opinions with examples.

1. Preventing further spread of the epidemic, especially by giving young people the knowledge and power to protect themselves.

2. Reducing HIV transmission from mother to child, which he called "the cruelest, most unjust" infections of all.

3. Ensuring that care and treatment are within reach of all.

4. Delivering scientific breakthroughs. Finding a cure and vaccine for HIV/AIDS must be given increased priority in scientific budgets.

5. Protecting those made most vulnerable by the epidemic, especially orphans.

To achieve these five goals, Annan called world leaders to help finance the campaign against AIDS, tuberculosis, and malaria in Africa. In April 2001, he said, "a war chest of 7 billion to 10 billion U.S. dollars is needed annually, over an extended period of time, to wage an effective global campaign against AIDS. [This number has now been raised to $12 billion to $18 billion.] Current spending on AIDS in developing countries totals around $1 billion annually." This is many billions of dollars less than they spend on their military. Although Annan's figure of $10 billion for combating AIDS, tuberculosis, and malaria seems like a large sum, it is equivalent to:

• Four days of global military spending.

• Ten days of running the Organization for Economic Cooperation and Development (OECD).

• The cost of 100 Eurofighters (jet fighter planes).

A contribution of $10 billion a year would be equivalent to the amount of money spent in 60 days in the United States on soft drinks or in 35 days on fast foods.

Annan also wants all antiretroviral drugs to be sold to underdeveloped nations at 5% of the cost to people in the developed world. The current U.N. Secretary-General is Ban Ki-moon.

How Far Will Ten Billion Dollars Go in Africa?

Should Africa alone receive $10 billion annually from the developed world, it would average out that each living HIV-infected African would receive about $455 per year ($10 billion divided by 22 million HIV infected) for as long as the money was provided. This would occur only if the money was actually given to the people. This money, along with free or very low drug costs could be of considerable help, especially since many African countries spend less than $5 to $10 per person a year on public health. But, used in this way, this large sum of money would not be available to build needed medical facilities or import the thousands of doctors necessary to treat the HIV infected. That will take a few hundred billion more dollars.

An article on "Estimating the Cost of Expanded AIDS Treatment in Africa," that appeared in the June 2001 issue of *Topics in HIV Medicine*, states that it would cost $1.12 billion each year to treat 1 million HIV-infected Africans. Ending 2009 there will be an estimated 23 million Africans living with HIV. The cost, based on information presented in the article, would be about $25 billion a year if all were to be treated equally.

Comments Relative to the Global Fund War Chest

Why Is AIDS Exceptional?—This is the title to Peter Piot's arguments on why AIDS should be in a category all by itself. And why the world should fund the Global AIDS Fund. Piot said, "Is the AIDS pandemic so exceptional a threat that it is in a league altogether different to other infectious diseases or causes of ill health? Is the pandemic so exceptional a threat that its control should not be just one of many Millennium Development Goals (MDGs) but rather an overarching priority, a prerequisite to achieving the MDGs? Is the threat so exceptional that it

THE GLOBAL FUND TO FIGHT HIV/AIDS, TB, AND MALARIA

The Global Fund is set up as a public-private partnership that is independent of the United Nations and is funded by governments around the world, foundations, nonprofit corporations, and select individuals. Its purpose is to attract, manage, and disburse resources to fight AIDS, TB, and malaria.

HIV/AIDS, TB, and malaria kill over 6 million people annually with an additional 350 million people suffering from these diseases. This fund was set up in response to widespread public criticism of governments' apathy to the health crisis in developing countries, especially concerning HIV/AIDS. The health status of the poor, women, men, and children is deteriorating in many parts of the world, and the fund is a unique opportunity to mobilize international political will and resources to address this crisis in a new way, rather than continuing with business as usual.

Of the new disease-fighting projects funded in developing countries, 66% are in Africa, 13% are in Asia, 13% are in the Middle East, and 5% are in Latin America. AIDS projects represented 48% of the total; malaria 42%; and TB 10%.

The Global Fund was initiated through the United Nations General Assembly Special Session on AIDS (UNGASS) in June 2001. The year 2001 has been recorded in AIDS history as the year when political commitment to the disease moved to center stage.

The goal of the 189 countries at the UNGASS 2001 was to reverse the global AIDS pandemic by 2015. On May 31 through June 2, 2006, the UN General Assembly held its second-ever UNGASS to review what changes, if any, occurred because of the global strategy against AIDS adopted by world governments in 2001. The review clearly showed failure to progress toward UNGASS 2001 goals, including HIV prevention, the availability of ART, and HIV education for 90% of those living in underdeveloped nations. Peter Piot, executive director of UNAIDS, said of the work done over the five-year period, "We've failed, we've failed." The new goals seek to find $23 billion per year by 2010 in order to fund AIDS treatment, care, prevention, and health infrastructure and to bring recognition to the rights of all HIV-infected people to receive help. But it appears that the final Declaration from UNGASS 2006 did not specify help for homosexuals, prostitutes, and drug addicts.

Reporting to UNGASS

Every two years, in compliance with the Declaration of Commitment on HIV/AIDS signed by UN member states in June 2001, countries report to UNAIDS on their progress made in the response to the AIDS epidemic. As of March 2008, 147 out of 192 countries had submitted their reports. Submission rates stand significantly at 100% of the Caribbean, 95% of Eastern Europe and Central Asia, 95% of Latin America and 94% of sub-Saharan Africa. However, by the same date only 50% of North America, 53% of Western and Central Europe and 50% of North Africa and Middle East has submitted their reports. East Asia reporting stands at 60% and Oceania 57%.

demands a binding first call on the attention of political leaders as well as on finances? So exceptional that it demands that we undertake fundamental changes on many fronts if we are to succeed? Ladies and Gentlemen: AIDS is that exceptional. The [financial] response to AIDS needs to be equally exceptional."

The Global Fund: Countries Pledge, But Do They Pay?—The UN proposed that contributions to the Fund should be made according to an *Equitable Contributions Framework,* in which donor countries contribute in relation to the sizes of their economies. But, many nations refuse to pledge money because there is no mechanism in place to handle corruption. They also ask who besides Africa will receive how much of the fund, and how the money will be spent. For example, there remains a large division among the 184 countries of the United Nations General Assembly over whether most of the money should be spent on prevention rather than antiretroviral drugs. Many members of the General Assembly said that about half the $10 billion should be spent on drugs for Africa and the other half be spent on prevention programs in Asia and the former Soviet nations where the epidemic is expanding out of control. Clearly there are no easy choices, but choices must be made. The United States was the first and only country by mid-2001 to offer Annan $200 million toward his global AIDS fund. Twenty-nine other nations have followed. By U.S. law, the American share of the Global Fund can total no more than 33% of all contributions to the fund. Total financial pledges from all countries and private foundations, etc., through 2008 amount to about $10 billion. But will the pledges be fulfilled? The financial goal for 2006 is $7.1 billion, but the fund was $3.4 billion short. No single nation has committed more money to this fund toward the African HIV/AIDS problem than the United States.

Entering 2009, 40 nations have pledged $10 billion to the Global Fund. However, most donor nations pledge year by year. There are no long-term or multi-year pledges. It is only optimism that the money will be made available. Insufficient funding undermines the Millennium Development Goal of halving or reversing the spread of HIV and other communicable diseases by 2015.

Progress of the Global Fund

A five-year progress report (2001–2006) shows that the lives of about 1.5 million people with HIV/AIDS, TB, and malaria worldwide have been saved/extended as a result of activities supported by the Global Fund. Lives are being saved/extended at a rate of 3000 daily. And the report finds that 1.5 million AIDS and TB cases have been prevented because of Global Fund programs; 770,000 people with access to antiretroviral therapy will live an estimated total of 290,000 additional years; and 33 million malaria episodes have been prevented.

A total of about $10 billion has been pledged and/or contributed for 2009 to the Global Fund. But at least $22.1 billion is needed!

FORMS OF U.S. MONETARY ASSISTANCE FOR HIV/AIDS

A U.S. Congressman once said, "A billion dollars here, a billion dollars there, it begins to add up." With respect to U.S. HIV/AIDS support, those hundreds of millions and billions of dollars have indeed added up. The United States has provided and continues to provide more money globally to foreign governments and nongovernmental organizations (NGOs) than any country on earth. The U.S. federal government has donated billions of dollars, through a variety of organizations, directly to people in need and to the Global AIDS, TB, and Malaria Fund. Direct spending for international HIV/AIDS activities by the U.S. began in 1986 with a $1.1 million investment, through several U.S. agencies that had already started international HIV/AIDS projects. Spending increased steadily and has reached $2.8 billion per year.

International Global Fund—In 2002, the G8 countries (United States, Russia, Great Britain, France, Germany, Italy, Japan, and Canada) organized a new International Global Fund, which became operational in January 2002. Through 2009, the U.S. will have contributed an estimated $4 billion to this fund. These international global funds are also to be used to support programs for HIV/AIDS (20%), TB (50%), and malaria (30%). This fund should not be confused with the Global AIDS, TB, and Malaria Fund.

During the 2008 G8 meeting in Germany, G8 members agreed to provide $60 billion to fight HIV/AIDS. Eighty-three percent of this money, or $50 billion, will come from President Bush's 2008 five-year extension of his PEPFAR program! But, even with over half the financial burden being picked up by the U.S., the remaining $10 billion is not a firm pledge from the G8 because some countries want to be cautious about increasing spending on HIV/AIDS.

Past President George W. Bush's Emergency Plan for AIDS Relief (PEPFAR) through the International Global Fund: January 28, 2003 Through 2013

Then-President Bush announced in the State of the Union address the Emergency Plan for AIDS Relief, a five-year, $15 billion initiative to turn the tide in combating the global HIV/AIDS pandemic. "To meet an urgent crisis abroad, tonight I propose the Emergency Plan for AIDS Relief (PEPFAR)—a work for mercy beyond all current international efforts to help the people of Africa. I ask the Congress to commit $15 billion over the next five years, including nearly $10 billion in new money to turn the tide against AIDS in the most afflicted nations of Africa and the Caribbean." This commitment of resources is helping the 15 most afflicted countries in Africa and the Caribbean (Haiti, Guyana, and Vietnam).

PEPFAR calls for treating two million people in 15 countries over five years (2×5) and should not be confused with the World Health Organization's plan to treat three million HIV infected in 38 countries by 2005 (3×5). The 3×5 plan failed. In addition, PEPFAR targets call for the prevention of seven million infections and providing care for 10 million people.

The $15 billion in funding for this initiative virtually triples the U.S. commitment to international AIDS assistance. Funding began with $2 billion in fiscal year 2004, and increased thereafter. The $15 billion included $1 billion for the Global Fund To Fight HIV/AIDs, Tuberculosis, and Malaria, conditioned on whether or not the fund shows results.

An important aspect of Bush's Emergency Plan is that it issues a challenge to every other member of the G8 countries to follow suit. In a sense he has placed a moral burden on these countries. On May 26, 2003, President Bush signed into law the $15 billion program that he called "a great mission to rescue." This program is the largest monetary commitment for an international public health initiative involving a specific disease in history! From 2004 through 2008, all of the $15 billion was spent.

The $15 billion original PEPFAR fund expired in September 2008. Congress extended the program for an additional five years, and to increase its funding to $48 billion. This will increase the number of people receiving antiretroviral drugs through PEPFAR from 1.4 million to 3 million. By 2013, there will be about 18 million people who will urgently need antiretroviral therapy!

To achieve universal access to antiretroviral drugs by 2010, officials at UNAIDS say an additional $42 billion will have to be found. If this money is forthcoming, another $54 billion will be necessary, by 2015, just to maintain those placed on ART back in 2010 and those added through 2014. Where will these monies be coming from and for how long?

Some Results of PEPFAR

Ending-2008, PEPFAR provided antiretroviral drugs to over 1.4 million people in the 15 target countries and has prevented over 100,000 mother-to-child HIV transmissions. According to Mark Dybul, who administers PEPFAR, the number of those receiving antiretrovirals is increasing at the rate of about 50,000 a month.

In 2006, UNAIDS said that the cost of AIDS across the globe is increasing dramatically. For 2006, U.S. $15 billion was needed, $18.5 billion for 2007, and $22 billion for 2008, and $42 billion by 2010.

Problems—**First,** pledges of money to the UN Global Fund do not equal what the fund receives. Certain of the countries do not give, and for those that pledge not all deliver on their pledges. In fact, the Global Fund is close to broke. It may not be able to fund 2009 grant requests, a first since the Global Fund was established. The fund needs about $6 to 8 billion. **Second,** a number of countries in Africa lack the infrastructure to disburse the money they receive.

DISCUSSION QUESTIONS—The UN Global Fund, for 2006 through 2008, needed $55.5 billion or on average, $18.5 billion a year. Even if the Global Fund had received this money, is $18.5 billion a year or more sustainable and for how long?

Comments—A report from the London-based Panos Institute entitled "Missing The Message—Twenty Years Of Learning From HIV/AIDS," says "After years of neglect, more money and political interest are being directed towards AIDS than ever before." However, it says spending large sums of money in hopes of achieving rapid results has often brought "disappointing or short lived" results. Implying that lessons haven't been learned means that the total world response to HIV/AIDS isn't panning out in the way that one would possibly hope that it could. That is, money in and of itself will not solve the AIDS crises in Africa or in any other developing nation. Whether it is $5 billion or $50 billion—pick a number—the money is useless if those funds do not reach the vulnerable, the HIV infected,

---

POINT OF INFORMATION 14.4

HIV/AIDS: MONEY MATTERS

Over the past decade, funding for HIV/AIDS research and treatment in low- and middle-income countries has exploded, jumping more than 20-fold to $10 billion [in 2007]. The U.S. National Institutes of Health (NIH), the largest funder of basic research, also doubled its budget to nearly $3 billion.

In a 6-month investigation, *Science* correspondent Jon Cohen followed the money, looking at how these dollars have been divvied up, what they have accomplished, and how countries have dealt with this sudden influx of cash, who's minding the store and what happens when [monetary] abuses occur.

Cohen found that the billions of dollars the major funders have spent have been concentrated in a few countries—often for legitimate reasons—but not necessarily in the countries with the worst epidemics. And despite the massive influx of funds, the number of people in need of anti-HIV drugs continues to climb: a reflection of the treatment's success but also of the failure of prevention efforts. All of this raises unsettling questions about whether resources can keep up with future demands. It is clear from these articles that poor choices and poor coordination have led to wasted effort! (Roberts et al., 2008).

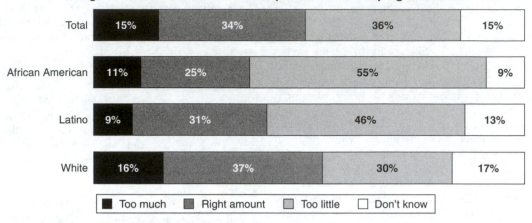

Do you think the U.S. is now spending too much, too little, or about the right amount on foreign aid to deal with the HIV/AIDS problem in developing countries?

	Too much	Right amount	Too little	Don't know
Total	15%	34%	36%	15%
African American	11%	25%	55%	9%
Latino	9%	31%	46%	13%
White	16%	37%	30%	17%

FIGURE 14-13 Views of U.S. Spending on Foreign Aid to Fight HIV/AIDS in Developing Countries. *"Kaiser Family Foundation Survey of Americans on HIV/AIDS, Part Three—Experiences and Opinions by Race/Ethnicity and Age," (#7140), The Henry J. Kaiser Family Foundation, August 2004. The information was reprinted with permission from the Henry J. Kaiser Family Foundation. The Kaiser Family Foundation, based in Menlo Park, California, is a nonprofit, independent national healthcare philanthropy and is not associated with Kaiser Permanente or Kaiser Industries. (Conducted March 15–May 11, 2004.) National random sample of 2902 respondents age 18 and older.*

the dying and whole communities that need them. Institutions and policies must be firmly in place to assure that the allocated funds can be well spent. To demand less would be irresponsible. We can all agree that the AIDS pandemic is a horror of unimaginable proportions, but spending vast sums of money without accountability never, ever works. It does not bring about solutions, but it does bring about disorder and discord. Stephen Lewis, the former United Nations Special Envoy, HIV/AIDS for Africa, said in his presentation at the Fourteenth International AIDS Conference in Durban, South Africa, "What is wrong with the world? People are dying in numbers that are the stuff of science fiction. Millions of human beings are at risk. Communities, families, mothers, fathers, children are like shards of humanity caught in a maelstrom of destruction. They're flesh and blood human beings, for God's sake; is that not enough to ignite the conscience of the world? Why should we have to produce all these tortured rationales to drive home such an obvious point? This pandemic has done something dreadful to the instinct for compassion. I don't really understand what's happening; I don't really understand why the simple act of saving or prolonging human life isn't sufficient anymore. It's irrational to need a balance

sheet of geometric calculation and economic architecture. It's sick."

United States Spending on HIV/AIDS in Developing Countries

In 2004, the Kaiser Family Foundation surveyed people in the United States as to their views on the U.S. government's spending money on developing countries to fight HIV/AIDS (Figure 14-13). The survey asked, does it make a difference—will this money slow the spread of HIV/AIDS in those countries receiving monetary help from the United States (Figure 14-14)? About 32% think the spending is about right, and 42% think not enough is being spent. A significant number (38%) do not think spending more money will help.

The Problem in Perspective: Wealth, Poverty, and AIDS

The relationship between poverty and HIV transmission is not simple. If it were, South Africa might not have Africa's largest epidemic, for South Africa is rich by African standards. Botswana is also relatively rich, yet this country has the highest levels of infection in the world. While most people with HIV/AIDS are

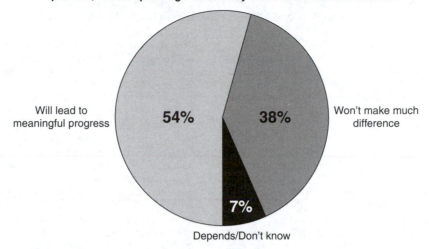

In general, do you think that spending more money on HIV/AIDS prevention in DEVELOPING COUNTRIES will lead to meaningful progress in slowing the epidemic, or that spending more money won't make much difference?

Will lead to meaningful progress — 54%

Won't make much difference — 38%

7%

Depends/Don't know

FIGURE 14-14 Will Spending on HIV/AIDS Prevention in Developing Countries Lead to Progress? *"Kaiser Family Foundation Survey of Americans on HIV/AIDS, Part Three—Experiences and Opinions by Race/Ethnicity and Age," (#7140), The Henry J. Kaiser Family Foundation, August 2004. The information was reprinted with permission from the Henry J. Kaiser Family Foundation. The Kaiser Family Foundation, based in Menlo Park, California, is a nonprofit, independent national healthcare philanthropy and is not associated with Kaiser Permanente or Kaiser Industries. (Conducted March 15–May 11, 2004.) National random sample of 2902 respondents age 18 and older.*

poor, many of the infected are not poor. Undernourishment; lack of clean water, sanitation, and hygienic living conditions; generally low levels of health, compromised immune systems, high incidence of other infections including genital infections and exposure to diseases such as tuberculosis and malaria; inadequate public health services; illiteracy and ignorance; pressures encouraging high-risk behavior, from labor migration to alcohol abuse and gender violence; an inadequate leadership response to either HIV/AIDS or the problems of the poor; and finally, lack of confidence or hope for the future—all companions of poverty promote HIV infection!

The cycle of poverty intensifies as individuals, households, and communities living with HIV/AIDS find that lost earnings, lost crops, and missing treatment make them weaker, make their poverty deeper, and push the vulnerable into poverty. Inequality sharpens the impact of poverty, and a mixture of poverty and inequality may be driving the epidemic. A South African truck driver is not well paid compared to the executives who run his company, but he is rich in comparison to the people in the rural areas he drives through. For the woman at a truck stop, a

man with 50 rand ($10) is wealthy; her desperate need for money to feed her family may buy him unprotected sex, even though she knows the risks.

According to the UNAIDS chief epidemiologist, by the end of 2009 there will be 35 million living HIV-infected people globally. About 33 million of these people live on less than $2 a day. In many of the high HIV incidence countries in Southern Africa, like Kenya, Botswana, Zambia, Malawi, Nigeria, Swaziland, and Uganda, about 50% of their populations live on a dollar or less per day! An HIV-positive American can focus on his T cell counts; an HIV-positive African in a rural village still has to focus on finding clean water and food.

Politicians, economists, and AIDS specialists rarely say this bluntly, but the truth is that most of those 33 million people have simply been written off because the first priority for the first few billion dollars is prevention, not treatment. An economist who studies AIDS in South Africa said, "You can't give up on the infected because of the message it sends. But if he had $1 billion to spend most wisely, I would spend it on giving women more power, caring for orphans, and getting them education."

ARE DEVELOPED NATIONS OVERFUNDING HIV/AIDS NEEDS?
SHOULD THE UNITED STATES RETHINK ITS HIV/AIDS FUNDING POLICIES?

It has been over 27 years since HIV/AIDS began crossing planet Earth. This disease has been called the largest threat to international health ever! As the numbers of HIV/AIDS cases grew, so, too, have the monetary donations—billions upon billions of dollars with no end in sight to the pandemic and likewise the continued need for AIDS dollars. But, many HIV/AIDS scientists and politicians internationally are now asking why all this money for one disease, when there are so many other diseases to treat and fundamental health care issues to be met in every country on planet Earth, especially those countries in the developing nations.

Recently in December of 2007, with the announcement by WHO and UNAIDS epidemiologists that their numbers of HIV/AIDS cases have been seriously overinflated, many voices are now being added to the chorus calling for a shift of HIV/AIDS dollars into basic health issues like providing clean water, family planning, and the treatment of global cases of diarrhea. It has been estimated that 4000 children die each day, or about 1.5 million annually, because of using unclean or unsanitary water. About 900 children die daily from AIDS-related complications. In addition, over one billion people lack a sanitary water supply. How many adults and adolescents die each year because of the lack of clean water? Problems like malnutrition and a variety of diseases other than AIDS are responsible for many more deaths annually than HIV/AIDS.

Aside from southern Africa, most of the continent has relatively low rates of HIV and much higher rates of easily treatable diseases like diarrhea and respiratory illnesses. Yet much of the money from the West, especially from the United States, goes into HIV/AIDS. Richard Halperin, senior research scientist at Harvard School of Public Health, recently wrote a commentary in the *New York Times* (January 1, 2008) on the imbalance of spending billions of dollars on one disease while other serious life-threatening diseases go unfunded or underfunded. Halperin said he was astounded at the response to his article. Most were positive, he said, with many AIDS experts agreeing it was time to re-examine spending. (Read Roger England, 2007)

Halperin points out that former President Bush's $15 billion PEPFAR (the President's plan for AIDS Relief) program to fight HIV/AIDS in 15 under-developed countries over five years was an unprecedented amount of money aimed at a single disease. Meanwhile, other public health issues were ignored. This $15 billion program ended in September 2008 but was then continued by a newly approved $48 billion congressional allocation which continues to ignore basic global health issues. To this end, Richard Horton, editor of *Lancet*, said, "AIDS [spending] has grossly distorted our [a] limited budget." He went on to say that undernutrition is the largely preventable cause of over a third or 3.5 million of all child deaths. Stunting, severe wasting, and intrauterine growth restriction are among the most important problems. There is a golden interval for intervention: from pregnancy to two years of age. After age two, undernutrition will have caused irreversible damage for future development towards adulthood. Incredibly, 80% of the undernourished children live in just 20 countries across four regions—Africa, Asia, western Pacific, and the Middle East. Countries that are receiving billions of HIV/AIDS dollars. These are the priority nations for action. Undernutrition can have substantial negative effects on societies. A recent study by World Food Program and the Economic Commission for Latin America and the Caribbean estimated that economic losses due to undernutrition among children in just seven nations are a staggering $6.6 billion a year—six percent of the gross domestic product. (The February 2008 issue of *Lancet*, Volume 371, ran a series of five articles dealing with the above topics.) Halperin says, "The AIDS experience has demonstrated that poor countries can make complex treatments accessible to many people. Regimens that are much simpler to administer than antiretroviral drugs—like antibiotics for respiratory illnesses, oral rehydration for diarrhea, immunizations and contraception—could also be made widely available. But as there isn't a global fund for safe water, child survival, and family planning, countries cannot directly tackle their real problems without pegging them to the big three diseases: AIDS, malaria, and tuberculosis. Halperin asks, "With [over] ten million children and half a million mothers in developing countries dying annually of largely preventable conditions, should we multiply AIDS spending while giving a pittance for initiatives like safe-water projects?" The Global Fund's director's response to Halperin and others who believe that HIV/AIDS money should be redistributed for basic health care was, "We are not a global fund that funds local health."

In Defense of Continued Spending Only For HIV/AIDS

Kevin De Cock, director of the AIDS department at the World Health Organization says, "We cannot let the pendulum swing back to a time when we didn't spend a lot on AIDS, we now have millions of people on treatment and we can't just stop that." And Tom Coates, a professor of global AIDS research at the University of California said, "Let's not drag AIDS care and prevention down to the level of every other disease, but let's bring everything else up to the level of AIDS."

Author's Comments: Regardless of intent, there is just so much money available to help all those who need treatment, care, nutrition, and various kinds of environmental protection. It seems unusual, odd, or at least curious or peculiar that it took 27 years into this pandemic before a discussion or argument has begun for the integration of HIV/AIDS into basic antenatal care, family planning, and child-adolescent-adult health care and health prevention services. It would appear that rather than to create parallel programs for funding health care needs, all countries should strengthen existing health care systems, and create or strengthen the infrastructure necessary to spend the fewest dollars in the most efficient way.

PRESENT YOUR VIEWS ON GLOBAL SPENDING ON HIV/AIDS VERSUS OTHER HEALTH CARE NEEDS.

FINALLY, THE QUESTION: How much would it cost to contain the global AIDS pandemic? The answer is: How much have you got? How much would it cost to banish ignorance, to deaden lust, to shame rape, to stop war, to enrich the poor, to empower women, to defend children, to make decent medical care as globally ubiquitous as Coca-Cola—in short, to get rid of all the underlying causes of the pandemic in the developing nations. Much of the world at risk for HIV/AIDS can't read. Most of the world at risk has never used a condom. Most of the world at risk has never heard of ACT UP. And most of the world with AIDS thinks it doesn't have the disease and doesn't know anyone who does, because 95% of those infected in the developing nations have never been tested. (Most estimates come from anonymous testing at prenatal clinics.) Most of the world cannot afford the antiretroviral drugs.

Summary

In 1981, the CDC announced a new disease affecting the homosexual population. This disease was later called AIDS. Many religious people believed this was a sign that homosexuality should be punished. The few facts available at that time gave rise to a great deal of fantasy and fear. Affected people were either seen as innocent victims or it was felt that they deserved the disease. Contracting AIDS labeled a person as less than desirable, a homosexual, or one who practiced deviant forms of sexual behavior. But even the so-called innocent victims, the children, the hemophiliacs, and the recipients of blood transfusions were not spared social ostracism. If you had AIDS, you were twice the victim—first of the virus and second of the social discrimination.

Children were barred from attending school, adults from their jobs, and both from adequate medical care. For example, there are still relatively few dentists who will treat AIDS patients and a significant number of surgeons refuse to operate on AIDS patients. Years have passed, but many misconceptions about HIV/AIDS linger on.

Fear is being casually transmitted rather than the virus. A significant number of people, after years of broad-scale education, still believe that the AIDS virus can be casually transmitted from toilet seats, drinking glasses, and even by donating blood.

The fallout from the fear of the AIDS pandemic has been a major change in sexual language in TV advertisements, magazines, and radio. Condoms, once spoken about only in hushed tones and kept under the counter in most drug stores, are now spoken of everywhere as a means of safer sex. AIDS, perhaps more than any other disease, has demonstrated that ignorance leads to fear and knowledge can lead to compassion.

To achieve understanding and compassion, people must be educated as to their HIV risk status and how they can keep it low. Many hundreds of millions of dollars have been spent to inform the public of the kinds of behavior that either place them at risk or reduce their risk for HIV infection. The problem is that although people are getting the information, too many refuse to act on it. Former Surgeon General C. Everett Koop's office mailed 107 million copies of the brochure "Understanding AIDS" to households in the United States. Fifty-one percent of those who received it said they never read it. Even among those who read the brochure are those who refuse to change their sexual behavior. Old habits are difficult to break.

To date, the hard evidence shows that only the homosexual population has significantly modified their sexual behavior as evidenced by the drop in the number of new cases of AIDS among them from 1988 into 2009.

A major problem looming on the horizon is the prospect of HIV being spread in the young adult population. Large numbers of them use drugs and alcohol, have multiple sex partners, and believe they are invulnerable to infection.

The AMA stated in 1988 that physicians may not refuse to care for patients with AIDS because of actual risk or fear of contracting the disease. Some physicians get around this through referral to other physicians who will treat AIDS patients. There is one area of medicine that takes issue at having to treat AIDS patients: surgery. Because it is difficult not to accidently get cut during surgery, surgeons have been the leading advocates for HIV testing of all surgical patients so they will know their risks before performing surgery.

On the other hand, patients say they have a right to know if their physician, especially a surgeon, is HIV infected. Surveys indicate that most people would not want to be treated by an HIV-infected physician.

On June 25, 1998, the U.S. Supreme Court ruled that the Americans with Disabilities Act protected HIV-infected people. Even when they experience no symptoms, they are to be treated as handicapped.

A number of developed and developing nations now believe that HIV/AIDS is, or will soon be, a threat to their national security. Does the next quarter-century mark the endgame of this struggle between death and hope, or more repetitions of the cycle? Can treatment actually be delivered to all who need it? Will effective biological tools to prevent HIV infection be found? How will millions of deaths affect orphans, vulnerable youth, fragile cultures, and global security? It does not bode well that patients in many states within our own borders languish on waiting lists for HIV medication. The struggle between death and hope wages on.

Review Questions

(Answers to the Review Questions are on page 430.)

1. Name three major sources of information that contributed to the early panic and hysteria about the spread of AIDS.

2. Give three examples of unfounded public reactions to AIDS infection.

3. Fear of the casual transmission of AIDS parallels what other earlier STD epidemic?

4. What evidence is there that it is difficult to get people to change their behavior even though they know it is harmful to their well-being?

5. What is the major thrust of AIDS education in the United States?

6. If education is the key to preventing HIV infection and new cases of AIDS, and most people interviewed say they have been educated, why is it not working?

7. Why are today's young adults in danger of contracting and spreading HIV?

8. Yes or No: Do physicians have a right to refuse to treat AIDS patients? Support your answer.

9. Do patients have a right to know if their physician is HIV infected or has AIDS?

10. What is the primary means of offsetting the bias toward people with AIDS in the workplace?

11. Who is the current secretary of the United Nations and how much money does he believe is needed to fight AIDS globally each year?

12. About how much money was pledged to the Global AIDS Fund in 2009?

13. Compared with the money the federal government spends on research and treatment to combat other health and medical problems such as heart disease and cancer, do you think federal spending on AIDS research and treatment is too high, too low, or about right? Support your choice with credible evidence.

Answers to Review Questions

CHAPTER 1

1. Acquired Immune Deficiency Syndrome
2. No. AIDS is a syndrome. A syndrome is made up of a collection of signs and symptoms of one or more diseases. AIDS patients have a collection of opportunistic infections and cancers. Collectively these are mistakenly referred to as the AIDS disease.
3. In 1983 by Luc Montagnier
4. 1981
5. LAV
6. Five; 1982, 1983, 1985, 1987, and 1993
7. It allows HIV-infected persons earlier access into federal and state medical and social programs.

CHAPTER 2

1. The unbroken transmission of HIV infection from an HIV-infected person to an uninfected person.
2. The answer to both questions is unknown at this time.
3. AIDS dissidents
4. Mother, Christine Maggiore. Daughter, Eliza Jane
5. Peter Duesberg
6. Thabo Mbeki
7. No, because HIV indirectly influences one's health it is difficult to show in laboratory test tubes that HIV causes AIDS. But the postulates have been satisfied by following infection/transmission cycles in a population of humans.
8. Depends on whose research you believe. However, as presented in this chapter, most of the evidence indicates that HIV is a "new" virus.
9. SIV
10. Beatrice Hahn
11. The Congo in 1959

CHAPTER 3

1. Because it contains RNA as its genetic message and a reverse transcriptase enzyme to make DNA from RNA.
2. GAG-POL-ENV; at least six
3. Because HIV has demonstrated an unusually high rate of genetic mutations: (1) the reverse transcriptase enzyme in HIV is highly error prone (makes transcription errors), and (2) a variety of HIV mutants have been found within a single HIV-infected individual.
4. The reverse transcriptase enzyme is highly error prone, making at least one, and in many cases more than one, deletion, addition, or substitution per round of proviral replication.
5. b
6. e
7. c
8. a
9. b
10. c
11. GAG, POL, ENV
12. About 1,000 plus or minus
13. vif produces a protein that destroys the cell's APOBEC protein and causes HIV to produce inactive copies of itself.
14. The processes of gene mutation and gene recombination.
15. 11; B; C; C/E

CHAPTER 4

1. Not really, because there is no way as yet to remove the provirus from the cell's DNA.
2. A physiological measurement that serves as a substitute for a major clinical event.

3. March; 30

4. 8

5. Becoming incorporated into DNA as it is being synthesized, thereby stopping reverse transcriptase from attaching the next nucleotide.

6. (a) Clinical biological side effects; (b) the selection of drug-resistant HIV mutants.

7. (a) The number of copies of HIV RNA present in the plasma. (b) This number indicates the reproductive activity of HIV at the time and, if therapy is being used, the effect of the therapy on the reproductive ability of the virus.

8. Saquinavir mesylate, saquinavir (Fortovase), ritonavir, indinavir, nelfinavir, amprenavir, atazanavir, fosamprenavir, tipranavir.

9. They physically interact with the reverse transcriptase enzyme and interfere with its function.

10. To suppress HIV replication, thereby reducing the number of mutant RNA strands produced.

11. A

12. B

13. To be determined by the instructor.

14. D

15. D

16. C

17. D

18. False

19. A

20. False

21. D

22. D

23. Selzentry or maraviroc

24. True

25. E

CHAPTER 5

1. T4 helper cells; because T4 cells are crucial for the production of antibodies, a depletion of T4 cells results in immunosuppression, which results in OIs.

2. CD4 is a receptor protein (antigen) secreted by certain cells of the immune system, for example, monocytes, macrophages, and T4 helper cells. It becomes located on the exterior of the cellular membrane and happens to be a compatible receptor for the HIV to attach and infect the CD4-carrying cell.

3. The question of true latency after HIV infection has not been settled. Most HIV/AIDS investigators currently believe there is a latent period, a time of few if any clinical symptoms and low levels of HIV in the blood. Other scientists, currently the minority, believe there is no true latency. The virus hides out in the lymph nodes, slowly reproducing, and slowly killing off the T4 cells. The virus is always present, increasing slowly in numbers over time.

4. True

5. False

6. True

7. False

8. False

9. True

10. False

11. True

12. True

13. True

14. B, assessing risk of disease progression.

15. CD4, macrophage, monocytes.

CHAPTER 6

1. OI is caused by organisms that are normally within the body and held in check by an active immune system. When the immune system becomes suppressed, for whatever reason, these agents can multiply and produce disease.

2. *Pneumocystis jiroveci;* lungs, pneumonia

3. *Isospora belli*

4. *Mycobacterium avium intracellulare*

5. False. HIV has not been found in KS tissue. KS is believed to develop as a result of a suppressed immune system and not the virus *per se.*

6. Classic KS, as described by Moritz Kaposi; and KS associated with AIDS

7. False. KS normally affects gay males. It is highly unusual to find KS in hemophiliacs, injection-drug users, and female AIDS patients.

8. True

9. True

10. True (Answer provided in POI 6.1)

Opportunistic Infections

MATCHING: Left side to Right side

1. 1997
2. Candidiasis
3. Cryptococcosis
4. Cryptosporidum
5. Cytomegalovirus
6. HAART
7. Encephalitis
8. Fungal pathogen
9. Herpes Virus
10. HIV disease
11. Kaposi's
12. Most infections
13. Mycobacterium
14. Opportunistic infection
15. *P. jiroveci*
16. Suppression
17. Tuberculosis
18. Weight loss

___8___ endemic in the Mississippi and Ohio River Valleys

___18___ associated with Wasting Syndrome and chronic diarrhea, fever, or weakness

___15___ causes extensive damage to the alveoli of the lung

___10___ suppresses the immune system

___3___ symptomatic disease most often represents infection of the central nervous system

___17___ coinfects 14% of AIDS patients

___14___ most commonly diagnosed infections among HIV/AIDS population

___4___ causes profuse watery diarrhea

___11___ Sarcoma, rare tumor in U.S., the most frequent neoplasm affecting HIV-infected individuals

___16___ of immune system, allows harmless agents become harmful opportunistic infection

___12___ considered opportunistic are not reportable

___5___ (CMV) considered the most common infectious cause of mental retardation

___13___ tuberculosis, TB

___9___ coinfects 95% of HIV infected

___7___ caused by *Toxoplasma gondii* entering and infecting the human brain causing encephalitis

___2___ quite common to the body, associated with yeast infections

___6___ prophylaxis cornerstone of treatment for AIDS patients

___1___ first time AIDS-related OI's fell in number from the previous year's total

CHAPTER 7

1. The 6-stage Walter Reed System and the 4-group CDC system
2. About 30%; about 90%
3. AIDS Dementia Complex
4. Skin—Kaposi's sarcoma
   Eyes—CMV retinitis
   Mouth—thrush or hairy leukoplakia
   Lungs—*Pneumocystis* pneumonia
   Intestines—diarrhea
5. True
6. False. The average time is 6 to 18 weeks.
7. False. HIV infection leads to HIV disease. AIDS is the result of a weakened immune system that allows opportunistic infections to occur.
8. False. The average length of time is about 10 to 11 years.
9. Instructor's evaluation
10. E, all of the above.
11. D, any of the above.
12. D, blindness
13. E, all of the above.

CHAPTER 8

1. False. The United States currently *reports* most of the world's AIDS cases.
2. Cases of AIDS-related death, according to the CDC definition, can be traced back to 1952 in the United States and to the mid-1950s in Africa.
3. HIV-1 and HIV-2 show a 40% to 50% genetic relationship to each other.
4. False. HIV-1 and HIV-2 are both transmitted via the same routes. HIV-2 is spreading globally in similar fashion to HIV-1.
5. True. All scientific and empirical evidence to date indicates that HIV is *not* casually transmitted.

6. Through sexual activities: exchange of certain body fluids—blood and blood products, semen, and vaginal secretions; and from mother to fetus or newborn by breast milk.

7. False. There is only one documented case of HIV infection caused by deep kissing. HIV has been found in the saliva of infected people in very low concentration, and saliva has been shown to have anti-HIV properties.

8. True; but this assertion has been proven to be untrue. Insects, in particular mosquitoes, have not been shown to transmit HIV successfully.

9. False. According to studies involving the sexual partners of injection-drug users and hemophiliacs, HIV transmission from male to female is the more efficient route. This is believed to be due to a greater concentration of HIV found in semen than in vaginal fluid.

10. The answer may be true or false. There have been cases in which a single act of intercourse has resulted in HIV infection. However, the majority of surveys on the sexual partners of injection-drug users and hemophiliacs indicate that the number of sexual encounters may increase the risk of HIV infection but does not guarantee infection. Sexual partners of infected people have remained HIV-free after years of unprotected penis-vagina or penis-anus intercourse.

11. The percentage of fetal risk varies widely in a number of hospital studies. At the moment, the risk as reported without zidovudine therapy varies from less than 30%. For Africa the figures most commonly used are 30% to 50%. With the use of zidovudine therapy, the risk has been cut to about 8%. Using zidovudine and a cesarean section reduces HIV transmission to about 2%.

12. E, all of the above.

13. True
14. True
15. True
16. True
17. True
18. False

19. True
20. True
21. False
22. True
23. True
24. True

25. B, mosquito bites.

26. False

27. D, none of the above.

28. True

29. B, sweat.

30. They can transmit HIV without knowing they are infected.

CHAPTER 9

1. Latex condoms. They are known to stop the transmission of viruses. This may not be true for animal intestine condoms.

2. Water-based lubricants. Oil-based lubricants weaken the latex rubber, causing them to leak or break under stress.

3. Safer sex is having sexual intercourse with an *uninfected* partner while using a condom.

4. The answer may be true or false. There have been cases where a single act of intercourse resulted in HIV infection. However, the majority of surveys completed by sexual partners of injection-drug users and hemophiliacs indicate that the number of sexual encounters may increase the risk of HIV infection but does not guarantee infection. Sexual partners of infected persons have remained HIV-free after years of unprotected penis-vagina intercourse.

5. No. IDUs exist between "fixes." They lose things, they may not care to pick up new equipment—they need the "fix" now, it may be easier to share. Circumstances vary considerably among the IDUs. Just giving them free equipment is no assurance that they will use it.

6. Between 1 in 39,000 and 1 in 200,000.

7. Have several students read their answers for promoting class discussion. Compare their response to that given in the text (that they should be punished).

8. Because attenuated HIV may mutate to a virulent form, causing an HIV infection; there is no absolute guarantee that 100% of HIV are inactivated.

9. Because at no time will a whole HIV be present in the vaccine. Only a specific subunit of the HIV will be present in pure form so the vaccine should be free of any contaminating proteins that might prove toxic to one or more persons receiving the vaccine.

10. Universal precautions are a list of rules and regulations provided by the CDC to help prevent HIV and other bloodborne diseases infection in healthcare workers.

11. False
12. True
13. True
14. True

15. False
16. False
17. False, 1998
18. Instructor evaluation

CHAPTER 10

1. B, 1959.

2. Because their social and sexual behaviors and medical needs place some people at a greater risk for HIV exposure than those not practicing these behaviors or who do not need blood or blood products.

3. False. Studies show that the time for progression from HIV infection to AIDS is about the same regardless of parameters.

4. 52%

5. Two per 1000 students; more: the rate for military personnel is 1.4 per 1000.

6. College students 2/1000, general population 0.2/1000; this means the rate of HIV infection on college campuses is about 10 times higher than in the general population.

7. One in 250 to 300

8. Needle stick injuries

9. Hepatitis B virus

10. Worldwide about 24 million, United States about 613,000.

11. 54% $\dfrac{594,000}{1,105,000}$ (53.7%)

12. About 35 million.

13. About 2.5 million.

14. No. The use of HAART is slowing the progression to AIDS in the HIV infected.

CHAPTER 11

1. Approximately 17.5 million women and 17.5 million men

2. About 50%

3. Injection-drug use, being a sexual partner of an IDU, and through heterosexual contact.

4. IDU

5. 1 million; about 1 million

6. Leading; 25 and 34; fifth; all; 25 and 44; second leading; 25 to 44

7. An estimated 6000

8. None, all states now have reported pediatric cases.

9. Virtually all—100%

10. (1) Maternal viral load; (2) route of delivery, and (3) duration of early membrane rupture.

11. Most orphaned AIDS children have mothers who are IDUs and are themselves HIV infected. They are AIDS orphans because (1) their parents abandon them due to illness or death; and (2) these children

are HIV infected or demonstrate AIDS and therefore no one wants them.

12. A

13. B (about 4.7 million)

14. D

15. A

16. True

17. False

CHAPTER 12

1. 2

2. Over 50%

3. 11.5 million

4. About 50%

5. 77%, 39%, 28%, 70%

6. 70%

7. Having sex after school and before our parents come home.

8. Engaging in sexual activity without the knowledge of safer sex choices.

9. Over $1.5 billion.

10. 85%

11. 29 million

12. About 40%

13. 13 to 24

14. 20

15. True

CHAPTER 13

1. ELISA; enzyme linked immunosorbent assay

2. That the body will produce antibody against antigenic components of the HIV virus after infection occurs.

3. No; a positive antibody result must be repeated in duplicate and if still positive, a confirmatory test is performed prior to telling people they are HIV infected.

4. No; AIDS is medically diagnosed after certain signs and symptoms of specific diseases occur.

5. Western Blot

6. Indirect immunofluorescent assay

7. By a color change in the reaction tube; the peroxidase enzyme oxidizes a clear chromogen into color

formation. This occurs if the HIV antibody–antigen enzyme complex is present in the reaction tube.

8. False. Some newborns receive the HIV antibody passively during pregnancy. About 30% to 50% of HIV-positive newborns are truly HIV positive; it is unknown whether all HIV-positive newborns go on to develop AIDS. Not all have been discovered and it has not been determined whether 100% of HIV-infected adults or babies will develop AIDS.

9. They are not 100% accurate.

10. Determining that positive and negative tests are truly positive and negative and not falsely positive or negative.

11. Using either too high or too low cut-off points in the spectrophotometer and the presence of cross-reacting antibodies.

12. The percentage of false positives will increase as the prevalence of HIV-infected people in a population decreases.

13. It is a screening test value that represents the probability that a positive HIV test is truly positive; because screening tests are not 100% accurate.

14. Western Blot

15. There is no standardized WB test interpretation. Different agencies use different WB results (reactive bands) to determine that the test sample is positive.

16. Because the PCR allows for the detection of proviral DNA in cells before the body produces detectable HIV antibody; PCR reactions can be used to determine if high-risk (or anybody), antibody-negative people are HIV infected but not producing antibodies and whether newborns are truly HIV positive or passively HIV positive.

17. 20 minutes

18. 3 minutes

19. False. The FDA-approved two home-use HIV antibody test kits in 1996, but one was withdrawn from the market.

20. Between 6 and 18 weeks after HIV infection.

21. As early as two weeks after infection.

22. (1) Changes in their lifestyles that reduce stress on their immune systems may delay the onset of illness.
(2) They can practice safer sex and hopefully not transmit the virus to others.
(3) The earlier the detection, the earlier they can enter into preventive therapy.

23. Mandatory with confidentiality; voluntary with confidentiality, anonymous, and blinded.

24. For anonymous testing no personal information is given; in blind tests, the name is deleted but the demographic data remain.

25. Because there are many examples of breaches of confidence, which destroys trust and subjects people to social stigma.

26. False

27. True

CHAPTER 14

1. Newspapers, TV, radio, magazines, etc.

2. Barring children from public schools, police wearing rubber gloves during arrests, not going to a restaurant because someone who works there has AIDS, firing AIDS employees, etc.

3. Syphilis

4. Use of tobacco products, alcohol, drugs; nonuse of seat belts and motorcycle helmets, etc.

5. The ways by which one can become HIV infected and how not to become HIV infected.

6. Because most of the new cases of HIV infection and AIDS occur in high-risk groups that will not or cannot change sexual and drug practices.

7. Because a larger percentage of young adults are sexually active with more than one partner, use drugs, use alcohol, and think they are invulnerable to infection and death.

8. According to the AMA, no. Physicians may not refuse to care for patients with AIDS because of actual risk or fear of contracting the disease.

9. The CDC and AMA state that a patient's right to that information should be determined on a case-by-case basis where surgery will be performed. There is no legal requirement for physicians to tell their patients of their HIV status.

10. Worker information sessions that explain how the virus can and cannot be transmitted.

11. Ban Ki-moon; about 22.1 billion

12. About 10 billion.

13. Review students' evidence—share with class.

Glossary

ACRONYMS

ACTG AIDS Clinical Trial Group

ADA Americans with Disabilities Act

AIDS Acquired Immune Deficiency Syndrome

AZT Azathioprine (a misnomer for zidovudine or azidothymidine)

CD Cluster Differentiating Antigen

CD4 a protein imbedded on the surface of a T lymphocyte to which HIV most often binds—a CD4+ or T4 cell.

CD8 a protein imbedded on the surface of a T lymphocyte suppressor cell—a T8 cell.

CDC Centers for Disease Control and Prevention (part of PHS)

DHHS Department of Health and Human Services

DNA deoxyribonucleic acid

d4T stavudine; nucleoside analog

ddC dideoxycytosine; nucleoside analog

ddI dideoxyinosine; nucleoside analog

FDA Food and Drug Administration (part of PHS)

HAART Highly Active Antiretroviral Therapy

HIV Human Immunodeficiency Virus

IDU Injection-Drug User

LAV lymphadenopathy-associated virus

NCI National Cancer Institute (part of NIH)

NIAID National Institute of Allergy and Infectious Diseases (part of NIH)

NIH National Institutes of Health (part of PHS)

NNRTI Non-nucleoside reverse transcriptase inhibitor

PCR (polymerase chain reaction) a very sensitive test used to detect the presence of HIV

PHS Public Health Service (part of DHHS)

PLWA Person Living With AIDS

RNA ribonucleic acid

3TC lamivudine; nucleoside analog

ZDV zidovudine; major drug in treating HIV/AIDS; nucleoside analog

For the newest anti-HIV drugs, names, and use, see Chapter 4.

TERMS

Acquired Immune Deficiency Syndrome (AIDS): A life-threatening syndrome caused by a virus and characterized by the breakdown of the body's immune defenses. (See AIDS.)

Acute: Sudden onset, short-term with severe symptoms.

Acyclovir (Zovirax): Antiviral drug for herpes 1 and 2 and herpes zoster.

Adjuvant: The active ingredient in vaccines that improves the human immune system response by attracting immune cells into the region where the vaccine is injected.

AIDS (Acquired Immune Deficiency Syndrome): A disease caused by a retrovirus called HIV and characterized by a deficiency of the immune system. The primary defect in AIDS is an acquired, persistent, quantitative functional depression within the T4 subset of lymphocytes. This depression often leads to infections caused by opportunistic microorganisms in HIV-infected individuals. A rare type of cancer (Kaposi's sarcoma) usually seen in elderly men or in individuals who are severely immunocompromised may also occur.

AIDS dementia: Neurological complications affecting thinking and behavior; intellectual impairment.

AIDSVAX: Trade name for all formulations of VAXGEN's vaccine.

Analog (analogue): A chemical molecule that closely resembles another one but which may function differently, thus altering a natural process.

Anal sex: A type of sexual intercourse in which a man inserts his penis in his partner's anus. Anal sex can be insertive or receptive.

Anemia: Low number of red blood cells.

Antibiotic: A chemical substance capable of destroying bacteria and other microorganisms.

Antibody: A blood protein produced by mammals in response to a specific antigen.

Antigen: A large molecule, usually a protein or carbohydrate, which when introduced into the body stimulates the production of an antibody that will react specifically with that antigen.

Antigenemia: Presence of viral proteins (antigens).

Antigen-presenting cells: B cells, cells of the monocyte lineage (including macrophages and dentritic cells), and various other body cells that present antigen in a form that T cells can recognize.

Antiretroviral therapy: Treatment with drugs designed to prevent HIV from replicating in HIV-infected persons. Highly active antiretroviral therapy (HAART) is an antiretroviral regimen that includes multiple classifications of antiretroviral drugs.

Antiserum: Serum portion of the blood that carries the antibodies.

Antiviral: Means against virus; drugs that destroy or weaken virus.

Apoptosis: Cellular suicide, also known as programmed cell death. A possible mechanism used by HIV to suppress the immune system. HIV may cause apoptosis in both HIV-infected and HIV-uninfected immune system cells.

Asymptomatic carrier: A host that is infected by an organism but does not demonstrate clinical signs or symptoms of the disease.

Asymptomatic seropositive: HIV positive without signs or symptoms of HIV disease.

Attenuated: Weakened. See Live/attenuated vaccine.

Atypical: Irregular; not of typical character.

Autoimmunity: Antibodies made against self tissues.

B and T cell lymphomas: Cancers caused by proliferation of the two principal types of white blood cells—B and T lymphocytes.

B lymphocytes or B cells: Lymphocytes that produce antibodies. B lymphocytes proliferate under stimulation from factors released by T lymphocytes.

Bacterium: A microscopic organism composed of a single cell. Many but not all bacteria cause disease.

Blood count: A count of the number of red and white blood cells and platelets.

Bone marrow: Soft tissue located in the cavities of the bones. The bone marrow is the source of all blood cells.

Canarypox: A virus that infects birds and is used as a live vector for HIV vaccines. It can carry a large quantity of foreign genes. Canarypox virus cannot grow in human cells, an important safety feature.

Cancer: A large group of diseases characterized by uncontrolled growth and spread of abnormal cells.

Candida albicans: A fungus; the causative agent of vulvovaginal candidiasis or yeast infection.

Candidiasis: A fungal infection of the mucous membranes (commonly occurring in the mouth, where it is known as thrush) characterized by whitish spots and/or a burning or painful sensation. It may also occur in the esophagus. It can also cause a red and itchy rash in moist areas, for example, the vagina.

Capsid: The protein coat of a virus particle.

CC-CKR-5 (CKR-5): Receptor for human chemokines and a necessary receptor for HIV entrance into a macrophage.

CD: Cluster differentiating-type antigens found on T lymphocytes. Each CD is assigned a number: CD1, CD2, etc.

CD4 (T4 cell): White blood cell with type 4 protein embedded in the cell surface—target cell for HIV infection.

CD8 cell: Suppressor white blood cell with type 8 protein embedded in the cell surface.

Cell-mediated immunity: The reaction to antigenic material by specific defensive cells (macrophages) rather than antibodies.

Cellular immunity: A collection of cell types that provide protection against various antigens.

Chain of infection: A series of infections that are directly or immediately connected to a particular source.

Chemokines: Chemicals released by T cell lymphocytes and other cells of the immune system to attract a variety of cell types to sites of inflammation.

Chemotherapy: The use of chemicals that have a specific and toxic effect upon a disease-causing pathogen.

Chlamydia: A species of bacterium, the causative organism of *Lymphogranuloma venereum,* chlamydial urethritis, and most cases of newborn conjunctivitis.

Chromosomes: Physical structures in the cell's nucleus that house the genes. Each human cell has 22 pairs of autosomes and two sex chromosomes.

Chronic: Having a long and relatively mild course.

Clade: Related HIV variants classified by degree of genetic similarity; nine are known for HIV.

Cleavage site: One of nine sites (peptide bond) within the *gag-pol* polyprotein (peptide precursor) that is cleaved by HIV-1 protease to form functional subunits of GAG (p17, p7, p24) and POL (protease, reverse transcriptase, integrase).

Clinical latency: Infectious agent developing in a host without producing clinical symptoms.

Clinical manifestations: The signs of a disease as they pertain to or are observed in patients.

CMV: See cytomegalovirus.

Cofactor: Factors or agents that are necessary or that increase the probability of the development of disease in the presence of the basic etiologic agent of that disease.

Cohort: A group of individuals with some characteristics in common.

Communicable: Able to spread from one diseased person or animal to another, either directly or indirectly.

Condylomata acuminatum (venereal warts): Viral warts of the genital and anogenital area.

Confidential HIV test: An HIV test for which a record of the test and the test results are recorded in the client's chart.

Confirmatory test: A highly specific test designed to confirm the results of an earlier (screening) test. For HIV testing, a Western Blot or, less commonly, an immunofluorescence assay (IFA) is used as a confirmatory test.

Congenital: Acquired by the newborn before or at the time of birth.

Core proteins: Proteins that make up the internal structure or core of a virus.

Cross-resistance: Development of resistance to one agent as an antibotic, that results in resistance to other, usually similar agents.

Cryptococcal meningitis: A fungal infection that affects the three membranes (meninges) surrounding the brain and spinal cord. Symptoms include severe headache, vertigo, nausea, anorexia, sight disorders, and mental deterioration.

Cryptococcosis: A fungal infectious disease often found in the lungs of AIDS patients. It characteristically spreads to the meninges and may also spread to the kidneys and skin. It is due to the fungus *Cryptococcus neoformans.*

Cryptosporidiosis: An infection caused by a protozoan parasite found in the intestines of animals. Acquired in some people by direct contact with the infected animal, it lodges in the intestines and causes severe diarrhea. It may be transmitted from person to person. This infection seems to be occurring more frequently in immunosuppressed people and can lead to prolonged symptoms that do not respond to medication.

Cutaneous: Having to do with the skin.

CXCR-4 (FUSIN):   Receptor for human chemokines and a necessary receptor for HIV entrance into T4 cells.

Cytokines: Powerful chemical substances secreted by cells. Cytokines include lymphokines produced by lymphocytes and monokines produced by monocytes and macrophages.

Cytomegalovirus (CMV):   One of a group of highly host-specific herpes viruses that affect humans and other animals. Generally produces mild flu-like symptoms but can be more severe. In the immunosuppressed, it may cause pneumonia.

Cytopathic: Pertaining to or characterized by abnormal changes in cells.

Cytotoxic: Poisonous to cells.

Cytotoxic T cells: A subset of T lymphocytes that carry the T8 marker and can kill body cells infected by viruses or transformed by cancer.

Dementia: Chronic mental deterioration sufficient to significantly impair social and/or occupational function. Usually patients have memory and abstract thinking loss.

Dendritic cells: White blood cells found in the spleen and other lymphoid organs. Dendritic cells typically use thread-like tentacles to "hold" the antigen, which they present to T cells.

Didanosine: Also known as Videx; see ddI—inhibits HIV replication.

Dissemination: Spread of disease throughout the body.

DNA (deoxyribonucleic acid):   A linear polymer, made up of deoxyribonucleotide repeating units. It is the carrier of genetic information in living organisms and some viruses.

DNA vaccine (nucleic acid vaccine):   Direct injection of a gene(s) coding for a specific antigenic protein(s), resulting in direct production of such antigen(s) within the vaccine recipient in order to trigger an appropriate immune response.

DNA viruses: Contain DNA as their genetic material.

Dysentery: Inflammation of the intestines, especially the colon, producing pain in the abdomen and diarrhea containing blood and mucus.

Efficacy: Effectiveness.

ELISA test: A blood test that indicates the presence of antibodies to a given antigen. Various ELISA tests are used to detect a variety of infections. The HIV ELISA test does not detect AIDS but only indicates if viral infection has occurred.

Endemic: Prevalent in or peculiar to a community or group of people.

Enteric infections: Infections of the intestine.

ENV: HIV gene that codes for protein gp160.

Envelope proteins: Proteins that comprise the envelope or surface of a virus, gp120 and gp41.

Enzyme: A catalytic protein that is produced by living cells and promotes the chemical processes of life without itself being altered or destroyed.

Epidemic: Affecting many persons at once, outbreak or rapid, sudden growth or development.

Epidemiology: Science that deals with the incidence, distribution, and control of disease in a population.

Epitope: A specific site on an antigen that stimulates specific immune responses, such as the production of antibodies or activation of immune cells.

Epivir: See 3TC.

Epstein–Barr virus (EBV):   A virus that causes infectious mononucleosis. It is spread by saliva. EBV lies dormant in the lymph glands and has been associated with Burkitt's lymphoma, a cancer of the lymph tissue.

Etiologic agent: The organism that causes a disease.

Etiology: The study of the cause of disease.

Extracellular: Found outside the cell wall.

Factor VIII: A naturally occurring protein in plasma that aids in the coagulation of blood. A congenital deficiency of Factor VIII results in the bleeding disorder known as hemophilia A.

Factor VIII concentrate: A concentrated preparation of Factor VIII that is used in the treatment of individuals with hemophilia A.

False negative: Failure of a test to demonstrate the disease or condition when present.

False positive: A positive test result caused by a disease or condition other than the disease for which the test is designed.

Fellatio: Oral sex involving the penis.

Fitness: The ability of an individual virus to replicate successfully under defined conditions.

Follicular dendritic cells: Found in germinal centers of lymphoid organs.

Fomite: An inanimate object that can hold infectious agents and transfers them from one individual to another.

Fortovase: A more easily assimilated form of saquinavir.

Fulminant: Rapid onset, severe.

Fungus: Member of a class of relatively primitive organisms. Fungi include mushrooms, yeasts, rusts, molds, and smuts.

FUSIN: See CXCR-4.

Gammaglobulin: The antibody component of the serum.

Ganciclovir (DHPG):   An experimental antiviral drug used in the treatment of CMV retinitis.

Gene: The basic unit of heredity; an ordered sequence of nucleotides. A gene contains the information for the synthesis of one polypeptide chain (protein).

Gene expression: The production of RNA and cellular proteins.

Genitourinary: Pertaining to the urinary and reproductive structures; sometimes called the GU tract or system.

Genome: A complete set of genes in a cell or virus.

Genotype: The sequence of nucleotide bases that constitutes a gene.

Globulin: That portion of serum that contains the antibodies.

Glycoproteins: Proteins with carbohydrate groups attached at specific locations.

Gonococcus: The specific etiologic agent of gonorrhea discovered by Neisser and named *Neisseria gonorrhoeae*.

gp41:   Glycoprotein found in envelope of HIV.

gp120:   Glycoprotein found in outer level of HIV envelope.

gp160: Precursor glycoprotein to forming gp41 and gp120.

Granulocytes: Phagocytic white blood cells filled with granules containing potent chemicals that allow the cells to digest microorganisms. Neutrophils, eosinophils, basophils, and mast cells are examples of granulocytes.

Hemoglobin: The oxygen-carrying portion of red blood cells that gives them a red color.

Hemophilia: A hereditary bleeding disorder caused by a deficiency in the ability to synthesize one or more of the blood coagulation proteins, for example, Factor VIII (hemophilia A) or Factor IX (hemophilia B).

Hepatitis: Inflammation of the liver; due to many causes including viruses, several of which are transmissible through blood transfusions and sexual activities.

Hepatosplenomegaly: Enlargement of the liver and spleen.

Herpes simplex virus I (HSV-I): A virus that results in cold sores or fever blisters, most often on the mouth or around the eyes. Like all herpes viruses, it may lie dormant for months or years in nerve tissues and flare up in times of stress, trauma, infection, or immunosuppression. There is no cure for any of the herpes viruses.

Herpes simplex virus II (HSV-II): Causes painful sores on the genitals or anus. It is one of the most common sexually transmitted diseases in the United States.

Herpes varicella zoster virus (HVZ): The varicella virus causes chicken pox in children and may reappear in adulthood as herpes zoster. Herpes zoster, also called shingles, is characterized by small, painful blisters on the skin along nerve pathways.

Histoplasmosis: A disease caused by a fungal infection that can affect all the organs of the body. Symptoms usually include fever, shortness of breath, cough, weight loss, and physical exhaustion.

HIV (Human Immunodeficiency Virus): A newly discovered retrovirus that is said to cause AIDS. The target organ of HIV is the T4 or CD4 subset of T lymphocytes, which regulate the immune system.

HIV positive: Presence of the human immunodeficiency virus in the body.

Homophobia: Negative bias toward or fear of individuals who are homosexual.

Human leukocyte antigens (HLA): Protein markers of self used in histocompatibility testing. Some HLA types also correlate with certain autoimmune diseases.

Humoral immunity: The production of antibodies for defense against infection or disease.

Immunity: Resistance to a disease because of a functioning immune system.

Immune complex: A cluster of interlocking antigens and antibodies.

Immune response: The reaction of the immune system to foreign substances.

Immune status: The state of the body's natural defense to diseases. It is influenced by heredity, age, past illness history, diet, and physical and mental health. It includes production of circulating and local antibodies and their mechanism of action.

Immunoassay: The use of antibodies to identify and quantify substances. Often the antibody is linked to a marker such as a fluorescent molecule, a radioactive molecule, or an enzyme.

Immunocompetent: Capable of developing an immune response.

Immunoglobulins: A family of large protein molecules, also known as antibodies.

Immunostimulant: Any agent that will trigger a body's defenses.

Immunosuppression: When the immune system is not working normally. This can be the result of illness or certain drugs (commonly those used to fight cancer).

Incidence: The total number of new cases of a disease in a defined population within a specified time, usually one year.

Incubation period: The time between the actual entry of an infectious agent into the body and the onset of disease symptoms.

Indeterminate test result: A possible result of a Western Blot, which might represent a recent HIV infection or a false positive.

Indinavir: Crixivan, a protease inhibitor drug.

Infection: Invasion of the body by viruses or other organisms.

Infectious disease: A disease that is caused by microorganisms or viruses living in or on the body as parasites.

Inflammatory response: Redness, warmth, and swelling in response to infection; the result of increased blood flow and a gathering of immune cells and secretions.

Injection-drug use: Use of drugs injected by needle into a vein or muscle tissue.

Innate immunity: Inborn or hereditary immunity.

Inoculation: The entry of an infectious organism or virus into the body.

Integrase: HIV enzyme used to insert HIV DNA into host cell DNA.

Interferon: A class of glycoproteins important in immune function and thought to inhibit viral infection.

Interleukins: Chemical messengers that travel from leukocytes to other white blood cells. Some promote cell development, others promote rapid cell division.

Intracellular: Found within the cell wall.

In utero: In the uterus.

In vitro: "In glass"—pertains to a biological reaction in an artificial medium.

In vivo: "In the living"—pertains to a biological reaction in a living organism.

IV: Intravenous.

Kaposi's sarcoma: A multifocal, spreading cancer of connective tissue, principally involving the skin; it usually begins on the toes or the feet as reddish blue or brownish soft nodules and tumors.

Lamivudine: Nucleoside analog inhibits HIV replication.

Langerhans cells: Dendritic cells in the skin that pick up antigen and transport it to lymph nodes.

Latency: A period when a virus or other organism is in the body but in an inactive state.

Latent viral infection: The virion becomes part of the host cell's DNA.

Lentiviruses: Viruses that cause disease very slowly. HIV is believed to be this type of virus.

Lesion: Any abnormal change in tissue due to disease or injury.

Leukocyte: A white blood cell.

Leukopenia: A decrease in the white blood cell count.

Live or attenuated vaccine: A vaccine in which an active virus is weakened through chemical or physical processes in order to produce an immune response without causing the severe effects of the disease. Attenuated vaccines currently licensed in the United States include measles, mumps, rubella, polio, yellow fever, and varicella.

Live-vector vaccine: A vaccine that uses a non-disease-causing organism (virus or bacterium) to transport HIV or other foreign genes into the body, thereby stimulating an effective immune response to the foreign products. This type of vaccine is important because it is particularly capable of inducing cytotoxic leukocyte activity. Examples of organisms used as live vectors in HIV vaccines are canarypox and vaccinia.

Log: 10-fold difference.

Lymph: A transparent, slightly yellow fluid that carries lymphocytes, bathes the body tissues, and drains into the lymphatic vessels.

Lymphadenopathy: Enlargement of the lymph nodes.

Lymphadenopathy syndrome (LAS): A condition characterized by persistent, generalized, enlarged lymph nodes, sometimes with signs of minor illness such as fever and weight loss, which apparently represents a milder reaction to HIV infection.

Lymphatic system: A fluid system of vessels and glands that is important in controlling infections and limiting their spread.

Lymph nodes: Gland-like structures in the lymphatic system that help to prevent spread of infection.

Lymphocytes: Specialized white blood cells involved in the immune response.

Lymphoid organs: The organs of the immune system where lymphocytes develop and congregate. They include the bone marrow, thymus, lymph nodes, spleen, and other clusters of lymphoid tissue.

Lymphokines: Chemical messengers produced by T and B lymphocytes. They have a variety of protective functions.

Lymphoma: Tumor of lymphoid tissue, usually malignant.

Lymphosarcoma: A general term applied to malignant neoplastic disorders of lymphoid tissue, not including Hodgkin's disease.

Lytic infection: When a virus infects the cell, the cell produces new viruses and breaks open (lyse), releasing the viruses.

Macrophage: A large and versatile immune cell that acts as a microbe-devouring phagocyte, an antigen-presenting cell, and an important source of immune secretions.

Major histocompatibility complex (MHC): A group of genes that controls several aspects of the immune response. MHC genes code for self markers on all body cells.

Malaise: A general feeling of discomfort or fatigue.

Malignant tumor: A tumor made up of cancerous cells. The tumors grow and invade surrounding tissue, then the cells break away and grow elsewhere.

Messenger RNA (mRNA): RNA that serves as the template for protein synthesis; it carries the information from the DNA to the protein synthesizing complex to direct protein synthesis.

Microbes: Minute living organisms including bacteria, viruses, fungi, and protozoa.

Microorganisms: Microscopic plants or animals.

Molecule: The smallest amount of a specific chemical substance that can exist alone. To break a molecule down into its constituent atoms is to change its character. A molecule of water, for instance, reverts to oxygen and hydrogen.

Monoclonal antibody: Custom-made, identical antibody that recognizes only one epitope.

Monocyte: A large phagocytic white blood cell which, when it enters tissue, develops into a macrophage.

Monokines: Powerful chemical substances secreted by monocytes and macrophages. They help direct and regulate the immune response.

Morbidity: The proportion of people with a disease in a community.

Morphology: The study of the form and structure of organisms.

Mortality: The number of people who die as a result of a specific cause.

Mucosal immunity: Resistance to infection across mucous membranes.

Mucous membrane: The lining of the canals and cavities of the body that communicate with external air, such as the intestinal tract, respiratory tract, and the genitourinary tract.

Mucous patches: White, patchy growths, usually found in the mouth, that are symptoms of secondary syphilis and are highly infectious.

Mucus: A fluid secreted by membranes.

Mutant: A new strain of a virus or microorganism that arises as a result of change in the genes of an existing strain.

Natural killer cells (also called NK cells): Immune cells that kill infected cells directly within four hours of contact. NK cells differ from other killer cells, such as cytotoxic T lymphocytes, in that they do not require contact with antigen before they are activated.

Neisseria gonorrhoeae: The bacterium that causes gonorrhea.

Neonatal: Pertaining to the first four weeks of life.

Neoplasm: A new abnormal growth, such as a tumor.

Neuropathy: Group of nerve disorders—symptoms range from tingling sensation and numbness to paralysis.

Neutralizing antibody: The kind of antibody that prevents a virus from entering a cell. It is hoped that a vaccine will produce neutralizing antibody because if HIV is prevented from entering cells, it cannot replicate and dies in the bloodstream within a few hours.

Nevirapine: Non-nucleoside analog inhibits HIV replication.

Notifiable disease: A notifiable disease is one that, when diagnosed, health providers are required, usually by law, to report to state or local public health officials. Notifiable diseases are those of public interest by reason of their contagiousness, severity, or frequency.

Nucleic acids: Large, naturally occurring molecules composed of chemical building blocks known as nucleotides. There are two kinds of nucleic acid, DNA and RNA.

Nucleoside analog: Synthetic compounds generally similar to one of the bases of DNA.

Nucleotide of DNA: Made up of one of four nitrogen-containing bases (adenine, cytosine, guanine, or thymine), a sugar, and a phosphate molecule.

Oncogenic: Anything that may give rise to tumors, especially malignant ones.

Opportunistic disease: Disease caused by normally benign microorganisms or viruses that become pathogenic when the immune system is impaired.

p24 antigen: A protein fragment of HIV. The p24 antigen test measures this fragment. A positive test result suggests active HIV replication and may mean the individual has a chance of developing AIDS in the near future.

Pandemic: Occurring over a wide geographic area and affecting a high proportion of the population.

Parenteral: Not taken in through the digestive system or lungs (intravenous, intramuscular, subcutaneous).

Parasite: A plant or animal that lives, grows, and feeds on another living organism.

Pathogen: Any disease-producing microorganism or substance.

Pathogenic: Giving rise to disease or causing symptoms of an illness.

Pathogenicity: Capable of causing a disease.

Pathology: The science of the essential nature of diseases, especially of the structural and functional changes in tissues and organs caused by disease.

Perianal glands: Glands located around the anus.

Perinatal: Occurring in the period during or just after birth.

Pestilence: A virulent, devastating contagious disease that is caused by a bacterium, for example, *Yersina pestis,* which causes the plague.

Phagocytes: Large white blood cells that contribute to the immune defense by ingesting microbes or other cells and foreign particles.

Phenotype: A defined behavior; specifically drug susceptibility with regard to HIV drug resistance.

PID (pelvic inflammatory disease): Inflammation of the female pelvic organs; often the result of gonococcal or chlamydial infection.

Placebo: An inactive substance against which investigational treatments are compared to see how well the treatment worked.

Plague: A calamity; an epidemic of disease causing a high rate of mortality.

Plasma: The fluid portion of the blood that contains all the chemical constituents of whole blood except the cells.

Plasma cells: Derived from B cells, they produce antibodies.

Platelets: Small oval discs in blood that are necessary for blood to clot.

PLWA: Person Living With AIDS.

***Pneumocystis carinii pneumonia* (PCP):** A rare type of pneumonia primarily found in infants and now common in patients with AIDS.

Polymerase chain reaction: Method to detect and amplify very small amounts of DNA in a sample.

Positive HIV test: A sample of blood that is reactive on an initial ELISA test, reactive on a second ELISA run of the same specimen, and reactive on Western Blot, if available.

Prenatal: During pregnancy.

Prevalence: The total number or percentage of cases of a disease existing at any time in a given area.

Primary immune response: Production of antibodies about 7 to 10 days after an infection.

Prime-boost: In HIV vaccine research, administration of one type of vaccine, such as a live-vector vaccine, followed by or together with a second type of vaccine, such as a recombinant subunit vaccine. The intent of this combination regimen is to induce different types of immune responses and enhance the overall immune response, a result that may not occur if only one type of vaccine were to be given for all doses.

Prophylactic treatment: Medical treatment of patients exposed to a disease before the appearance of disease symptoms.

Protease: Enzyme that cuts proteins into peptides (breaks down proteins).

Protease inhibitors: Compounds that inhibit the action of protease.

Proteins: Organic compounds made up of amino acids. Proteins are one of the major constituents of plant and animal cells.

Protocol: Standardization of procedures so that results of treatment or experiments can be compared.

Protozoa: A group of one-celled animals, some of which cause human disease including malaria, sleeping sickness, and diarrhea.

Provirus: The genome of an animal virus integrated into the chromosome of the host cell, and thereby replicated in all the host's daughter cells.

Quasispecies: A complex mixture of genetic variants of an RNA virus.

Race: Beginning in 1976 the federal government's data systems classified individuals into the following racial groups: American Indian or Alaskan Native, Asian or Pacific Islander, black, and white.

Rapid HIV test: A test to detect antibodies to HIV that can be collected and processed within a short interval of time (approximately 3–30 minutes).

Rate: A rate is a measure of some event, disease, or condition in relation to a unit of population, along with some specification of time.

Receptors: Special molecules located on the surface membranes of cells that attract other molecules to attach to them. (For example, CD4, CD8, and CCCKR-5).

Recombinant DNA: DNA produced by joining pieces of DNA from different sources.

Recombinant DNA techniques: Techniques that allow specific segments of DNA to be isolated and inserted into a bacterium or other host (like yeast or mammalian cells) in a form that will allow the DNA segment to be replicated and expressed as the cellular host multiplies.

Remission: The lessening of the severity of disease or the absence of symptoms over a period of time.

Retroviruses: Viruses that contain RNA and produce a DNA analog of their RNA using an enzyme known as reverse transcriptase.

Reverse transcriptase: An enzyme produced by retroviruses that allows them to produce a DNA analog of their RNA, which may then incorporate into the host cell.

Ritonavir: Norvir, a protease inhibitor drug.

RNA (ribonucleic acid): Any of various nucleic acids that contain ribose and uracil as structural components and are associated with the control of cellular chemical activities.

RNA viruses: Contain RNA as their genetic material.

Sarcoma: A form of cancer that occurs in connective tissue, muscle, bone, and cartilage.

Saquinavir: Invirase, a protease inhibitor drug.

Secondary immune response: On repeat exposure to an antigen, there is an accelerated production of antibodies.

Sensitivity: The probability that a test will be positive when the infection is present.

Septicemia: A disease condition in which the infectious agent has spread throughout the lymphatic and blood systems, causing a general body infection.

Seroconversion: The point at which an individual exposed to HIV has detectable antibodies to HIV in their serum.

Serologic test: Laboratory test made on serum.

Serum: The clear portion of any animal liquid separated from its more solid elements, especially the clear liquid that separates in the clotting of blood (blood serum).

Shigella: A bacterium that can cause dysentery.

Specificity: The probability that a test will be negative when the infection is not present.

Spirochete: A corkscrew-shaped bacterium; for example, *Treponema pallidum.*

Spleen: A lymphoid organ in the abdominal cavity that is an important center for immune system activities.

Squamous: Scaly or plate-like; a type of cell.

STARHS: HIV test to differentiate infections from older infections.

Statistical significance: The probability that an event or difference occurred as the result of the intervention (vaccine) rather than by chance alone. This probability is determined by using statistical tests to evaluate collected data.

Stavudine: Also known as Zerit; See d4T—inhibits HIV replication.

STD (sexually transmitted disease): Any disease that is transmitted primarily through sexual practices.

Subclinical infections: Infections with minimal or no apparent symptoms.

Subtype: Also called a clade. With respect to HIV isolates, a classification scheme based on genetic differences.

Subunit vaccine: A vaccine that uses only one component of an infectious agent rather than the whole to stimulate an immune response.

Suppressor T cells: A subset of T cells that carry the T8 marker and turn off antibody production and other immune responses.

Surrogate marker: A substitute; a person or agent that replaces another, an alternate.

Surveillance: The process of accumulating information about the incidence and prevalence of disease in an area.

Susceptible: Inability to resist an infection or disease.

Syndrome: A set of symptoms that occur together.

Systemic: Affecting the body as a whole.

T8 cells: A subset of T cells that may kill virus-infected cells and suppress immune function when the infection is over.

T cell growth factor (TCGF, also known as interleukin-2): A glycoprotein that is released by T lymphocytes on stimulation by antigens and that functions as a T cell growth factor by inducing proliferation of activated T cells.

T helper cells (also called T4 or CD4 cells): A subset of T cells that carry the CD4 marker and are essential for turning on antibody production, activating cytotoxic T cells, and initiating many other immune responses.

T lymphocytes or T cells: Lymphocytes that mature in the thymus and that mediate cellular immune reactions. T lymphocytes also release factors that induce proliferation of T lymphocytes and B lymphocytes.

Therapeutic HIV vaccine: A vaccine designed to boost the immune response to HIV in a person already infected with the virus. Also referred to as an immunotherapeutic vaccine.

Thrush: A disease characterized by the formation of whitish spots in the mouth. It is caused by the fungus *Candida albicans* during times of immunosuppression.

Thymus: A primary lymphoid organ high in the chest where T lymphocytes proliferate and mature.

Titer: Level or amount.

Tolerance: A state of nonresponsiveness to a particular antigen or group of antigens.

Toxic reaction: A harmful side effect from a drug; it is dose dependent, that is, becomes more frequent and severe as the drug dose is increased. All drugs have toxic effects if given in a sufficiently large dose.

Toxoplasmosis: An infection with the protozoan *Taxoplasma gondii,* frequently causing focal encephalitis (inflammation of the brain). It may also involve the heart, lungs, adrenal glands, pancreas, and testes.

Transcription: The synthesis of messenger RNA on a DNA template; the resulting RNA sequence is complementary to the DNA sequence. This is the first step in gene expression.

Translation: The process by which the genetic code contained in a nucleotide sequence of messenger RNA directs the synthesis of a specific order of amino acids to produce a protein.

Treponema pallidum: The bacterial spirochete that causes syphilis.

Tropism: Involuntary turning, curving, or attraction to a source of stimulation.

Tumor: A swelling or enlargement; an abnormal mass that can be malignant or benign. It has no useful body function.

V3 loop: Section of the gp120 protein on the surface of HIV; appears to be important in stimulating neutralizing antibodies.

Vaccine: A preparation of dead organisms, attenuated live organisms, live virulent organisms, or parts of microorganisms that is administered to artificially increase immunity to a particular disease.

V.D.:   Contagious disease usually acquired through sexual intercourse.

Vector: The means by which a disease is carried from one human to another.

Venereal: Venus = love, sexual desire; involves the sexual organs and related to sexual pleasure; comes through contact of sexual organs.

Venereal warts: Viral *Condylomata acuminata* on or near the anus or genitals.

Viral load: The total amount of virus in a person's blood.

Viremia: The presence of virus in the blood.

Virulence: The quality of expression or the expression of the disease.

Virus: Any of a large group of submicroscopic agents capable of infecting plants, animals, and bacteria; characterized by a total dependence on living cells for reproduction and by a lack of independent metabolism.

Western Blot: A blood test used to detect antibodies to a given antigen. Compared to the ELISA test, the Western Blot is more specific and more expensive. It can be used to confirm the results of the ELISA test.

Wild type: A genotype or phenotype circulating prior to selection of drug resistance.

X-ray: Radiant energy of extremely short wavelength used to diagnose and treat cancer.

Zalcitabine: Also known as HIVID; see ddC—inhibits HIV replication.

Zidovudine: Also known as Retrovir; see ZDV—inhibits HIV replication. Mistakenly referred to as AZT.

References

CHAPTER 1

BARRE-SINOUSSI, FRANCOISE, et al. (1983). Isolation of a T lymphocyte retrovirus from a patient at risk for acquired immune deficiency syndrome (AIDS). *Science,* 220:868–871.

GALLO, ROBERT C. (1987). The AIDS virus. *Sci. Am.,* 256:47–56.

HAHN, BEATRICE, et al. (2000). AIDS as a zoonosis: Scientific and public health implications. *Science,* 287:607–614.

MARLINK, RICHARD. (1996). Lessons from the second AIDS virus HIV-2. *AIDS,* 10:689–699.

MASUR H., et al. (1981). An outbreak of community-acquired *Pneumocystis catinii* pneumonia: Initial manifestations of cellular immune dysfunction. *N. Eng. J. Med.,* 305(24):1431–1438.

MASUR, HENRY, et al. (1982). Opportunistic infection in previously healthy women. Initial manifestations of a community-acquired cellular immunodeficiency. *Annals of Internal Medicine,* 97(4): 533–539.

Morbidity and Mortality Weekly Report. (1981a). Follow-up on Kaposi's sarcoma and Pneumocystis pneumonia. 30:409–10.

Morbidity and Mortality Weekly Report. (1981b). Pneumocystis pneumonia Los Angeles, 30:250–252.

Morbidity and Mortality Weekly Report. (1982). Update on acquired immune deficiency syndrome (AIDS) United States, 31:507–508, 513–514.

Morbidity and Mortality Weekly Report. (1990). Surveillance for HIV-2 infection in blood donors—United States, 1987–1989, 39:829–831.

Morbidity and Mortality Weekly Report. (1993). 1993 revised classification system for HIV infection and expanded surveillance case definition for AIDS among adolescents and adults, 41:1–19.

Morbidity and Mortality Weekly Report. (1994). Update: Impact of the expanded AIDS surveillance case definition for adolescents and adults on case reporting—United States, 1993, 43:160–170.

SPRECHER, LORRIE. (1991). Women with AIDS: Dead but not disabled. *The Positive Woman,* 1:4.

STADTMAUER, GARY, et al. (1997). Primary Immune Deficiency Disorders that mimic AIDS. *Infections in Medicine,* 4:899–905.

WAIN-HOBSON, SIMON, et al. (1991). LAV revisited: Origins of the early HIV-1 isolates from Institut Pasteur. *Science,* 252:961–965.

CHAPTER 2

ANDREWS, CHARLA. (1995). "The Duesberg Phenomenon." What does it mean? *Science,* 267:157.

BAILES, ELIZABETH, et al. (2003). Hybrid origin of SIV in chimpanzees. *Science,* 300:1713.

BALTER, MICHAEL. (1998). Virus from 1959 sample marks early years of HIV. *Science,* 279:801.

BAUM, RUDY. (1995). HIV link to AIDS strengthened by epidemiological study. *Chem. Eng. News,* 74:26.

BOGART, LAURA M., et al. (2005). Are HIV/AIDS Conspiracy Beliefs A Barrier To Prevention Among African Americans *AIDS,* 38:213–218.

CDC Weekly. (1988). Extremists seek to blame AIDS on Jews. July 11.

CHERRY, MIKE. (1999). AZT critics swayed South African president. *Nature,* 402:225.

COHEN, JON. (1993). Keystone's blunt message: "It's the virus, Stupid." *Science,* 260:292–293.

CONNOR, EDWARD. (1994). Reduction of maternal infant transmission of HIV with zidovudine treatment (ACTG 076). *N. Engl. J. Med.,* 331:1173–1180.

CULLITON, BARBARA J. (1992). The mysterious virus called "Isn't." *Nature,* 358:619.

DARBY, SARAH, et al. (1995). Mortality before and after HIV infection in the complete UK population of haemophiliacs. *Nature,* 377:79–82.

DUESBERG, PETER H. (1990). Duesberg replies [to the charges of Weiss and Jaffe]. *Nature,* 346:788.

DUESBERG, PETER H. (1993). HIV and AIDS. *Science,* 260:1705–1708.

DUESBERG, PETER H. (1995a). The Duesberg Phenomenon: Duesberg and other voices. *Science,* 267:313.

DUESBERG, PETER H. (1995b). Duesberg on AIDS causation: the culprit is noncontagious risk factors. *The Scientist,* 9:12.

DUESBERG, PETER H., et al. (1998). The AIDS Dilemma: drug diseases blamed on a passenger virus. *Genetica,* 104:85–132.

Editorial. (1995). More conviction on HIV and AIDS. *Nature,* 377:1.

GEVISSER, MARK (2007). Thabo Mbeki: The Dream Deferred. Jeppestown (Johannesburg): Jonathan Ball.

GIBBS, WAYT. (2001). Dissident or Don Quixote? *Scientific American,* 285:30–32.

GRMEK, MIRKO. (1990). *History of AIDS: Emergence and Origin of a Modern Pandemic.* Princeton, NJ: Princeton University Press.

HAHN, BEATRICE, et al. (1999). Origin of HIV-1 in the chimpanzee *Pan troglodytes troglodytes. Nature,* 397:436–441.

HAHN, BEATRICE, et al. (2000). AIDS as a zoonosis: scientific and public health implications. *Science,* 287:607–614.

HARRIS, STEVEN. (1995). The AIDS heresies: A case study in skepticism taken too far. *Skeptic,* 3, No. 2:42–58.

HIRSCH, VANESSA, et al. (1995). Phylogeny and natural history of the primate lentiviruses, SIV and HIV. *Current Opinion Genetic Development,* 5:798–806.

HOLDER, CONSTANCE. (1988). Curbing Soviet disinformation. *Science,* 242:665.

KALISH, MARSHA, et. al. (2005). Central African Hunters Exposed to Simian Immunodeficiency Virus. *Emerging Infectious Diseases,* 11:1928–1930.

KOPROWSKI, HILARY. (1992). AIDS and the polio vaccine. *Science,* 257:1024–1026.

LEVY, JAY. (1995). *HIV and the Pathogenesis of AIDS.* Washington, D.C.: ASM Press.

MOORE, JOHN. (1996). À Duesberg, adieu! *Nature,* 380:293–294.

National Institute of Allergy and Infectious Diseases. (1995). The relationship between the human immunodeficiency virus and the acquired immunodeficiency syndrome. *National Institutes of Health,* 1–61.

PEETERS, MARTINE, et al. (2002). Risk to human health from a plethora of simian immunodeficiency viruses in primate bushmeat. *Emerging Infectious Diseases,* 8:451–457.

ROOT-BERNSTEIN, ROBERT. (1993). *Rethinking AIDS.* New York: Free Press.

SANTIAGO, MARIO, et al. (2002). SIVcpz in wild chimpanzees. *Science,* 795:465.

SANTIAGO, MARIO, BEATRICE HAHN, et al. (2003). Amplification of a complete simian immunodeficiency virus gnome from fecal RNA of a wild chimpanzee. *Virology,* 77:2233–2242.

SULLIVAN, JOHN, et al. (1995). HIV and AIDS. *Nature,* 378:10.

THOMAS, M., P. GILBERT et al. (2007). The Emergence of HIV/AIDS in the Americas and Beyond. Proc. Natl. Acad. Sci. USA 10:1073/pnas 0705329104

VANGROENWEGHE, DANIEL. (2001). The earliest cases of human immunodeficiency virus type 1 group M in Congo-Kinshasa, Rwanda and Burundi and the origin of acquired immune deficiency syndrome. *Philos. Trans. R. Soc. Lond. B. Biol. Sci.;* 356 (1410):923–925.

VIDAL, NICOLE, et al. (2000). Unprecented degree of HIV-1 Group M genetic diversity in the Democratic Republic of Congo suggests HIV-1 pandemic originated in Central Africa. *J. Virology* 74:10,498–10,507.

WEISS, ROBIN A., et al. (1990). Duesberg, HIV and AIDS. *Nature,* 345:659–660.

WOROBEY, MICHAEL, et al. (2007). Exodus and genesis: The emergence of HIV-1 group M subtype B. Fourteenth Conference on Retroviruses and Opportunistic Infections, abstract 149, Los Angeles.

CHAPTER 3

BONHOEFFER, SEBASTIAN, et al. (1995). Causes of HIV diversity. *Nature,* 376:125.

BRIGGS, J. A., et al. (2006). The Mechanism of HIV-1 core assembly: Insights from three-dimensional reconstructions of authentic visions. *Structure* 14, 15–20.

BRIX, DEBORAH, et al. (1996). Summary of track A: Basic science. *AIDS,* 10 (suppl. 3): S85–S106.

BRODINE, STEPHANIE, et al. (1997). Genotypic variation and molecular epidemiology of HIV. *Infect. Med.,* 14:739–748.

COHEN, JON. (2008). HIV gets by with a lot of help from human host. *Science,* 319:143–144 www.sciencemag.org.

COHEN, JON. (1997). Looking for leads in HIV's battle with immune system. *Science,* 276:1196–1197.

COHEN, MITCHELL, et al. (1994). When bugs outsmart drugs. *Patient Care,* 28:135–146.

COLLINS, KATHLEEN, et al. (1998). HIV-1 Nef protein protects infected primary cells against killing by cytotoxic T Lymphocytes. *Nature,* 391:397–401.

DELWART, ERIC, et al. (1993). Genetic relationships determined by a DNA heteroduplex mobility assay: Analysis of HIV *env* Genes. *Science,* 262:1257–1262.

DERDEYN, CYNTHIA, et al. (2004). Envelope-constrained naturalization-sensitive HIV-1 after heterosexual transmission. *Science,* 303:2019–2022.

DEVEREUX, HELEN, et al. (2002). In vitro HIV-1 compartmentalisation: drug resistance associated mutation distribution. *J. Med. Virology,* 66:8–12.

DIAZ, RICARDO, et al. (1997). Divergence of HIV quasispecies in an epidemiology cluster. *AIDS,* 11:415–422.

DIMMROCK, N.J., and S.B. PRIMROSE, (1987). *Introduction to Modern Virology,* 3rd ed. Oxford: Blackwell Scientific Publications.

ELLEDGE, STEPHEN J. et al. (2008). Identification of host proteins required for HIV infection through a functional genomic screen. www.scienceexpress.org/ 10 January 2008:1–10.

FIELDS, BERNARD. (1994). AIDS: Time to turn to basic science. *Nature,* 369:95–96.

FISCHL, MARGARET. (1984). Combination retroviral therapy for HIV infection. *Hosp. Pract.,* 29:43–48.

FOLKS, THOMAS, et al. (2004). Recombinant viruses and early global HIV-1 epidemic. *Emerging Infectious Diseases,* 10: 1227–1233.

FRITZ, CHRISTIAN, et al. (1995). A human nucleoprotein-like protein that specifically interacts with HIV-Rev. *Nature,* 376:530–533.

GARRUS, JENNIFER, et al. (2001). Tsg 101 and the vacuolar protein sorting pathway are essential for HIV-1 budding. *Cell,* 107:55–65.

GREENE, WARNER. (1993). AIDS and the immune system. *Sci. Am.,* 269:99–105.

HILDRETH, JAMES. (2001). Adhesion molecules, lipid rafts and HIV pathogenesis. HIV Pathogenesis Keystone Symposium, March 28–April 3, Presentation 038.

HU, DALE, et al. (1996). The emerging genetic diversity of HIV. *JAMA,* 275:210–216.

JETZT, AMANDA, et al. (2000). High rate of recombination throughout the HIV genome. *Journal of Virology,* 74:1234–1240.

KOHLEISEN, MARKUS, et al. (1992). Cellular localization of Nef expressed in persistently HIV-1 infected low-producer astrocytes. *AIDS,* 6:1427–1436.

LENNOX, JEFFREY. (1995). Approaches to gene therapy. *International AIDS Society—USA,* 3:13–16.

LI, CHIANG. (1997). Tat protein perpetuates HIV-1 infection. *Proc. Natl. Acad. Sci. USA,* 94:8116–8120.

LUM, JULIAN, et al. (2003). Vpr R77Q is associated with long-term nonprogressive HIV and impaired induction of apoptosis. *J. Clin. Invest.,* 111:1547–1554.

MARX, PRESTON, et al. (2001). Serial human passage of simian immunodeficiency Virus by unsterile injections and the emergence of epidemic HIV in Africa. *Philos. Trans. R. Soc. Lond. B. Biol. Sci.,* 356:911–920.

MATSUYA, HIROAKI, et al. (1990). Molecular targets for AIDS therapy. *Science,* 249:1533–1543.

MOORE, JOHN, et al. (1994). The who and why of HIV vaccine trials. *Nature,* 372:313–314.

Morbidity and Mortality Weekly Report. (1993). Nosocomial enterococci resistant to Vancomycin—United States, 1989–1993, 42:597–599.

NOWAK, MARTIN A. (1990). HIV mutation rate. *Nature,* 347:522.

NOWAK, MARTIN A., et al. (1991). Antigenic diversity thresholds and the development of AIDS. *Science,* 254:963–969.

NOWAK, RACHEL. (1995). How the parasite disguises itself. *Science,* 269:755.

Parada, et al. (1996).

PATRUSKY, BEN. (1992). The Intron story. *Mosaic,* 23:20–33.

POTASH, MARY JANE, et al. (1998). Peptid inhibitors of HIV-1 protease and viral infection of peripheral blood lymphocytes based on HIV-1 ViF. *Proc. National Academy of Science,* 95:13,865–13,868.

ROBERTSON, DAVID, et al. (1995). Recombination in HIV-1. *Nature,* 374:124–126.

ROSEN, CRAIG A. (1991). Regulation of HIV gene expression by RNA-protein interactions. *Trends Genet.,* 7:9–14.

SAGG, MICHAEL S., et al. (1988). Extensive variation of human immunodeficiency virus Type-1 *in vivo. Nature,* 334:440–444.

SAGG, MICHAEL S., et al. (1995). Improving the management of HIV disease. *Advanced Causes in HIV Pathogenesis,* pp. 1–30. February 25, Swissotel, Atlanta (Michael Sagg, Program Chair).

SIMON, FRANCOIS, et al. (1998). Identification of a new human immunodeficiency virus Type I distinct from Group M and Group O. *Nature Medicine,* 4:1032.

SOMASUNDARAN, M., et al. (1988). Unexpectedly high levels of HIV-1 RNA and protein synthesis in a cytocidal infection. *Science,* 242:1554–1557.

SOTO-RAMIREZ, LUIS, et al. (1996). HIV-Langerhans' cell tropism associated with heterosexual transmission of HIV. *Science,* 271:1291–1293.

STEVENSON, MARIO. (1998). Basic Science: Highlights of the 5th Retrovirus Conference. *Improving the Management of HIV Disease,* 6:4–10.

TAYLOR, BARBARA et al. (2008). The challenge of HIV-1 subtype diversity. *NEJM* 358: 1590–1602.

TORRES, YOLANDA, et al. (1996). Cytokine network and HIV syncytium-inducing phenotype shift. *AIDS,* 10:1053–1055.

WILLS, JOHN W., et al. (1991). Form, function and use of retroviral *gag* protein. *AIDS,* 5:639–654.

Workshop Report from the European Commission/Joint United Nations Program on HIV/AIDS. (1997). HIV-1 subtypes: Implications for epidemiology, pathogenicity, vaccines, and diagnostics. *AIDS,* 11:17–36.

WU, YUNTAO, et al. (2001). Selective transcription and modulation of resting T cell activity by preintegrated HIV DNA. *Science,* 293:1503–1506.

CHAPTER 4

AUTRAN, BRIGITTE, et al. (1997). Positive effects of combined antiretroviral therapy on CD4+ T cell homeostasis and function in advanced HIV disease. *Science,* 277:112–116.

BACK, DAVID. (2001). Pharmacology to the fore. *PRN Notebook,* 6:11–14.

BARTHWELL, ANDREA. (1997). Substance use and the puzzle of adherence. *Focus,* 12:1–4.

BANGSBERG, DAVID, et al. (2006). Adherence-resistance relationships for protease and non-nucleoside reverse transcriptase inhibitors explained by virological fitness. *AIDS* 20: 223–231.

BEEKER, AMANDA STEPHEN, et al. (2002). Young HIV-infected adults are at greater risk for medication nonadherence. *Medscape HIV/AIDS eJournal* B(4).

BOZZETTE, SAMUEL, et al. (2001). Expenditures for the care of HIV-infected patients in the era of HAART. *N. Eng. J. Med.,* 344: 817–823.

British Guidelines Coordinating Committee. (1997). British HIV Association guidelines for antiretroviral treatment of HIV seropositive individuals. *Lancet,* 349:1086–1091.

BURMAN, WILLIAM, et al. (1998). The Case for Conservative Management of Early HIV Disease. *JAMA,* 280:93–95.

CARPENTER, CHARLES, et al. (1997). Antiviral therapy for HIV infection in 1997. *JAMA,* 277:1962–1969.

CARPENTER, CHARLES, et al. (2000). Antiretroviral therapy for adults: Updated recommendations of the International AIDS society—USA Panel. *JAMA,* 283:381–390.

Cascade Collaboration (2000). Survival after the introduction of HAART in people with known duration of HIV-1 infection. 355:1158–1159.

CASPER, TONY. (2000). How to make billions out of the misery of millions. Online. Available: http://www.dispatch.co.2a [2000, May 18].

CHEN, RAY V. et al. (2006). Distribution of healthcare expenditures for HIV-infected patients. *Clinical Infectious Diseases,* 42:1003–1010.

CLARK, DAWN, et al. (1999). T cell renewal impaired in HIV-1 infected individuals. Presented at: Sixth Conference on Retroviruses and Opportunistic Infections; January 31– February 4, Chicago. Abstract 22.

CLOUGH, LISA, et al. (1999). Factors that predict incomplete virological response to protease inhibitors-based antiretroviral therapy. *Clinical Infections Diseases.* 29:75–81.

CLUMECK, NATHAN. (1995). Summary to the use of saquinavir for HIV therapy. *AIDS,* 9(Suppl. 2):533–534.

COFFIN, JOHN. (1995). HIV population dynamics *in vivo:* Implications for genetic variation, pathogenesis and therapy. *Science,* 267:483–489.

DANNER, SVEN, et al. (1995). Short-term study of the safety, pharmacokinetics and efficacy of ritonavir. *N. Engl. J. Med.,* 333:1528–1533.

DEEKS, STEVEN, et al. (1997). Genotypic-resistance assays and antiretroviral therapy. *Lancet,* 349:1489–1490.

DEEKS, STEVEN, et al. (1999). HIV RNA and CD4 cell count response to protease inhibitor therapy in an urban AIDS clinic: Response to both initial and salvage therapy. *AIDS,* 13:F35–F43.

DE MARTINO, MAURIZIO. (1995). Redox potential status in children with perinatal HIV-1 infection treated with zidovudine. *AIDS,* 9:1381–1383.

DICKOVER, RUTH, et al. (1996). Identification of levels of maternal HIV RNA associated with risk of perinatal transmission. *JAMA,* 275:599–605.

DOBKIN, JAY. (1997). Fortovase: Son of Invirase. *Infections in Medicine.* 14:926, 934.

D'SOUZA, M. PATRICIA, et al. (2000). Current evidence and future directions for targeting HIV entry. *JAMA,* 284: 215–222.

DUBEÉ, MICHAEL, et al. (1997). Protease associated hyporglycaemia. *Lancet,* 350:713–714.

ERICKSON, JOHN, et al. (1990). Design, activity, and 2.8 angstrom crystal structure of a C_2 symmetric inhibitor complexed to HIV protease. *Science,* 249:527–533.

FLEXNER, CHARLES. (1996). Pharmacokinetics and pharmacodynamics of HIV protease inhibitors. *Infect. Med.,* 13:16–23.

FRATER, ALEXANDER, et al. (2002). Comparative response of African HIV-1 infected individuals to highly active antiretroviral therapy. *AIDS,* 16:1139–1146.

FREEDBERG, KENNETH, et al. (2001). The cost effectiveness of combination antiretroviral therapy for HIV disease. *N. Eng. J. Med.,* 344:824–831.

GERBER, JOHN. (1996). Drug interactions with HIV protease inhibitors. *Improv. Manage. HIV Dis.,* 4:20–23.

GOLDSCHMIDT, RONALD, et al. (1995). Antiretroviral strategies revisited. *J. Am. Board Fam. Pract.,* 8:62–69.

GOLDSCHMIDT, RONALD, et al. (1998). Individualized strategies in the era of combination antiretroviral therapy. *J.A.M. Board Family Practice,* 11:158–164.

HELLERSTEIN, MARC, et al. (1999). Directly measured kinetics of circulating T lymphocytes in normal and HIV-infected humans. *Nat. Med.,* 5:83–89.

HENDERSON, DAVID, et al. (2001). HIV postexposure prophylaxis in the 21st Century. *Emerging Infectious Diseases,* 7:254–258.

HENRARD, DENIS, et al. (1995). Natural history of HIV cell-free viremia. *JAMA,* 274:554–558.

HIRSCHEL, BERNARD, et al. (1998). Progress and problems in the fight against AIDS. *N. Engl. J. Med.,* 338:906–908.

HO, DAVID, et al. (1995). Rapid turnover of plasma virions and CD4 lymphocytes in HIV-1 infection. *Nature,* 373:123–126.

HOGG, WOOD, et al. (2003). Effect of medication adherence on survival of HIV-infected adults who start HAART when the CD4+ cell count is 200 to 350. *Ann. Intern. Med.,* 139:810–816.

HU, DALE, et al. (1996). The emerging genetic diversity of HIV. *JAMA,* 275:210–216.

JURRIAANS, SUZANNE, et al. (1994). The natural history of HIV infection: Virus load and virus phenotype independent determinants of viral course? *Virology,* 204:223–233.

Kaiser Family Foundation. (1999). National monitoring project: *Annual Report* 1–45 and Appendix 1–14.

KAUFMANN, DANIEL, et al. (1998). CD4 cell count in HIV-1 infected individuals remaining viraemic with HAART. (Swiss HW Cohort Study) *Lancet,* 351:723–724.

KENYON, GEORGE. (2001). Resistance study to re-evaluate HAART, *Nature,* 7:515.

KIRCHHOFF, FRANK, et al. (2007). Discovery and optimization of a natural HIV-1 entry inhibitor targeting the gp41 fusion peptide. *Cell,* 129:263–275.

LAURENCE, JEFFREY. (1996). The clinical promise of HIV protease inhibitors. *AIDS Reader,* 6:39–41, 71.

LEE HUANG, SYLVIA, et al. (1999). Lysozyme and RNases as anti-HIV components in beta-core preparations of human chorionic gonadotropin. *Proceedings of the National Academy of Sciences.* 96:2678–2681.

MARGOLIS, DAVID. (2007). Confronting proviral HIV infection. *Current HIV/AIDS reports,* 4:60–64.

MARKOWITZ, MARTIN, et al. (1995). A preliminary study of ritonavir, an inhibitor of HIV protease. *N. Engl. J. Med.,* 333:1534–1539.

MAYERS, DOUGLAS. (1996). Rational approaches to resistance: Nucleoside analogues. *AIDS,* 10 (Suppl. 1):S9–S13.

MELLORS, JOHN, et al. (1995). Quantitation of HIV-1 RNA in plasma predict outcome after seroconversion. *Ann. Intern. Med.,* 122:573–579.

MELLORS, JOHN. (1996). Clinical implications of resistance and cross-resistance to HIV protease inhibitors. *Infect Med.,* 13:32–38.

MERRICK, SAMUEL. (1997). Managing antiretrovirals in HIV-infected patients. *AIDS Reader,* 7:16–27.

MILLER, KIRK, et al. (1998). Visceral abdominal-fat accumulation associated with use of indinavir. *Lancet,* 351:871–875.

Morbidity and Mortality Weekly Report. (1994). Zidovudine for the prevention of HIV transmission from mother to infant 43:285–287.

Morbidity and Mortality Weekly Report. (1998). Guidelines for the use of antiretroviral agents in pediatric HIV infection, 47:1–38 No. RR-4.

O'BRIEN, MEGAN, et al. (2003). Patterns and correlates of discontinuation of the initial HAART regimen in an urban outpatient cohort. *AIDS,* 34:407–414.

PALELLA, FRANK, et al. (1998). Declining morbidity and mortality among patients with advanced HIV infection. *N. Engl. J. Med.,* 338:853–860.

PALMER, SARAH, et al. (2008). Low-level viremia persists for at least 7 years in patients on suppressive antiretroviral therapy. PNAS 105:3879–3884.

PERRIN, LUC, et al. (1998). HIV treatment failure: Testing for HIV resistance in clinical practice. *Science,* 280:1871–1873.

PIATAK, MICHAEL, et al. (1993). High levels of HIV-1 in plasma during all stages of infection determined by competitive PCR. *Science,* 259:1749–1754.

PINKERTON, STEVEN, et al. (2004). Cost effectiveness of post exposure prophylaxis after sexual or injection drug exposure to HIV. *Arch. Intern. Med.,* 164:46–54.

RICH, JOSIAH, et al. (1999). Misdiagnosis of HIV infection by HIV plasma viral load testing: A case series. *Annals of Internal Medicine Online* (1/5/99), 130:37.

RODRIGUEZ, BENIGNO, et al, (2006) Predictive value of plasma HIV RNA level on rate of CD4 T cell decline in untreated HIV infection. *JAMA,* 296: 1498–1506.

SAKSELA, KALLE, et al. (1994). Human immunodeficiency virus type 1 mRNA expression in peripheral blood cells predicts disease progression independently of the number of CD_4+ lymphocytes. *Proc. Natl. Acad. Sci. USA,* 91:1104–1108.

SARKAR, INDRANI, et al. (2007). HIV-1 proviral DNA excision using an evolved recombinase. *Science,* 316:1912–1915.

SCHACKMAN, BRUCE, et al. (2006). The lifetime cost of current HIV care in the United States. *Medical Care.* 44(11):990–997.

SCHMIT, JEAN-CLAUDE, et al. (1996). Resistance-related mutations in the HIV protease gene of patients treated for 1 year with protease inhibitor ritonavir. *AIDS,* 10:995–999.

SIMBERKOFF, MICHAEL. (1996). Long-term follow-up of symptomatic HIV-infected patients originally randomized to early vs. later zidovudine treatment: Report of a Veterans Affairs cooperative study. *AIDS,* 11:142–150.

SIMONI, JANE, et al. (2003). Antiretroviral adherence interventions: A review of current literature and ongoing studies. *Topics in HIV Medicine,* 11:185–198.

STEPHENSON, JOAN. (1996). New anti-HIV drugs and treatment strategies buoy AIDS researchers. *JAMA,* 275:579–580.

TELENTI, AMALIO, et al. for the Swiss HIV Cohort Study. (1998). CD_4 T cell counts in HIV-infected individuals remaining viraemic with highly active antiretroviral therapy followed in the Swiss HIV Cohort Study (SHCS). *Antiviral Ther.,* 3(Suppl. 1):53.

VALDEZ, HERNAN, et al. (1999). Human immunodeficiency virus 1 protease inhibitors in clinical practice. Archives of *Internal Medicine.* 159:1771–1776.

VAN COMPERNOLLE, SCOTT, et al. (2005). Antimicrobial peptides from amphibian skin potently inhibit HIV infection and transfer of virus from dendritic cells to T cells. *J. Virology,* 79:11598–11606.

VELLA, STEFANO. (1995). Clinical experience with saquinavir. *AIDS,* 9(suppl. 2):S21–S25.

VELLA, STEFANO. (1997). Clinical implications of resistance to antiretroviral drugs. *AIDS Clin. Care,* 9:45–47, 49.

VELLA, STEFANO, et al. (1996). HIV resistance to antiretroviral drugs. *Improv. Manage. HIV Dis.,* 4:15–18.

VIGAN, ALESSANDRA, et al. (2003). Increased lipodystrophy is associated with increased exposure to highly active antiretroviral therapy in HIV-infected children. *J. Acq. Immune Def. Syndromes,* 15; 32:482–489.

WAIN-HOBSON, SIMON. (1995). Virologies mayhem [editorial]. *Nature,* 373:102.

WALENSKY, ROCHELLE, et al. (2006). The survival benefits of AIDS Treatment in the United States. *JID* 194:11–19.

WALKER, BRUCE, et al. (1998). Treat HIV infection like other infections—Treat it. *JAMA,* 208:91–93.

WEI, XIPING, et al. (1995). Viral dynamics in human immunodeficiency virus type 1 infection. *Nature,* 373:117–122.

WILLIAMS, CAROLYN, et al. (2004). Persistent GB virus C infection and survival in infected men. *N. Engl. J. Med.,* 350:981–990.

CHAPTER 5

AMEISEN, JEAN CLAUDE. (1994). Programmed cell death apoptosis and cell survival regulation: relavance to cancer. *AIDS,* 8:1197–1213.

AMIGORENA, SEBASTIAN, et al. (1994). Transient accumulation of new class II MHC molecules in a novel endocytic compartment in B lymphocytes. *Nature,* 369:113–120.

BAKKER, LEENDERT J., et al. (1992). Antibodies and complement enhance binding and uptake of HIV-1 by human monocytes. *AIDS,* 6:35–41.

BARR, PHILIP, et al. (1994). Apoptosis and its role in human disease. *BioTechnology,* 12:487–494.

BELMONTE, LILIANA et al. (2007). The intestinal mucosa as a reservoir of HIV-1 infection after successful HAART. *AIDS* 2106–2108.

BENCHLEY, JASON, et al. (2004). CD4+ T cell depletion during all stages of HIV disease occurs predominantly in the gastrointestinal tract. *J. Experimental Medicine.* 200:749–759.

BLEUL, CONRAD, et al. (1996). The lymphocyte chemoattractant SDF-1 is a ligand for LESTR/FUSIN and blocks HIV entry. *Nature,* 382:829–833.

CALLEBAUT, CHRISTIAN, et al. (1993). T cell activation antigen, CD26 as a cofactor for entry of HIV in CD4+ cells. *Science,* 262:2045–2050.

CHUGH, PAULINE, et al. (2008). Akt inhibitors as an HIV-1 infected macrophage-specific anti-viral therapy. *Retrovirology,* 5:11 doi 10–1186/1742–4690–5–11.

COHEN, JON. (1993). Keystone's blunt message: "It's the virus, Stupid." *Science,* 260:292–293.

COHEN, JON. (1997). Exploiting the HIV-chemokine nexus. *Science,* 275:1261–1264.

CONNER, RUTH, et al. (1994). Human immunodeficiency virus type 1 variants with increased replicative capacity develop during the asymptomatic stage before disease progression. *J. Virol.,* 68: 4400–4408.

DEAN, MICHAEL, et al. (1996). Genetic restriction of HIV infection and progression to AIDS by a deletion allele of the CKR-5 structural gene. *Science,* 273:1856–1861.

DEEM, MICHAEL. (2003). Sequence space localization in the immune system response to vaccination and disease. *Phys. Rev. Lett.* Aug. 8; 91(6):068101

DOHERTY, PETER. (1995). The keys to cell-mediated immunity. *JAMA,* 274:1067–1068.

DOUEK, DANIEL. et al. (2005). Making sense of HIV pathogenesis. *PRN Notebook.* 10:9–12.

EDGINGTON, STEPHEN M. (1993). HIV no longer latent, says NIAID's Fauci. *BioTechnology,* 11:16–17.

EMBRETSON, JANET, et al. (1993). Massive covert infection of helper T lymphocytes and macrophages by HIV during the incubation period of AIDS. *Nature,* 362:359–362.

EUGEN-OLSEN, JESPER, et al. (1997). Heterozygosity for a deletion in the CKR-5 gene leads to prolonged AIDS-free survival and slower CD4 T cell decline. *AIDS,* 11:305–310.

FAUCI, ANTHONY, et al. (1995). Trapped but still dangerous. *Nature,* 337:680–681.

FOX, CECIL. (1996). How HIV causes disease. *Carolina Tips,* 59:9–11.

GEIJTENBEEK, TEUNIS, et al. (2000). Identification of DC-SIGN, a novel dendritic cell specific ICAM-3 receptor that supports primary immune response. *Cell,* 100:575–585.

GELDERBLOM, H. R., et al. (1985). Loss of envelope antigene of HTLV III/LAV, a factor in AIDS pathogenesis. *Lancet,* 2: 1016–1017.

GUADALUPE, MORAIMA, et al. (2006). Viral suppression and immune restovation in the gastrointestinal mucosa of human immunodeficiency virus type 1-infected patients initiating therapy during primary or chronic infection. Journal of Virology, 80:8236–8347.

HAASE, ASHLEY. (1999). Population biology of HIV-1 infection: Viral and CD4+ T cell demographics and dynamics in lymphatic tissues. *Annu. Rev. Immunol.,* 17:625–656.

HAASE, ASHLEY, et al. (1996). Quantitative image analysis of HIV infection in lymphoid tissue. *Science,* 274:985–990.

HEATH, SONYA, et al. (1995). Follicular dendritic cells and HIV infectivity. *Nature,* 377:740–744.

HILL, MARK, et al. (1996). Natural resistance to HIV. *Nature,* 382:668–669.

HO, DAVID. (1995). Pathogenesis of HIV infection. *International AIDS Society–USA,* 3:9–12.

HO, DAVID, et al. (1995). Rapid turnover of plasma virons and CD4 lymphocytes in HIV infection. *Nature,* 373:123–126.

HUANG, JIALING, et al. (2007). Cellular microRNAs contribute to HIV latency in resting primary CD4+ T lymphocytes. *Nature Medicine* 13:1241–1247.

KLEIN, JAN, et al. (2000a). The HLA System: Part I. *NEJM,* 343:702–709.

KLEIN, JAN, et al. (2000b). The HLA System: Part II. *NEJM,* 343:782–786.

KNIGHT, STELLA. (1996). Bone-marrow-derived dendritic cells and the pathogenesis of AIDS. *AIDS,* 10:807–817.

KUNAL, SAHA, et al. (2001). Isolation of primary HIV-1 that target CD8+ lymphocytes using CD8 as a receptor. *Nature Medicine,* 7:65–72.

KWONG, PETER, et al. (1998). Structure of an HIV gp120 envelope glycoprotein in complex with the CD4 receptor and a neutralizing human antibody. *Nature:* 648–659.

LEE, SANG KYUNG. (2002). The functional CD8 T cell response to HIV becomes type–specific in progressive disease. *J. Clin. Invest.,* 110:1339–1347.

LIU, RONG, et al. (1996). Homozygous defect in HIV-1 coreceptor accounts for resistance of some multiple-exposed individuals to HIV-1 infection. *Cell,* 86:367–377.

MARMOR, MICHAEL, et al. (2001). Homozygous and heterozygous CCR-5-32 genotypes are associated with resistance to HIV infection. *J. Acq. Immune Def. Syndromes,* 27:472–481.

MCDERMOTT, DAVID, et al. (2000). Chemokine promoter polymorphism affects risk of both HIV infection and disease progression in Multicenter AIDS Cohort Study. *AIDS,* 14:2671–2678.

MOIR, SUSAN, et al. (2000). B cells of HIV-1 infected patients bind virons through CD21-complement interactions and transmit infectious virus to activated T cells. *J Exp Med,* 192:637–646. Published online August 28, at http://www.jem.org.

MOIR, SUSAN, et al. (2001). HIV induces phenotypic and functional perturbations of B cells in chronically infected individuals. *PNAS,* 98:10,362–10,367.

MOORE, JOHN. (1997). Coreceptors: Implications for HIV pathogenesis and therapy. *Science,* 276:51–52.

Mountain-Plains Regional HIV/AIDS Curriculum, 4th ed. (1992). Mountain-Plains Regional AIDS Office, University of Colorado Health Sciences Center, Denver, CO 80262.

NOWAK, MARTIN, et al. (1995). HIV results in the frame: Results confirmed. *Nature,* 375:193.

O'BRIEN, STEPHEN. (1998). AIDS: A role for host genes. *Hospital Practice,* 33:53–79.

OLINGER, GENE, et al. (2000). CD4-negative cells bind HIV-1 and efficiently transfer virus to T cells. *J. Virol.,* 74:8550–8557.

PENNISI, ELIZABETH. (1994). A room of their own. *Science News,* 145:335.

PIANZ, OLIVER, et al. (1996). Specific cytotoxic T cells eliminate cells producing neutralizing antibodies. *Nature,* 382:726–729.

POPE, MELISSA. (2002). Dendritic cells: Immune activators or virus facilitators? *PRN Notebook,* 7:8–10.

RIZZUTO, CARLO, et al. (1998). A conserved HIV gp120 glycoprotein structure involved in chemokine receptor binding. *Science,* 280:1949–1953.

SAMSON, MICHEL, et al. (1996). Resistance to HIV-1 infection in caucasian individuals bearing mutant alleles of the CCR 5 chemokine gene. *Nature,* 382:722–725.

SCHMID, SANDRA, et al. (1994). Making class II presentable. *Nature,* 369:103–104.

SINHA, ANIMESH, et al. (1990). Autoimmune diseases: The failure of self-tolerance. *Science,* 248:1380–1387.

SPRENT, JONATHAN, et al. (1994). Lymphocyte life span and memory. *Science,* 265:1395–1400.

STEINMAN, RALPH. (2000). DC-SIGN: A guide to some mysteries of dendritic cells. *Cell,* 100:491–494.

STROMINGER, JACK, et al. (1995). The Class I and Class II proteins of the human major histocompatibility complex. *JAMA,* 274:1074–1076.

SUBBRAMANIAN, RAMU, et al. (2002). The presence of ADCC—but not NA—antibodies in serum was associated with viral neutralization in the presence of complement (Comparison of human immunodeficiency virus (HIV)-specific infection enhancing and inhibiting antibodies in AIDS patients.) *J. of Clin. Micro.,* 40:2141–2146).

TULP, ABRAHAM, et al. (1994). Isolation and characterization of the intracellular MHC class II compartment. *Nature,* 369:120–126.

UNANUE, EMIL. (1995). The concept of antigen processing and presentation. *JAMA,* 274:1071–1073.

WEI, XIPING, et al. (1995). Viral dynamics in HIV type I infection. *Nature,* 373:117–122.

WEI, XIPING, et al. (2003). Antibody neutralization and escape by HIV-1. *Nature,* 422:307–312.

WEIJING, HE, et al. (2008) Duffy antigen receptor for chemokines mediates trans-infection of HIV-1 from red blood cells to target cells and affects HIV-AIDS susceptibility. *Cell Host and Microbe,* 4:52-62.

WEISS, ROBIN, et al. (1996). Hot fusion of HIV. *Nature,* 381:647–648.

WYATT, RICHARD, et al. (1998). The antigenic structure of the HIV gp120 envelope glycoprotein. *Nature,* 705–711.

ZHU, TOUFU. (1993). Genotypic and phenotypic characterization of HIV-1 patients with primary infection. *Science,* 261:1179–1181.

ZINKERNAGEL, ROLF. (1995). MHC-restricted T cell recognition: The basis of immune surveillance. *JAMA,* 274:1069–1071.

CHAPTER 6

AMIN, NAVIN M. (1987). Acquired immunodeficiency syndrome, Part 2: The spectrum of disease. *Fam. Pract. Recert.,* 9:84–118.

AWE, ROBERT J. (1988). Benefits, promises and limitations of zidovudine (AZT). *Consultant,* 28:57–72.

BALFOUR, HENRY. (1995). Cytomegolovirus retinitis in persons with AIDS. *Postgrad. Med.,* 97:109–118.

BUCHANAN, KENT, et al. (1998). What makes *Cryptococcus neoformans* a pathogen? *Emerg. Infect. Dis.,* 4:71–83.

CHANG, YUAN, et al. (1994). Identification of Herpes virus-like DNA sequences in AIDS-Associated Kaposi's Sarcoma. *Science,* 266:1865–1869.

CHIN, DANIEL. (1992). Mycobacterium avium complex infection. *AIDS File: Clin. Notes,* 6:7–8.

Coalition News. (1993). Pet guidelines for people with HIV. 2:4–5.

CURRIER, JUDITH, et al. (1997). Pathogenesis, prevention and treatment of opportunistic complications. *Improv. Manage. HIV Dis.,* 4: S17–S18.

DALEY, CHARLES L. (1992). Epidemiology of tuberculosis in the AIDS era. *AIDS File: Clin. Notes,* 6:1–2.

DANNENBERG, ARTHUR M. (1993). Immunopathogenesis of pulmonary tuberculosis. *Hosp. Pract.,* 28:51–58.

DEWIT, STEPHANE, et al. (1991). Fungal infections in AIDS patients. *Clin. Adv. Treatment Fungal Infect.,* 2:1–11.

Emergency Medicine. (1989). Fighting opportunistic infections in AIDS. 21:24–38.

ERNST, JEROME. (1990). Recognize the early symptoms of PCP. *Med. Asp. Hum. Sexuality,* 24:45–47.

GANEM, DONALD. (1996) Kaposi's sarcoma-associated herpesvirus. *Improv. Manage. HIV Dis.,* 4(3):8–10.

GOTTLIEB, MICHAEL S., et al. (1987). Opportunistic viruses in AIDS. *Patient Care,* 23:139–154.

GROSSMAN, RONALD J., et al. (1989). PCP and other protozoal infections. *Patient Care,* 23:89–116.

GRULICH, ANDREW. (2000). Cancer risk in persons with HIV/AIDS in the era of combination antiretroviral therapy. *AIDS Reader,* 10:341–346.

GUARINO, M., et al. (1995). Progressive multifocal leucoencephalopathy in AIDS: Treatment with cytosine arabinoside. *AIDS,* 9:819–820.

Guidelines, U.S. Public Health Service. (1995). Preventing OIs in persons with HIV disease. *AIDS Reader,* 5:172–179.

HARDEN, C.L., et al. (1994). Diagnosis of central nervous system toxoplasmosis in AIDS patients confirmed by autopsy. *AIDS,* 8:1188–1189.

HARRIS, CHARLES. (1993). TB and HIV: The boundaries collide. *Medical World News,* 34:63.

Harvard AIDS Institute. (1994). *Special Report—Opportunistic Infections.* Fall issue: 1–14.

HERNDIER, BRIAN, et al. (1994). Pathogenesis of AIDS lymphomas. *AIDS,* 8:1025–1049.

HESSOL, NANCY. (1998). The changing epidemiology of HIV related cancers. *The AIDS Reader,* 8:45–49.

HESSOL, NANCY, et al. (2007). The impact of HAART on non–AIDS-defining cancers among adults with AIDS. *Am J. Epidemiology,* 165:1143–1153.

HUGHES, WALTER. (1994). Opportunistic infections in AIDS patients. *Postgrad. Med.,* 95:81–86.

JACOBSON, MARK A., et al. (1988). Serious cytomegalovirus disease in the acquired immunodeficiency syndrome (AIDS): Clinical findings, diagnosis, and treatment. *Ann. Intern. Med.,* 108:585–594.

JOINER, K.A., et al. (1990). *Toxoplasma gondii:* Fusion competence of parasitophorous vacuoles in Fe receptor-transfected fibroblasts. *J. Cell Biol.,* 109:2771.

KLEDAL, THOMAS, et al. (1997). A broad spectrum chemokine antagonist encoded by KS-associated herpesvirus. *Science,* 277:1656–1659.

KOEHLER, CHRISTOPHER. (2002). Consumption, the great killer. *Modern Drug Discovery,* 5:47–48.

LAURENCE, JEFFREY. (1995). Evolving management of OIs. *AIDS Reader,* 5:187–188, 208.

LAURENCE, JEFFREY. (1996). Where do we go from here? *AIDS Reader,* 6:3–4, 36.

LEDERGERBER, BRUNO, et al. (1999). AIDS-related OI occurring after initiation of potent antiretroviral therapy: A Swiss cohort study. *JAMA,* 282:2220–2226.

LOONEY, DAVID, (1996). Kaposi's sarcoma. *Improv. Manage. HIV Dis.,* 4:21–24.

LYNCH, JOSEPH P. (1989). When opportunistic viruses infiltrate the lung. *J. Resp. Dis.,* 10:25–30.

MCGRATH, MICHAEL, et al. (1994). Identification of a common clonal human immunodeficiency virus integration site in human immunodeficiency virus-associated lymphomas. *Cancer Res.,* 54:2069.

MEDOFF, GERALD, et al. (1991). Systemic fungal infections: An overview. *Hosp. Pract,* 26:41–52.

MONETTE, PAUL. (1988). *Borrowed Time: An AIDS Memoir.* New York: Avon Books.

MONFORTE, ANTONELLA D'ARMINIO, et al. (1992). AIDS-defining diseases in 250 HIV-infected patients: A comparative study of clinical and autopsy diagnoses. *AIDS,* 6:1159–1164.

Morbidity and Mortality Weekly Report. (1995a). 1995 revised guidelines for prophylaxis against PCP for children infected with or perinatally exposed to HIV. 44:1–10.

Morbidity and Mortality Weekly Report. (1995b). USPHS/IDSA guidelines for the prevention of opportunistic infections in persons infected with HIV: A summary. 44:1–34.

Morbidity and Mortality Weekly Report. (2004). Treating opportunistic infections among HIV-infected adults and adolescents. 53:1–112.

MURPHY, ROBERT. (1994). Opportunistic infection prophylaxis. *Int. AIDS Soc.–USA,* 2:7–8.

NEWCOMB-FERNANDEZ, JENNIFER. (2003) Cancer in the HIV-infected population. *RITA,* 9:5–10.

NEWTON, HERBERT. (1995). Common neurologic complications of HIV infection and AIDS. *Am. Fam. Phys.,* 51:387–398.

PATEL, PRAGNA, et al. (2008). Incidence of types of cancer among HIV-infected persons compared with the general population of the United States, 1992–2003. *Annals of Internal Medicine* 148 (10): 728–736.

PHAIR, JOHN, et al. (1990). The risk of *Pneumocystis carinii* among men infected with HIV-1. *N. Engl. J. Med.,* 322:161–165.

POWDERLY, WILLIAM, et al. (1998). Recovery of the immune system with antiretroviral therapy: the end of opportunism? *JAMA,* 280:72–77.

POWDERLY, WILLIAM G., et al. (1992). Molecular typing of *Candida albicans* isolated from oral lesions of HIV-infected individuals. *AIDS,* 6:81–84.

RINALDO, CHARLES, et al. (2001). Primary human herpesvirus 8 infection generates a broadly specific CD8+ T cell response to viral lytic cycle proteins. *Blood,* 97:2366–2373.

ROSSITCH, EUGENE, et al. (1990). Cerebral toxoplasmosis in patients with AIDS. *Am. Fam. Pract.,* 41:867–873.

RUSSELL, JAMES. (1990). Study focuses on eyes and AIDS. *Baylor Med,* 21:3.

SAID, JONATHAN, et al. (1997). KS-associated herpesvirus/ human herpesvirus type 8 encephalitis in HIV-positive and -negative individuals. *AIDS,* 11:1119–1122.

SCADDEN, DAVID. (2002). Lymphoma in the setting of HIV disease. *PRN Notebook,* 7:21–25.

SEPKOWITZ, KENT. (1998). Effect of HAART on natural history of AIDS-related opportunistic disorders. *Lancet,* 351:228–230.

SIBLEY, L. DAVID. (1992). Virulent strains of *Toxoplasma gondii* comprise single clonal linage. *Nature,* 359:82–85.

SMALL, PETER. (1996). Tuberculosis research: Balancing the portfolio. *JAMA,* 276:1512–1513.

SOLOWAY, BRUCE. (1998). Report on the Fifth Conference on Retroviruses and Opportunistic Infections. *AIDS Clinical Care,* 10:27–29.

STRINGER, JAMES, et al. (2002). A new name (*Pneumocystis jiroveci*) for pneumocystis from humans. *Emerging Infectious Diseases,* 8:891–896.

TUAZON, CARMELITA, et al. (1991). Diagnosing and treating opportunistic CNS infections in patients with AIDS. *Drug Therapy,* 21:43–53.

United States Public Health Service and Infectious Diseases Society of America. (2001). Guidelines for the prevention of opportunistic infections in persons infected with human immunodeficiency virus. *MMWR,* November 28, 1–65.

WALLACE, MARK R., et al. (1993). Cats and toxoplasmosis risk in HIV-infected adults. *JAMA,* 269:76–77.

WHEAT, L. JOSEPH. (1992). Histoplasmosis in AIDS. *AIDS Clin. Care,* 4:1–4.

CHAPTER 7

ABOULKER, JEAN-PIERRE, et al. (1993). Preliminary analysis of the Concorde trial. *Lancet,* 341:889–890.

ANDERSON, ROBERT E., et al. (1991). CD8 T lymphocytes and progression to AIDS in HIV-infected men: Some observations. *AIDS,* 5:213–215.

BALTER, MICHAEL. (1998). Chemokine mutation slows progression. *Science,* 279:327.

BALTIMORE, DAVID. (1995). Lessons from people with nonprogressive HIV infection. *N. Engl. J. Med.,* 332:259–260.

BARNHART, HUIMAN, et al. (1995). *Abstracts of the 2nd National Conference on Human Retroviruses,* Washington, D.C., p. 161, Abstr. 575.

BARTLETT, JOHN, et al. (1998). Primary care of HIV infection. *Hospital Practice,* 33:53–55.

BOLOGNESI, DANI P. (1989). Prospects for prevention of and early intervention against HIV. *JAMA,* 261:3007–3013.

BRYSON, YVONNE J., et al. (1995). Clearance of HIV infection in a prenatally infected infant. *N. Engl. J. Med.,* 332:833–838.

BUCHBINDER, SUSAN P., et al. (1992). Healthy long-term positives: Men infected with HIV for more than 10 years with CD4 counts of 500 cells. *Eighth International Conference on AIDS,* Amsterdam, July 1992, abstr. TUCO572.

BUCHBINDER, SUSAN P., et al. (1994). Long-term HIV infection without immunologic progression. *AIDS,* 8:1123–1128.

BUCY, R. PAT. (1999). Viral and cellular dynamics in HIV-1 disease. *Improving Management of HIV Disease,* 7:8–11.

BURCHAM, JOYCE, et al. (1991). CD4 % is the best predictor of development of AIDS in a cohort of HIV-infected homosexual men. *AIDS,* 5:365–372.

CAO, YUNZHEN, et al. (1995). Virologic and immunologic characterization of long-term survivors of human immunodeficiency virus type 1 infection. *N. Engl. J. Med.,* 332:201–208.

CATALAN, JOSÉ, et al. (2001). The changing picture of HIV: A chronic illness, again? *Focus,* 16:1–4.

Centers for Disease Control and Prevention. (2001). Report of NIH panel to define principles of therapy of HIV infection and guidelines for the use of antiretroviral agents in HIV-infected adults and adolescents. Updated February 5, as a living document: www.hivatis.org.

CHUN, TAE-WOOK, et al. (1998). Early establishment of a pool of latently infected, resting CD4+ T cells during primary HIV-1 infection. *PNAS,* 95:8869–8873.

CLERICI, MARIO, et al. (2003). Mucosal and systemic HIV specific immunity in HIV exposed but uninfected heterosexual men. *AIDS,* 17:531–539.

COCCHI, FIORNZA, et al. (1995). Identification of RANTES, MIP-la and MIP-lb as the major HIV-suppressive factors produced by CD8+ T cells. *Science,* 270:1811–1815.

COFFIN, JOHN M. (1995). HIV population dynamics in vivo: Implications for genetic variation, pathogenesis and therapy. *Science,* 267:483–489.

COHEN, JON. (1993). Keystone's blunt message: "It's the virus, Stupid." *Science,* 260:292–293.

COHEN, JON. (1995). High turnover of HIV in blood revealed by new studies. *Science,* 267:179.

COLLMAN, RONALD. (1997). Effect of CCR 2 and CCR 5 variants on HIV disease. *JAMA,* 278:2113–2114.

CONANT, MARCUS. (1995). The current face of the AIDS epidemic. *AIDS Newslink,* 6(Fall):1–9.

COULIS, PAUL A., et al. (1987). Peptide-based immunodiagnosis of retrovirus infections. *Am. Clin. Prod. Rev.*, 6:34–43.

DAVIS, SUSAN, et al. (1995). Prevalence and incidence of vertically acquired HIV infection in the U.S.A. *JAMA*, 274:952–955.

DEACON, NICHOLAS, et al. (1995). Genomic structure of an attenuated quasi species of HIV from a blood transfusion donor and recipients. *Science*, 270:988–991.

DENTON, PAUL, et al. (2008). Antiretroviral pre-exposure prophylaxis prevents vaginal transmission of HIV-1 in humanized BLT mice. Pages 1–13 http://medicine.plosjournal.org. doi 10.1371.

ENSOLI, F., et al. (1990). Proviral sequences detection of human immunodeficiency virus in seronegative subjects by polymerase chain reaction. *Mol. Cell Probes*, 4:153–161.

ENSOLI, F., et al. (1991). Plasma viraemia in seronegative HIV-1 infected individuals. *AIDS*, 5:1195–1199.

ESCAICH, SONIA, et al. (1991). Plasma viraemia as a marker of viral replication in HIV-infected individuals. *AIDS*, 5:1189–1194.

FAUCI, ANTHONY S. (1988). The scientific agenda for AIDS. *Issues Sci. Technol.*, 4:33–42.

FENG, YU, et al. (1996). HIV-1 entry cofactor: Functional cDNA cloning of a seven-transmembrane, G protein-coupled receptor. *Science*, 272:872–877.

FREED, ERIC, et al. (1994). HIV infection of non-dividing cells. *Nature*, 369:107–108.

FRENKEL, LISA, et al. (1998). Genetic evaluation of suspected cases of transient HIV infection of infants. *Science*, 280:1073–1077.

GEGNEY, THOMAS. (2000). Long-term nonprogressors: The study of HIV infection without progression to AIDS. Research Initiative Treatment Alert (RITA), 6, No. 2. June 2000. http://www.aegis.org/pubs/rita/2000/RI00064.html.

GOLDSCHMIDT, RONALD, et al. (1997). Treatment of AIDS and HIV-related conditions—1997. *J. Am. Board Fam. Pract.*, 10:144–167.

GRUBMAN, SAMUEL, et al. (1995). Older children and adolescents living with perinatally acquired HIV infection. *Pediatrics*, 95:657–663.

HAAS, DAVID, et al. (2000). Evidence of a source of HIV-1 within the central nervous system by ultraintensive sampling of cerebrospinal fluid and plasma. *AIDS Res. Hum. Retroviruses*, 16:1491–1502.

HAYNES, BARTON, et al. (1996). Toward an understanding of the correlates of protective immunity to HIV infection. *Science*, 271:324–328.

HENRARD, DENIS, et al. (1995). Natural history of HIV cell-free viremia, *JAMA*, 274:554–558.

HIRBOD, TADA, et al. (2008). HIV-neutralizing immunoglobulin A and HIV-specific proliferation are independently associated with reduced HIV acquisition in Kenyan sex workers. *AIDS*, 22:727–735.

HO, DAVID. (1996). HIV pathogenesis. *Improv. Manage. HIV Dis.*, 4:4–6.

HO, DAVID, et al. (1995). Rapid turnover of plasma virons and CD4 lymphocytes in HIV infection. *Nature*, 373:123–126.

HORSBURG, C.R., et al. (1989). Duration of HIV infection before detection of antibody. *Lancet*, ii:637–639.

IMAGAWA, D.T., et al. (1989). Human immunodeficiency virus type I infection in homosexual men who remain seronegative for prolonged periods. *N. Engl. J. Med.*, 320:1458–1462.

Italian Register for HIV Infection in Children. (1994). *Lancet*, 343:191–195.

KATZENSTEIN, TERESE, et al. (1996). Longitudinal Serum HIV RNA quantification: Correlation to viral phenotype at seroconversion and clinical outcome. *AIDS*, 10:167–173.

KELLY, MAUREEN, et al. (1991). Oral manifestations of human immunodeficiency virus infection. *Cutis*, 47:44–49.

KIRCHHOFF, FRANK, et al. (1995). Brief report: Absence of intact Nef sequences in a long-term survivor with nonprogressive HIV-1 infection. *N. Engl. J. Med.*, 332:228–232.

KLINE, MARK. (1995). Long-term survival in vertically acquired HIV infection. *AIDS Reader*, 5:153.

LEARMONT, JENNIFER, et al. (1999). Immunological and virologic status after 14 to 18 years of infection with an attenuated strain of HIV-1. *N. Engl. J. Med.*, 340:1715–1722.

LEVY, JAY. (1995). HIV and long-term survival. *Int. AIDS Soc. USA*, 3:10–12.

LIPTON, STUART. (1997). Treating AIDS dementia. *Science*, 276:1629–1630.

MCARTHUR, JUSTIN. (1999). Declining incidence of neurologic complications of HIV disease. *Hopkins HIV Report*, 11:8.

MCGUIRE, DAWN. (1993). Pathogenesis of brain injury in HIV disease. *Clin. Notes*, 7:1–11.

MERIGAN, THOMAS, et al. (1996). The prognostic significance of viral load, codon 215-reverse transcriptase mutation and CD4+ T cells on HIV disease progression. *AIDS*, 10:159–165.

MIGUELES, STEPHEN, et al. (2000). HLA B5701 is highly associated with restriction of virus replication in a subgroup of HIV-infected long-term nonprogressors. *Pro. Natl. Acad. Sci. USA*, 97:2709–2714.

MIGUELES, STEPHEN, et al. (2002). HIV-specific CD8+ T cell proliferation is coupled to perforin expression and maintained in nonprogressors. *Nature Immunology*, 3:1061–1068.

MISHRAHI, MICHELINE, et al. (1998). CCR 5 chemokine receptor variant in HIV-1 mother-to-child transmission and disease progression. *JAMA*, 279:277–280.

Morbidity and Mortality Weekly Report. (1996). Persistent lack of detectable HIV-antibody in a person with HIV infection—Utah, 1995. 45:181–185.

Morbidity and Mortality Weekly Report. (1997). Revised guidelines for performing CD4+ T cell determinations in persons infected with HIV. 46:1–4.

National Institute of Allergy and Infectious Diseases. (1989). Tests confirm lack of mental impairment in asymptomatic HIV-infected homosexual men. June: 1–2.

NEWELL, MARIE, et al. (1996). Detection of virus in vertically exposed HIV-antibody-negative children. *Lancet,* 347:213–215.

NIELSON, CLAUS, et al. (1993). Biological properties of HIV isolates in primary HIV infection: Consequences for the subsequent course of infection. *AIDS,* 7:1035–1040.

NOWAK, M.A., et al. (1990). The evolutionary dynamics of HIV-1 quasispecies and the development of immunodeficiency disease. *AIDS,* 4:1095–1103.

PANTALEO, GUISEPPE, et al. (1993). The immunopathogenesis of HIV infection. *N. Engl. J. Med.,* 328:327–335.

PANTALEO, GUISEPPE, et al. (1995). Studies in subjects with long-term nonprogressive human immunodeficiency virus infection. *N. Engl. J. Med.,* 332:209–216.

PEDERSEN, C., et al. (1989). Clinical course of primary HIV infection: Consequences for subsequent course of infection. *Br. Med. J.,* 299:154–157.

PERELSON, ALAN, et al. (1996). HIV dynamics in vivo: Viron clearance rate, infected cell life span and viral generation time. *Science,* 271:1582–1586.

PHILLIPS, ANDREW N., et al. (1991a). p24 Anti-genaemia, CD4 lymphocyte counts and the development of AIDS. *AIDS,* 5:1217–1222.

PHILLIPS, ANDREW N., et al. (1991b). Serial CD4 lymphocyte counts and development of AIDS. *Lancet,* 337:389–392.

PHILLIPS, ANDREW, et al. (1994). A sex comparison of rates of new AIDS-defining disease and death in 2554 AIDS cases. *AIDS,* 8:831–835.

PRICE, RICHARD W. (1988). The brain in AIDS: Central nervous system HIV infection and AIDS dementia complex. *Science,* 239:586–593.

QUINN, THOMAS. (1997). Acute primary HIV infection. *JAMA,* 278:58–62.

RANKI, A., et al. (1987). Long latency precedes overt seroconversion in sexually transmitted human immunodeficiency virus infection. *Lancet,* ii:589–593.

RANKI, ANNAMARI, et al. (1995). Abundant expression of HIV Nef and Rev proteins in brain astrocytes *in vivo* is associated with dementia. *AIDS,* 9:1001–1008.

REYNES, JACQUES, et al. (2001). CD4 T cell surface CCR 5 density as a host factor in HIV-1 disease progression. *AIDS,* 15:1627–1634.

ROQUES, PIERRE, et al. (1995). Clearance of HIV infection in 12 perinatally infected children: Clinical, virological and immunological data. *AIDS,* 9:F19–F26.

ROSENBERG, PHILIP, et al. (1994). Declining age at HIV infection in the United States. *N. Engl. J. Med.,* 330:789–790.

ROYCE, RACHEL A., et al. (1991). The natural history of HIV-1 infection: Staging classifications of disease. *AIDS,* 5:355–364.

SAX, PAUL, et al. (1995). Potential clinical implications of inter-laboratory variability in CD4+ T lymphocyte counts of patients infected with human immunodeficiency virus. *Clin. Infect. Dis.,* 21:1121–1125.

SCHONNING, KRISTIAN, et al. (1998). Chemokine receptor polymorphism and autologous neutralizing antibody response in long-term HIV infection. *J. acquired immune deficiency syndrome and Human Retrovirology,* 18:195–202.

SHERNOFF, MICHAEL. (1997). A history of hope: The HIV roller coaster. *Focus,* 12:5–7.

SHIFENG, SUN, et al. (2008). Intrarectal transmission, systemic infection, and CD4+ T cell depletion in humanized mice infected with HIV-1. J Experimental Medicine. www.jem.org (accessed February 13, 2008).

SKURNICK, JOAN, et al. (2002). Correlates of nontransmission in U.S. women at high risk of HIV-1 infection through sexual exposure. *J. Infect. Dis.,* 185:428–438.

SOLOWAY, BRUCE, et al. (2000). Antiretroviral failure: A biopsychosocial approach. *AIDS Clinical Care,* 12:23–25, 30.

STRAMER, SUSAN L., et al. (1989). Markers of HIV infection prior to IgG antibody seropositivity. *JAMA,* 262:64–69.

The European Collaborative Study. (1994). *Pediatrics,* 94:815–819.

THOMPSON, PAUL, et al. (2005). Thinning of the cerebral cortex visualized in HIV/AIDS reflects CD4+ T lymphocyte decline. 102:15647–15752.

VANHEMS, PHILLIPPE, et al. (1999). Recognizing primary HIV infection. *Infections in Medicine,* 16:104–108, 110.

VOELKER, REBECCA. (1995). New studies say viral burden tops CD4 as a marker of HIV disease progression. *JAMA,* 275:421–422.

WAINBERG, MARK, et al. (2007). High rates of forward transmission events after acute/early HIV-1 infection. *J. of Infectious Diseases,* 195:951–959.

WAIN-HOBSON, SIMON. (1995). Virological mayhem. *Nature,* 373:102.

WEI, XIPING, et al. (1995). Viral dynamics in HIV type 1 infection. *Nature,* 373:117–122.

WINKLER, CHERYL, et al. (1998). Genetic restriction of AIDS pathogenesis by an SDF-1 chemokine gene variant. *Science,* 279:389–393.

YAN XU, et al. (2004). HIV-1 mediated apoptosis of neuronal cells: Proximal molecular mechanisms of HIV-1 induced encephalopathy. *PNAS,* 101:7070–7075.

YU, KALVIN, et al. (2000). Primary HIV infection. *Postgraduate Medicine,* 107:114–122.

CHAPTER 8

ABBOTT, ALISON. (1995). Murder charges brought in German HIV blood products case. *Nature,* 376:628.

ABBOTT, ALISON. (1996). Japan agrees to pay HIV blood victims. *Nature,* 380:278.

ALDHOUS, PETER. (1991). France will compensate. *Nature,* 353:425.

AMIRKHANIAN, YURI, et al. (2001). AIDS knowledge, attitudes and behavior in Russia: Results of a population based, random-digit telephone survey in St. Petersburg. *Int. J. STD AIDS,* 12:50–57.

ARCHIBALD, D.W., et al. (1990). *In vitro* inhibition of HIV-1 infectivity by human salivas. *AIDS Res. Human Viruses,* 6:1425–1431.

BARON, SAMUEL, et al. (1999). Why is HIV rarely transmitted by oral secretions? Saliva can disrupt orally shed, infected leukocytes. *Archives of Internal Medicine,* 159:303–310.

BENNETT, AMANDA, et al. (1996). AIDS fight is skewed by federal campaign exaggerating risks. *Wall Street Journal,* May 1, A1.

BOLLING, DAVID R. (1989). Anal intercourse between women and bisexual men. *Med. Asp. Human Sexuality,* 23:34.

BOYER, PAMELA J., et al. (1994). Factors predictive of maternal-fetal transmission of HIV. *JAMA,* 271:1925–1930.

BREO, DENNIS L. (1991). The two major scandals in France's AIDS-GATE. *JAMA,* 266:3477–3482.

BUCHBINDER, K., et al. (2001). Per-contact risk of HIV transmission between male sexual partners. *American Journal of Epidemiology,* 150:306–311.

BUJAN, LOUIS, et al. (2007). Safety and efficacy of sperm washing in HIV-1 serodiscordant couples when the male is infected: results from the European CREAThE network. *AIDS,* 21:1909–1914.

BURKETT, ELINOR. (1995). The gravest show on earth: America in the age of AIDS. Boston: Houghton Miflin.

BUTLER, DAVID, et al. (2007). Serosorting can potentially increase HIV transmission. *AIDS* 21(9):1218–1220.

BUTLER, DECLAN. (1994a). Allain freed to face new charges? *Nature,* 370:404.

BUTLER, DECLAN. (1994b). Blood scandal raises spectre of Dreyfus case. *Nature,* 371:548.

CAMERON, WILLIAM D. (1989). Female to male transmission of human immunodeficiency virus type 1: risk factors for seroconversion in men. *Lancet,* ii:403–407.

CDC (Centers for Disease Control and Prevention). (1990). *HIV/AIDS Surveillance Report,* Oct.:1–18.

Centers for Disease Control and Prevention. AIDS among persons aged > 50 years—U.S. 1991–1996. *MMWR,* 47:21–27.

CHU, S.Y., et al. (1990). Epidemiology of reported cases of AIDS in lesbians, United States, 1980–89. *Am. J. Public Health,* 80:1380.

COHEN, J.B., et al. (1989). Heterosexual transmission of HIV. *Immunol. Ser.,* 44:135–137.

COHEN, JON. (1995). Bringing AZT to poor countries. *Science,* 269:624–626.

CONANT, MARCUS. (1995). The current face of the AIDS epidemic. *AIDS Newslink,* 6:14–18.

COOMBS, ROBERT W., et al. (1989). Plasma viremia in HIV infection. *N. Engl. J. Med.,* 321:1526.

COTTONE, JAMES A., et al. (1990). The Kimberly Bergalis case: An analysis of the data suggesting the possible transmission of HIV infection from a dentist to his patient. *Phys. Assoc. AIDS Care,* 2:267–270.

COUTSOUDIS, ANNA, et al. (1999). Influence of infant-feeding patterns on early mother-to-child transmission of HIV-1 in Durban, South Africa: a prospective cohort study. *Lancet,* 354:9177, 9471.

COUTSOUDIS, ANNA, et al. (2001). Method of feeding and transmission of HIV-1 from mothers to children by 15 months of age prospective cohort study from Durban, South Africa. *AIDS,* 15:379–387.

CURRAN, JAMES W., et al. (1988). Epidemiology of HIV infection and AIDS in the United States. *Science,* 239:610–616.

DEMARTINO, MAURIZIO, et al. (1992). HIV-1 transmission through breast milk: Appraisal of risk according to duration of feeding. *AIDS,* 6:991–997.

DES JARLAIS, DON, et al. (2000). HIV incidence among injection-drug users in New York City, 1992–1997; Evidence for a declining epidemic. *Am. J. Public Health,* 90:352–359.

DES JARLAIS, DON, et al. (1995). Maintaining low HIV-seroprevalence in populations of injecting-drug users. *JAMA,* 274:1226–1231.

DES JARLAIS, DON C., et al. (1989). AIDS and IV-drug use. *Science,* 245:578.

DEVINCENZI, I., et al. (1989). Risk factors for male-to-female transmission of HIV. *Br. Med. J.,* 298:411–415.

DILLON, BETH, et al. (2000). Primary HIV infections associated with oral transmission. Program and abstracts of the Seventh Conference on Retroviruses and Opportunistic Infections; January 30–February 2; San Francisco, Calif. Abstract 473.

DORFMAN, ANDREA. (1991). Bad blood in France. *Time,* 138:48.

DROTMAN, PETER. (1996). Professional boxing, bleeding, and HIV testing. *JAMA,* 276:193.

EDWARDS, SARA, et al. (1998). Oral sex and the transmission of viral STD's. *J. Infect. Dis.,* 74:6–10.

ELSON, JOHN. (1991). The dangerous world of wannabes. *Time,* 138:77–80.

Emergency Cardiac Care Committee, American Heart Association. (1990). Risk of infection during CPR training and rescue: Supplemental guidelines. *JAMA,* 262:2714–2715.

European Mode of Delivery Collaboration, The. (1999). Elective Cesarean section versus vaginal delivery in prevention of vertical HIV-1 transmission: A randomized clinical trial. *Lancet,* 353:1035–1039.

FOX, PHILIP. (1991). Saliva and salivary gland alterations in HIV infection. *J. Am. Dental Assoc.,* 122:46–48.

FRIEDLAND, GERALD H. (1991). HIV transmission from healthcare workers. *AIDS Clin. Care,* 3:29–30.

GAUR, ADITYA, et al. (2008). Practice of offering a child premasticated (pre-chewed) food: an unrecognized possible risk factor of HIV transmission. Fifteenth Conference on Retroviruses and Opportunistic Infections, Boston, Abstract 613b.

GAUTHIER, DEANN et al. (1999). Bareback sex, bugchasers and the gift of death. *Deviant Behavior,* 20:85–100.

GIBBONS, MARY. (1994). Childhood sexual abuse. *Am. Fam. Phys.,* 49:125–136.

Global AIDSNEWS. (1994). A new approach to STD control and AIDS prevention. 4:13–14, 20.

GODDARD, JEROME. (1997). Why mosquitoes cannot transmit the AIDS virus. *Infect. Med.,* 14:353–354.

GOLDEN, MATHEW. (2006). HIV serosorting among men who have sex with men: implications for prevention. Thirteenth Conference on Retroviruses and Opportunistic Infections, Denver, Abstract 163.

GOTO, Y., et al. (1991). Detection of proviral sequences in saliva of patients infected with human immunodeficiency virus type 1. *AIDS Res. Hum. Retroviruses,* 7:343–347.

GRAY, RONALD, et al. (2007). Randomized trial of male circumcision for HIV prevention in Rakai, Uganda. Fourteenth Conference on Retroviruses and Opportunistic Infection, Los Angeles, abstract 155aLB.

GRIVEL, JEAN-CHARLES, et al. (2007). HIV-1 pathogenesis differs in rectosigmoid and tonsillar tissues infected ex vivo with CCR5- and CXCR4-tropic HIV-1. *AIDS* 21(10):1263–1272.

GROSSKURTH, HEINER, et al. (1995). Impact of improved treatment of sexually transmitted diseases on HIV infection in rural Tanzania. *Lancet,* 346:530–536.

GUINAN, MARY. (1995). Artificial insemination by donor: Safety and secrecy. *JAMA,* 273:890–891.

HARRISON, LEE, et al. (2000). Drugs cut HIV in semen: Safe sex still crucial. *Ann. Int. Med.,* 133:280–284.

HAWTHORNE, PETER. (1999). An epidemic of rapes. *Time,* 154, No. 18: p 59.

HECHT, FREDERICK, et al. (1998). Sexual transmission of an HIV-1 variant resistant to multiple reverse-transcriptase and protease inhibitors. *N. Eng. J. Med.,* 339:307–311.

HELPERIN, DANIEL, et al. (1999). Viewpoint: male circumcision and HIV infection: 10 years and counting. *Lancet,* 354(9192): 1813–1815.

HIV/AIDS Surveillance Report. (December 1996). 8:1–39.

HIV/AIDS Surveillance Report. (December 1997). 9:1–43.

HIV/AIDS Surveillance Report. (December 1999). 10:1–44.

HIV/AIDS Surveillance Report. (June 2001). 13:1–41.

HOLDEN, CONSTANCE. (1994). Switzerland has its own blood scandal. *Science,* 264:1254.

HOLMSTROM, PAUL, et al. (1992). HIV antigen detected in gingival fluid. *AIDS,* 6:738–739.

HOLTGRAVE, DAVID (2004). Estimation of annual HIV transmission rates in the United States, 1978–2000. *JAIDS,* 35:89–92.

HOOKER, TRACEY. (1996). HIV/AIDS: Facts to consider: 1996 National Conference of State Legislators, Denver, Colorado, February. 1–64.

HORN, TIM. (2001). Safety and efficacy of solid organ transplantation in HIV-positive patients. *PRN Notebook,* 6:19–24.

HU, DALE J., et al. (1992). HIV infection and breast-feeding: Policy implications through a decision analysis model. *AIDS,* 6:1505–1513.

JACKSON, BROOKS. (1999). Progress in reducing mother-to-infant HIV transmission. *The Hopkins Report,* 11:2–3.

JAFFE, HOWARD, et al. (2007). The re-emerging HIV/AIDS epidemic in men who have sex with men. *JAMA,* 298:2412–2414.

JAYARAMAN, KRISHNAMURTHY. (1995). HIV scandal hits Bombay blood centre. *Nature,* 376:285.

JOSEPH, STEPHEN C. (1993). Dragon within the gates: The once and future AIDS epidemic. *Med. Doctor,* 37:92–104.

JOVAISAS, E., et al. (1985). LAV/HTLV III in 20-week fetus. *Lancet,* 2:1129.

KAHN, JAMES, et al. (1998). Acute HIV-1 Infection. *N. Eng. J. Med.,* 339:33–40.

KAISER, JOCELYN. (1996). Pasteur implicated in blood scandal? *Science,* 272:185.

KALICHMAN, SETH, et al. (2008). Human immunodeficiency virus load in blood plasma and semen: review and implications of empirical findings. *Sexually Transmitted Diseases,* 35:55–60.

KATNER, H.P., et al. (1987). Evidence for a Euro-American origin of human immunodeficiency virus. *J. Natl. Med. Assoc.,* 79:1068–1072.

KIND, CHRISTIAN, et al. (1998). Prevention of vertical HIV transmission: Additive protective effect of elective cesarean section and zidovudine prophylaxis. *AIDS,* 12:205–210.

KINGSLEY, L.A., et al. (1990). Sexual transmission efficiency of hepatitis B virus and human immunodeficiency virus among homosexual men. *JAMA,* 264:230–234.

KLEIN, HARVEY. (2000). Will blood transfusion ever be safe enough? *JAMA,* 284:238–240.

KUHN, LOUISE, et al. (1994). Maternal–infant HIV transmission and circumstances of delivery. *Am. J. Public Health*, 84:1110–1115.

LACAYO, RICHARD. (1997). Assault with a deadly virus. *Time*, 149:82.

LAGA, MARIE. (1991). HIV infection and sexually transmitted diseases. *Sexually Transmitted Dis. Bull.*, 10:3–10.

LAGA, MARIE, et al. (1993). Non-ulcerative STDs as risk factors for HIV transmission in women: Results from a cohort study. *AIDS*, 7:95–102.

LEWIS, S.H., et al. (1990). HIV-1 introphoblastic villous Hofbauer cells and haematological precursors in eight-week fetuses. *Lancet*, 335:565.

LICHTMAN, STUART M., et al. (1991). Greater attention urged for HIV in older patients. *Infect. Dis. Update*, 2:5.

MARLINK, RICHARD, et al. (1994). Reduced rate of disease development after HIV infection as compared to HIV-1. *Science*, 265:1587–1590.

MCGOWAN, JOHN, et al. (2004). Risk behavior for transmission of human immunodeficiency virus (HIV) among HIV-seropositive individuals in an urban setting. *Clin. Infect. Dis.*, 38:122–127.

MIIKE, LAWRENCE. (1987). Do insects transmit AIDS? Office of Technological Assessment, Sept. 1:43.

MONZON, O.T., et al. (1987). Female-to-female transmission of HIV. *Lancet*, 2:40–41.

Morbidity and Mortality Weekly Report. (1988). Update: Universal precautions for prevention of transmission of human immunodeficiency virus, hepatitis B virus, and other blood-borne pathogens in healthcare settings. 37:377–382, 387–388.

Morbidity and Mortality Weekly Report. (1990a). Possible transmission of HIV to a patient during an invasive dental procedure. 39:489–493.

Morbidity and Mortality Weekly Report. (1990b). HIV infection and artificial insemination with processed semen. 39:249–256.

Morbidity and Mortality Weekly Report. (1991a). Update: Transmission of HIV infection during an invasive dental procedure—Florida. 40:21–27, 33.

Morbidity and Mortality Weekly Report. (1991b). Drug use and sexual behaviors among sex partners of injecting-drug users—U.S. 40:855–860.

Morbidity and Mortality Weekly Report. (1992). Childbearing and contraceptive-use plans among women at high risk for HIV infection—Selected U.S. sites, 1989–1991. 41:135–144.

Morbidity and Mortality Weekly Report. (1994a). Human immunodeficiency virus transmission in household settings—United States. 43:347, 353–357.

Morbidity and Mortality Weekly Report. (1994b). Guidelines for preventing transmission of HIV through transplantation of human tissue and organs. 43:1–15.

Morbidity and Mortality Weekly Report. (1994c). Medical-care expenditures attributable to cigarette smoking—United States, 1993. 43:469–472.

Morbidity and Mortality Weekly Report. (1994d). Zidovudine for the prevention of HIV transmission from mother to infant. 43:285–287.

Morbidity and Mortality Weekly Report. (1997). Transmission of HIV possibly associated with exposure of mucous membrane to contaminated blood. 46:620–623.

Morbidity and Mortality Weekly Report. (1998). AIDS among people aged 50 years—United States, 1991–1996. 47:21–27.

MUNZER, ALFRED. (1994). The threat of secondhand smoke. *Menopause Manage.*, 3:14–17.

NEWELL, MARIE-LOUISE, et al. (1990). HIV-1 infection in pregnancy: Implications for women and children. *AIDS*, 4:S111–S117.

NOWAK, RACHEL. (1995). Rockefeller's big prize for STD test. *Science*, 269:782.

OLESKE, JAMES M. (1994). The many needs of HIV-infected children. *Hosp. Pract.* 29:81–87.

OMETTO, LUCIA, et al. (1995). Viral phenotype and host-cell susceptibility to HIV infection as risk factors for mother-to-child HIV transmission. *AIDS*, 9:427–434.

PADIAN, NANCY S., et al. (1991). Female-to-male transmission of HIV. *JAMA*, 266:1664–1667.

PADIAN, NANCY, et al. (1997). Heterosexual transmission of HIV in northern California: Results from a ten-year study. *Am. J. Epidemiol.*, 146:350–357.

PATHELA, PREET, et al., (2006). Discordance between sexual behavior and self-reported sexual identity: A population-based survey of New York City men. *Annuals of Internal Medicine*, 145:416–425.

PATTERSON, JULIE, et al. (1995). Basic and clinical considerations of HIV infection in the elderly. *Infect. Dis.*, 3:21–34.

PECKHAM, CATHERINE, et al. (1995). Mother-to-child transmission of HIV. *N. Engl. J. Med.*, 333:298–302.

PETERMAN, THOMAS A., et al. (1988). Risk of human immunodeficiency virus transmission from heterosexual adults with transfusion-associated infections. *JAMA*, 259:55–58.

PETO, RICHARD. (1992). Statistics of chronic disease control. *Nature*, 356:557–558.

PILCHER, CHRISTOPHER, et al. (2007). Amplified transmission of HIV-1: Comparison of HIV-1 concentrations in semen and blood during acute and chronic infection. *AIDS*, 21:1723–1730.

POURTOIS, M., et al. (1991). Saliva can contribute in quick inhibition of HIV infectivity. *AIDS*, 5:598–599.

QUINN, THOMAS, et al. (2000). Viral load and heterosexual transmission of human HIV-1. *N. Engl. J. Med.*, 342:921–929.

REICHHARDT, TONY. (1995). Top aide to face charges in French HIV blood scandal. *Nature*, 375:349.

ROGERS, DAVID, et al. (1993). AIDS policy: Two divisive issues. *JAMA*, 270:494–495.

ROSS, MICHAEL W., et al. (2006). Conspiracy beliefs about the origin of HIV/AIDS in four racial/ethnic groups. *J. Acquired Immune Deficiency Syndrome*, 41:342–344.

ROTHENBERG, RICHARD, et al. (1998). Oral Transmission of HIV. *AIDS*, 12:2095–2105.

ROZENBAUM, W., et al. (1988). HIV transmission by oral sex. *Lancet*, 1:1395.

SCHACKER, TIMOTHY, et al. (1998). Frequent recovery of HIV from genital herpes simplex virus lesions in HIV-infected men. *JAMA*, 280:61–66.

Science in California. (1993). AIDS: I want a new drug. *Nature*, 362:396.

SCOTT, G.B., et al. (1985). Mothers of infants with the acquired immunodeficiency syndrome: Evidence for both symptomatic and asymptomatic carriers. *JAMA*, 253:363–366.

SEGARS, JAMES H. (1989). Heterosexual anal sex. *Med. Asp. Human Sexuality*, 23:6.

SELWYN, PETER A. (1986). AIDS: What is now known. *Hosp. Pract.*, 21:127–164.

SHERNOFF, MICHAEL. (1988). Integrating safer-sex counseling into social work practice. *Social Casework: J. Contemp. SocialWork*, 69:334–339.

SPITZER, P.G., et al. (1989). Transmission of HIV infection from a woman to a man by oral sex. *N. Engl. J. Med.*, 320:251.

SPURGEON, DAVID. (1994). Canadian AIDS suit raises hope for HIV blood victims. *Nature*, 281.

SPURGEON, DAVID. (1996). Canadian inquiry points the finger. *Nature*, 663.

ST. LOUIS, MICHAEL E., et al. (1993). Risk for perinatal HIV transmission according to maternal immunologic, virologic and placental factors. *JAMA*, 269:2853–2860.

STRYKER, JEFF, et al. (1993). AIDS policy: Two divisive issues. *JAMA*, 270:2436–2437.

SWENSON, ROBERT M. (1988). Plagues, History and AIDS. *Am. Scholar*, 57:183–200.

SWINBANKS, DAVID. (1993). American witnesses: Testify in Japan about AIDS risks. *Nature*, 364:181.

TOBIAN, AARON, et al. (2008). Trial of male circumcision: prevention of HSV-2 in men and vaginal infections in female partners, Rakai, Uganda. Fifteenth Conference on Retroviruses and Opportunistic Infections, Boston. Abstract 28LB.

TURNER, ABIGAIL, et al. (2007). Men's circumcision status and women's risk of HIV acquisition in Zimbabwe and Uganda. *AIDS*, 21:1779–1789.

UNAIDS. (1997). Implications of HIV variability for transmission: Scientific and policy issues. *AIDS*, 11:S1–S15.

VAN DE PERRE, PHILIPPE, et al. (1993). Infective and anti-infective properties of breast milk from HIV-infected women. *Lancet*, 341:914–918.

VERNAZZA, PIETRO, et al. (2008). Les personnes seropositives ne souffrant d'aucune autre MST et suivant un traitement anti-retroviral efficace ne transmettent pas le VIH par voie sexuelle. *Bulletin des medecins suisses*, 89(5).

VITTECOQ, D., et al. (1989). Acute HIV infection after acupuncture treatments. *N. Engl. J. Med.*, 320:250–251.

VOELKER, REBECCA. (1996). HIV guide for primary care physicians stresses patient-centered prevention. *JAMA*, 276:85–86.

WAWER, MARIA, et al. (2007). Effects of male circumcision on genital ulcer disease and urethral symptoms, and on HIV acquisition: An RCT in Rakai, Uganda. Fourteenth Conference on Retroviruses and Opportunistic Infections, Los Angeles, abstract 155bLB.

WAWER, MARIA et al. (2008). Trial of circumcision in HIV+ men in Rakai, Uganda: Effects in HIV+ men and women partners. Fifteenth Conference on Retroviruses and Opportunistic Infections, Boston. Abstract 33LB.

WEBB, PATRICIA, et al. (1989). Potential for insect transmission of HIV: Experimental exposure of *Cimex hemipterous* and *Toxorhynchites amboinensis* to human immunodeficiency virus. *J. Infect. Dis.*, 160:970–977.

WILL, GEORGE F. (1991). Foolish choices still jeopardize public health. *Private Pract.*, 24:46–48.

Women's AIDS Network. (1988). Lesbians and AIDS: What's the connection? San Francisco AIDS Foundation, 333 Valencia St., 4th Floor, P.O. Box 6182, San Francisco, CA 94101-6182.

WOOLLEY, ROBERT J. (1989). The biologic possibility of HIV transmission during passionate kissing. *JAMA*, 262:2230.

ZIGLER, J.B., et al. (1985). Postnatal transmission of AIDS-associated retrovirus from mother to infant. *Lancet*, 1:896–897.

CHAPTER 9

ABDALA, NADIA, et al. (1999). HIV-1 can survive in syringe for more than 4 weeks. *J. Acq. Imm. Def. Syndromes*, 20:73–80.

ABDALA, NADIA, et al. (2001). Use of bleach to disinfect HIV-1 contaminated syringes. *Am. Clinical Lab.*, 20:26–28.

ANDERSON, FRANK W.J. (1993). Condoms: A technical guide. *Female Patient*, 18:21–26.

BARBER, HUGH R.K. (1990). Condoms (not diamonds) are a girl's best friend. *Female Patient*, 15:14–16.

BAYER, RONALD, et al. (1992). HIV Prevention and the two faces of partner notification. *Am. J. Public Health*, 82:1158–1164.

BOLOGNESI, DANIEL, et al. (1998). Viral envelope fails to deliver? *Nature*, 391:638–639.

BURNETT, JOSEPH. (1995). Fundamental basic science of HIV. *Cutis*, 55:84.

BURRIS, SCOTT, et al. (1996). Legal strategies used in operating syringe-exchange programs in the United States. *Am. J. Public Health*, 86:1161–1166.

BURRIS, SCOTT, et al. (2000). Physician prescribing of sterile injection equipment to prevent HIV infection: Time for action. *Ann. Intern. Med.,* 133:218–226.

CIVIC, DIANE, et al. (2002). Ineffective use of condoms among young women in managed care. *AIDS,* 14:779–788.

Consumer Reports. (1989). Can you rely on condoms? 54:135–141.

DESROSIERS, RONALD. (2008). Scientific obstacles to an effective HIV vaccine. Fifteenth Conference on Retroviruses and Opportunistic Infections, Boston, plenary presentation 91.

DRUCKER, LURIE, et al. (1997). An opportunity lost: HIV infection associated with lack of a national needle-exchange program in the USA. *Lancet,* 349:604–608.

ETZIONI, AMITAI. (1993). HIV sufferers have a responsibility. *Time,* 142:100.

EZZELL, CAROL. (1987). Hospital workers have AIDS virus. *Nature,* 227:261.

FENTON, KEVIN, et al. (1997). HIV partner notification: Taking a new look. *AIDS,* 11:1535–1546.

FINDLAY, STEVEN. (1991). AIDS: The second decade. *U.S. News World Rep.,* 110:20–22.

FISHER, PETER. (1990). A report from the underground. *International Working Group on AIDS and IV-Drug Use,* 5:15–17.

FREZIERES, RON, et al. (1999). Evaluation of the efficacy of a polyurethane condom: Results from a randomized, controlled clinical trial. *Family Planning Perspectives,* 31:81–87.

GERBERDING, JULIE LOUISE. (1991). Reducing occupational risk of HIV infection. *Hosp. Pract.,* 26:103–118.

GOSTIN, LAWRENCE, et al. (1998). HIV infection and AIDS in the public health and healthcare systems: The role of law and litigation. *JAMA,* 279:1108–1113.

GRIMES, DAVID A.(1992). Contraception and the STD epidemic: Contraceptive methods for disease prevention. *The Contraception Report: The Role of Contraceptives in the Prevention of Sexually Transmitted Diseases,* III:1–15.

HAGEN, HOLLY. (1991). Studies support syringe exchange. *Focus,* 6:5–6.

HEARST, NORMAN, et al. (2004). Condom promotion for AIDS prevention in the developing world: Is it working? *Studies in Family Planning,* 35:39–47.

HOOKER, TRACEY. (1996). HIV/AIDS: Facts to consider, 1996. *National Conference of State Legislature.* Denver, February, 1–64.

HOTGRAVE, DAVID. (2002). Estimating the effectiveness and efficiency of U.S. HIV prevention efforts using scenario and cost-effectiveness analysis. *AIDS,* 16:2347–2350.

HOXWORTH, TAMARA, et al. (2003). Changes in partnerships and HIV risk behaviors after partner notification. *Sexually Transmitted Diseases,* 30:83–88.

JUDSON, FRANKLYN N. (1989). Condoms and spermicides for the prevention of sexually transmitted diseases. *Sexually Transmitted Dis. Bull.,* 9:3–11.

KAPLAN, EDWARD, et al. (1993). Let the needles do the talking! Evaluating the New Haven needle exchange. *Interfaces,* 23:7–26.

KISSINGER, PATRICIA, et al. (2003). Partner notification for HIV and syphilis: Effects on sexual behaviors and relationship stability. *Sexually Transmitted Diseases,* 30:75–82.

KORBER, BETTE, et al. (2007). Founder effects in the assessment of HIV polymorphisms and HLA allele associations. *Science,* 315:1583–1586.

KWONG, PETER, et al. (2007). Structural definition of a conserved neutralization epitope on HIV-1 gp120. *Nature,* 445:732–737.

LEWIS, DAVID. (1995). Resistance of microorganisms to disinfection in dental and medical devices. *Nature Med.,* 1:956–958.

LURIE, PETER, et al. (1994). Ethical behavioral and social aspects of HIV vaccine trials in developing countries. *JAMA,* 271:295–302.

LURIE, PETER, et al. (1998). A sterile syringe for every drug user injection: How many injections take place annually and how might pharmacists contribute to syringe distribution? *J. Acquired Immune Defic. Syndr. Hum. Retrovirol,* 18:545–551.

Morbidity and Mortality Weekly Report. (1988). Partner notification for preventing human immunodeficiency virus (HIV) infection—Colorado, Idaho, South Carolina, Virginia. 37:393–396; 401–402.

Morbidity and Mortality Weekly Report. (1989). Guideline for prevention of transmission of HIV and hepatitis B virus to healthcare workers. 38:3–17.

Morbidity and Mortality Weekly Report. (1992). Sexual behavior among high school students—United States, 1990. 40:885–888.

Morbidity and Mortality Weekly Report. (1993). Update: Barrier protection against HIV infection and other sexually transmitted diseases. 42:589–591.

Morbidity and Mortality Weekly Report. (1995). Notification of syringe-sharing and sex partners of HIV-infected persons—Pennsylvania, 1993–1994. 44:202–204.

Morbidity and Mortality Weekly Report. (1996). School-based HIV-prevention education—United States, 1994. 45:760–764.

Morbidity and Mortality Weekly Report. (1997). Update: Syringe-exchange programs—United States, 1996. 46:565–568.

Morbidity and Mortality Weekly Report. (2000a). Cluster of HIV-Infected adolescents and young adults—Mississippi, 1999. 49:861–864.

Morbidity and Mortality Weekly Report. (2000b). Notice to readers: CDC statement on study results of product containing nonoxynol-9. 49:717.

NATHANSON, NEAL. (2008). AIDS vaccine at the crossroads. Fifteenth Conference on Retroviruses and Opportunistic Infections, Boston, plenary presentation 92.

Office Nurse. (1995). Contraception: how today's options stack up. 8:13–14.

PARRAN, THOMAS, P. (1937). *Shadow on the Land: Syphilis.* New York: Reynal and Hitchcock.

RAYMOND, CHRIS ANNE. (1988). U.S. cities struggle to implement needle exchanges despite apparent success in European cities. *JAMA,* 260:2620–2621.

RENZI, CRISTINA, et al. (2003). Safety and acceptability of the Reality condom for anal sex among men who have sex with men. *AIDS,* 17:727–731.

RUTHERFORD, GEORGE W. (1988). Contact tracing and the control of human immunodeficiency virus infection. *JAMA,* 259:3609–3670.

SATTAR, SYED, A., et al. (1991). Survival and disinfectant inactivation of HIV: A critical review. *Rev. of Infect. Dis.,* 13:430–447.

SMOAK, NATALIE, et al. (2006). Sexual risk reduction interventions do not inadvertently increase the overall frequency of sexual behavior: a meta-analysis of 174 studies with 116, 735 participants.. *JAIDS* 41 (3), 374–384.

SPRUYT, ALAN, et al. (1998). Identifying condom users at risk for breakage and slippage; Findings from three International Sites. *Am. J. Public Health,* 88:239–240.

STIMSON, GERRY V., et al. (1989). Syringe exchange. *International Working Group on AIDS and IV-Drug Use,* 4:15.

STRATHDEE, STEFFANIE, et al. (2002). Sex differences in risk factors for HIV seroconversion among injection-drug users: A 10-year perspective. *Archives of Internal Medicine,* 161:1281–1288.

Time. (1992). Closed: Needle Park. 139:53.

U.S. Public Health Service. (1994). Counseling to prevent unintended pregnancy. *Am. Fam. Phys.,* 50(5):971.

WEINSTEIN, STEPHEN P., et al. (1990). AIDS and cocaine: A deadly combination facing the primary care physician. *J. Fam. Prac.,* 31:253–254.

WODAK, ALEX. (1990). Australia smashes international needle and syringe exchange record. *International Working Group on AIDS and IV-Drug Use,* 5:28–29.

CHAPTER 10

BOOTH, WILLIAM. (1989). Asking America about its sex life. *Science,* 243:304.

CATANIA, JOSEPH, et al. (2001). The continuing HIV epidemic among gay men. *Am. J. Public Health,* 91:907–914.

CHIN, J., et al. (1990). Projections of HIV infections and AIDS cases to the year 2000. *Bull. WHO,* 68:1–11.

COUTINHO, ROEL, et al. (1996). Summary of Track C: Epidemiology and public health. *AIDS* 10(suppl. 3):S115–S121.

DE GROOT, ANNE, et al. (1996). Barriers to care of HIV-infected inmates: A public health concern. *AIDS Reader,* 6:78–87.

DOLAN, KATE, et al. (1995). AIDS behind bars: Preventing HIV spread among incarcerated drug infections. *AIDS,* 9:825–832.

EL-SADR, WAFFA, et al. (1994). *Managing Early HIV Infection: Quick Reference Guide for Clinicians.* Agency for Healthcare Policy and Research. Publication #94–0573, Rockville, MD.

FAY, ROBERT E., et al. (1989). Prevalence and patterns of same-gender sexual contact among men. *Science,* 243:338–348.

FELDMAN, MITCHELL, et al. (1994). The growing risk of AIDS in older patients. *Patient Care,* 28:61–72.

FILLIT, HOWARD, et al. (1989). AIDS in the elderly: A case and its implications. *Geriatrics,* 44:65–70.

GAYLE, HELENE. (1988). Demographic and sexual transmission differences between adolescent and adult AIDS patients, U.S.A. *Fourth International Conference on AIDS.*

GOSTIN, LAWRENCE, et al. (1997). National HIV case reporting for the United States. *N. Engl. J. Med.,* 337:1162–1167.

HALL, IRENE, et al. (2008). Estimation of HIV incidence in the United States. *J Amer Med Assoc* 300: 520–529.

HENDERSON, DAVID, et al. (1990). Risk for occupational transmission of human immunodeficiency virus type 1 (HIV-1) associated with clinical exposures. *Ann. Intern. Med.,* 113:740.

HIRSCHHORN, LISA. (1995). HIV infection in women: Is it different? *AIDS Reader,* 5:99–105.

HIV/AIDS Surveillance Report. (December 1996). 8:1–36.

HIV/AIDS Surveillance Report. (December 1997). 9:1–43.

HIV/AIDS Surveillance Report. (December 1999). 11:1–45.

HOOKER, TRACEY. (1996). HIV/AIDS: Facts to consider—1996. National Conference of State Legislatures, Denver. pp. 1–64.

LEMP, GEORGE. (1991). The young men's survey: Principal findings and results. A presentation to the San Francisco Health Commission, June 4.

MacKELLAR, DUNCAN, et al. (2005). Unrecognized HIV Infection, Risk Behaviors and Perceptions of Risk Among Young Men Who Have Sex With Men: Opportunities for Advancing HIV Prevention in the Third Decade of HIV/AIDS, 38:603–614.

MARCUS, R., et al. (1988). AIDS: Healthcare workers exposed to it seldom contract it. *N. Engl. J. Med.,* 319:1118–1123.

MARTORELL, REYNALDO, et al. (1995). Vitamin A supplementation and morbidity in children born to HIV-infected women. *Am. J. Public Health,* 85:1049–1050.

MICHAELS, DAVID, et al. (1992). Estimates of the number of motherless youth orphaned by AIDS in the United States. *JAMA,* 268:3456–3461.

MILLER, PATTI, et al. (1997). Compensation for occupationally acquired HIV needs revamping. *Am. J. Public Health,* 87:1558–1562.

MOLOTILOV, VICTOR, et al. (2003). Rapid increases in HIV rates–Orel Oblast, Russian Federation, 1999–2001. *Morbidity and Mortality Weekly Report,* 52:657–660.

Morbidity and Mortality Weekly Report. (1990). HIV prevalence, projected AIDS case estimates. Workshop, October 31–November 1, 1989. 39:110–119.

Morbidity and Mortality Weekly Report. (1991). The HIV/AIDS epidemic: The first 10 years. 40:357–368.

Morbidity and Mortality Weekly Report. (1992). Surveillance for occupationally acquired HIV infection—United States, 1981–1992. 41:823–824.

Morbidity and Mortality Weekly Report. (1993). Update: Mortality attributable to HIV infection among persons aged 25–44 years—United States, 1991 and 1992. 42:869–873.

Morbidity and Mortality Weekly Report. (1994). Heterosexually acquired AIDS—United States, 1993. 43:155–160.

Morbidity and Mortality Weekly Report. (1995). First 500,000 AIDS cases—United States, 1995. 44:849–853.

Morbidity and Mortality Weekly Report. (1996a). AIDS associated with injection-drug use—United States, 1995. 45:392–398.

Morbidity and Mortality Weekly Report. (1996b). HIV/AIDS education and prevention programs for adults in prisons and jails and juveniles in confinement facilities—United States, 1994. 45:268–271.

Morbidity and Mortality Weekly Report. (1996c). Update: Mortality attributable to HIV infection among persons aged 25–44 years—United States, 1994. 45:121–125.

Morbidity and Mortality Weekly Report. (2000). HIV/AIDS among racial/ethnic minority men who have sex with men—United States, 1989–1998.

Nations Health Report. (1995). Women learn of progress, share deep concerns on HIV/AIDS issues. XXV:10.

OSBORNE, JUNE E. (1993). AIDS policy advisor foresees a new age of activism. *Fam. Prac. News,* 23:1, 45.

REISMAN, JUDITH. (1990). *Kinsey, Sex and Fraud: The Indoctrination of a People.* Lafayette, LA: Huntington House Press.

ROSENBERG, PHILIP. (1995). Scope of the AIDS epidemic in the United States. *Science,* 270:1372–1376.

RUBEL, JOHN, et al. (1997). HIV-related mental health in correctional settings. *Focus,* 12:1–4.

RYDER, ROBERT, et al. (1994). AIDS orphans in Kinshasa, Zaire: Incidence and socioeconomic consequences. *AIDS,* 8:673–679.

SPAULDING, ANNE, et. al. (2002). Human Immunodeficiency Virus in Correctional Facilities: A Review. *Clinical Infectious Diseases,* 35:305–312.

UNAIDS. (1997). The HIV/AIDS situation in 1997: Global and regional highlights, Geneva 27, Switzerland, pp. 1–14.

VLAHOV, D., et al. (1991). Prevalence of antibody to HIV-1 among entrants to U.S. correctional facilities. *JAMA,* 265:1129.

WALENSKY, ROCHELLE, et al. (2007). Antiretroviral treatment rollout in South Africa: Alternative scenarios and outcomes. HIV Implementers' meeting, Kigali, Rwanda, abstract 1755.

WEISFUSE, ISAAC C., et al. (1991). HIV-1 infection among New York City inmates. *AIDS,* 5:1133–1138.

WILSON, J., et al. (1990). Keeping your cool in a time of fear. *Emergency Medical Services,* 19:30–32.

WOLITSKI, RICHARD, et al. (2001). Are we headed for a resurgence of the HIV epidemic among gay men? *Am. J. Pub. Health,* 91:883–888.

CHAPTER 11

AGGLETON, PETER, et al. (1994). Risking everything? Risk behavior, behavior change, and AIDS. *Science,* 265:341–345.

ALLEN, J. R., et al. (1988). Prevention of AIDS and HIV infection: Needs and priorities for epidemiologic research. *Am. J. Public Health,* 78:381–386.

BARDEGUEZ, ARLENE. (1995). Managing HIV infection in women. *AIDS Reader, Suppl.,* Nov/Dec, pp. 2–3.

BECKERMAN, KAREN PALMORE. (2002). Mothers, orphans, and prevention of pediatric AIDS *The Lancet,* vol. 359, issue 9313, 1168-1169.

BESSINGER, RUTH, et al. (1997). Pregnancy is not associated with the progression of HIV disease in women attending an HIV outpatient program. *Am J. Epidemiol.,* 147:434–440.

Bloomberg School of Public Health and Johns Hopkins University. (2001). Youth and HIV/AIDS: Can We Avoid Catastrophe? http://www.jhuccp.org/pr/112/112print.shtml.

BUTLER, DECLAN. (1993). Whose side is focus of AIDS research? *Nature,* 366:293.

CHU, SUSAN, et al. (1994). Female-to-female sexual contact and HIV transmission. *JAMA,* 272:433.

COHEN, JON. (1995). Women: Absent term in the AIDS research equation. *Science,* 269:777–780.

COTTON, PAUL. (1994). U.S. sticks head in sand on AIDS prevention. *JAMA,* 272:756–757.

CU-RIN, SUSAN. (1999). Antiretroviral treatment during pregnancy. *Improving Management of HIV Disease,* 7:14–18.

CURRAN, JAMES W., et al. (1988). Epidemiology of HIV infection and AIDS in the United States. *Science*, 239:610–616.

DICKINSON, GORDON M. (1988). Epidemiology of AIDS. *Int. Ped.*, 3:30–32.

EHRHARDT, ANKE A. (1992). Trends in sexual behavior and the HIV pandemic. *Am. J. Public Health*, 82:1459–1464.

FARZADEGAN, HOMAYOON, et al. (1998). Sex differences in HIV-1 viral load and progression to AIDS. *Lancet*, 352:1510–1514.

GRAY, GLENDA, et al. (2008) Breast-feeding, antiretroviral prophylaxis, and HIV. *NENGJM*, 359:089-191.

HADER, SHANNON, et al. (2001). HIV infection in women in the United States. *JAMA*, 285:1186–1192.

Health. (1996). AIDS still spreading rapidly among young gay men. *Am. Med. News*, 39:30.

HIV/AIDS Surveillance Report. (1995). Year end, 7:1–36.

HIV/AIDS Surveillance Report. (1996). Year end, 8:1–39.

HIV/AIDS Surveillance Report. (1997). December, 9:1–34.

HOLDEN, CONSTANCE. (1998). World-AIDS; The worst is yet to come. *Science*, 278:1715.

IOANNIDIS, JOHN, et al. (1999). Maternal viral load and the risk of perinatal transmission of HIV-1. *NEJM*, 341:1698.

JOHNSON, TIMOTHY, et al. (1995). Current issues in the primary care of women with HIV. *Female Patient*, 20:51–58.

JOSEPH, STEPHEN C. (1993). The once and future AIDS epidemic. *Med. Doctor*, 37:92–104.

KUHN, LOUISE, et al. (2008) Effects of early, abrupt weaning for HIV-free survival of children in Zambia. *NEJM*, 10.1056/NEJMoa073788

KWAKWA, HELENA, et al. (2003). Female-to-female transmission of human immunodeficiency virus. *Clinical Infectious Diseases*, 36:e40–e41.

MANDELBROT, LAURENT, et al. (1997). Natural conception in HIV-negative women with HIV-infected partners. *Lancet*, 349:850–851.

MANDELBROT, LAURENT, et al. (1998). Perinatal HIV-1 Transmission. *J. Am. Med. Assoc.*, 280:55–60.

MIOTTI, PAOLO, et al. (1999). HIV transmission through breast-feeding. *JAMA*, 282:744–749.

Morbidity and Mortality Weekly Report. (1993). Update: Acquired immunodeficiency syndrome—United States, 1992. 42:547–557.

Morbidity and Mortality Weekly Report. (1994). Update: Impact of the expanded AIDS surveillance case definition for adolescents/adults on case reporting—United States, 1993. 43:160–170.

Morbidity and Mortality Weekly Report. (1996a). HIV testing among women aged 18–44 years—United States, 1991 and 1993. 46:733–736.

Morbidity and Mortality Weekly Report. (1996b). Update: Mortality attributable to HIV infection among persons aged 25–44 years—United States, 1994:45:121–125.

Morbidity and Mortality Report. (1999). Surveillance for AIDS-defining opportunistic illnesses, 1992–1997. 48:1–20.

Morbidity and Mortality Weekly Report. (2003). Pregnancy in perinatally HIV-infected adolescents and young adults—Puerto Rico, 2002. 52:149–151.

NEWELL, MICHAEL, et al. (1997). Immunological markers in HIV-infected pregnant women: The European Collaborative Study and the Swiss HIV Pregnancy Cohort. *AIDS*, 11:1859–1865.

NEWTON, KUMWENDA, et al. (2008). Extended antiretroviral prophylaxis to reduce breast milk HIV-1 transmission.

Office of National AIDS Policy. (1996). Youth and HIV/AIDS: An American agenda. *Report to the President*, pp. 1–14.

PFEIFFER, NAOMI. (1991). AIDS risk high for women; care is poor. *Infect. Dis. News*, 4:1,18.

ROTHERAM-BORUS, M., et al. (1991). Sexual risk behaviors, AIDS knowledge, and beliefs about AIDS among runaways. *Am. J. Public Health*, 81:208–210.

SCHABLE, BARBARA, et al. (1996). Characteristics of women 50 years of age or older with heterosexually acquired AIDS. *Am. J. Public Health*, 86:1616–1618.

SELWYN, PETER A., et al. (1989). Knowledge of HIV antibody status and decisions to continue or terminate pregnancy among intravenous-drug users. *JAMA*, 261;3567–3571.

STERLING, TIMOTHY, et al. (2001). Initial plasma HIV-1 RNA levels and progression to AIDS in women and men. *N. Engl. J. Med.*, 344:720–725.

TAHA & TAHA, et al. (2000). Morbidity among HIV-1 infected and uninfected African children. *Pediatrics*, 106: http://www.pediatrics.org/cgi/content/full/106/6/e77.

THOMAS, PATRICIA. (1988). Official estimates of epidemic's scope are grist for political mill. *Med. World News*, 29:12–13.

THOMAS, PATRICIA. (1989). The epidemic. *Med World News*, 30:41–49.

TOWSEND, CLAIRE, et al. (2008). Low rates of mother-to-child transmission of HIV following effective pregnancy interventions in the United Kingdom and Ireland, 200-2006. *AIDS*, 22(8): 973-981.

UNAIDS, (1997). Global summary of the HIV/AIDS epidemic. *Report on the global HIV/AIDS epidemic*. December 1997:1–25.

VAN BENTHEM, BIRGIT, et al. (2002). The impact of pregnancy and menopause on CD4 lymphocyte counts in HIV-infected women. *AIDS,* 16:919–924.

World Health Organization, Geneva. (1994). *Women's Health,* p. 18.

WORTLEY, PASCALE, et. al. (1997). AIDS in women in the United States. *JAMA,* 278:911–916.

YAO, FAUSTIN K. (1992). Youth and AIDS: A priority for prevention education. *AIDS Health Promotion Exchange No. 2,* Royal Tropical Institute, The Netherlands: 1–3.

ZIERLER, SALLY, et al. (2000). Violence victimization after HIV infection in a U.S. probability sample of adult patients in primary care. *Am. J. Pub. Health,* 90:208–215.

ZIJENAH, LYNN, et al. (2004). Timing of mother-to-child transmission of HIV-1 and infant mortality in the first six months of life in Harare, Zimbabwe. *AIDS,* 18:273–280.

CHAPTER 12

COLLINS, CHRIS, et al. (1997). Outside the prevention vacuum: Issues in HIV prevention for youth in the next decade. *AIDS Reader,* 7:149–154.

DI CLEMENTE, RALPH. (1998). Preventing sexually transmitted infections among adolescents: A clash of ideology and science. *JAMA,* 279:1574–1575.

FUTTERMAN, DONNA, et al. (1992). Medical care of HIV-infected adolescents. *AIDS Clin. Care,* 4:95–98.

JEMMOT, JOHN, et al. (1998). Abstinence and safer sex high risk-reduction interventions for African American adolescents: A randomized controlled trial. *JAMA,* 279:1529–1536.

KIRBY, DOUGLAS, et al. (1997). The impact of the Postponing Sexual Involvement Curriculum among youths in California. *Fam. Plann. Perspect,* 29:100–108.

MARKS, ROBERT. (2003). Editorial: Just say know. *FOCUS,* 18:2.

Morbidity and Mortality Weekly Report. (1992). Selected behaviors that increase risk for HIV infection among high school students—United States, 1990. 41:236–240.

Paltiel et al. 2005.

ROSENBAUM, JANET, et al. (2006). Reborn a Virgin: Adolescent retracting of Virginily pledges and sexual histories. *Am. J. Pub. Health,* 96: 1098–1103.

Saunders et al. 2005.

SELLS, WAYNE, et al. (1996). Morbidity and mortality among U.S. adolescents: An overview of data and trends. *Am. J. Public Health,* 86:513–519.

WITKIN, ANDREA, et. al. (2003). Comprehensive versus abstinence-only sex education: What works? *FOCUS,* 18:1–4.

CHAPTER 13

AIDS, Health and Human Rights. (1995). Francois-Xavier Bagnoud Center for Health and Human Rights–Harvard School of Public Health, pp. 1–162.

ALLEN, BRADY. (1991). The role of the primary care physician in HIV testing and early stage disease management. *Fam. Pract. Recert,* 13:30–49.

ANDERSON, JOHN, et al. (1992). HIV antibody testing and post-test counseling in the United States: Data from the 1989 National Health Interview Study. *Am. J. Public Health,* 82:1533–1535.

ANGELL, MARCIA. (1991). A dual approach to the AIDS epidemic. *N. Engl. J. Med.,* 324:1498–1500.

BAYER, RONALD, et al. (1995). Testing for HIV infection at home (Sounding Board). *N. Engl. J. Med.,* 332:1296–1299.

BELONGIA, EDWARD A., et al. (1989). Premarital HIV screening. *JAMA,* 261:2198.

CORDES, ROBERT, et al. (1995). Pitfalls in HIV testing. *Postgrad. Med.,* 98:177–189.

DE LEJARAZ, RAUL ORTIZ, et al. (2008). HIV-1 infection in persistently HIV-1 seronegative individuals: More reasons for HIV RNA screening. *Clinical Infectious Disease* 46:785.

EL-SADR, W. et al. (1994). *Managing early HIV infection: quick reference guide for clinicians.* AHCPR Publication No. 94–0573. Rockville, MD.

EL-SADR, WAFAA, et al. (1994). Managing early HIV infection: Agency for Healthcare Policy and Research. *Clinical Practice Guideline on Evaluation and Management of Early HIV Infection.* January, 7:1–37.

FANG, CHYANG T., et al. (1989). HIV testing and patient counseling. *Patient Care,* 23:19–44.

GOSTIN, LAWRENCE, et al. (1997). National HIV case surveillance is urged. *N. Engl. J. Med.,* 337:1162–1167.

HARTLAUB, PAUL, et al. (1993). Obtaining informed consent: It is not simply asking "do you understand?" *J. Fam. Pract.,* 36:383–384.

HEGARTY, J.D., et al. (1988). The medical care costs of human immunodeficiency virus infected children in Harlem. *JAMA,* 260:1901–1905.

HOOKER, TRACEY. (1996). HIV/AIDS: Facts to consider—1996. Natural Conference of State Legislatures, February, pp. 1–64.

Intergovernmental AIDS Report. (1989). Illinois court overrules mandatory HIV testing for prostitutes and sex offenders, 2:1–18.

JANSSEN, ROBERT, et al. (1998). New testing strategy to detect early HIV-1 infection for use in incidence estimates and for clinical and prevention purposes. *JAMA,* 280:42–48.

JENNY-AVITAL, ELIZABETH, et al. (2001). Erroneously low or undetectable plasma HIV-1 RNA load, determined by PCR, in West African and American patients with non-B subtype HIV infection. *Clinical Infectious Diseases,* 32:1227–1230.

JOHNSON, CHRISTINE. (2000). Factors known to cause false positive HIV antibody test results. In *Alive and Well* [online]. Available: http://www.aliveandwell.org.

KELLER, G.H., et al. (1988). Identification of HIV sequences using nucleic acid probes. *Am. Clin. Lab.,* 7:10–15.

KRAMER, F.R., et al. (1989). Replicatable RNA reporters. *Nature,* 339:401–402.

MACKENZIE, WILLIAM R., et al. (1992). Multiple false positive serologic tests for HIV, HTLV-1 and hepatitis C following influenza vaccination, 1991. *JAMA,* 268:1015–1017.

MCFARLAND, WILLIAM, et al. (1999). Detection of early HIV infection and estimation of incidence using a sensitive/less sensitive enzyme immunoassay testing strategy at anonymous counseling and testing sites in San Francisco. *JAIDS,* 22:484–489.

MERCOLA, JOSEPH M. (1989). Premarital HIV screening. *JAMA,* 261:2198.

MIIKE, LAWRENCE. (1987). *AIDS Antibody Testing.* Office of Technological Assessment Testimony to the U.S. Congress. October: 1–21.

Morbidity and Mortality Weekly Report. (1996). U.S. Public Health Service Guidelines for testing and counseling blood and plasma donors for HIV type I antigen. 45:1–9.

Morbidity and Mortality Weekly Report. (1998b). Update: Counseling and testing using rapid tests—United States, 1995, 47:211–215.

Morbidity and Mortality Weekly Report (1999). HIV Testing—United States, 1996. 48:52–55.

MORE, DANIEL, et al. (2000). Utility of an HIV-1 RNA assay in the diagnosis of acute retroviral syndrome. *Southern Medical Journal,* 93:1004–1006.

MOSER, MICHAEL, (1998). Anonymous HIV testing. *Am. J. Pub. Health,* 88:683.

MULLIS, KARY B., et al. (1987). Process for amplifying, detecting, and/or, cloning nucleic acid sequences. (U.S. Patent No. 4,683,195). *Official Gazette of the U.S. Patient and Trademark Office,* vol. 1080, No. 4, July.

NASH, GRANT, et al. (1998). Health benefits and risks of reporting HIV-infected individuals by name. *Am. J. Pub. Health,* 88:876–879.

PASSANNANTE, MARIAN R., et al. (1993). Responses of healthcare professionals to proposed mandatory HIV testing. *Arch. Fam. Med.,* 2:38–44.

PHILLIPS, KATHRYN, et al. (1995a). Potential use of home HIV testing. *N. Engl. J. Med.,* 332:1308–1310.

PHILLIPS, KATHRYN, et al. (1995b). Who plans to be tested for HIV or would get tested if no one could find out the results? *Am. J. Prevent. Med.,* 11(3):156.

REIMER, LARRY, et al. (1997). Undetectable antibody reported in a patient with typical HIV. *Clin. Infect. Dis.* 25:98–103.

RHAME, FRANK S., et al. (1989). The case for wider use of testing for HIV infection. *N. Engl. J. Med.,* 320:1242–1254.

RICH, JOSIAH, et al. (1999). Misdiagnosis of HIV infection by HIV-1 Plasma Viral load testing: A case series. *Annals of Internal Medicine,* 130:37–39.

SAMET, JEFFREY, et al. (1998). Trillion Niron delay: Time from testing positive for HIV to presentation for primary care. *Arch. Int. Med.,* 158:734–740.

SCHEFFEL, J.W. (1990). Retrocell HIV-1 passive haemagglutination assay for HIV-1 antibody screening. *J. Acquired Immune Deficiency Syndromes,* 3:540–545.

WAKE, WILLIAM T. (1989). How many patients will die because we fear AIDS? *Med. Econ.,* 66:24–30.

WOFOY, C.B. (1987). HIV infection in women. *JAMA,* 257:2074–2076.

WOLF, LESLIE et al. (2007). Implementing routine HIV testing: The role of state law. PLOS ONE 2(10) E1005. DOI: 10.1371/Journal. Pone. 0001005.

CHAPTER 14

American Medical Association News. (1991). Ruling fuels debate over HIV-infected doctors. May, 1: 41–43.

BURRIS, SCOTT. (1996). Human immunodeficiency virus-infected healthcare workers. *Arch. Fam. Med.,* 5:102–106.

CRAVEN, DONALD, et al. (1994). Fictitious HIV Infection. *Ann. Intern. Med.,* 121:763–766.

EICKHOFF, THEODORE C. (1989). Public perceptions about AIDS and HIV infection. *Infect. Dis. News,* 2:6.

ENGLAND, ROGER. (2007). Are we spending too much on HIV? *BMJ* 334:(17 February) DOI:10.1136/36/bmj.39113.402361.94

FISHER, J.D., et al. (1992). Changing AIDS risk behavior. *Psychol. Bull.,* 111:455–474.

FOURNIER, A.M., et al. (1989). Preoperative screening for HIV infection. *Arch. Surg.,* 124:1038–1040.

GERBERT, BARBARA, et al. (1988). Why fear persists: Healthcare professionals and AIDS. *JAMA,* 260:3481–3483.

GOSTIN, LAWRENCE, et al. (1998). HIV infection and AIDS in the public health and healthcare systems: The role of law and litigation. *JAMA,* 279:1108–1113.

GOUJAN, CHRISOPHE, et al. (2000). Phylogenetic analysis indicates an atypical nurse to patient transmission of HIV-1. *J. Virology,* 74:2525–2532.

HAGEN, M.D., et al. (1988). Routine preoperative screening for HIV: Does the risk to the surgeon outweigh the risk to the patient? *JAMA,* 259:1357–1359.

HEGARTY, JAMES D., et al. (1988). The medical care costs of HIV-infected children in Harlem. *JAMA,* 260:1901–1909.

HEREK, GREGORY M., et al. (1993). Public reaction to AIDS in the United States: A second decade of stigma. *Am. J. Public Health,* 83:574–577.

J. Virology, 74:2525–2534.

JAPENGA, ANN. (1992). The secret. *Health,* 6:43–52.

KIRBY, D. (1988). The effectiveness of educational programs to help prevent school-age youth from contracting AIDS: A review of relevant research. United States Congress.

LEFKOWITZ, MATHEW. (1990). A healthcare system in crisis: The possible restriction against HIV-infected healthcare workers. *PAACNotes,* 2:175–176.

MCCARTHY, GILLIAN, et al. (1999). Factors associated with refusal to treat HIV-infected patients: The results of a National Survey of Dentists in Canada. *Am. J. of Public Health,* 89:541–545.

MCNEILL, WILLIAM H. (1976). *Plagues and People,* Garden City, NJ: Anchor Press.

MICHAELS, DAVID, et al. (1992). Estimates of the number of youth orphaned by AIDS in the United States. *JAMA,* 268:3456–3461.

MILENO, MARIA, et al. (2001). Factitious HIV syndrome in young women. *The AIDS Reader,* 11:263–268.

Morbidity and Mortality Weekly Report. (1990). HIV-related knowledge and behavior among high school students—Selected U.S. cities, 1989. 39:385–396.

NARY, GORDON. (1990). An editorial. *PAACNotes,* 2:170.

PHILLIPS, KATHRYN A. (1993). Subjective knowledge of AIDS and Use of HIV testing. *Am. J. Public Health,* 83:1460–1462.

POLDER, JACQUELYN A., et al. (1989). AIDS precautions for your office. *Patient Care,* 23:161–171.

POWELL, JOHN H. (1965). *Bring Out Your Dead.* New York: Time-Life Inc.

RHAME, FRANK S., et al. (1989). The case for wider use of testing for HIV infection. *N. Engl. J. Med.,* 320:1242–1254.

ROBERTS, LESLIE, et al. (2008). HIV/AIDS: Money Matters. *Science,* 321: 511 Special Issue DOI:10. 1126/Science, 321.5888.511.

ROWE, MONA, et al. (1987). *A Public Health Challenge: State Issues, Policies and Programs, Volume 2.* Intergovernmental Health Policy Project, George Washington University.

STRYKER, JEFF, et al. (1995). Prevention of HIV infection. *JAMA,* 273:1143–1148.

VOELKER, REBECCA. (1989). No uniform policy among states on HIV/AIDS education. *Am. Med. News,* September 3:28–29.

WEISS, RICK. (1999). Thousands of deaths linked to medical errors. Online. Available: http://www.washingtonpost.com (November 30).

ZUGER, ABIGAIL. (1995). The high cost of living. *Sci. Am.* 273:108.

Index

Page references followed by *f* or *t* indicate material in figures or tables, respectively.

T

T4 lymphocytes
  in acute disease stage, 152–154
  apoptosis of, 122
  in asymptomatic HIV disease,
      154–155
  count
    in AIDS definition, 4, 28
    correlation with
        complications, 155
    importance of, 166–167
    normal, 110
    regular measurement of,
        111, 166–167
    understanding results of, 111
    uses of, 111
  depletion of
    cofactors and, 122
    impact of, 111, 122–123, 123f
    mechanisms of, 122
  disconnect with viral load, 67
  gender differences in, 319
  HIV infection and, 23–24, 66,
      111, 118, 122, 180, 181f
  HIV infection sites for, 124
  HIV life cycle in, 53f
  human leukocyte antigen
      and, 106
  normal, 23f
  and progression to AIDS,
      163–167
  receptor sites for, filling of, 122
  response to HAART, 155
  resting state of, 116
  as surrogate markers for
      therapy, 67
  in symptomatic HIV disease,
      155
  syncytia and, 122
  and treatment guidelines, 91–93
T4 percentage, 110
T8 lymphocytes, in
    nonprogressors, 165
T-20, 70t
Tacoma, Washington, needle
    exchange program in, 246
Taiwan, fear of HIV, 389
Tampa Hillsborough Action Plan
    (THAP), 415
Tanox, 70t
Tanzania
  cleansers in, 309
  HIV and schools in, 299
  HIV-infected women
      in, 308, 322
tat gene, 55, 55f, 56–57

Tattoos, and HIV transmission, 208
Taylor, Elizabeth, 14, 401
TB. See Tuberculosis
T cell(s), 107–113. See also T4
    lymphocytes
  cluster differentiation in, 108f
  cytotoxic or killer, 106,
      108–111, 152
  function of, 107
  helper, 108–111
  naïve or unexposed, 115, 116f
T cell antigen receptor (TCR), 107
T cell receptor, 106
T cell zone, in lymph nodes,
    163–167
Teachers, African, HIV and, 298–299
Tears, HIV in, 180
Technical Meeting on Male
    Circumcision-Global, 185
Television programs depicting
    AIDS, 25
Telling the truth, 398–399
Temin, Howard, 51f
Tenet, George, 344
Tennessee, HIV testing in
    pregnancy, 328
Tenofovir (Viread), 70t
  cellular targets of, 70f
  mechanism of action, 73f
  for pre-exposure prophylaxis, 86
  in vaginal microbicide, 243
Terry Higgins Trust, 21
Testicular cancer, 144
Testing, 347–382, See also specific tests
  age and, 372t
  anonymous, 376, 380–381
  athlete, 374
  barriers to, addressing, 372
  blinded, 381
  candidates/indications for, 371
  CDC recommendations on,
      378–379, 381–382
  competency for, 374–375
  compulsory, 376–379
  confidential, 379–380, 382
  confirmatory, 352, 357,
      368–371, 381
  counseling before and after, 363
  current practice versus more,
      377, 377t
  emotional reactions to, 356, 381
  errors in, 356
  false negative in, 352
  false positive in, 356–357, 360
  history of, 351
  home, 348, 367–368

immigrant, 372–374
importance of, 348
indeterminate results in, 359–361
informed consent for, 375,
    379–380
locations for, 381
mandatory, 376
mistaken diagnoses without, 356
misunderstanding and lack
    of, 350
named, 376
negative results in, 358t
newborn, 376
partner deception in, 380
positive results in, 358t
in pregnancy, 328, 371, 376
problems with, 363
race and, 3
rapid, 348, 363–367, 364t,
    381–382
reasons for, 349, 371
reasons for not undergoing,
    349, 350f
requests for, 348–349
results of, meaning of, 358t
routine, need for, 349–350,
    377–379, 381
stigma and, 377
timing of, 371–372
universal, 377–379
unnamed or anonymous, 376
urine-based, 348, 362, 381
viral load, 88, 92, 361
voluntary, 376, 381
without consent, 375
Tetanus vaccine, 257
Texas
  HIV-infected young adults
      in, 338
  HIV prevalence data in, 285t
  HIV testing in pregnancy, 328
Thailand
  HIV-infected women
      in, 308, 323
  HIV subtypes in, 61
  opportunistic infections in, 132
  prevention education in, 227
  sex trade in, 207
  "women's diseases" in, 308
"That's What Friends Are For," 220
Therapeutic vaccine, 256–257
Third line regimens, 86–87
Thomas E. Starlz Transplantation
    Institute, 208
Thompson, Paul, 168
Thompson, Tommy, 255